Obesity Epidemiology

Obesity Epidemiology

Frank B. Hu, MD, PhD
Associate Professor of Nutrition and Epidemiology
Harvard School of Public Health
Associate Professor of Medicine
Harvard Medical School
Boston, Massachusetts

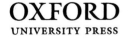
UNIVERSITY PRESS

2008

OXFORD

UNIVERSITY PRESS

Oxford University Press, Inc., publishes works that further
Oxford University's objective of excellence
in research, scholarship, and education.

Oxford New York
Auckland Cape Town Dar es Salaam Hong Kong Karachi
Kuala Lumpur Madrid Melbourne Mexico City Nairobi
New Delhi Shanghai Taipei Toronto

With offices in
Argentina Austria Brazil Chile Czech Republic France Greece
Guatemala Hungary Italy Japan Poland Portugal Singapore
South Korea Switzerland Thailand Turkey Ukraine Vietnam

Published by Oxford University Press, Inc.
198 Madison Avenue, New York, New York 10016

www.oup.com

Oxford is a registered trademark of Oxford University Press

Library of Congress Cataloging-in-Publication Data

Hu, Frank.
Obesity epidemiology / Frank Hu.
p. ; cm.
Includes bibliographical references.
ISBN 978-0-19-531291-1 (cloth: alk. paper)
1. Obesity—United States—Epidemiology. 2. Obesity—Complications—United States.
3. Obesity—Risk factors—United States. I. Title.
[DNLM: 1. Obesity—epidemiology—United States. 2. Epidemiologic Methods—United States.
3. Obesity—complications—United States. 4. Risk Factors—United States. WD 210 H874o 2008]
RA645.O23H8 2008
362.196'39800973—dc22   2007029027

9 8 7 6 5 4 3 2

Printed in the United States of America
on acid-free paper

To Lisa

▩ Acknowledgments

I am deeply indebted to many colleagues for the discussions, ideas, and concepts that I have included in this book. I am particularly grateful to Dr. Walter Willett for his initial encouragement, intellectual inspiration, and continued support. Dr. Willett read many chapters of the book and provided invaluable comments. Other colleagues, including Drs. Eduardo Villamor, Meir Stampfer, Donna Speigelman, Rob van Dam, Matthias Schulze, Cuilin Zhang, Lu Qi, Vasanti Malik, Russell de Souza, JoAnn Manson, Peter Kraft, Marilyn Cornelis, James Meigs, Steve Heymsfield, and George Bray, reviewed specific chapters and provided many constructive comments. Students in my obesity epidemiology class also provided valuable feedback. Much of the work owes a great deal to the support and advice of many other colleagues and collaborators, including Drs. Frank Speizer, Sue Hankinson, David Hunter, Eric Rimm, Simin Liu, Edward Giovannucci, Eric Ding, Dariush Mozaffarian, Hannia Campos, Alberto Ascherio, Teresa Fung, Frank Sacks, David Ludwig, Steve Gortmaker, Christos Mantzorous, Alessandro Doria, and George Blackburn. Furthermore, I am extremely grateful to Drs. Eugenia Calle, Ichiro Kawachi, Daniel Kim, Graham Colditz, Y. Claire Wang, Sanjay Patel, Gary Bennett, Dustin Duncan, Kathleen Wolin, Matthew Gillman, and Alison Field for contributing individual chapters in a timely and scholarly fashion.

Some of the data described in various chapters of the book were derived from ongoing, large cohort studies (the Nurses' Health Study and the Health Professionals' Follow-up Study) at Harvard School of Public Health and Channing Laboratory, Brigham and Women's Hospital and Harvard Medical School. Over the past 11 years, I have had the great fortune to play a small part in conducting and contributing to these studies. These cohorts have not only produced unparalleled resources in studying causes and consequences of obesity and its related conditions but have also created a collegial and intellectually stimulating environment for young investigators to grow in and develop.

I would like to thank Rita Buckley and Paul Guttry for excellent editorial help, Vanessa Boulanger for generating some of the graphs and tables, and Bill Lamsback and Carrie Pedersen at Oxford University Press for critical support in the production of this book. Finally, special thanks to my wife, Lisa, for her encouragement, love, and unwavering support over the years, and also to our children, Emily and Peter, for their understanding and patience over the many months that were consumed by this project.

Frank B. Hu
Boston, Massachusetts

Preface

Sparked by a surging epidemic of obesity worldwide, epidemiologic research on the determinants and consequences of obesity has dramatically increased over the past several decades. The vast amount of new data has not only advanced our understanding of health consequences and environmental causes of obesity but has also raised many methodological issues in the conduct and interpretation of epidemiologic research on obesity. Obesity is a complex variable. It can be characterized by a variety of methods and analyzed as an exposure, outcome, confounding variable, or mediator in biological pathways that link environmental factors and disease risk. Many epidemiologic studies of obesity and morbidity and mortality have methodological limitations that may have contributed to inconsistencies in the literature and confusion among the general public. It is, therefore, critical that we bring a better understanding of these issues to the interpretation of epidemiologic reports of obesity. We also need to address the unique challenges in the design, analysis, and interpretation of genetic association studies of obesity, a rapidly evolving research area.

This book describes in detail the epidemiologic methods used to conduct obesity research, analyze and interpret epidemiologic data, and summarize current literature on the consequences and determinants of obesity. There are many obesity-related books, but none have focused on epidemiologic methods nor have any conducted in-depth reviews of social, behavioral, and biological determinants of obesity. This book aims to fill those gaps by emphasizing sound epidemiologic methods and principles throughout. In doing so, my hope is that it will advance study design, analysis, and data interpretation in obesity research; improve understanding of the causes and consequences of obesity; and identify needs and future directions for obesity research.

The book is divided into three parts. The first focuses primarily on study designs and measurement issues. Chapter 1 is an introduction to the field of obesity epidemiology. It describes the historical context of epidemiology and obesity research and the major research domains of obesity epidemiology. Chapter 2 covers national and international obesity trends, and Chapter 3 reviews epidemiologic study designs commonly used in obesity research. Chapter 4 discusses conceptual and analytic issues related to causal inferences in obesity epidemiologic research. Chapter 5 examines the validity and application of various methods used to assess body fatness in epidemiologic studies, and Chapter 6 provides a critical review of methods for measuring individual dietary components and total energy intake in nutritional epidemiologic studies. Chapter 7 discusses methods for measuring physical activity, including their validity and application in epidemiologic studies of obesity.

The second part of the book focuses on the health and societal consequences of obesity. Chapter 8 reviews metabolic and physiological consequences of obesity. Chapter 9 describes current evidence on the relationship between obesity and cardiovascular outcomes, including coronary heart disease, stroke, and heart failure. Chapter 10, written by Dr. Eugenia Calle, provides a concise state-of-the-art summary of the vast literature on obesity and cancer. Chapter 11 discusses common methodological problems in obesity and mortality studies, including reverse causation, confounding by smoking, and survival biases. It also covers methods to deal with these problems in study design and data analyses. Chapter 12, written by Drs. Daniel Kim and Ichiro Kawachi, reviews current evidence on the effects of obesity and weight gain on health-related quality of life as well as methodological issues concerning measurements and analyses of quality of life in epidemiological studies. Chapter 13, written by Drs. Graham Colditz and Y. Claire Wang, provides an updated analysis of direct and indirect costs of obesity.

The final part of the book deals with determinants of obesity. Chapters 14 and 15 review the large and complex literature on the relationships between diet and physical activity and obesity and age-related weight gain. In Chapter 16, Dr. Sanjay Patel and I consider emerging data suggesting that sleep deprivation has important metabolic effects that may predispose to weight gain. Together we examine biological mechanisms and current evidence from epidemiologic studies of sleep duration and subsequent weight gain and obesity. In Chapter 17, Dr. Gary Bennett and colleagues provide a comprehensive review of social determinants of obesity, including race/ethnicity, socioeconomic status, education, neighborhood characteristics, stress, and social support. Chapter 18 discusses current literature on metabolic and hormonal predictors of obesity, including basal metabolic rate, fat oxidation, insulin resistance, and leptin and other adipokines. Chapter 19, written by Dr. Matthew Gillman, provides a conceptual framework for the developmental origins of obesity and summarizes key findings from this relatively new and exciting area of research. Chapter 20, written by Dr. Alison Field, examines dietary and lifestyle predictors of childhood obesity and unique methodological issues in studies of childhood obesity. The final two chapters review recent developments and future directions in genetic studies of obesity and gene-environment interactions in the development of obesity.

To assure a coherent presentation of epidemiologic methods in the context of obesity research, I wrote most of the book. Colleagues with greater expertise in specific areas authored a few chapters. Chapter citations have been selected from a vast and rapidly growing body of literature; I apologize to colleagues for the omission of many important papers. In addition, I regret that some important areas in obesity epidemiologic research have been omitted due to space limitations. These include the impact of obesity on renal, pulmonary, neurodegenerative, and skeletal muscular conditions, and on reproductive health. To maintain an epidemiologic focus, I did not cover medical or surgical treatment of obesity, but excellent resources are available on those subjects.

This volume is intended as a textbook for a graduate-level course in obesity epidemiology, but it can be used by a wider audience, including obesity and chronic disease researchers, national and international organizations, and researchers and practitioners in nutrition, exercise, and public health. Most chapters require some elementary epidemiologic and statistical knowledge for understanding of concepts and methods; only a few chapters require a deeper background in biology and genetics. Because of its comprehensive coverage of social, behavioral, and biological determinants of obesity, this book can be used as a resource for designing prevention and intervention programs and public health policies on obesity.

As the worldwide obesity epidemic continues to grow, epidemiologic methods will continue to be the primary tool for the study of trends, consequences, and causes of obesity. There is a clear need for a book that focuses on epidemiologic methods in obesity research. I hope this volume satisfies that need.

Contents

List of Invited Contributors

GARY G. BENNETT   Department of Society, Human Development and Health, Harvard School of Public Health, Boston, Massachusetts

EUGENIA E. CALLE   Department of Epidemiology and Surveillance Research, American Cancer Society, Atlanta, Georgia

GRAHAM A. COLDITZ   Siteman Cancer Center, Washington University School of Medicine, St. Louis, Missouri

DUSTIN T. DUNCAN   Center for Community-Based Research, Dana-Farber Cancer Institute, Boston, Massachusetts

ALISON E. FIELD   Children's Hospital Boston, Division of Adolescent Medicine, Harvard Medical School, Boston, Massachusetts

MATTHEW W. GILLMAN   Department of Ambulatory Care and Prevention, Harvard Medical School and Harvard Pilgrim Health Care, Boston, Massachusetts

ICHIRO KAWACHI   Department of Society, Human Development and Health, Harvard School of Public Health, Boston, Massachusetts

DANIEL KIM   Department of Society, Human Development and Health, Harvard School of Public Health, Boston, Massachusetts

SANJAY R. PATEL   Division of Pulmonary, Critical Care and Sleep Medicine, University Hospital and Case Western Reserve University, Cleveland, Ohio

Y. CLAIRE WANG   Department of Health Policy and Management, Columbia Mailman School of Public Health, New York

KATHLEEN Y. WOLIN   Center for Community-Based Research, Dana-Farber Cancer Institute, Boston, Massachusetts

Obesity Epidemiology

Part I

Study Designs and Measurements

1

Introduction to Obesity Epidemiology

Frank B. Hu

The last three decades have witnessed an alarming increase in obesity rates in the United States and other industrialized countries. Many developing countries, where there has been a dramatic shift from undernutrition to overnutrition, are also experiencing a marked rise in obesity and obesity-related diseases, including hypertension, type 2 diabetes, and cardiovascular disease. In parallel with the rising obesity epidemic, the number of epidemiologic studies on consequences and determinants of obesity has grown exponentially. This unprecedented interest in obesity research has spurred the formation of a relatively new branch of epidemiology focused on obesity.

Obesity epidemiology uses epidemiologic approaches to examine the causes and consequences of obesity in human populations. It includes the study of multiple, broad, interrelated domains such as (a) the distributions, patterns, and dynamics of obesity in populations; (b) health and other consequences of obesity; (c) the determinants or causes of obesity; and (d) the development and validation of body composition measurement methods used in epidemiologic studies. Knowledge gained is eventually applied to public health initiatives to prevent and control obesity and related health conditions.

The adverse effects of obesity have been described for millennia (discussed below). However, systematic studies of the relationships between obesity and body composition and health outcomes are a relatively recent phenomenon. Large epidemiologic surveys and cohort studies to monitor trends and examine nutritional and lifestyle predictors of chronic diseases have been conducted only since the middle of the 20th century. The methodology of obesity epidemiology, however, dates back to the 19th century, when Quetelet[1] developed the concept of body mass index (BMI) to evaluate adiposity in populations (see below). Like most other branches of epidemiology, this relatively new field has deep roots in classical epidemiologic methods. It couples modern epidemiologic thinking with a biological understanding of obesity and its sequelae. Therefore, recounting the historical developments of epidemiologic methods and obesity research provides some perspective on how these elements have converged to form the field of obesity epidemiology.

Historical Developments in Epidemiology

The earliest epidemiology took place more than 2000 years ago, when Hippocrates used clinical observation to identify environmental causes of a disease, thereby dispelling the notion that health depends on magical influences.[2] The earliest systematic attempts to quantify the health of populations date back to John Graunt (London, 1620-1674),[3] who used demographic approaches to investigate patterns of mortality rates in specific populations. These efforts led to subsequent development of the first life table.[4] They also set the stage for England to emerge as the first country to collect vital statistics in large populations and apply them to public health policy.[5-9]

Milestones in classic epidemiology took place during the Industrial Revolution. These included William Farr's (1807-1883) introduction in 1838 of a national cause-of-death recording system[10] and John Snow's (1813-1858) classic study of the role of polluted water in the spread of cholera,[11] which led to suppression of outbreaks 44 years before the discovery of *Vibrio cholerae*, the causal agent.[12] Another classic epidemiologic observation of that time was the discovery by Joseph Goldberger (1874-1927) that pellagra was not caused by germs, but by deficiency of niacin, a B-complex vitamin.[13]

Near the end of the 19th century, the discovery of microorganisms ushered in the era of infectious disease epidemiology.[10] In 1882, Robert Edward Koch (1843-1910) published a seminal paper on the tubercle bacillus[14] and developed criteria for establishing causality in infectious disease epidemiology. His work resulted in environmental (e.g., improved sanitation and living conditions) and medical interventions to interrupt transmission of certain microorganisms.[10] Over a short and dramatic period, toward the end of the 19th century microorganisms were discovered and established as causes of syphilis, diphtheria, and other epidemic diseases.[15] During the same era, Rudolf Virchow's concept of "social medicine" laid the groundwork for today's public health science and social epidemiology.[16]

During the 20th century, especially during its second half, epidemiology shifted focus from infectious to chronic diseases, and the field came to "shape public health discourses and practices to an unprecedented extent."[17] In 1912, Janet Elizabeth Lane-Claypon first used the retrospective (historical) cohort design to study weight gain during the first year of life among 204 infants who were fed boiled cows' milk compared with 300 infants who were fed human breast milk.[18,19] Subsequent major developments in chronic disease epidemiology were brought about by a series of landmark studies on tobacco and health. In 1938, Pearl[20] used insurance data to show that life expectancies of smokers were substantially reduced relative to nonsmokers. In 1950, three hospital-based case-control studies[21-23] showed almost simultaneously that smoking was linked to lung cancer. One year later, Doll and Hill initiated the first major prospective cohort study of British doctors to examine the relation between tobacco smoking, lung cancer, and other chronic diseases.[24]

The transition from infectious to chronic disease epidemiology led to the rethinking of causal inferences and the publication of Hill's criteria for establishing causality in modern epidemiology.[25] The subsequent development and evolution of other key epidemiologic methods and concepts, including confounding, bias, effect modification, and causal inference, can be traced via a series of classic textbooks in epidemiology.[26] These include those by Morris,[27] MacMahon and Pugh,[28] Lilienfeld and Lilienfeld,[29] Miettinen,[30] and Rothman.[31]

Over the past two decades, the intersection of epidemiologic methods and substantive areas has led to the development of specialized areas within epidemiology, such as clinical,[32] nutritional,[33] genetic,[34] social,[35] environmental,[36] occupational,[37] cancer,[38,39] life course,[40,41] psychiatric,[42] spatial,[43] and injury[44] epidemiology. Obesity epidemiology, a new area of specialization, is coming of age in a time of escalating obesity epidemic and rapid advances in obesity research.

Historical Context of Obesity Research

In the *Handbook of Obesity*,[45] Bray gives an authoritative account of the historical context of obesity research. Obesity was documented in ancient civilizations.[46] Cases of massive obesity were identified in Stone Age drawings;[47] portrayals of obese women date back thousands of years.[48] Hippocrates observed that "sudden death is more common in those who are naturally fat than in the lean,"[49] and described obesity as "not only a disease itself, but the harbinger of others."[50]

A booklet by Short[51] was the earliest monograph on the subject of obesity treatment through exercise and other "natural means." It was followed by Flemyng's description of four causes of obesity, one of them overeating.[52] William Banting's *A Letter on Corpulence Addressed to the Public*,[53] published in 1863, is considered the first popular "diet book." It was a 21-page pamphlet written by an obese patient treated with a high-protein diet to lose weight.

Some of the concepts that are the current basis for research in the field of obesity had their origins in the 18th century.[47] In 1720, Santorio, a professor of medicine at Padua, Italy, developed a balance for weighing himself, a scale used daily to monitor his weight changes as he ate and exercised.[54] In 1777, Lavoisier made fundamental contributions to the concept of energy balance by measuring human oxygen consumption and demonstrating that metabolism is similar to combustion.[55] It would take another century before Atwater showed that the Law of Conservation of Energy applied to humans,[56] and Quetelet,[1] a mathematician in Belgium, developed an index of weight minimally correlated with height to evaluate an individual's body size. Called the Quetelet Index and widely known as BMI (weight in kilograms divided by the square of height in meters), it remains the most widely used measure of obesity to this day.

During the 20th century, there were major advances in experimental approaches to obesity research at cellular, genetic, and individual levels, as well as applications of modern technology to obesity research: dual-energy x-ray absorptiometry (DXA), computed tomography (CT), and magnetic resonance imaging (MRI) to provide quantitative estimates of percentage of body fat and regional fat distribution;[55] and the doubly labeled water method to measure energy expenditure.[57] These breakthroughs formed the basis of the modern discipline of obesity research, which has led to our current understanding of the pathophysiology of this condition and substantial progress in the behavioral, pharmacological, and surgical treatment of obesity.

One of the milestones of the 20th century was the discovery of leptin, a hormone that regulates appetite and energy metabolism.[58] Although this watershed event did not lead to a cure for obesity, it did open the door to research on other adipocyte-derived hormones and cytokines such as resistin and adiponectin. This line of research has led to the widespread acceptance of adipose tissue as an endocrine organ.[59,60]

In the past several decades, researchers have launched a series of large prospective studies on the relationship among diet, obesity, and chronic diseases. These epidemiologic studies have produced unprecedented amounts of data on the health consequences and determinants of obesity. They have also generated enormous controversy regarding optimal weight for health and longevity. In the 21st century, rapid advances in genomic, proteomic, and metabolomic technologies have already presented new opportunities and challenges for obesity epidemiology.

Epidemiologic Models of Obesity

The Epidemiologic Triad

The traditional model of infectious disease causation has been represented as a triangle consisting of three components: an external agent (e.g., bacteria), a susceptible host, and a facilitating environment that connects the host and agent (e.g., climate, sanitation, insects). The triad has proven to be a robust model in infectious disease epidemiologic research[61,62] and has also been successfully applied in noninfectious disease settings, such as injury prevention.[63] However, it is considered too simplistic for chronic diseases.

An integrated approach to the epidemiology and prevention of obesity has been developed by Egger and colleagues.[61] Known as the obesity ecological model, it identifies host factors (e.g., genetics, behaviors, attitudes, medications), vectors (energy-dense and nutrient-poor foods or beverages, large portion sizes, energy-saving devices), and environmental variables (physical, sociocultural, political, economic) (Fig. 1.1). The model takes policy, legislation, food services, and city planning into account and is therefore considered a comprehensive approach for use in the development of intervention strategies aimed at both societal and individual factors.

Life-Course Model and Developmental Origins of Obesity

There is increasing evidence that obesity and many chronic diseases start early in life (see Chapter 19). Intrauterine factors, especially low birth weight, have been associated with a wide range of chronic diseases in adulthood, including hypertension, diabetes, cardiovascular diseases, and some cancers.[40] The intrauterine environment and early childhood factors may influence adult onset of obesity through multiple pathways, including fetal metabolic programming, maternal diet during pregnancy, breast-feeding, postnatal growth, adiposity rebound, and early childhood behaviors. A conceptual framework for the life-course model puts a great deal of emphasis on the developmental origins of health and disease, with a particular focus on the long-term health effects of exposures during prenatal period and infancy (see Chapter 19).

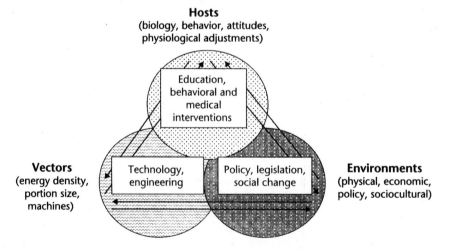

Figure 1.1 The epidemiological triad as it applies to obesity. Reproduced with permission from Egger G, Swinburn B, Rossner S. Dusting off the epidemiological triad: could it work with obesity? *Obes Rev.* 2003;4:115-119.[62]

A life-course approach to obesity prevention requires the identification of intervening risk factors across different life stages, including intrauterine exposures, infant feeding practice, parental influences, school environment, and adult-life transitions. Several birth cohort studies have been established to examine age-specific risk factors for obesity and associated chronic diseases. Results from these studies are particularly valuable in identifying risk factors for infant and childhood obesity, which can then be used to guide preventive efforts during critical periods of development.

A Multilevel Pathway Model of Obesity

Kim and Popkin[64] proposed a multilevel pathway model to depict multifactorial causation of obesity as well as multiple health consequences engendered by obesity. In this model, overweight and obesity are considered intermediate outcomes in the causal pathway that links dietary factors, physical activity, fetal/infant development, genetics, and sociocultural variables to development of chronic diseases, including diabetes, cardiovascular diseases, and cancers. Effects of overweight and obesity on chronic diseases are mediated through metabolic disorders, including hypertension, dyslipidemia, and insulin resistance.

This model highlights the dynamic nature and complexity of obesity epidemiology. It has important implications for analysis and interpretation of data on the causes of obesity and the relationship to mortality. For example, in many studies of obesity and mortality, controlling for blood cholesterol, hypertension, and diabetes attenuates or even eliminates the effects of BMI on cardiovascular disease and total mortality.[65] However, the results of such analyses should be interpreted carefully, because high cholesterol, hypertension, and diabetes are biological intermediates—factors that mediate, in part, the effects of obesity on chronic disease and mortality.

Domains of Obesity Epidemiology Research

The goal of obesity epidemiology is to identify the determinants and consequences of obesity, thereby informing prevention and intervention strategies. By definition, obesity epidemiology encompasses a variety of research activities. These include monitoring population trends, identifying genetic and environmental risk factors, examining health and other consequences of obesity, and carrying out intervention studies on prevention or treatment. As shown in a conceptual model similar to that used in physical activity research,[66] the different domains of obesity research are interrelated; findings from each inform the others (Fig. 1.2). For example, population trends detected in descriptive epidemiology may prompt analytic epidemiologic studies of risk factors. These reports may, in turn, guide obesity prevention and intervention research.

Results from epidemiologic studies of obesity in relation to disease outcomes and mortality are crucial to the development of healthy weight guidelines and recommendations. Basic or mechanistic research on obesity, although not part of obesity epidemiology, plays an important role in understanding biological mechanisms, causes, and consequences of obesity. This knowledge can help with the interpretation of findings from epidemiologic and intervention studies and guide further in-depth investigations of novel risk factors and treatment modalities. Sound study design, analysis, and interpretation, as well as valid measurements of body fatness and energy balance, are crucial to all epidemiologic research. In subsequent chapters, we will discuss each of these topics in detail. We briefly summarize key research domains in obesity epidemiology in the following pages.

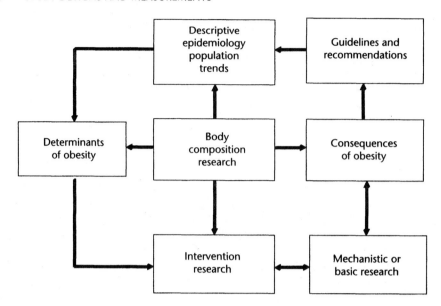

Figure 1.2 Conceptual framework for the interrelationships among obesity epidemiology research domains. Adapted from Welk GJ. Introduction to physical activity research. In: Welk GJ, ed. *Physical Activity Assessments for Health-Related Research*. Champaign, IL: Human Kinetics, 2000:3-18.[66]

Monitoring Obesity Trends in Populations

Descriptive epidemiologic surveys are instrumental in identifying obesity patterns and secular trends in populations. Since 1960, the Centers for Disease Control and Prevention (CDC) has conducted a series of national surveys of population trends in obesity, nutrition, and physical activity in the U.S. population. The National Health and Nutrition Examination Survey (NHANES) is now an ongoing survey designed to collect information about nutrition, physical activity, weight, and health conditions (http://www.cdc.gov/nchs/about/major/nhanes). Since the 1970s, the NHANES surveys have revealed dramatic increases in the prevalence of adult and childhood obesity across socioeconomic and ethnic groups (see Chapter 2). Recent NHANES surveys (2001-2002 and 2003-2004) have included more refined measurements of body composition, physical fitness, and diet in subsamples of the population. However, the development of instruments to measure nutrition and physical activity that can be readily and efficiently administered to large populations is an ongoing challenge. Meanwhile, the lack of systematic surveys in many developing countries also presents a challenge.

Health and Other Consequences of Obesity

The literature on health consequences of obesity has increased exponentially in the past decades. One reason is the growing obesity epidemic; another is the widespread availability of body size or adiposity measurements in almost all epidemiologic or clinical studies. These studies have substantially improved our understanding of the relationships between adiposity and various health outcomes. However, many questions and controversies remain. These include continuing debate on the impact of obesity on mortality; the relative importance of fatness versus fitness; the relative predictive powers of BMI versus waist circumference or waist-to-hip ratio; and the effects of voluntary versus involuntary weight loss on health. All of these issues require careful consideration of epidemiologic study design, analyses, and interpretation. Most of these concerns will be discussed in Part II of this book.

Determinants or Predictors of Obesity

The cause of obesity is deceptively simple—energy intake that exceeds energy expenditure. However, the regulation of body weight and adiposity is an exceedingly complex process that involves genetic, endocrine/regulatory, behavioral, psychosocial, and environmental factors. In the past several decades, numerous epidemiologic studies have examined a wide range of risk factors for the development of obesity. While considerable progress has been made in understanding the causes of obesity, the specific relationships and interrelationships among the many contributing factors have yet to be elucidated. As with studies on the health consequences of obesity, epidemiologic research on the determinants of obesity is fraught with methodological problems that include confounding, reverse causation, and imprecise measurement of diet and physical activity. Obesity is a complex outcome to study because many potential confounders such as dietary restraints and fidgeting are difficult to measure. Also, because body weight is a visible outcome that can alter eating behavior, epidemiologic studies of diet and obesity, especially cross-sectional analyses, are prone to reverse causation bias. Understanding these methodological issues is critical to the interpretation of the vast literature on this topic. In Part III of this book, we will discuss behavioral, psychosocial, biochemical, and genetic predictors of obesity.

The Development and Validation of Body Composition Measurement Methods

Accurate body composition measurements are central to obesity epidemiologic research, regardless of whether obesity is used as an exposure or an outcome. The past several decades have witnessed major advances in the field of body composition research, including the development of multicomponent body composition models and highly accurate imaging techniques such as DXA, CT, and MRI to quantify percentage of body fat and locations of fat at tissue-organ levels. Despite these advances, anthropometric measures, particularly weight and height, remain the most widely used method for assessing adiposity in epidemiologic studies. Further validation and refinement of anthropometric measures and the application of newly developed body composition methods to epidemiologic studies remain an important area for research in obesity epidemiology. We will discuss a variety of methods for assessing adiposity and body composition in Chapter 5.

The ultimate goal of obesity research is to prevent the condition and treat those who suffer from it. Obesity intervention research includes trials of dietary strategies and lifestyle modifications at individual, school, community, and societal levels; clinical studies of behavioral, pharmacological, and surgical approaches to weight control; and clinical trials on the effects of weight loss and maintenance on health outcomes such as diabetes and cardiovascular disease. In recent years, the growing prevalence of childhood obesity has drawn attention to the role of social and environmental factors, such as school lunch programs, physical education facilities and curriculum, vending machine products, and family support.

Despite a large number of studies that have improved insight into the prevention and treatment of obesity, sufficiently effective intervention strategies are yet to be identified and widely implemented. Sound epidemiologic research on determinants and consequences of obesity are essential to the design and interpretation of intervention trials and the development of public health policy and guidelines. Although intervention is an important area in obesity research, a detailed discussion of this topic is beyond the scope of this book. Readers interested in more specific details about prevention and treatment of obesity should consult a variety of other excellent resources.[67-73]

References

1. Quetelet A. Sur l'homme et le developpement de ses facultes, ou essai de phsyique sociale. Paris: Bachelier, 1835.
2. Hippocrates. *On Airs, Waters and Places.* 400 B.C.E. The Internet Classics Archive. http://classics.mit.edu//Hippocrates/airwatpl.html.
3. Grandjean P, Klein G. Epidemiology and precaution 150 years before Snow. *Epidemiology.* 2005;16:271-272.
4. Susser M. *Causal Thinking in the Health Sciences: Concepts and Strategies of Epidemiology.* New York: Oxford University Press; 1973.
5. Eyler JM. *Social Medicine: The Ideas and Methods of William Farr.* Baltimore: Johns Hopkins University Press; 1979.
6. Susser M, Adelstein A, eds. *Vital Statistics: A Memorial Volume of Sections from the Reports and Writings of William Farr.* Metuchen: The Scarecrow Press; 1975.
7. Lambert R. *Sir Jon Simon (1816-1904) and English Social Administration.* London: MacGibbon & Kee; 1963.
8. Hamlin C. *Public Health and Social Justice in the Age of Chadwick.* Cambridge: Cambridge University Press; 1998.
9. Brockington CF. *Public Health in the Nineteenth Century.* London: E&S Livingstone; 1965.
10. Susser E, Bresnahan M. Origins of epidemiology. *Ann N Y Acad Sci.* 2001;954:6-18.
11. Snow J. *On the Mode of Communication of Cholera.* London: John Churchill, New Burlington Street, England; 1855.
12. Buck C, Llopis A, Najera E, Terris M, eds. *The Challenge of Epidemiology.* Washington, DC: Pan American Health Organization; 1988.
13. Goldberger J, Wheeler GA. *The Experimental Production of Pellagra in Human Subjects by Means of Diets.* Washington, DC: Goverment Printing Office; 1920.
14. Koch RE. Die Aetiologie der Tuberculose. *Berliner klinische Wochenschrift.* 1882;19:221-230.
15. Winslow CEA. *The Conquest of Epidemic Disease: A Chapter in the History of Ideas.* Madison, WI: The University of Wisconsin Press; 1943.
16. Berkman LF. Seeing the forest and the trees: new visions in social epidemiology. *Am J Epidemiol.* 2004;160:1-2.
17. Berlivet L. "Association or causation?" The debate on the scientific status of risk factor epidemiology, 1947-c. 1965. *Clio Med.* 2005;75:39-74.
18. Lane-Claypon JE. *Report to the Local Government Board upon the Available Data in Regard to the Value of Boiled Milk as a Food for Infants and Young Animals, No 63.* London: His Majesty's Stationary Office; 1912:1-60.
19. Winkelstein W, Jr. Vignettes of the history of epidemiology: three firsts by Janet Elizabeth Lane-Claypon. *Am J Epidemiol.* 2004;160:97-101.
20. Pearl R. Tobacco smoking and longevity. *Science.* 1938;87:216-217.
21. Doll R, Hill AB. Smoking and carcinoma of the lung; preliminary report. *Br Med J.* 1950;2:739-748.
22. Wynder EL, Graham EA. Tobacco smoking as a possible etiologic factor in bronchiogenic carcinoma; a study of 684 proved cases. *JAMA.* 1950;143:329-336.
23. Levin M, Goldstein H, Gerhardt P. Cancer and tobacco smoking: a preliminary report. *JAMA.* 1950;143:336-338.
24. Doll R, Hill AB. The mortality of doctors in relation to their smoking habits; a preliminary report. *Br Med J.* 1954;4877:1451-1455.
25. Hill AB. The environment and disease: association or causation? *Proc R Soc Med.* 1965;58:295-300.

26. Zhang FF, Michaels DC, Mathema B, et al. Evolution of epidemiologic methods and concepts in selected textbooks of the 20th century. *Soz Praventivmed.* 2004;49:97-104.
27. Morris JN. *Uses of Epidemiology.* Edinburgh: E&S Livingstone; 1964.
28. MacMahon B, Pugh TF. *Epidemiology: Principles and Methods.* Boston, MA: Little, Brown and Company; 1970.
29. Lilienfeld AM, Lilienfeld DE. *Foundations of Epidemiology.* New York: Oxford University Press; 1976.
30. Miettinen OS. *Theoretical Epidemiology: Principles of Occurrence Research in Medicine.* New York: John Wiley & Sons; 1985.
31. Rothman KJ. *Modern Epidemiology.* Boston, MA: Little, Brown and Company; 1986.
32. Fletcher RH, Fletcher SW. *Clinical Epidemiology: The Essentials.* 4th ed. Philadelphia, PA: Lippincott, Williams & Wilkins; 2004.
33. Willett WC. *Nutritional Epidemiology.* 2nd ed. New York: Oxford University Press; 1998.
34. Khoury MJ, Beaty TH, Cohen BH. *Fundamentals of Genetic Epidemiology.* New York: Oxford University Press; 1993.
35. Berkman LF, Kawachi I. *Social Epidemiology.* New York: Oxford University Press; 2000.
36. Talbott E, Craun GF. *An Introduction to Environmental Epidemiology.* Boca Raton, FL: CRC Press; 1995.
37. Monson RR. *Occupational Epidemiology.* 2nd ed. Boca Raton, FL: CRC Press; 1990.
38. Schottenfeld D, Fraumeni J. *Cancer Epidemiology and Prevention.* 3rd ed. New York: Oxford University Press; 2006.
39. Adami H-O, Hunter D, Trichopoulos D. *Textbook of Cancer Epidemiology.* New York: Oxford University Press; 2006.
40. Kuh D, Ben Shlomo Y. *A Life Course Approach to Chronic Disease Epidemiology.* 2nd ed. New York: Oxford University Press; 2004.
41. Pickles A, Maughan B, Wadsworth M. *Epidemiological Methods in Life Course Research.* New York: Oxford University Press; 2007.
42. Susser E, Schwartz S, Morabia A, et al. *Psychiatric Epidemiology: Searching for the Causes of Mental Disorders.* New York: Oxford University Press; 2006.
43. Elliott P, Wakefield J, Best N, Briggs D. *Spatial Epidemiology: Methods and Applications.* New York: Oxford University Press; 2001.
44. Robertson L. *Injury Epidemiology: Research and Control Strategies.* 3rd ed. New York: Oxford University Press; 2007.
45. Bray G, Bouchard C, James P, eds. *Handbook of Obesity: Etiology and Pathophysiology.* New York: Marcel Dekker, Inc.; 2004.
46. Boriani F, Taveggia A, Cravero L. Obesity and body contouring: contemporary lessons from a historical example. *Obes Surg.* 2005;15:1218.
47. Bray GA. Obesity: historical development of scientific and cultural ideas. *Int J Obes.* 1990;14:909-926.
48. Gourevitch D, Grmek M. *L'obesite et ses representations figurees dans l'Antiquite. Archeologie et Medecine VIIemes Rencontres Internationales d'Archeologie et d'Histoire.* Juan-les-Pins, France: A.P.D.C.A., 1987:355-367.
49. Bray GA. Risks of obesity. *Endocrinol Metab Clin North Am.* 2003;32:787-804.
50. Bain C. Commentary: What's past is prologue. *Int J Epidemiol.* 2006;35:16-17.
51. Short T. *Discourse concerning the causes and effects of corpulency together with the method for its prevention and cure.* London: J. Roberts; 1727.
52. Flemyng M. *A Discourse on the Nature, Causes, and Cure of Corpulency.* Illustrated by a remarkable case, read before the Royal Society, November 1757 and now first published. London: L. Davis and C. Reymers; 1760.
53. Banting W. *A Letter on Corpulence Addressed to the Public.* London: Harrison and Sons (Reprinted in *Obes Res,* 1993;1:153-156); 1863.
54. Santorio S. Medica Statica. Being the Aphorisms of Sanctorius (Translated into English with large explanations). London: W. and J. Newton, A. Bell, W. Taylor and J. Osborne; 1720.

55. Heymsfield SB. Rhoads Lecture. Heat and life: the ongoing scientific odyssey. *JPEN J Parenter Enteral Nutr.* 2002;26:319-332, vii.
56. Bray GA. *A Brief History of Obesity.* New York, NY: The Guilford Press; 2002.
57. Schoeller DA, Ravussin E, Schutz Y, Acheson KJ, Baertschi P, Jequier E. Energy expenditure by doubly labeled water: validation in humans and proposed calculation. *Am J Physiol Regul Integr Comp Physiol* 1986;250:R823-R830.
58. Zhang Y, Proenca R, Maffei M, Barone M, Leopold L, Friedman JM. Positional cloning of the mouse obese gene and its human homologue. *Nature* 1994;372:425-432.
59. Hauner H, Hochberg Z. Endocrinology of adipose tissue. *Horm Metab Res.* 2002;34:605-606.
60. Prins JB. Adipose tissue as an endocrine organ. *Best Pract Res Clin Endocrinol Metab.* 2002;16:639-651.
61. Egger G, Swinburn B. An "ecological" approach to the obesity pandemic. *BMJ.* 1997;315:477-480.
62. Egger G, Swinburn B, Rossner S. Dusting off the epidemiological triad: could it work with obesity? *Obes Rev.* 2003;4:115-119.
63. Hadden W. Advances in the epidemiology of injuries as a basis for public policy. *Public Health Rep.* 1980;95:411-421.
64. Kim S, Popkin BM. Commentary: understanding the epidemiology of overweight and obesity—a real global public health concern. *Int J Epidemiol.* 2006;35:60-67.
65. Manson JE, Stampfer MJ, Hennekens CH, Willett WC. Body weight and longevity. A reassessment. *JAMA.* 1987;257:353-358.
66. Welk GJ. Introduction to physical activity research. In: Welk GJ, ed. *Physical Activity Assessments for Health-Related Research.* Champaign, IL: Human Kinetics; 2002:3-18.
67. *NHLBI Obesity Education Initiative Expert Panel on the Identification, Evaluation, and Treatment of Overweight and Obesity in Adults.* Bethesda, MD: National Institutes of Health. National Heart, Lung, and Blood Institute; 1998.
68. *Obesity: Preventing and Managing the Global Epidemic.* Report of a WHO Consultation. World Health Organization. Geneva; Technical Report Series World Health Organization, 2000:1-253.
69. Clinical guidelines on the identification, evaluation, and treatment of overweight and obesity in adults. The evidence report. *Obes Res* 1998;6(suppl):51S-209S.
70. Wadden TA, Stunkard AJ, eds. *Hankbook of Obesity Treatment.* New York: The Guilford Press; 2002.
71. Bray GA, Bouchard C, eds. *Handbook of Obesity—Clinical Applications,* 2nd ed. New York: Marcel Dekker, Inc.; 2004.
72. Crawford D, Jeffery RW, eds. *Obesity Prevention and Public Health.* New York: Oxford University Press; 2005.
73. Kumanyika S, Brownson RC, eds. *Handbook of Obesity Prevention. A Resource for Health Professionals.* New York: Springer; 2007.

2

Descriptive Epidemiology of Obesity Trends

Frank B. Hu

Epidemiologic studies are typically divided into three categories: descriptive (identifying the pattern and trends of health conditions), analytic (examining associations between exposures and health outcomes), and experimental (intervention studies to test specific preventive or treatment strategies in clinical or community settings).[1] In descriptive or analytic studies, also termed "observational epidemiology," researchers observe outcomes rather than experiment with interventions. The term "observational epidemiology" encompasses a variety of research designs—from ecological to prospective cohort—with different levels of evidence for causal inference. When reviewing the literature, it is more informative to refer to specific study designs (e.g., cross-sectional vs. case-control vs. cohort study) than generic research categories (e.g., observational studies).

As discussed in the earlier chapter, a central goal of obesity epidemiology is to use epidemiologic methods to examine health consequences and determinants of obesity. Thus, analytic study designs for obesity research consider obesity as one of two variables: either as an exposure/predictor or as an outcome. Typically, epidemiologic studies progress from descriptive to analytic epidemiology and then to experimental studies. In this chapter, we describe population obesity trends from descriptive epidemiologic studies. In the next chapter, we discuss analytic epidemiologic study designs and research into the consequences and determinants of obesity, and in Chapter 4, we discuss key issues related to causal inference in obesity epidemiology, including the role of randomized clinical trials, confounding, reverse causation, generalizability, and causal criteria.

Tracking of Obesity Trends

Descriptive epidemiology typically describes health conditions according to time, place, and person. Surveillance studies, a special type of descriptive epidemiologic research, are employed to detect and track meaningful epidemiologic trends of certain health conditions (e.g., obesity and diabetes) from a representative sample of a population. Such studies are typically repeated cross-sectional surveys conducted in nationally representative samples. In the past several decades, the U.S. Centers for Disease Control and Prevention (CDC) have conducted several national surveys to track the nutrition and health status of the U.S. population. Among them, National Health and Nutrition Examination Survey (NHANES; http://www.cdc.gov/nchs/nhanes.htm) and the annual Behavioral Risk Factor

Surveillance Survey (BRFSS; http://www.cdc.gov/brfss) are the most important. These studies have provided extremely valuable information on secular obesity trends in the United States. As discussed in the subsequent text, only a few other countries have conducted systematic surveys to monitor obesity trends.

NHANES describes the health and nutritional status of a cross-sectional, nationally representative sample of the U.S. noninstitutionalized population. Information for each participant is obtained from an in-home interview followed by a medical evaluation and physical examination in a mobile examination center (MEC). The study design is a stratified, multistage probability sample. From 1960 to 1994, seven NHANES were completed. Beginning in 1999, the survey has been conducted continuously. The NHANES 1999-2000 and 2001-2002 surveys, for example, included approximately 5,000 people examined at 15 locations, with oversampling of African Americans, Mexican Americans, adolescents, older persons, and low-income non-Hispanic whites. The sample size is smaller than NHANES III and the number of geographic units is also smaller. In addition, the sample design, weighting, and variance estimation methodology also differ from NHANES III. However, the procedures for conducting the interviews and examinations were similar to those for earlier surveys.[2,3] Recent data from NAHES 2005-2006 indicate a small increase in obesity prevalence from since 2003-2004 (http://origin.cdc.gov/nchs). In 2005-2006, the prevalence of obesity has reached 33.3% for men and 35.3% for women.

The BRFSS is an ongoing, state-based cross-sectional telephone survey of U.S. adults aged 18 years or older. Its purpose is to monitor state-level prevalence of the major behavioral risks associated with premature morbidity and mortality. By 1994, all states, the District of Columbia, and three territories were participating in the BRFSS.[4] The survey uses a multistage cluster design based on random digit dialing methods to select a representative sample from each state's noninstitutionalized residents. Approximately 2,000 to 4,000 adults are interviewed in each state. Data are pooled to produce nationally representative estimates.[5]

Obesity Trends in U.S. Adults

The World Health Organization (WHO)[6] and U.S. National Institutes of Health (NIH)[7] define overweight as a BMI $\geq$ 25 kg/m^2 and obesity as a BMI $\geq$ 30 kg/m^2. According to these criteria and NHANES 2003-2004 data, the prevalence of overweight and obesity in U.S. adults is estimated at 66.3% and 32.2%, respectively.[8] The prevalence of morbid obesity (BMI $\geq$ 40 kg/m^2) is approximately 4.8%. There has been a marked upward trend in obesity over the past several decades in both men and women (Fig. 2.1), although there is some indication that the prevalence of obesity in women has stabilized around 33% from 1999 to 2004. In 2005-2006, the prevalence of obesity increased slightly to 33.3% in men and 35.3% in women (http://origin.cdc.gov/nchs).

The increase in morbid obesity is particularly dramatic. On the basis of data from the BRFSS, from 1986 to 2000 the prevalence of individuals with a BMI $\geq$ 40 kg/m^2 quadrupled, and the prevalence of those with a BMI $\geq$ 50 kg/m^2 quintupled.[9] In 2001-2002, the number of people with severe obesity, who carry more than 100 lbs (or 45 kg) of excess weight (equivalent to BMI $\geq$ 40 kg/m^2), grew to nearly 11 million people.[10]

Estimates of overweight and obesity generated from self-reported BRFSS weight and height data are known to underestimate true prevalence[11] and are substantially lower than those from NHANES surveys. However, the BRFSS offers the advantage of annual state-by-state data on secular trends of obesity according to geographic locations. These data are well depicted in the CDC obesity maps,[12] which show very high prevalence of obesity in the Midwest and southern region of the country, with somewhat lower rates in the

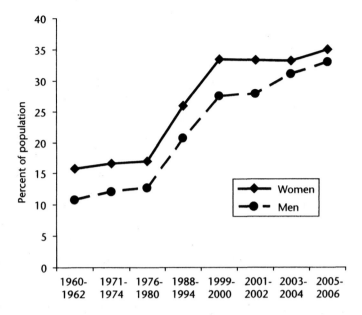

Figure 2.1 Age-adjusted prevalence of obesity in Americans aged 20 to 74 by sex and survey. NHES: 1960-1962; NHANES: 1971-1974, 1976-1980, 1988-1994, 1999-2000, 2001-2002, 2003-2004, and 2005-2006 (http://origin.cdc.gov/nchs). With permission from Ogden CL, Carroll MD, Curtin LR, McDowell MA, Tabak CJ, Flegal KM. Prevalence of overweight and obesity in the United States, 1999-2004. *JAMA*. 2006;295:1549-1555.[8]

western region. To account for underreporting of self-reported BMI data, Ezzati et al.[13] obtained statistically corrected obesity estimates from BRFSS by using measured height and weight data from the NHANES. As expected, the corrected prevalence of obesity was substantially higher than the original BRFSS estimates for all states. Because there is no overlap between the BRFSS and NHANES participants, the statistical corrections were done at group level stratified by age and sex. As discussed by the authors, underreport of obesity in BRFSS is likely to result from two sources. First, telephone interviews in BRFSS may have resulted in greater underreporting of weight and overreporting of height than other modes of self-report such as in-person interviews or data collected by mail. Second, the nonresponse rate is much higher in BRFSS (approximately 55%) than in NHANES medical examinations (approximately 25%).[13] Thus, lower estimates of obesity in BRFSS may also have resulted from a greater nonresponse rate in obese individuals than those who are normal weight.

Ethnic and Socioeconomic Status Disparities

Although the increase in the prevalence of obesity is a population-wide phenomenon, with relatively similar upward trends in men and women, substantial disparities in obesity prevalence exist.[14] According to the 2003-2004 NHANES data, compared with non-Hispanic white (30.2%) and Mexican American women (42.3%), non-Hispanic black women had the highest prevalence of obesity (53.9%) (Fig. 2.2). The prevalence of extreme obesity (BMI $\geq$ 40) was 5.8% for non-Hispanic white women, 7.8% for Mexican American women, and 14.7% for non-Hispanic black women.[8] According to the 2001 BRFSS data, the two groups with the highest prevalence of obesity were African-American women (38.4%) and American Indian/Alaska Natives (31.9%). Asian women

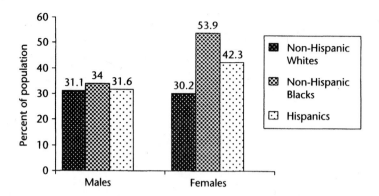

Figure 2.2 Obesity by sex and race/ethnicity (NHANES 2003-2004). With permission from Ogden CL, Carroll MD, Curtin LR, McDowell MA, Tabak CJ, Flegal KM. Prevalence of overweight and obesity in the United States, 1999-2004. *JAMA*. 2006;295:1549-1555.[8]

had the lowest rate (7.8%).[15] In men, the prevalence of obesity did not differ significantly across different racial/ethnic groups.[16,17]

Using self-reported data from the 2000 National Health Interview Survey, Goel et al.[18] reported a lower prevalence of obesity in immigrants (16%) compared with U.S.-born individuals (22%). However, the prevalence among immigrants living in the United States for at least 15 years approached that of U.S.-born adults.[18] Lauderdale and Rathouz[19] found similar results among Asian American ethnic groups. The longer foreign-born individuals lived in the United States, the higher their risk of being overweight or obese.

There has been a close association between socioeconomic status (SES) and obesity, particularly in women.[20] In general, low-SES groups in industrialized countries are more likely to be obese than their high-SES counterparts, whereas in developing nations, high-SES groups are more likely to be obese.[21-23] However, the link between SES and obesity in the United States has weakened, even as the prevalence of obesity has dramatically increased.[20] In other words, although obesity is still more common in individuals with a lower SES, disparities in obesity rates have declined over the past three decades.[24] The relative difference in the prevalence of obesity between low- and high-SES groups decreased from 50% in NHANES I (1971-1974) to 14% in NHANES (1999-2000). These data are consistent with findings of a greater increase in obesity in the high-SES group, resulting in a modest association between low-SES and obesity in most gender and ethnic groups.[20] Among black women, those with middle incomes experienced the largest increase in the prevalence of obesity; for black men, the largest increase was seen in the high-income group.[24]

Increase in Central Obesity

The National Cholesterol Education Program (NCEP) includes elevated waist circumference (>40 in./102 cm in men; >35 in./88 cm in women), a measure of central obesity, as one of the five abnormalities that define the metabolic syndrome.[25] Li et al.[26] examined secular trends in waist circumference in U.S. adults based on the NHANES conducted between 1988 and 2004. Between the periods of 1988-1994 and 2003-2004, the age-adjusted mean waist circumference increased from 96.0 to 100.4 cm in men and from 89.0 to 94.0 cm in women. The age-adjusted abdominal or central obesity increased from 29.5% to 42.4% in men and from 47.0% to 61.3% in women. In 2003-2004, over half of U.S. adults had abdominal obesity as defined by the NCEP criterion. In men, whites appeared to have the highest prevalence of abdominal obesity, whereas in women, African Americans had the highest prevalence of abdominal obesity. Increase in abdominal obesity has occurred in all socioeconomical groups, but people with higher education levels experienced the largest relative increase.

Incidence of Obesity

Longitudinal studies of the same individuals over time are needed to examine incidence of obesity. Among 4,117 white participants aged 30 to 50 years in the Framingham Offspring Study 1971-2001,[27] the 4-year rates for developing overweight varied from 14% to 19% in normal-weight women and 26% to 30% in normal-weight men, depending on age. Four-year rates for developing obesity ranged from 5% to 7% in nonobese women and 7% to 9% in nonobese men. The long-term (30-year) risk estimates were similar for men and women. Overall, the risk exceeded 1 in 2 persons for developing overweight, 1 in 4 individuals for developing obesity, and 1 in 10 people for developing severe obesity (BMI $\geq$ 35 kg/m²) across different age groups.

Obesity Trends in U.S. Children

According to NHANES 2003-2004, approximately 17.1% of children and adolescents aged 2 to 19 years are overweight[8] based on the 95th percentile or higher of BMI values in the 2000 CDC growth chart for the United States.[28] The prevalence of overweight is highest among 6- to 11-year-old children (18.8%), followed by adolescents 12 to 19 years old (17.4%) and children 2 to 5 years old (13.9%). This represents a 3- to 4-fold increase in prevalence of overweight from the early 1970s (Fig. 2.3). The prevalence of at-risk of overweight (defined as BMI for age at 85th percentile or higher) was 26.2% for 2- to 5-year-olds, 37.1% for 6- to 11-year-olds, and 34.3% for 12- to 19-year-olds. The prevalence of overweight is substantially higher among minorities, especially Hispanic boys (25.3%) and non-Hispanic black girls (26.5%) (Fig. 2.4).

In parallel with the increase in BMI, waist circumference and waist-to-height ratio have increased dramatically in US children and adolescents in the past two decades.[29]

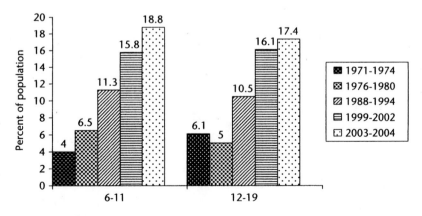

Figure 2.3 Prevalence of overweight among children aged 6 to 19 years. Adapted with permission from Ogden CL, Carroll MD, Curtin LR, McDowell MA, Tabak CJ, Flegal KM. Prevalence of overweight and obesity in the United States, 1999-2004. *JAMA.* 2006;295:1549-1555.[8]

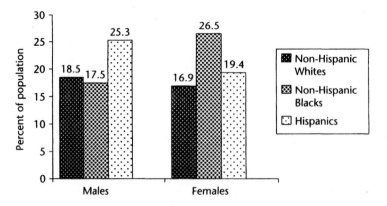

Figure 2.4 Prevalence of overweight among children 6 to 11 years old by sex and race/ethnicity in 2003-2004. Adapted with permission from Ogden CL, Carroll MD, Curtin LR, McDowell MA, Tabak CJ, Flegal KM. Prevalence of overweight and obesity in the United States, 1999-2004. *JAMA*. 2006;295:1549-1555.[8]

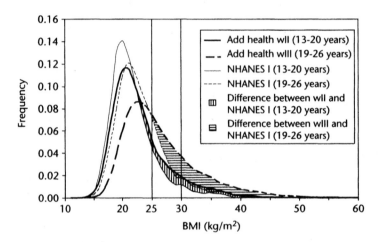

Figure 2.5 Distribution frequency of BMI from the National Longitudinal Study of Adolescent Health (Add Health) waves II and III. NHANES, National Health and Nutrition Examination Survey. With permission from Gordon-Larsen, P, Adair LS, Nelson MC, Popkin BM. Five-year obesity incidence in the transition period between adolescence and adulthood: the National Longitudinal Study of Adolescent Health. *Am J Clin Nutr*. 2004;80:569-575.[30]

The increase in the mean waist circumference occurred consistently across different gender, racial/ethnic, and age subgroups.

Gordon-Larsen et al.[30] used nationally representative, longitudinally measured height and weight data from U.S. adolescents in waves II (1996; aged 13 to 20 years) and III (2001; 19 to 26 years) of the National Longitudinal Study of Adolescent Health (*n* = 9,795) to examine obesity trends through the transition to adulthood. On the basis of International Obesity Task Force (IOTF) cutoff points,[31] incidence of obesity over the 5-year study was 12.7%; 9.4% of the participants remained obese; and 1.6% shifted from obese to non-obese. Obesity incidence was highest in non-Hispanic black females (18.4%). Figure 2.5 compares the NHANES I and National Longitudinal Study of Adolescent Health distributions of BMI for adolescents and young adults in the same age group. The shift in the distribution of BMI (with a long right tail in adolescents) corresponds to an increase in BMI in adults, indicating increasing prevalence of severe or morbid obesity.

International Obesity Trends

The obesity epidemic first started in the United States and other industrialized nations before spreading to developing countries, especially their urban areas. Data from national surveys in Great Britain show that since 1980, the prevalence of obesity in adults had almost tripled, with a similar rise in childhood obesity.[32] The First Israeli National Health and Nutrition Survey 1999-2001 showed a prevalence of overweight at 39.3% of the adult population, with obesity prevalence at 22.9%.[33] In Turkey, the prevalence of obesity in adults increased from 18.6% in 1990 to 21.9% in 2000.[34] Korea carried out national health and nutrition surveys of adults and children in 1995, 1998, and 2001 and found substantial increase in prevalence of obesity over time. The data from 2001 indicated an overall prevalence of adult overweight (BMI $\geq$ 25 kg/m^2) of 30.6% (32.4% in men and 29.4% in women).[35] Between 1992 and 2002, the prevalence of overweight in Chinese adults increased from 14.6% to 21.8%.[36] In a cross-sectional survey of a nationally representative sample of 15,540 Chinese adults aged 35 to 74 years in 2000-2001, the age-standardized prevalence of overweight was 26.9% in men and 31.1% in women.[37] The prevalence of overweight was higher in northern than in southern China, and higher in urban than rural residents. Epidemiologic surveys from other countries including Australia,[38] Japan (National Nutrition Survey),[39] and Malaysia[40] have also found a rapid increase in prevalence of obesity over the past two decades.

Accumulating data notwithstanding, few nations have conducted systematic surveys to assess and monitor obesity trends over a long period of time (e.g., several decades). Katzmarzyk[41] analyzed Canadian population surveys since 1953 to examine secular trends in stature and BMI over time. Median stature increased 1.4 cm/decade in men and 1.1 cm/decade in women, whereas median body weight increased 1.9 kg/decade in men and 0.8 kg/decade in women. The average weight-for-height increased 5.1% in men and 4.9% in women. The respective prevalence of overweight (BMI 25-29.9 kg/m^2) and obesity (BMI $\geq$ 30 kg/m^2) increased from 30.3% and 9.7% in 1970-1972 (based on measured BMI values) to 35.8% and 14.9% in 1998 (based on self-reported BMI values) for men and women, respectively. More recent self-reported data on the adult ($\geq$18 years) population showed a continued increase in the prevalence of overweight and obesity.[42] Data show a shift to the right in the entire distribution of BMI since 1970-1972, particularly in men. This trend is similar to that seen in the U.S. population.

Prentice[43] compiled data on the prevalence of obesity across the world and made several observations: (a) very high rates of obesity in several of the Pacific Islands, with record rates in Nauru, where prevalence in some populations approached 80%; (b) generally lower prevalence of obesity in Asian nations, but with rapidly increasing rates in China, India, and other countries, especially in urban areas; (c) a higher prevalence of obesity in North America than in Europe, but with the gap quickly narrowing (more than half of the 15 original members of the European Union had a prevalence of obesity in excess of 20% in 2002);[44] (d) high prevalence of obesity in many Middle Eastern countries, with rates similar to those of the United States in some, such as Bahrain; and (e) generally low prevalence of obesity in Africa, but with great heterogeneity (for instance, Ghana has a 3% prevalence of obesity compared with 21% in South Africa).

Because many developing countries are in the midst of rapid economic, epidemiologic, and nutrition transitions, the global obesity epidemic is likely to accelerate. Underweight, which used to be the most important form of malnutrition in developing countries, is being replaced by overweight and obesity. In low- and middle-income countries, this shift is creating the paradoxical coexistence of obesity and underweight in the same population. For example, Villamor et al.[45] observed that among 73,689 women aged 14 to 52 years, who attended antenatal care clinics in the city of Dar es Salaam, Tanzania, the prevalence of obesity increased rapidly from 3.6% in 1995 to 9.1% in 2004, while underweight (defined as BMI < 18.5 kg/m^2) showed a modest decline from 3.3% in 1995 to 2.6% in 2004, with no change in the prevalence of wasting (defined as midupper arm circumference <22 cm). In this population, obesity was positively associated with age, parity, and SES, and inversely associated with HIV infection, whereas underweight was inversely related to SES and positively to HIV status.

Mendez et al.[46] analyzed 1992-2000 data from nationally representative cross-sectional surveys of women aged 20 to 49 years ($n = 148,579$) in 36 developing countries. They found that the prevalence of overweight exceeded underweight in most countries, with a median ratio of overweight to underweight 5.8 in urban areas and 2.1 in rural ones. In countries with more economic development, overweight among low-SES women was particularly high in both rural (38%) and urban (51%) areas.

Use of varied criteria for defining obesity in children and lack of systematic surveys in nationally representative samples make it difficult to track trends in international childhood obesity. The interpretation of survey data on obesity in children and adolescents is complicated by several methodological issues, including those related to sampling, sexual maturation, secular trends in growth and development, stunting, adiposity rebound, and measurement errors[47] (see Chapter 20). Nonetheless, available data from various countries clearly show a growing epidemic of childhood obesity in both developing and developed countries.

In a comprehensive review, Lobstein et al.[47] made several observations about the global obesity epidemic in children: (a) unequal global distribution of childhood obesity, with the highest rates in North America and the lowest in Sub-Saharan Africa, which also has the highest poverty and HIV infection rates. Among children and adolescents aged 5 to 17 years, the overall global prevalence of overweight defined by the IOTF criteria was approximately 10%, with a 2% to 3% prevalence of obesity; (b) a concentration of childhood obesity among the poor in industrialized countries and in the more economically developed areas of poorer countries; and (c) more rapid increase in childhood obesity in some developing countries (e.g., urban areas of Brazil and China) than in developed countries.

Summary

Descriptive epidemiology has played an essential role in uncovering the accelerating worldwide obesity epidemic and describing its patterns and trends. However, few countries are conducting systematic surveillance of obesity and its associated comorbidities over time. Nonetheless, there is clear evidence that obesity has reached epidemic proportions in many parts of the world and is increasing rapidly in developing countries. In many populations, the entire distribution of BMI values has shifted to the right, indicating a dramatic increase in morbid obesity. The growth in childhood obesity is more rapid and particularly disturbing. The dual burden of malnutrition and overweight currently observed in many developing countries reflects a transitional stage of the epidemic. If current trends continue, it is projected that by 2025, the prevalence of obesity will exceed 40% in the United States, 30% in England, and 20% in Brazil.[48,49]

Lack of high quality, comparable data from different countries hinders the tracking of obesity trends, especially in developing nations undergoing rapid economic and epidemiologic transitions. Nationally representative samples, standardized survey methodology, and measured body mass are needed across different populations to monitor the global epidemic of obesity. The need is even more crucial for tracking childhood obesity. Although many industrialized countries, especially the United States have collected representative data on childhood obesity, systematic data from developing countries are limited. The use of consistent criteria for defining childhood obesity is needed to facilitate international comparisons. Because of the evolving nature of the obesity epidemic, collection of longitudinal data in the same individuals over a long period of time is of great value in tracking the development of obesity across different life stages and in determining critical points for intervention.

References

1. Rothman KJ. *Epidemiology. An Introduction.* New York: Oxford University Press; 2002.
2. National Center for Health Statistics. Plan and Operation of the Third National Health and Nutrition Examination Survey, 1988-94. Series 1: programs and collection procedures. *Vital Health Stat* 1 1994;21:1-407.
3. Carroll MD, Lacher DA, Sorlie PD, et al. Trends in serum lipids and lipoproteins of adults, 1960-2002. *JAMA.* 2005;294:1773-1781.
4. United States Department of Health and Human Services. Centers for Disease Control and Prevention. National Center for Chronic Disease Prevention and Health Promotion. About the BRFSS. United States Department of Health and Human Services.
5. Nelson DE, Holtzman D, Waller M, Leutzinger CL, Condon K. Objectives and Design of the Behavioral Risk Factor Surveillance System. Proceedings of the Section on Survey Methods of the American Statistical Association National Meeting. August 10, 1998. Dallas, TX; 1998.
6. Obesity: preventing and managing the global epidemic: report of a WHO consultation. Geneva, Switzerland: World Health Organization; 1999.
7. Clinical Guidelines on the Identification, Evaluation, and Treatment of Overweight and Obesity in Adults. The Evidence Report. *Obes Res.* 1998;6(Suppl 2):51S-209S.
8. Ogden CL, Carroll MD, Curtin LR, McDowell MA, Tabak CJ, Flegal KM. Prevalence of overweight and obesity in the United States, 1999-2004. *JAMA.* 2006;295:1549-1555.
9. Sturm R. Increases in clinically severe obesity in the United States, 1986-2000. *Arch Intern Med.* 2003;163:2146-2148.
10. Commonwealth of Massachusetts Betsy Lehman Center for Patient Safety and Medical Error Reduction. Expert Panel on Weight Loss Surgery. Executive Report. *Obes Res.* 2005;13:205-26.
11. Yun S, Zhu BP, Black W, Brownson RC. A comparison of national estimates of obesity prevalence from the behavioral risk factor surveillance system and the National Health and Nutrition Examination Survey. *Int J Obes (Lond).* 2006;30:164-170.
12. Mokdad AH, Bowman BA, Ford ES, Vinicor F, Marks JS, Koplan JP. The continuing epidemics of obesity and diabetes in the United States. *JAMA.* 2001;286:1195-1200.
13. Ezzati M, Martin H, Skjold S, Vander Hoorn S, Murray CJ. Trends in national and state-level obesity in the USA after correction for self-report bias: analysis of health surveys. *J R Soc Med.* 2006;99:250-257.
14. Baskin ML, Ard J, Franklin F, Allison DB. Prevalence of obesity in the United States. *Obes Rev.* 2005;6:5-7.

15. Sundaram AA, Ayala C, Greenlund KJ, Keenan NL. Differences in the prevalence of self-reported risk factors for coronary heart disease among American women by race/ethnicity and age behavioral risk factor surveillance system, 2001. *Am J Prev Med.* 2005;29(5 Suppl):25-30.
16. Borders TF, Rohrer JE, Cardarelli KM. Gender-specific disparities in obesity. *J Community Health.* 2006;31:57-68.
17. Hedley AA, Ogden CL, Johnson CL, Carroll MD, Curtin LR, Flegal KM. Prevalence of overweight and obesity among U.S. children, adolescents, and adults, 1999-2002. *JAMA.* 2004;291:2847-2850.
18. Goel MS, McCarthy EP, Phillips RS, Wee CC. Obesity among US immigrant subgroups by duration of residence. *JAMA.* 2004;29:2860-2867.
19. Lauderdale DS, Rathouz PJ. Body mass index in a US national sample of Asian Americans: effects of nativity, years since immigration and socioeconomic status. *Int J Obes Relat Metab Disord.* 2000;24:1188-1194.
20. Zhang Q, Wang Y. Trends in the association between obesity and socioeconomic status in U.S. adults: 1971 to 2000. *Obes Res.* 2004;12:1622-1632.
21. Du S, Lu B, Zhai F, Popkin BM. A new stage of the nutrition transition in China. *Public Health Nutr.* 2002;5:169-174.
22. Monteiro CA, Conde WL, Popkin BM. Is obesity replacing or adding to undernutrition? Evidence from different social classes in Brazil. *Public Health Nutr.* 2002;5:105-112.
23. Wang Y, Monteiro C, Popkin BM. Trends of obesity and underweight in older children and adolescents in the United States, Brazil, China, and Russia. *Am J Clin Nutr.* 2002;75:971-977.
24. Chang VW, Lauderdale DS. Income disparities in body mass index and obesity in the United States, 1971-2002. *Arch Intern Med.* 2005;165:2122-2128.
25. Executive Summary of the Third Report of The National Cholesterol Education Program (NCEP) Expert Panel on Detection, Evaluation, and Treatment of High Blood Cholesterol in Adults (Adult Treatment Panel III). *JAMA.* 2001;285:2496-2497.
26. Li C, Ford ES, McGuire LC, Mokdad AH. Increasing trends in waist circumference and abdominal obesity among US adults. *Obesity (Silver Spring).* 2007;15:216-224.
27. Vasan RS, Pencina MJ, Cobain M, Freiberg MS, D'Agostino RB. Estimated risks for developing obesity in the Framingham Heart Study. *Ann Intern Med.* 2005;143:473-480.
28. National Center for Health & Statistics. CDC Growth Charts US Department of Health & Human Services, 2000.
29. Li C, Ford ES, Mokdad AH, Cook S. Recent trends in waist circumference and waist-height ratio among US children and adolescents. *Pediatrics.* 2006;118:e1390-e1398.
30. Gordon-Larsen P, Adair LS, Nelson MC, Popkin BM. Five-year obesity incidence in the transition period between adolescence and adulthood: the National Longitudinal Study of Adolescent Health. *Am J Clin Nutr.* 2004;80:569-575.
31. Cole TJ, Bellizzi MC, Flegal KM, Dietz WH. Establishing a standard definition for child overweight and obesity worldwide: international survey. *BMJ.* 2000;320:1240-1243.
32. Rennie KL, Jebb SA. Prevalence of obesity in Great Britain. *Obes Rev.* 2005;6:11-612.
33. Kaluski DN, Berry EM. Prevalence of obesity in Israel. *Obes Rev.* 2005;6:115-116.
34. Yumuk VD. Prevalence of obesity in Turkey. *Obes Rev.* 2005;6:9-10.
35. Kim DM, Ahn CW, Nam SY. Prevalence of obesity in Korea. *Obes Rev.* 2005;6:117-121.
36. Wang Y, Mi J, Shan XY, Wang QJ, Ge KY. Is China facing an obesity epidemic and the consequences? The trends in obesity and chronic disease in China. *Int J Obes (Lond).* 2007;31:177-188.
37. Gu D, Reynolds K, Wu X, et al. Prevalence of the metabolic syndrome and overweight among adults in China. *Lancet.* 2005;365:1398-1405.
38. Thorburn AW. Prevalence of obesity in Australia. *Obes Rev.* 2005;6:187-189.

39. Yoshiike N, Seino F, Tajima S, et al. Twenty-year changes in the prevalence of overweight in Japanese adults: the National Nutrition Survey 1976-95. *Obes Rev.* 2002;3:183.
40. Ismail MN, Chee SS, Nawawi H, Yusoff K, Lim TO, James WP. Obesity in Malaysia. *Obes Rev.* 2002;3:203-208.
41. Katzmarzyk PT. The Canadian obesity epidemic: an historical perspective. *Obes Res.* 2002;10:666-674.
42. Belanger-Ducharme F, Tremblay A. Prevalence of obesity in Canada. *Obes Rev.* 2005;6:183-186.
43. Prentice AM. The emerging epidemic of obesity in developing countries. *Int J Epidemiol.* 2006;35:93-99.
44. Fry J, Finley W. The prevalence and costs of obesity in the EU. *Proc Nutr Soc.* 2005;64:359-362.
45. Villamor E, Msamanga G, Urassa W, et al. Trends in obesity, underweight, and wasting among women attending prenatal clinics in urban Tanzania, 1995-2004. *Am J Clin Nutr.* 2006;83:1387-1394.
46. Mendez MA, Monteiro CA, Popkin BM. Overweight exceeds underweight among women in most developing countries. *Am J Clin Nutr.* 2005;81:714-721.
47. Lobstein T, Baur L, Uauy R, IASO International Obesity Task Force. Obesity in children and young people: a crisis in public health. *Obes Rev.* 2004;5(Suppl 1):4-104.
48. Kopelman PG. Obesity as a medical problem. *Nature.* 2000;404:635-643.
49. Wang Y, Beydoun MA. The obesity epidemic in the United States—gender, age, socioeconomic, racial/ethnic, and geographic characteristics: a systematic review and meta-regression analysis. *Epidemiolog Rev.* 2007;29:6-28.

3

Analytic Epidemiologic Designs in Obesity Research

Frank B. Hu

Descriptive epidemiology, as discussed in the previous chapter, concerns itself with distributions and patterns of health conditions without inferences about etiology. Analytic epidemiology, which examines relationships between exposure variables and health outcomes, involves the testing of hypotheses, the examination of determinants or risk factors for certain health outcomes, and the search for possible causal relationships.[1] Analytic epidemiologic study designs typically include ecological or cross-cultural comparisons, case-control studies, and prospective cohort studies. In epidemiologic research, obesity can be studied as an exposure or outcome variable. Similar study designs are used in both cases, but analytic strategies, methodological issues, and interpretations sometimes differ.

In the hierarchy of evidence for determining causal relationships, randomized clinical trials are widely accepted as the "gold standard." However, large multiyear trials are often infeasible because of high costs, lack of long-term compliance by subjects, and ethical issues (see Chapter 4). Classic case-control studies are useful in examining obesity as a risk factor for rare diseases, but the high likelihood of recall bias and the problem of reverse causation (discussed below) make the design unsuitable for the study of risk factors of obesity. In prospective cohort studies, exposure takes place before the assessment of health outcomes, minimizing the risk of biases from the selection of healthy controls and retrospective reporting of diet and lifestyle factors. For these reasons, the prospective cohort study is considered the strongest nonrandomized study design. As a result, most of the data on health consequences and determinants of obesity discussed in this book are from prospective cohort studies. Nevertheless, such studies are not immune from biases and methodological problems. In our examination of the strengths and weaknesses of different study designs, we will start with ecological research and then progress to case-control and cohort studies.

Ecological Studies

Ecological studies correlate disease rates with frequencies of exposure variables across different populations. The unit of observation is not the individual, but groups or populations; for example, countries, towns, and communities. Although ecological data have provided evidence for the importance of environmental factors in the development of chronic diseases, they require cautious interpretation. The most serious problem with ecological data is intractable confounding by different genetic backgrounds, diets, other lifestyle factors, and economic development across populations. Other widely recognized problems include "ecological fallacy" (erroneous conclusions drawn from applying aggregate data from groups to individuals) and the use of food disappearance data, which are more likely to reflect food waste than actual consumption.[2]

Confounding can easily lead to spurious correlations in ecological studies. For example, a strong positive association between the proportion of energy from fat (from food disappearance data) and prevalence of overweight has been observed across 20 countries,[3] with a higher prevalence of obesity in affluent nations compared with poor ones. Such contrasts, however, could easily be explained by differences in physical activity, food availability, and economic development. Indeed, subsequent prospective studies have not found an appreciable association between dietary fat intake as percentage of energy and incidence of obesity, and most dietary intervention trials have not supported significant benefits of low-fat diets on long-term weight loss.[4]

Confounding in ecological studies can also obscure true relationships. For example, initial cross-population comparisons in the Seven Countries Study[5] showed no relationship between obesity rates and risk of coronary heart disease (CHD) across the populations. However, subsequent prospective analyses of individual-level data indicated a strong association between obesity and risk of CHD and mortality.[6]

Correlational studies of time trends in prevalence of obesity and changes in environmental factors at the population level may provide some clues to the risk factors that are responsible for obesity epidemic. For example, in the United States, fat intake as percentage of energy has decreased in the past two to three decades even as the prevalence of obesity has increased dramatically,[7] suggesting that fat reduction may not be effective in preventing obesity. Interestingly, time trend analyses indicate a strong correlation between rising obesity in the United States and increases in consumption of refined carbohydrates[8] and high-fructose corn syrups in sugar-sweetened beverages.[9] These data suggest that refined carbohydrates and added sugar may contribute to the obesity epidemic. However, these relationships may be confounded by other simultaneous changes in diet and lifestyle (especially automation-related decreased physical activity and increased use of television and automobiles). A time trend analysis from the United Kingdom[10] suggested that less physical activity and more sedentary lifestyles played a larger role in the obesity epidemic than changes in diet. However, lack of detailed measurements at the individual level made it impossible to tease out independent effects of diet and physical activity.

The study of migrant populations is a special type of ecological analysis that can separate the effects of environmental and genetic factors. There is strong evidence that the prevalence of obesity among different immigrant subgroups is associated with number of years of residence in the United States,[11] a finding that points to changes in diet and lifestyle as primary causes of obesity. The Ni-Ho-San Study, which compared cardiovascular disease (CVD) rates and lifestyle factors among Japanese men living in Japan, Hawaii, and California, found that gradients in CVD mortality in the three populations paralleled changes in overweight, diet, and lifestyle. In particular, a dramatic increase in total and saturated fat intake appeared to have contributed to higher risk of obesity and CVD among Japanese men living in the United States than those living in Japan (percentage of energy from fat was twice as high in Hawaii and California compared with Japan).[13] However, confounding by other lifestyle factors (e.g., decreased alcohol intake and physical activity) made it impossible to establish causal relationships. While such analyses suggest that increased risk of obesity and CVD among immigrant populations is largely due to environmental rather than genetic factors, interactions between genetic susceptibility and environmental changes are also likely to play a role (see Chapter 22).

Despite methodological limitations, ecological studies are useful for generating hypotheses. Newer generations of ecological analyses could be built on existing multi-population cohort studies. Aggregate data analyses using multilevel analytic techniques can also be conducted in the context of traditional within-population analyses.[14] The combination of individual- and aggregate-level data can be particularly advantageous in elucidating macroenvironmental and societal risk factors for obesity.[15] However, collecting detailed diet and lifestyle data in a uniform and comparable manner across diverse populations is challenging.[14]

Cross-Sectional Studies

Cross-sectional studies examine associations between exposure variables and health outcomes within populations at a given time point or during a specific time interval. Although the National Health and Nutrition Examination Survey I (NHANES I) became a follow-up study when the same participants were reexamined after 10 years, the NHANES are cross-sectional in design. Such repeated surveys are useful in estimating population trends of health conditions, but their role in studying nutritional and lifestyle factors for obesity is limited. The main reason is an inability to establish a temporal relationship between exposure and obesity because diet, lifestyle, and weight are measured simultaneously. Reverse causation (e.g., weight gain leads to changes in diet) is even more problematic. For example, overweight individuals may stop consuming certain foods or beverages (e.g., sugary sodas), or switch to diet soda as part of a weight-loss strategy, changes that can lead to a spurious positive association between overweight and diet soda consumption.

Unlike heart disease or cancer, body weight is an endpoint that is readily apparent to participants, who can alter their diet and lifestyle in response to changes in weight status.[7] This can lead to reverse causation bias that is typical in retrospective studies. Besides the potentially spurious association between diet soda and obesity mentioned earlier, another example of such bias is the relationship between fat intake and obesity. Several cross-sectional studies have found an association between lower dietary fat and reduced prevalence of obesity.[16] However, this correlation could reflect changes made by lean and health-conscious individuals to reduce fat intake and modify other aspects of diet and lifestyle. Such factors are difficult to control for in statistical analyses.

Case-Control Studies

A classic case-control study compares levels of exposure in a group of people with disease (cases) to levels of exposure in a similar, disease-free group (controls). Although such a design can be used to study both determinants and consequences of obesity, it is more commonly used to investigate the relationship between measures of adiposity and less common disease outcomes such as cancer. In case-control studies, data are not typically available to calculate the incidence rate of the disease or the absolute risk. The measure of association between exposure and disease risk in case-control studies is the odds ratio—the ratio of odds of exposure in cases to the odds of exposure in controls.[17] In a properly designed case-control study, the odds ratio is an unbiased estimate of the parameter of interest, the incidence rate ratio. The selection of the controls is critical because case-control studies are typically vulnerable to selection bias. The controls can be selected from the general population or a special population (e.g., relatives of the cases or other patients from the same hospitals where the cases are ascertained). In population-based case-control studies, a random sample of cases in the target population is ascertained during a certain period of time. The controls are then randomly selected from the same "study base" or source population.

In many situations, a clear study base is difficult to define unless all cases are known to come from a well-defined geographic area or population.[17] This is especially true in hospital-based studies that select both cases and controls from hospitals. The problem of selection bias can arise when controls are drawn from an unknown study base or source population or when participation rates differ according to case-control or exposure status, leading to systematic differences in characteristics between those who are included in the study and those who are not. Another problem, which is common to retrospective studies, is recall bias, which results when cases and controls report past exposure inaccurately and the degree of inaccuracy differs between cases and controls. Compared with healthy controls, cases who tend to report exposure more accurately could also exaggerate it. Such bias can often lead to differential misclassifications of exposure variables (i.e., the degree of misclassifications of exposure differ between cases and controls) and biased associations. For example, in case-control studies, total energy consumption was frequently related to a higher risk of colon cancer. This relationship, however, was not substantiated by large prospective studies.[18] It is possible that in case-control studies, patients with colon cancer were more likely to overreport dietary intakes than healthy controls. In another classic example,[19] the analyses using retrospectively reported diet showed a significant association between total and saturated fats and risk of breast cancer, but the analyses using prospective diet in the same cohort did not find such a relationship. It is suspected that in the retrospective case-control study, patients with breast cancer reported spuriously high intakes of total and saturated fats.

The main advantage of a classic case-control design is its efficiency in exploring rare outcomes. Also, such studies can usually be carried out quickly and at relatively low cost. Though case-control studies still have a role in examining the relationship between obesity and rare health outcomes, they are being replaced by large cohort studies. The high prevalence of obesity in the general population, along with the potential for selection and recall biases, make the classic case-control study less desirable for research on diet and lifestyle determinants of obesity. However, such studies can be useful in research on biological markers. For example, Wu et al.[20] found an inverse association between *Helicobacter pylori* infection and morbid obesity in a hospital-based case-control study of obese and lean subjects with comparable socioeconomic status. In this study, because infection status was assessed by the laboratory, recall bias was not an issue. However, a temporal relationship between the infection and obesity could not be established and thus, it is unclear whether the infection was the consequence or cause of obesity.

Advances in genetic epidemiology and genotyping technology have led to widespread use of the case-control design in genetic association studies of obesity. These studies are unaffected by problems with temporal relationship or recall bias, but they require careful selection of controls and matching on key demographic variables, especially ethnicity, to minimize potential bias by genetic stratification (see Chapter 21). Survival bias can be a problem when prevalent cases are used and genes of interest are related to conditions that affect survival.

A nested case-control study draws cases and controls from a defined population in a cohort study.[21] The design is an efficient form of a cohort study. The study base is clearly delineated, avoiding the problem of selection bias. In the frequently used sampling scheme called risk set sampling or incidence-density sampling, all incident cases are ascertained and controls are randomly selected without replacement at the time when each case occurs from cohort members still at risk but free of the disease of interest when the corresponding case is diagnosed.[21] Here, as in other case-control studies using incidence-density sampling, the odds ratios are unbiased estimates of incident rate ratios or relative risk (RR). It is worth noting that controls for early occurring cases may themselves become cases at a later time and thus a subject can serve as both a control and a case in the same study. In obesity research, the nested case-control design is valuable in studying predictor variables that are expensive to assess, such as biochemical markers. A major advantage of such a design is the effective matching on sample storage time through matching on length of follow-up. Batch effects can also be removed by analyzing case-control pairs in the same batches.[22]

Cohort Studies

The classic cohort study follows subjects over time, comparing the outcome of interest in individuals who were exposed or not exposed at baseline.[1] A cohort design allows for a direct estimate of disease incidence and absolute risk. Typically, incidence rates are calculated by dividing the number of events by person-time of follow-up in the exposed and nonexposed groups. The RR is computed as the rate in the exposed group divided by that in the nonexposed group, with adjustment for age and other confounding variables.

Prospective cohort studies are usually considered the strongest nonrandomized study design. Compared with case-control studies, the cohort design is less susceptible to selection bias and differential recall bias between cases and noncases because exposure is assessed before the outcome. However, cohort studies of chronic conditions with low incidence, including heart disease and cancer, are expensive. They require large sample sizes and long follow-up, factors that also raise the risk of selection bias when individuals are lost to follow-up. Many large prospective cohort studies have been established over the past few decades to identify risk factors for major chronic diseases. Virtually all of these studies include some measures of adiposity, and they have been instrumental in identifying health consequences associated with overweight and obesity. Many of these studies have collected detailed information on diet and lifestyle, allowing longitudinal analyses of nutritional and lifestyle predictors of obesity. Below we discuss several important features of contemporary prospective cohort studies of diet, obesity, and chronic diseases.

Repeated Measurements of Body Weight and Diet

One major advantage of prospective cohort studies is the possibility of periodic collection of diet, weight, and other lifestyle data during follow-up. Traditionally, most cohort studies have collected exposure data only at baseline (Design I, Fig. 3.1). Such analyses assume that diets or weights are constant over time, or if changes occur, the rank order of diet or weight stays the same. This assumption, however, is hardly tenable; diets change over time and the change can be affected by weight status and disease conditions.[23] Although body weight generally tracks well across time, there are substantial differences between persons in weight gain or loss. While several previous studies have collected baseline data on multiple occasions (Design II, Fig. 3.1),[24] more contemporary cohort studies, such as the Nurses' Health Study (NHS), the Health Professionals' Follow-up Study (HPFS), the Multi-Ethnic Study of Atherosclerosis (MESA), the Atherosclerosis Risk in Communities (ARIC), the Coronary Artery Risk Development in Young Adults (CARDIA), the Framingham Heart Study, the Bogalusa Heart Study, and others have collected periodic diet, body

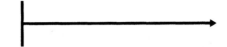

Design I. Single exposure measurement at baseline

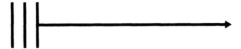

Design II. Multiple exposure measurements during baseline
period

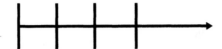

Design III. Multiple exposure measurements during follow-up
period

Figure 3.1 Three possible designs of prospective cohort studies with respect to exposure assessment. Used with permission from Hu FB, Stampfer MJ, Rimm E, et al. Dietary fat and coronary heart disease: a comparison of approaches for adjusting for total energy intake and modeling repeated dietary measurements. *Am J Epidemiol.* 1999;149:531-540.[23]

weight, and other lifestyle data during follow-up (Design III, Fig. 3.1). Although periodic collection of dietary and lifestyle data increases costs substantially, there is considerable return in improved validity and power of the study.

The repeated measures of body weight are useful in several ways. First, updated body weight data provide an opportunity to test whether remote or current weight is a better predictor of disease risk. In several studies, current weight has been shown to be more predictive of type 2 diabetes incidence,[25] whereas baseline weight is more predictive of CVD risk.[26] This is probably related to the fact that the induction and latency periods of CVD are much longer than those of diabetes. In prospective cohort studies, remote body mass index (BMI) is typically more predictive of mortality risk than current BMI because current weight is likely to be affected by the development of chronic diseases during follow-up.[27] Second, repeated measures of weight enable researchers to examine whether weight gain or loss, weight cycling, or weight fluctuations predict subsequent risk of chronic disease and mortality independent of baseline BMI (see Chapter 5). One study using updated measures of waist circumference found that increase in waist size was an important predictor of type 2 diabetes independent of weight gain.[28]

Repeated measures of diet and physical activity are useful in examining dietary and lifestyle predictors of incidence of obesity or chronic diseases. The use of updated lifestyle data in analyses not only allows for changes in dietary and exercise habits among participants but also reduces within-person random error. In a previous analysis of the NHS cohort, we calculated the cumulative average of dietary intake from all available dietary questionnaires up to the start of each 2-year follow-up interval.[23] For example, disease incidence 1980-1984 was related to the fat intake from the 1980 questionnaire, and disease incidence 1984-1986 was related to the average intake from the 1980 and 1984 questionnaires. We found that the analyses using cumulative averages of diet yielded stronger associations between dietary fats and CHD than did analyses that used only baseline or the most recent

Table 3.1 Choice of Approaches for Analyzing Repeated Dietary Assessments and Incident of Obesity and Chronic Diseases

Strategy	Hypothesis
Earliest measure only	Long latency
Most recent measure	Short latency
Consistently high versus consistently low	Cumulative exposure
Cumulative average measure	Cumulative exposure
Change in exposure, controlling for baseline	Relatively short latency

From Willett WC. *Nutritional Epidemiology.* 2nd ed. New York: Oxford University Press; 1998.[2]

dietary data.[23] Besides reducing measurement error caused by intraindividual variations over time, it is also possible that cumulative averages, which reflect long-term diets, are more relevant etiologically than recent diets because of a long latency of the disease. Whether this approach is more predictive of the development of obesity is yet to be tested.

Repeated measurements of diet can provide many opportunities to analyze various hypotheses of temporal relationships between dietary factors and onset of obesity or disease incidence (Table 3.1).[2] For example, the baseline measure can be used to test the long-term effects of exposure, while the most recent measure can be used to test short-term effects. Controlling for baseline exposure, one can also study the effects of change in dietary intakes over time on the development of obesity or a disease outcome.

Repeated measurements of diet and weight over time have commonly been used to examine the impact of specific changes in diet on weight gain. For example, Schulze et al.[29] evaluated the association between changes in soda consumption and mean changes in weight and BMI in adults over two 4-year time periods. They found the greatest weight gain in women who increased their soda consumption from ≤1 per week to ≥1 per day, and the least weight gain in women who decreased their intake. Controlling for baseline as well as dietary and lifestyle changes (e.g., physical activity, smoking, and alcohol use) is an important way to minimize confounding caused by changes in other diet and lifestyle factors during the course of a study. However, confounding by unmeasured variables is still possible.

In addition, analyses using repeated measures are not immune from the reverse causation bias that typically affects cross-sectional studies. Because individuals are aware of their weight status (dependent variable), they can respond by changing their diet and lifestyle (exposure variables). For example, Stellman and Garfinkel[30] found a positive association between artificial sweetener consumption and weight gain during 1 year of follow-up. However, that does not necessarily mean that artificial sweeteners cause weight gain. It is possible that people who were gaining weight began to use artificial sweeteners as a weight control strategy, leading to a positive association between artificial sweetener consumption and weight gain.

Long-Term Follow-Up

Extended follow-up is required to examine the long-term relationship between lifestyle factors and health outcomes. The advantage of large and long-running cohort studies is demonstrated by the British Doctors' Study,[31] which reported a more significant and stronger association between smoking and longevity with 50 years of follow-up than did earlier intermittent reports from the same cohort.[32]

Long-term follow-up is particularly important for the study of obesity and mortality. In that, reverse causation biases due to existing or subclinical diseases are most likely to occur in the first few years of follow-up, excluding early deaths can help to reduce such biases. In some situations, much longer follow-up is required to demonstrate the effects of obesity on mortality. For example, in the 25-year follow-up of the Chicago Heart Association Detection Project,[33] a stronger association between BMI and cardiovascular mortality was observed with a longer follow-up (>15 years) compared with that seen during a shorter follow-up (0 to 15 years). As a result, the association between BMI and 25-year cardiovascular mortality became much stronger after excluding deaths in the first 15 years. In the Framingham Heart Study,[34] a significant association between overweight and CHD incidence did not emerge until the 8-year follow-up, and it became stable through 26 years of follow-up. Compared with an earlier analysis of 16 years of follow-up of the NHS (established in 1976),[35] we noted an even stronger relationship between adiposity and mortality with longer follow-up of 24 years.[27] A long-term study with 55 years of follow-up demonstrated that obesity in adolescents was a significant predictor of adult mortality.[36] These reports demonstrate the importance of long-term follow-up in large and established cohorts.[37] Lack of long-term follow-up and an inability to exclude early deaths for a period sufficient to remove effects of disease on weight may thus have contributed to inconsistent associations between BMI and mortality in the literature.[33] This could in part explain a much weaker association between obesity and mortality observed in NHANES II (14 years of follow-up) and NHANES III (9 years of follow-up) than in NHANES I (19 years).[38]

Long-term follow-up is also important for examining dietary and lifestyle determinants of obesity and weight gain. For example, in a recent study, we examined the relationship between calcium and dairy intake and short-term (4 years), medium-term (8 years), and long-term (12 years) weight gain in the HPFS and found no evidence of an association at any of the time points, providing strong evidence against the benefit of dairy products in weight control.[39] Such analyses are useful in evaluating the effects of diet on the trajectory of body weight over a long period.

Biological Markers and Body Composition Measurements

Many contemporary cohort studies have collected and archived biological specimens. For example, in the NHS, blood samples and DNA from buccal cells as well as samples of toenail clippings and urine have been collected and stored.[40] These resources are extremely valuable for epidemiologic studies of obesity. For example, biomarkers of essential fatty acids (n-6 and n-3 fatty acids) and trans fatty acids measured in plasma and red blood cells can accurately reflect dietary intake over the past several months, and thus, can be used both as references for validating dietary questionnaires and as dietary exposure variables in nested case-control studies of disease risk (see Chapter 6). Plasma concentrations of adipocyte-derived hormones such as leptin and adiponectin are useful biomarkers of adiposity. The unique advantage of biomarkers is that their measurement errors are uncorrelated with errors in self-reported instruments (see Chapter 6). In addition, the integration of genetic markers into obesity epidemiologic studies has opened a new door for identifying genetic variants and gene-environment interactions that alter susceptibility to obesity (see Chapters 21 and 22).

The Health, Aging, and Body Composition (Health ABC) study is one of the few epidemiologic studies that include detailed measurements of body composition. It is a population-based prospective study of more than 3,000 men and women 70 to 79 years of age.[41] Besides standard anthropometric measurements, this study includes measures of body fat mass, percent body fat, and fat distribution assessed by dual-energy x-ray absorptiometry (DXA) and computed tomography (CT) scan. Analyses of these measures can provide important insights into the impact of change in body composition on physical function, morbidity, and mortality in the elderly. However, high cost and the need for special equipments make it infeasible to obtain body composition measures in large prospective cohorts involving hundreds of thousands of participants.

Multicenter Cohort Studies and Pooling Projects

Newer generations of cohort studies have employed a multicenter design to include diverse populations. For example, The European Prospective Investigation into Cancer and Nutrition (EPIC) cohort consists of subcohorts recruited from 22 centers in Denmark, France, Germany, Greece, Italy, the Netherlands, Norway, Spain, Sweden, and the United Kingdom, including more than half a million people aged 25 to 70 years.[42] Blood and DNA samples have been collected and stored, along with dietary habits and anthropometric measurements from the participants. Although the main focus of the cohort is diet and cancer, anthropometric measures allow the investigators to study obesity as a risk factor for both common and rare cancers and evaluate the heterogeneity of these associations across populations.

The Multiethnic Cohort Study (MCS), established between 1993 and 1996, includes more than 215,000 men and women (between the ages of 45 and 75) from California and Hawaii from 5 self-reported racial and ethnic groups: African Americans, Japanese Americans, Latinos, Native Hawaiians, and whites.[43] This is one of the few cohorts with sufficient power to test ethnic differences in the relationship between race/ethnicity and anthropometric measures on cancer risk. Other smaller cohort studies of multiracial groups, such as MESA,[44] the ARIC Study,[45] and the CARDIA Study,[46] have focused on obesity, the metabolic syndrome, and CVD outcomes. The Women's Health Initiative (WHI) Observational Cohort is a prospective, ethnically and racially diverse, multicenter observational study designed to address the major causes of illness and death in post-menopausal women ($n \approx 100,000$).[47] Body weight and waist circumferences were measured at baseline and during follow-up, allowing the examination of both determinants and consequences of obesity across different racial and ethnic groups.

The proliferation of prospective cohort studies has led to massive pooling projects of diet and chronic diseases. The Pooling Project of Prospective Studies of Diet and Cancer is a collaborative project by investigators from multiple international cohort studies. Its goal is to analyze diet and cancer associations using standardized criteria across studies.[48] Each cohort study was initiated independently and has either completed follow-up or follow-up is ongoing. A recent pooling analysis of dietary fiber and colon cancer included 13 prospective studies involving 725,628 men and women followed for 6 to 20 years.[49] In an earlier analysis, van den Brandt et al.[50] examined the association between anthropometric indices and the risk of breast cancer by pooling seven prospective cohort studies. In addition to increased power, the pooled analysis of original data from each cohort offers other advantages, in particular, the development of common definitions of the dietary exposure and analysis of the data using a standard approach. Compared to meta-analyses of the published literature, this approach provides more flexibility in examining dose-response relationships, confounding, and effect modification. However, it is much more costly and requires great effort to coordinate the data analyses.[48]

Summary

The goal of analytic epidemiology is to infer etiology regarding exposure variables and health outcomes. A range of analytic epidemiologic study designs can be used to examine the causes and consequences of obesity. Correlational or ecological analyses typically correlate per capita food consumption data with incidence of disease or mortality rates in different populations or cultures. Because of intractable confounding by other aspects of diet and lifestyle, these studies are the most useful as part of a hypothesis-generating process. Compared with correlational studies, cross-sectional and case-control designs can be used to examine the relationship between exposure and disease in more detail. However, because the exposure (e.g., diet) is typically assessed retrospectively, results from these studies are susceptible to recall bias.

Prospective cohort studies, in which exposure is assessed before the occurrence of disease, minimize risk of bias from retrospective reporting on diet and lifestyle factors, and are generally considered the strongest nonrandomized design. For this reason, results from prospective studies with detailed exposure assessment should be given more weight than findings from other analytic epidemiologic studies in the evaluation of evidence. In the past several decades, numerous large prospective studies of lifestyle and chronic diseases have been established worldwide. Contemporary cohort studies have the advantages of very large size, long-term follow-up, high rates of follow-up, availability of archived biological samples, and repeated measures of body weight and diet. These characteristics greatly increase the power of epidemiologic studies of obesity and chronic diseases and enhance the validity of the observed associations. However, this does not mean that large cohort studies are immune from biases. Although these studies have produced invaluable data on determinants and consequences of obesity, they have also generated controversy in some areas. In the next chapter, we will discuss methodological issues related to causal inference in obesity epidemiologic research.

References

1. Last JM. *A Dictionary of Epidemiology.* 4th ed. New York: Oxford University Press; 2001.
2. Willett WC. *Nutritional Epidemiology.* 2nd ed. New York: Oxford University Press; 1998.
3. Bray GA, Popkin BM. Dietary fat intake does affect obesity! *Am J Clin Nutr.* 1998;68:1157-1173.
4. Willett WC, Leibel RL. Dietary fat is not a major determinant of body fat. *Am J Med.* 2002;113(Suppl 9B):47S-59S.
5. Keys A. *Seven Countries: A Multivariate Analysis of Death and Coronary Heart Disease.* Cambridge, MA: Harvard University Press; 1980.
6. Visscher TL, Seidell JC, Menotti A, et al. Underweight and overweight in relation to mortality among men aged 40-59 and 50-69 years: the Seven Countries Study. *Am J Epidemiol.* 2000;151:660-666.
7. Willett WC. Is dietary fat a major determinant of body fat? *Am J Clin Nutr.* 1998;67 (3 Suppl):556S-562S.
8. Gross LS, Li L, Ford ES, Liu S. Increased consumption of refined carbohydrates and the epidemic of type 2 diabetes in the United States: an ecologic assessment. *Am J Clin Nutr.* 2004;79:774-779.
9. Bray GA, Nielsen SJ, Popkin BM. Consumption of high-fructose corn syrup in beverages may play a role in the epidemic of obesity. *Am J Clin Nutr.* 2004;79:537-543.
10. Prentice AM, Jebb SA. Obesity in Britain: gluttony or sloth? *BMJ.* 1995;311:437-439.
11. Goel MS, McCarthy EP, Phillips RS, Wee CC. Obesity among US immigrant subgroups by duration of residence. *JAMA.* 2004;29:2860-2867.
12. Benfante R. Studies of cardiovascular disease and cause-specific mortality trends in Japanese-American men living in Hawaii and risk factor comparisons with other Japanese populations in the Pacific region: a review. *Hum Biol.* 1992;64:791-805.

13. Curb JD, Marcus EB. Body fat and obesity in Japanese Americans. *Am J Clin Nutr.* 1991;53(6 Suppl):1552S-1555S.

14. Prentice RL, Willett WC, Greenwald P, et al. Nutrition and physical activity and chronic disease prevention: research strategies and recommendations. *J Natl Cancer Inst.* 2004;96:1276-1287.

15. Egger G, Swinburn B. An "ecological" approach to the obesity pandemic. *BMJ.* 1997;315:477-480.

16. Lissner L, Heitmann BL. Dietary fat and obesity: evidence from epidemiology. *Eur J Clin Nutr.* 1995;49:79-90.

17. Rothman KJ. *Epidemiology. An Introduction.* New York: Oxford University Press; 2002.

18. Giovannucci E, Goldin B. The role of fat, fatty acids, and total energy intake in the etiology of human colon cancer. *Am J Clin Nutr.* 1997;66(6 Suppl):1564S-1571S.

19. Giovannucci E, Stampfer MJ, Colditz GA, et al. A comparison of prospective and retrospective assessments of diet in the study of breast cancer. *Am J Epidemiol.* 1993;137:502-511.

20. Wu MS, Lee WJ, Wang HH, Huang SP, Lin JT. A case-control study of association of Helicobacter pylori infection with morbid obesity in Taiwan. *Arch Intern Med.* 2005;165:1552-1555.

21. Rothman KJ, Greenland S. *Modern Epidemiology.* 2nd ed. Philadelphia: Lippincott-Raven; 1998.

22. Rundle AG, Vineis P, Ahsan H. Design options for molecular epidemiology research within cohort studies. *Cancer Epidemiol Biomarkers Prev.* 2005;14:1899-1907.

23. Hu FB, Stampfer MJ, Rimm E, et al. Dietary fat and coronary heart disease: a comparison of approaches for adjusting for total energy intake and modeling repeated dietary measurements. *Am J Epidemiol.* 1999;149:531-540.

24. Shekelle RB, Rossof AH, Stamler J. Dietary cholesterol and incidence of lung cancer: the Western Electric Study. *Am J Epidemiol.* 1991;134:480-484.

25. Wang Z, Hoy WE. Waist circumference, body mass index, hip circumference and waist-to-hip ratio as predictors of cardiovascular disease in aboriginal people. *Eur J Clin Nutr.* 2004;58:888-893.

26. Li TY, Rana JS, Manson JE, et al. Obesity as compared with physical activity in predicting risk of coronary heart disease in women. *Circulation.* 2006;113:499-506.

27. Hu FB, Willett WC, Li T, Stampfer MJ, Colditz GA, Manson JE. Adiposity as compared with physical activity in predicting mortality among women. *New Engl J Med.* 2004;351:2694-2703.

28. Koh-Banerjee P, Chu NF, Spiegelman D, et al. Prospective study of the association of changes in dietary intake, physical activity, alcohol consumption, and smoking with 9-y gain in waist circumference among 16 587 US men. *Am J Clin Nutr.* 2003;78:719-727.

29. Schulze MB, Manson JE, Ludwig DS, et al. Sugar-sweetened beverages, weight gain, and incidence of type 2 diabetes in young and middle-aged women. *JAMA.* 2004;292:927-934.

30. Stellman SD, Garfinkel L. Artificial sweetener use and one-year weight change among women. *Prev Med.* 1986;15:195-202.

31. Doll R, Hill AB. The mortality of doctors in relation to their smoking habits; a preliminary report. *BMJ.* 1954;4877:1451-1455.

32. Doll R, Peto R, Boreham J, Sutherland I. Mortality in relation to smoking: 50 years' observations on male British doctors. *BMJ.* 2004;328:1519.

33. Dyer AR, Stamler J, Garside DB, Greenland P. Long-term consequences of body mass index for cardiovascular mortality: the Chicago Heart Association Detection Project in Industry study. *Ann Epidemiol.* 2004;14:101-108.

34. Hubert HB, Feinleib M, McNamara PM, Castelli WP. Obesity as an independent risk factor for cardiovascular disease: a 26-year follow-up of participants in the Framingham Heart Study. *Circulation.* 1983;67:968-977.

35. Manson JE, Willett WC, Stampfer MJ, et al. Body weight and mortality among women. *N Engl J Med.* 1995;333:677-685.

36. Must A, Jacques PF, Dallal GE, Bajema CJ, Dietz WH. Long-term morbidity and mortality of overweight adolescents. A follow-up of the Harvard Growth Study of 1922 to 1935. *N Engl J Med.* 1992;327:1350-1355.
37. Stampfer M. New insights from the British doctors study. *BMJ.* 2004;328:1507.
38. Flegal KM, Graubard BI, Williamson DF, Gail MH. Excess deaths associated with underweight, overweight, and obesity. *JAMA.* 2005;293:1861-1867.
39. Rajpathak SN, Rimm EB, Rosner B, Willett WC, Hu FB. Calcium and dairy intakes in relation to long-term weight gain in US men. *Am J Clin Nutr.* 2006;83:559-566.
40. Colditz GA, Hankinson SE. The Nurses' Health Study: lifestyle and health among women. *Nat Rev Cancer.* 2005;5:388-396.
41. Taaffe DR, Cauley JA, Danielson M, et al. Race and sex effects on the association between muscle strength, soft tissue, and bone mineral density in healthy elders: the Health, Aging, and Body Composition Study. *J Bone Miner Res.* 2001;16:1343-1352.
42. Riboli E, Hunt KJ, Slimani N, et al. European Prospective Investigation into Cancer and Nutrition (EPIC): study populations and data collection. *Public Health Nutr.* 2002;5:1113-1124.
43. Kolonel LN, Henderson BE, Hankin JH, et al. A multiethnic cohort in Hawaii and Los Angeles: baseline characteristics. *Am J Epidemiol.* 2000;151:346-357.
44. Nettleton JA, Steffen LM, Mayer-Davis EJ, et al. Dietary patterns are associated with biochemical markers of inflammation and endothelial activation in the Multi-Ethnic Study of Atherosclerosis (MESA). *Am J Clin Nutr.* 2006;83:1369-1379.
45. Harris MM, Stevens J, Thomas N, Schreiner P, Folsom AR. Associations of fat distribution and obesity with hypertension in a bi-ethnic population: the ARIC study. Atherosclerosis Risk in Communities Study. *Obes Res.* 2000;8:516-524.
46. Burke GL, Savage PJ, Manolio TA, et al. Correlates of obesity in young black and white women: the CARDIA Study. *Am J Public Health.* 1992;82:1621-1625.
47. McTigue K, Larson JC, Valoski A, et al. Mortality and cardiac and vascular outcomes in extremely obese women. *JAMA.* 2006;296:79-86.
48. Smith-Warner SA, Spiegelman D, Ritz J, et al. Methods for pooling results of epidemiologic studies: the Pooling Project of Prospective Studies of Diet and Cancer. *Am J Epidemiol.* 2006;163:1053-1064.
49. Park Y, Hunter DJ, Spiegelman D, et al. Dietary fiber intake and risk of colorectal cancer: a pooled analysis of prospective cohort studies. *JAMA.* 2005;294:2849-2857.
50. van den Brandt PA, Spiegelman D, Yaun SS, et al. Pooled analysis of prospective cohort studies on height, weight, and breast cancer risk. *Am J Epidemiol.* 2000;152:514-527.

4

Interpreting Epidemiologic Evidence and Causal Inference in Obesity Research

Frank B. Hu

In an ideal world, all exposure variables including diet and lifestyle factors would be evaluated in randomized controlled trials (RCTs), with perfect compliance and sufficient follow-up. In the real world, however, such an approach is often infeasible or even unethical. Typically, we have imperfect evidence from unsatisfactory dietary intervention trials (often due to short follow-up or low compliance) and nonexperimental data from obesity epidemiologic studies, making it difficult to draw definitive conclusions on the causes and consequences of obesity.

Challenges notwithstanding, epidemiologic evidence plays a valuable role in making causal judgments in obesity research. In this chapter, we will discuss key conceptual issues related to interpretation of epidemiologic evidence and inferences of causation in obesity research. We will start by discussing the role of RCTs, and then we will address several methodological issues in establishing causality, such as confounding, reverse causation, measurement errors, mediation and effect modification, validity versus generalizability, and the calculation and interpretation of population attributable risk (PAR). Finally, we will review commonly used criteria of causality in obesity epidemiology.

The Role of RCTs

Because random assignment of treatment eliminates known and unknown confounding, well-conducted RCTs with disease or mortality end points are considered the gold standard in evaluating causal relationships. In obesity research, RCTs have been used to evaluate weight loss medications and treatments, community-based prevention strategies, and diet and lifestyle interventions. Despite conceptual advantages, there are several methodological issues to consider when interpreting data from RCTs. High dropout rates resulting from loss of participants to follow-up or early termination before determination of outcome are common problems in dietary and lifestyle intervention trails.[1] In free-living populations, a 40% to 50% dropout rate from randomized dietary interventions of even 1-year duration is fairly common.[2,3] Such high attrition can lead to substantial selection bias because participants who stay often differ from those who drop out. Traditional methods of statistical analysis, such as last observation carried forward (LOCF) or imputation techniques, cannot easily correct for such bias.[4]

Noncompliance, when participants do not adhere to assigned dietary regimens or lifestyle interventions, is a related problem. The longer the follow-up period of a trial, the less likely participants are to adhere to the assigned intervention. For example, during 8 years of follow-up in the Women's Health Initiative (WHI), most of those randomized to the low-fat group were unable to achieve the target fat reduction goal of 20%.[5] Significant reductions in fat intake are usually reflected in a decrease in high-density lipoprotein (HDL) cholesterol and an increase in triglycerides.[6] Yet in the trial, there were no appreciable differences in blood levels of HDL cholesterol or triglycerides between the low-fat and usual diet groups, although there was a modest reduction in low-density lipoprotein (LDL) cholesterol in the low-fat group. These outcomes called into question the degree of fat reduction achieved in this study. Reduced compliance, which typically biases the results toward null, complicated the interpretation of the findings.

The long-term nature of RCTs puts even the best-designed interventions at risk of becoming obsolete. For example, when the WHI was designed in the early 1990s, a low-fat dietary pattern was the prevailing recommendation for weight loss and prevention of chronic diseases, such as cancer and coronary heart disease (CHD). During the course of the study, substantial clinical and epidemiologic evidence emerged showing that type of fat was more important than total amount of fat in reducing risk of CHD, and that substitution of fat for carbohydrates was unlikely to have appreciable effects on either weight loss or risk of CHD.[7] These new data weakened the original justification for the intervention, which could not be changed once the trial was underway.

Ethical, logistical, financial, and methodological constraints put large diet and exercise RCTs with hard disease end points such as CHD or mortality out of reach for most investigators. Thus, prospective cohort studies remain the mainstay of research on the consequences and determinants of obesity. Growing numbers of such studies and publicly available electronic databases offer unprecedented opportunities for obesity research. They also challenge investigators to apply sound epidemiologic principles and scientific rigor to study design, analyses, and interpretations of data. There are several threats to the internal validity of cohort studies, even those that are well powered and have minimal loss to follow-up. These include confounding, measurement error, and reverse causation. We will discuss each of these issues in the following sections.

Confounding

Confounding in Studies on the Consequences of Obesity

Confounding refers to distortion of the association between an exposure and disease, brought about by the association of a third variable that influences the outcome under investigation.[8] Typically, the confounder is correlated with both the exposure and the outcome, and is not on the causal pathway between exposure and disease. Confounding is one of the most important threats to the validity of nonrandomized studies. Although there is no formal statistical test to identify confounding, there is a rule of thumb— a 10% or greater change in the magnitude of the association between exposure and disease after controlling for the confounding variable.[9] Cigarette smoking is a classic example of confounding in studies of obesity and mortality. Smokers tend to be leaner and have increased risk of mortality. Adjustment for smoking, which is a strong negative confounder (i.e., confounding that leads to underestimation of the exposure effect), typically strengthens the relationship between body mass index (BMI) and mortality.[10]

Multivariate adjustment is the most popular way to control for confounding. But because it is impossible to remove all confounding through statistical control, there is room for residual confounding. One way to minimize residual confounding is to control for the confounder in more refined categories. For example, in addition to controlling for smoking status (never, past, and current), one can control for smoking more tightly by including the number of cigarettes smoked daily among current smokers. However, such analyses still cannot control for different brands of cigarettes and degrees of inhalation. Thus, when strong confounding is present, stratification is necessary to examine the associations separately in different strata of the confounder (especially among the group not exposed to the confounder). In the case of obesity and mortality, the best way to address confounding is to restrict the analyses to those who never smoked. In this way, the effects of obesity on mortality can be assessed without distortion by past or current smoking.

Confounding in Studies on Determinants of Obesity

Although longitudinal studies of determinants of obesity are better able to control for confounding than cross-sectional studies, they are still observational in nature and may not completely disentangle the effects of other aspects of diet and lifestyle from the effects of the dietary factor of interest on weight. Many studies have suggested that unhealthy lifestyle behaviors tend to cluster. For example, Schulze et al.[11] reported higher intakes of red and processed meats, higher prevalence of smoking, and low physical activity among those who consumed sugar-sweetened soda regularly. Therefore, when examining the association between soda consumption and weight gain, it is important to control for detailed measures of confounding variables. In addition to controlling for baseline weight, smoking, and alcohol use, Schulze et al.[11] also controlled for baseline and changes in physical activity and other lifestyle covariates, as well as for the intake of red meat, french fries, processed meat, sweets, and snacks (food items that cluster together in this study population in a "Western" dietary pattern).

Matching, an approach commonly used in case-control studies, is another way to address confounding.[12] Individual cases and controls can be pairwise or frequency matched for various factors, especially strong confounders. Conceptually, matching is equivalent to fine stratification (in which the matching factors are finely categorized), which leads to statistically analogous results when a conditional logistic model is used for matched analyses. Matching not only removes the influences of strong constitutional confounders, such as age, sex, and race, but also increases the efficiency of the study by balancing the number of cases and controls in each stratum. Matching is widely used in genetic association studies to reduce confounding by unobserved genetic admixture or stratification that results from different distributions of ethnicity or genetic background in cases and controls (see Chapter 21).

Overmatching, sometimes caused by matching on intermediate variables in the causal pathway between exposure and outcome, can reduce statistical power. For example, matching for BMI in a case-control study of obesity-related cytokines and risk of myocardial infarction (MI) can result in overmatching because cytokines are secreted by adipose tissue, and thus, BMI and adipocyte-derived cytokines are on the same causal pathway.

Use of propensity score methods to control for confounding in epidemiologic studies has also become increasingly popular. The propensity score is the conditional probability of being exposed given the observed covariates. It can be used to balance observed covariates between the exposed and nonexposed groups and to reduce confounding through matching, stratification, regression adjustment, or some combination of these.[13] This approach appears to be most useful in situations where there is a need to adjust for large numbers of covariates. However, most prospective cohort studies on health consequences of obesity have a relatively small number of covariates that are well suited to the traditional regression adjustment approach. In a systematic review of 78 exposure-outcome associations from 43 studies, adjusting for confounder bias using propensity scores generally produced similar results compared with traditional regression methods.[14]

Reverse Causation

Reverse causation, also known as "effect-cause," is a special type of bias that takes place when the exposure is affected by the outcome. For example, several earlier epidemiologic studies found an association between low serum cholesterol and increased cancer mortality.[15] In subsequent studies, however, the inverse association between serum cholesterol and cancer mortality decreased over time, whereas the association with serum cholesterol and cardiovascular mortality persisted.[16] RCTs have shown that aggressive cholesterol-lowering treatment reduces total mortality but does not lead to increased cancer risk.[17] These findings suggest that preexisting or preclinical cancer causes low cholesterol levels, rather than low cholesterol causing cancer.

Studies on Consequences of Obesity

Reverse causation—where low BMI or leanness results from, rather than causes, underlying illness—is probably the most serious problem in analyzing the relationship between obesity and mortality, especially in older adults. Artificially elevated mortality in the lean group caused by reverse causation can often lead to an underestimation of relative risks (RRs) of mortality in the overweight and obese groups. Obesity is a dynamic condition, as most people who are obese at age 25 to 64 die after age 70. By the time they reach an older age, many have already lost weight because of aging and underlying diseases. Weight loss can result from the direct effects of disease on weight, or sometimes from intentional weight loss motivated by a diagnosis of serious illness. Many conditions that cause weight loss, such as chronic obstructive pulmonary disease (COPD) and depression, may remain undiagnosed for years. Because populations of lean individuals include smokers, healthy active people, and those with chronic illness, disentangling various influences on cause and effect can be challenging. Strategies for meeting this challenge include the exclusion of individuals with known chronic diseases at baseline and those with recent substantial weight loss (see Chapter 11). Stratified analyses by physical activity levels have also proven useful. Analyses restricted to physically active people are less likely to be affected by reverse causation because prevalence of clinical and subclinical diseases in this subgroup is lower compared with physically inactive subjects.[18] All of these approaches, though useful, do not guarantee complete elimination of reverse causation.

Studies on Determinants of Obesity

Reverse causation in studies of determinants of obesity differs from that in studies on obesity and mortality. Cross-sectional research on dietary determinants of obesity is especially susceptible to reverse causation, because body weight is a visible outcome that can influence an individual's eating behavior and lifestyle. Depending on psychological and behavioral feedback, overweight individuals might, for example, consume low-fat or fat-free products to control weight.[19] Therefore, a cross-sectional analysis could find a positive relationship between low-fat products and body weight. While repeated measures of diet and weight are useful for reducing reverse causation bias (i.e., individuals changing their diets because of weight gain or loss), it is important to acknowledge that longitudinal analyses cannot eliminate this problem.

Measurement Issues

The internal validity of epidemiologic studies depends on obtaining accurate and reliable measurements of body fat, diet, and physical activity. In the next three chapters, we will discuss measurement issues for these variables. Here, we briefly summarize key methodological topics related to measurements in obesity epidemiologic research.

Adiposity is most commonly assessed by BMI, which in many large prospective studies is calculated by self-reported rather than by measured height and weight.[20] Although it is important to use measured height and weight to obtain accurate estimates of obesity prevalence in the population, whether self-reported BMI values are reliable enough for valid or unbiased predictions of health consequences has been a contentious issue. Validation studies have commonly found a high correlation between measured and self-reported weights, but differential reporting bias in self-reported BMI is of concern because obese people tend to underreport weight and shorter people tend to overreport height.[21] In Chapter 5, we will address the validity of self-reported BMI.

Obtaining accurate measurements of complex and multidimensional behaviors, such as diet and physical activity, is one of the most challenging aspects of obesity epidemiology research. Questionnaires are typically used to assess these behaviors, but they are prone to random and systematic errors that can attenuate and distort true exposure-outcome associations. The underreporting of calorie intake and the overreporting of physical activity levels by obese subjects compound these problems. In epidemiologic studies of dietary factors and obesity, observed associations can be simultaneously influenced by multiple sources of errors and biases: measurement errors of both dietary and body fat assessments, reverse causation, and confounding by other dietary and lifestyle factors. Addressing these issues in epidemiologic study design and statistical analyses is a major challenge. We will discuss measurement issues in Chapters 6 and 7.

The introduction of objective measurements for diet and physical activity represents a promising direction in epidemiologic research. Electronic activity trackers, such as heart rate monitors, accelerometers, and pedometers, have become increasingly popular in small- to medium-scale clinical trials and epidemiologic studies. However, use of such devices in large-scale cohort studies, with thousands of people, may be limited by logistic and economic considerations. Similarly, nutrient biomarkers promise to provide more accurate and objective records of dietary intake, but their use is limited by a lack of measurable biomarkers for important nutrients like fiber and carbohydrates. Rather than replace the questionnaire method of dietary assessment, researchers are more likely to augment it by calibrating and correcting measurement errors in self-reported dietary data and by using biomarkers to provide additional measures of exposure[22,23] (see Chapter 7).

Mediation and Effect Modification

It is important to distinguish a mediator from a confounder. Unlike a confounder, a mediator is the third variable that accounts, at least in part, for the relationship between exposure and outcome. In the study of obesity and mortality, for example, diabetes is considered a biological intermediate in the pathway. Controlling for diabetes, which is expected to reduce estimated risks of obesity and mortality, can lead to overcontrol and underestimation of obesity's effects. Similarly, obesity can serve as a mediator when studying the relationship between lifestyle factors, such as physical activity and television watching, and risk of type 2 diabetes.[24] The general test for mediation is a weakened association between exposure and outcome after the mediator is included in the model.[25] Theoretically, the proportion of the exposure-outcome association explained by the mediator can be quantified by comparing the estimates with and without the mediator in the models.[26] However such analyses require several assumptions, for example, continuous outcomes, the absence of confounding in the relationship between the intermediate variable and the outcome, and lack of interaction between the exposure and intermediate variable.[27] Violation of these assumptions may lead to biased estimates of the proportion of exposure-outcome association explained by the mediator.

An effect modifier or moderator is a variable that changes the direction and/or strength of the relationship between an exposure and the outcome variable.[25] For example, studies have found that the relationship between BMI and mortality varies by age group;[28] that is, the RR of mortality with increasing BMI tends to decline with age. However, this does not necessarily mean that obesity is less detrimental to older people than middle-aged ones. Assessing effect modification or the presence and extent of the interactions depends on the scale used. When a ratio measure (e.g., RR) is used, the interaction is assessed on the multiplicative scale; when an absolute risk measure (e.g., mortality rate) is used, the interaction is assessed on the additive scale. In some situations, measures of interactions on the additive and multiplicative scales may lead to divergent conclusions. For example, although the RR of death associated with obesity is lower in older people in than middle-aged individuals, the absolute increase in death rates associated with obesity is much greater in the elderly[29] (see Chapter 11). Thus, the decreased association between obesity and mortality with age does not diminish the importance of obesity in older individuals.

Rothman and Greenland[30] argued that the additive model is the best model for interaction if the goal is to predict "disease load" or public health burden in a population. On the other hand, the multiplicative model is more appropriate if the goal is to unravel etiological factors of the disease. It is sometimes important to assess both multiplicative and additive models when an interaction may have both public health and etiological implications.

Although the multiplicative interactions can be easily estimated using standard procedures such as the likelihood ratio test, methods for testing additive interactions are less well-developed. To assess interaction as a departure from joint additive effects, Rothman and Greenland[30] suggested the computation of a synergy index (S) based on model coefficients from a logistic regression. S compares the risk of disease or mortality in patients with joint exposures to those with a single exposure.

$$S = \frac{R_{11} - R_{00}}{(R_{10} - R_{00}) + (R_{01} - R_{00})} = \frac{RR_{11} - 1}{(RR_{10} - 1) + (RR_{01} - 1)}$$

RR_{11} is the relative risk of patients with joint exposures compared to those with neither exposure. RR_{10} is the relative risk of patients with the first exposure only compared to those with neither exposure, and RR_{01} is the relative risk of patients with the second exposure only compared to those with neither exposure.

A value greater than 1 implies synergism, and a value less than 1 implies antagonism. A 95% confidence interval may also be calculated.[31,32] Alternative measures of additive interactions, including relative excess risk due to interaction (RERI) and the attributable proportions due to interaction (AP), have also been used in the literature. The methodological superiority of these additive interaction measures is yet to be clearly established, but Skrondal[33] suggested that S be the method of choice when assessing additive interaction in multivariate settings.

Obesity can also modify the relationship between dietary factors and disease risk. For example, over 10 years of follow-up, Liu et al.[34] found a strong positive association between GL and risk of CHD, and the increased risk was more pronounced in overweight and obese women than in normal-weight women ($P < .01$ for interaction between BMI and GL). These results are consistent with metabolic studies showing that the adverse effects of a high GL diet are exacerbated by underlying insulin resistance.[35]

Because confounding threatens the validity of epidemiologic studies, the objective is always to remove confounding through appropriate study design and analyses. On the other hand, an important goal of epidemiologic studies is to identify biologically meaningful interactions or effect modifiers.[30] In obesity epidemiology, such analyses can enhance understanding of the biology that underlies the consequences and determinants of obesity and help identify high-risk populations for more effective prevention and treatment.

Validity versus Generalizability

The foremost goal of any scientific endeavor is to obtain valid results or the *truth*. In epidemiology, validity of a study means that the findings cannot be explained simply by confounding, bias, or chance. While validity is the overriding objective of the study, generalizability—the applicability of observed associations to other populations—is also of concern. While validity and generalizability are both needed to draw meaningful public health conclusions, the former is a prerequisite for the latter; if there is no confidence in the validity of the study, there is no reason to generalize associations to other populations.[36]

Because there is no formal statistical test for generalizability, the assessment of the generalizability of study results is, to some degree, a judgment call. Although it is commonly believed that generalizability requires correspondence between the basic characteristics of the study population and those of the larger target population, this is a fallacy. Whether results observed in a study population apply to the target population depends on whether the biological relationship between the exposure and disease is the same between the two populations.[37] In other words, generalizability means that the biological process operates the same way in the study population and the larger population, with no unmeasured effect modifications for the exposure-disease relationships. Nongeneralizability implies biological and statistical effect modification by population characteristics, that is, different associations for different subpopulations. Thus, generalizability is more concerned with underlying biological mechanisms than similarity of the population distributions of variables such as age, sex, race, and socioeconomic status

(SES). However, one can argue that biological processes are more likely to be the same in populations with similar demographic characteristics.

Although greater ethnic and SES diversity in study populations may increase generalizability, this approach typically increases the heterogeneity of the population, and thus, the chance for unmeasured or uncontrolled confounding. For example, it would be necessary to include smokers and those who are ill in a representative sample to estimate national obesity prevalence and trends, but inclusion of smokers and those who are ill in the analyses of obesity and mortality can lead to serious confounding by smoking and reverse causation by existing diseases, and thus, diminish the validity of the estimated associations between obesity and mortality. On the other hand, a more homogeneous cohort with respect to residence, education, or occupation would not represent a random sample of U.S. men and women. As a result, the distribution of dietary and other lifestyle characteristics may not reflect the general population. However, this does not mean that the identified associations do not apply to other populations. In fact, most cohort studies do not rely on national samples but draw on participants with similar educational, occupational, or geographic backgrounds. Compared with the general population, more homogeneous cohorts have relatively less unmeasured or uncontrolled confounding by SES and other variables, and therefore, enhanced internal validity. But if there were effect modification by a variable defining a cohort (e.g., educational levels, ethnicity), it would not possible to detect it, and thus, it would affect the generalizability of the results. On the other hand, although epidemiologic studies of obesity and mortality based on U.S. national datasets, such as the National Health and Nutrition Examination Surveys (NHANES), are considered more generalizable, the analyses are more likely to be confounded and are typically not sufficiently powered to characterize potential effect modifications by ethnicity, SES, or other covariates. Nonetheless, epidemiologic study designs still need to balance validity and generalizability, and improving generalizability without compromising validity is a challenge for epidemiologists.

Calculation and Interpretation of the Population Attributable Risk

The PAR is the fraction of disease in the population that is attributable to the exposure, and thus, the percent of cases that would be prevented if the exposure were to be removed.[38] Widely used in epidemiology and public health, the PAR is sometimes referred to as population attributable fraction, etiological fraction, or preventive fraction. In that, the PAR provides information about public health significance and burden of an exposure on disease, it can be useful in setting public health priorities.[38] The PAR has been used in obesity epidemiology to estimate the number of deaths attributable to obesity[39-41] and the fraction of obesity cases that could be prevented by adopting a healthy lifestyle, such as one that includes exercise.[24] In the absence of confounding, to calculate the PAR, one needs to estimate the association between a dichotomized exposure and disease (RR) (typically from a cohort study), and obtain the prevalence of exposure (P_e) in the population (typically from the specific cohort or population-based surveys, such as NHANES):

$$PAR = P_e(RR - 1)/(1 + P_e(RR - 1))$$

This equation can be generalized to an exposure variable with multiple categories, but could lead to a biased estimate in the presence of confounding and effect modification.[42] Benichou[43] discussed several methods for calculating the PAR in a multivariate setting that includes multiple risk factors with or without confounding. One method is the model-based approach for case-control studies proposed by Bruzzi.[44] Recently, Spiegelman et al.[45] extended this method to cohort studies with algorithms for obtaining point and interval estimates of full (all disease risk factors are eliminated) and partial PAR (some risk factors are eliminated). A SAS macro for implementing these algorithms has also been developed (see http://www.hsph.harvard.edu/faculty/spiegelman/par).

Another approach for calculating multivariate adjusted PAR is the weighted-sum method proposed by Walter.[46] This method was used by Flegal et al.[41] to calculate the number of deaths attributable to obesity. In this approach, unadjusted RRs from each category of a major confounder, for example, age group and prevalence of obesity by age group in the population, are used to calculate the age group-specific PAR, which is then multiplied by the number of deaths within each age group in the population to derive the number of deaths attributable to obesity. These numbers are summed across age groups to obtain the total number of deaths attributable to obesity in the population. This method becomes inefficient if there are many confounders in the data.[43]

In a hypothetical example, Flegal et al.[47] found that incomplete adjustment for confounding of the obesity-mortality relation by age and sex (simply plugging the multivariate RRs into the above equation) led to a 17% overestimation of deaths due to obesity compared with the weighted-sum method. On the other hand, the estimated number of deaths was particularly sensitive to the change in the estimated RR of mortality associated with obesity. For example, a small increment of 0.20 in the estimated RRs led to a 97% increase in the calculated number of deaths. Therefore, a key factor in determining the estimated PAR was a valid (unconfounded) estimate of the association of obesity with mortality, making it essential to obtain unbiased RRs from cohort studies for accurate assessment of the PAR. This is especially important for the estimation of the number of deaths due to obesity, because the association is prone to biases resulting from confounding by smoking and reverse causation (see Chapter 11).

One common misinterpretation of the PAR is that if the calculated PAR for one factor is $x\%$, then $(1 - x\%)$ of the disease must be due to "other factors." For example, it has been estimated that over 90% of diabetes is attributable to unhealthy diet and lifestyle.[48] However, that does not mean that less than 10% of diabetes is accounted for by other factors, including genetics. For diseases with multiple risk factors, the sum of PAFs can be more than 100% because of overlapping risk factors and interactions among them.[42]

From a public health point of view, it is of great interest to calculate PAR by considering a group of risk factors together.[49,50] In fact, Wacholder et al.[50] have advocated the use of a broad definition of exposure (low- vs. high-risk) when estimating the overall PAR from several risk factors whose effects are additive. Using data from the Nurses' Health Study, we estimated that excess weight (defined as a BMI ≥ 25 kg/m^2) and physical inactivity (<3.5 hours of exercise per week) together could account for 31% of all premature deaths, 59% of deaths from cardiovascular disease, and 21% percent of deaths from cancer among nonsmoking women.[51] Such analyses are useful, because the close relationship between physical inactivity and obesity may make it impossible to separate their effects. In a study using obesity and diabetes as outcomes, we estimated that 30% (95% CI: 24% to 36%) of new cases of obesity and 43% (95% CI: 32% to 52%) of new cases of diabetes could be prevented by adopting a relatively active lifestyle (<10 hours/week of TV watching and ≥ 30 minutes/day of brisk walking).[24] These analyses are useful in estimating combined effects of increasing exercise and reducing sedentary behaviors on obesity.

Causal Inference in Obesity Epidemiology

Thinking about causality in epidemiology has evolved from single- to multicausality. The classic Henle-Koch model for infectious disease causality requires one-to-one correspondence between cause and effect.[52] This applies to some infectious diseases but not to others. It certainly has little bearing on chronic disease epidemiology, because virtually all modern chronic diseases, including obesity and obesity-related health conditions, are multifactorial.

Common forms of obesity are a perfect example of a complex and multifactorial condition caused by genetic, metabolic, lifestyle, diet, environmental, and psychosocial factors. Individually, none of these variables are necessary or sufficient to cause obesity, but the combination of some of the factors could create conditions sufficient for the current obesity epidemic. A major goal of obesity epidemiology is to identify individual component causes of obesity as well as their interactions. As Rothman and Greendland[53] pointed out,

> The importance of multi-causality is that most identified causes are neither necessary nor sufficient to produce disease. Nevertheless, a cause needs not be either necessary or sufficient for its removal to result in disease prevention. If a component cause that is neither necessary nor sufficient is blocked, a substantial amount of disease may be prevented.

Causal inference about individual component causes of obesity is a process of reasoning based on incomplete and imperfect evidence. Sir Austin Bradford Hill proposed a set of criteria for making causal inferences.[54] These include strength of association, consistency across different studies, specificity of association (i.e., a one-to-one relationship between an exposure and a disease), temporality (i.e., exposure always precedes disease outcomes), gradient (i.e., a dose-response relationship between exposure and disease), biological plausibility, and experimental evidence. The criteria are widely recognized as a basis for making causal inferences in epidemiology. However, their usefulness has been debated, and some authors have warned against their use as a checklist for causal inference.[30] Others, on the other hand, have advocated "weakening the rules of inference accompanying the criteria." Such changes are purported to identify "minimum evidentiary conditions" for making causal inferences about the health effects of environmental pollutants.[55] The so-called Precautionary Principle reflects the "precautionary goal of earlier primary preventive intervention, that is, acting on insufficient evidence, the least amount, or minimum level of evidence for causation."[55]

Among the causal criteria proposed by Hill, only a temporal relationship is a prerequisite for a causal relationship. As Hill noted, "none of my nine viewpoints can bring indisputable evidence for or against the cause and effect hypothesis and none can be required as a sine qua non." For example, a strong association is less likely to be explained by confounding, but a modest association is also important if it can be replicated in multiple studies and the prevalence of exposure is relatively high in the general population. In epidemiologic studies of BMI and cancer incidence, the RRs associated with overweight range from 1.2 to 2.0 for most cancers (see Chapter 10). These associations are relatively weak compared to that linking smoking and lung cancer. Nonetheless, they are important from both etiological and public health perspectives because of the high prevalence of overweight in the U.S. population.

Understanding of biological mechanisms is usually limited by available knowledge but can still be very useful in interpreting epidemiologic data. For example, some studies observed a lower cardiovascular mortality among overweight persons than those with normal weight. These findings contradict with known adverse metabolic and physiological effects of overweight, and a positive association between overweight and incidence of cardiovascular disease observed in numerous epidemiologic studies.[56] This suggests that the inverse association between overweight and mortality may be due to alternative explanations, for example, methodological biases resulting from confounding and reverse causation (see Chapter 11).

Consistency of results from different epidemiologic studies is critically important in making inferences of causation. True replication of highly controlled experimental studies, especially tissue culture and animal studies, is relatively straightforward. However, it is not often possible to truly replicate epidemiologic studies, because they almost always involve different populations and conditions. Although underlying biological mechanisms are expected to be the same for the majority of the population, observed associations can be exaggerated or obscured by the characteristics of participants or their environment. Rather than using random allocation of exposure to eliminate confounding, epidemiologic studies typically rely on multivariate adjustment or other statistical methods. Thus, different confounding structures in different populations, and various degrees of adjustment, can also lead to divergent results. Therefore, in interpreting inconsistent results, one should try to differentiate between lack of replication or inconsistency as a result of inadequate study design and confounding from true effect modifications by population characteristics.

Nonreplication is considered to be one of the most serious problems in genetic association studies of complex conditions like obesity. Common reasons cited for nonreplication include population stratification (confounding by race or ethnicity), publication bias, heterogeneity of effect, multiple comparisons, and lack of statistical power (see Chapter 21). These problems are not unique to genetic association studies, nor is there a single optimal solution to all of them. Careful adherence to sound epidemiologic principles and methods can reduce the problem of nonreplication. Meta-analysis of published results or pooled analyses of individual-level data from multiple studies can also help by improving the power of the analyses providing weighted averages of estimates of effect, and assessing sources of heterogeneity. Although the quality of meta- or pooled analyses largely depends on that of the original studies, such methodology has a role in improving the quality of causal inference.[57]

Summary

In this chapter, we discussed key methodological issues related to interpretation of epidemiologic evidence and inferences of causation in obesity research. RCTs with hard outcomes are considered the strongest design in the hierarchy of evidence for the evaluation of causal relationships. However, in most circumstances, large, long-term trials are either infeasible or unethical. The next level of evidence comes from large and carefully conducted prospective cohort studies, which are less susceptible to recall or selection biases than studies with retrospective exposure assessment and difficulties in defining valid comparison groups. This does not mean, however, that cohort studies are immune from biases and methodological problems. In obesity epidemiologic studies, confounding and reverse causation are the most serious threats to validity. Because there is no perfect solution to these problems, it is critical to apply sound epidemiologic principles and scientific rigor to study design and data analyses. Imprecise measurements also represent a unique challenge to obesity epidemiology. This is because diet and lifestyle factors are measured with substantial errors that can be compounded by the obesity status of participants. Another challenge in epidemiologic studies is how to balance validity with

Table 4.1 Levels of Inference from Epidemiologic Evidence

Inference	*Requirements*
Statistical associations	Study sufficiently powered; measurements of exposure and outcomes reasonably accurate
Causal effect of exposure on disease in study population	Rule out confounding, bias, and chance; temporality between exposure and disease, consistency of the results, and biological plausibility
Causal effect of exposure on disease in external populations	No effect modification by population characteristics (generalizability)
Prevention of disease through elimination or reduction of exposure	Amenability of exposure to modification
Substantial public health impact for elimination or reduction of exposure	Large population attributable fraction (high exposure prevalence, relatively strong exposure effect)

Adapted from Savitz DA. *Interpreting epidemiologic evidence: strategies for study design and analysis.* New York: Oxford University Press; 2003.[58]

generalizability. We should bear in mind, however, that maximizing internal validity is always the highest priority for analytic epidemiologic studies.

Understanding cause and effect is the goal of analytic epidemiology, and knowledge of cause (albeit tentative) should be used to help devise intervention strategies, address risk factors, and reduce the health consequences of obesity. Causal inference is not a static process, but a dynamic one that progresses from pure statistical associations to cause-effect in the study population to population-level impact[58] (Table 4.1). Ultimately, we want to apply knowledge gained from epidemiologic studies to public health initiatives to prevent and control obesity and related health conditions. We should bear in mind that causal inference does not condone inaction before obtaining "definite proof." Sir Austin Bradford Hill's thoughts on causality more than 40 years ago still apply today:[54]

All scientific work is incomplete—whether it be observational or experimental. All scientific work is liable to be upset or modified by advancing knowledge. That does not confer upon us a freedom to ignore the knowledge we already have, or to postpone the action it appears to demand at a given time.

References

1. Hernan MA. A definition of causal effect for epidemiological research. *J Epidemiol Community Health.* 2004;58:265-271.
2. Stern L, Iqbal N, Seshadri P, et al. The effects of low-carbohydrate versus conventional weight loss diets in severely obese adults: one-year follow-up of a randomized trial. *Ann Intern Med.* 2004;140:778-785.
3. Dansinger ML, Gleason JA, Griffith JL, Selker HP, Schaefer EJ. Comparison of the Atkins, Ornish, Weight Watchers, and Zone diets for weight loss and heart disease risk reduction: a randomized trial. *JAMA.* 2005;293:43-53.
4. Ware JH. Interpreting incomplete data in studies of diet and weight loss. *N Engl J Med.* 2003;348:2136-2137.
5. Howard BV, Manson JE, Stefanick ML, et al. Low-fat dietary pattern and weight change over 7 years: the Women's Health Initiative Dietary Modification Trial. *JAMA.* 2006;295:39-49.

6. Mensink RP, Katan MB. Effect of dietary fatty acids on serum lipids and lipoproteins. A meta-analysis of 27 trials. *Arterioscler Thromb.* 1992;12:911-919.

7. Hu FB, Willett WC. Optimal diets for prevention of coronary heart disease. *JAMA.* 2002;288:2569-2578.

8. Last JM. *A Dictionary of Epidemiology.* 4th ed. New York: Oxford University Press; 2001.

9. Grayson DA. Confounding confounding. *Am J Epidemiol.* 1987;126:546-553.

10. Manson JE, Stampfer MJ, Hennekens CH, Willett WC. Body weight and longevity. A reassessment. *JAMA.* 1987;257:353-358.

11. Schulze MB, Manson JE, Ludwig DS, et al. Sugar-sweetened beverages, weight gain, and incidence of type 2 diabetes in young and middle-aged women. *JAMA.* 2004;292:927-934.

12. Schlesselman JJ. *Case-Control Studies. Design, Conduct, Analysis. (Monographs in Epidemiology and Biostatistics).* New York: Oxford University Press; 1982.

13. D'Agostino RB Jr. Propensity score methods for bias reduction in the comparison of a treatment to a non-randomized control group. *Stat Med.* 1998;17:2265-2281.

14. Shah BR, Laupacis A, Hux JE, Austin PC. Propensity score methods gave similar results to traditional regression modeling in observational studies: a systematic review. *J Clin Epidemiol.* 2005;58:550-559.

15. Neaton JD, Blackburn H, Jacobs D, et al. Serum cholesterol level and mortality findings for men screened in the Multiple Risk Factor Intervention Trial. Multiple Risk Factor Intervention Trial Research Group. *Arch Intern Med.* 1992;152:1490-1500.

16. Pekkanen J, Nissinen A, Punsar S, Karvonen MJ. Short- and long-term association of serum cholesterol with mortality. The 25-year follow-up of the Finnish cohorts of the seven countries study. *Am J Epidemiol.* 1992;135:1251-1258.

17. Strandberg TE, Pyorala K, Cook TJ, et al. Mortality and incidence of cancer during 10-year follow-up of the Scandinavian Simvastatin Survival Study (4S). *Lancet.* 2004;364:771-777.

18. Baik I, Ascherio A, Rimm EB, et al. Adiposity and mortality in men. *Am J Epidemiol.* 2000;152:264-271.

19. Willett WC. Is dietary fat a major determinant of body fat? *Am J Clin Nutr.* 1998;67(3 Suppl):556S-562S.

20. McAdams MA, Van Dam RM, Hu FB. Comparison of self-reported and measured BMI as correlates of disease markers in US adults. *Obesity (Silver Spring).* 2007;15:188-196.

21. Nyholm M, Gullberg B, Merlo J, Lundqvist-Persson C, Rastam L, Lindblad U. The validity of obesity based on self-reported weight and height: implications for population studies. *Obesity (Silver Spring).* 2007;15:197-208.

22. Bingham SA. Biomarkers in nutritional epidemiology. *Public Health Nutr.* 2002;5:821-827.

23. Willett WC. *Nutritional Epidemiology.* 2nd ed. New York: Oxford University Press; 1998.

24. Hu FB, Li TY, Colditz GA, Willett WC, Manson JE. Television watching and other sedentary behaviors in relation to risk of obesity and type 2 diabetes mellitus in women. *JAMA.* 2003;289:1785-1791.

25. Baron RM, Kenny DA. The moderator-mediator variable distinction in social psychological research: conceptual, strategic, and statistical considerations. *J Pers Soc Psychol.* 1986;51:1173-1182.

26. Lin DY, Fleming TR, De Gruttola V. Estimating the proportion of treatment effect explained by a surrogate marker. *Stat Med.* 1997;16:1515-1527.

27. Kaufman JS, Maclehose RF, Kaufman S. A further critique of the analytic strategy of adjusting for covariates to identify biologic mediation. *Epidemiol Perspect Innov.* 2004;1:4.

28. Stevens J, Cai J, Pamuk ER, Williamson DF, Thun MJ, Wood JL. The effect of age on the association between body-mass index and mortality. *N Engl J Med.* 1998;338:1-7.

29. Byers T. Overweight and mortality among baby boomers—now we're getting personal. *N Engl J Med.* 2006;355:758-760.

30. Rothman KJ, Greenland S. *Modern Epidemiology*. 2nd ed. Philadelphia: Lippincott-Raven; 1998.
31. Hosmer DW, Lemeshow S. Confidence interval estimation of interaction. *Epidemiology*. 1992;3:452-456.
32. Assmann SF, Hosmer DW, Lemeshow S, Mundt KA. Confidence intervals for measures of interaction. *Epidemiology*. 1996;7:286-290.
33. Skrondal A. Interaction as departure from additivity in case-control studies: a cautionary note. *Am J Epidemiol*. 2003;158:251-258.
34. Liu S, Willett WC, Stampfer MJ, et al. A prospective study of dietary glycemic load, carbohydrate intake, and risk of coronary heart disease in US women. *Am J Clin Nutr*. 2000;71:1455-1461.
35. Jeppesen J, Schaaf P, Jones C, Zhou MY, Chen YD, Reaven GM. Effects of low-fat, high-carbohydrate diets on risk factors for ischemic heart disease in postmenopausal women. *Am J Clin Nutr*. 1997;65:1027-1033.
36. Rothman KJ. *Epidemiology. An Introduction*. New York: Oxford University Press; 2002.
37. Willett WC, Blot WJ, Colditz GA, Folsom AR, Henderson BE, Stampfer MJ. Merging and emerging cohorts: not worth the wait. *Nature*. 2007;445:257-258.
38. Gefeller O. Comparison of adjusted attributable risk estimators. *Stat Med*. 1992;11:2083-2091.
39. Allison DB, Fontaine KR, Manson JE, Stevens J, VanItallie TB. Annual deaths attributable to obesity in the United States. *JAMA*. 1999;282:1530-1538.
40. Mokdad AH, Marks JS, Stroup DF, Gerberding JL. Actual causes of death in the United States, 2000. *JAMA*. 2004;291:1238-1245.
41. Flegal KM, Graubard BI, Williamson DF, Gail MH. Excess deaths associated with underweight, overweight, and obesity. *JAMA*. 2005;293:1861-1867.
42. Rockhill B, Newman B, Weinberg C. Use and misuse of population attributable fractions. *Am J Public Health*. 1998;88:15-19.
43. Benichou J. A review of adjusted estimators of attributable risk. *Stat Methods Med Res*. 2001;10:195-216.
44. Bruzzi P, Green SB, Byar DP, Brinton LA, Schairer C. Estimating the population attributable risk for multiple risk factors using case-control data. *Am J Epidemiol*. 1985;122:904-914.
45. Spiegelman D, Hertzmark E, Wand HC. Point and interval estimates of partial population attributable risks in cohort studies: examples and software. *Cancer Causes Control*. 2007;18:571-579.
46. Walter SD. The estimation and interpretation of attributable risk in health research. *Biometrics*. 1976;32:829-849.
47. Flegal KM, Graubard BI, Williamson DF. Methods of calculating deaths attributable to obesity. *Am J Epidemiol*. 2004;160:331-338.
48. Hu FB, Manson JE, Stampfer MJ, et al. Diet, lifestyle, and the risk of type 2 diabetes mellitus in women. *N Engl J Med*. 2001;345:790-797.
49. Rowe AK, Powell KE, Flanders WD. Why population attributable fractions can sum to more than one. *Am J Prev Med*. 2004;26:243-249.
50. Wacholder S, Benichou J, Heineman EF, Hartge P, Hoover RN. Attributable risk: advantages of a broad definition of exposure. *Am J Epidemiol*. 1994;140:303-309.
51. Hu FB, Willett WC, Li T, Stampfer MJ, Colditz GA, Manson JE. Adiposity as compared with physical activity in predicting mortality among women. *N Engl J Med*. 2004;351:2694-2703.
52. Evans AS. Causation and disease: the Henle-Koch postulates revisited. *Yale J Biol Med*. 1976;49:175-195.
53. Rothman KJ, Greenland S. Causation and causal inference in epidemiology. *Am J Public Health*. 2005;95(Suppl 1):S144-S150.
54. Hill AB. The environment and disease: association or causation? *Proc R Soc Med*. 1965;58:295-300.

55. Weed DL. Methodologic implications of the Precautionary Principle: causal criteria. *Int J Occup Med Environ Health*. 2004;17:77-81.
56. Manson JE, Bassuk SS, Hu FB, Stampfer MJ, Colditz GA, Willett WC. Estimating the number of deaths due to obesity: can the divergent findings be reconciled? *J Women's Health*. 2007;16:168-176.
57. Weed DL. Interpreting epidemiological evidence: how meta-analysis and causal inference methods are related. *Int J Epidemiol*. 2000;29:387-390.
58. Savitz DA. *Interpreting Epidemiologic Evidence. Strategies for Study Design & Analysis*. New York: Oxford University Press; 2003.

5

Measurements of Adiposity and Body Composition

Frank B. Hu

Accurate assessment of body composition is essential to obesity research. The past several decades have witnessed major conceptual and technological advances in the measurement of body composition. Traditionally, approaches based on the classic two-compartment model that divides body weight into fat mass (FM) and fat-free mass (FFM), such as underwater weighing (densitometry) and isotope dilution (hydrometry), have been used as reference methods for measuring body density and total body water (TBW), respectively; both are then used to calculate body composition.[1] Although the classic two-compartment model is still useful, multicompartment models that include direct measurements of TBW, bone mineral, protein, fat, and other body measurements can provide more accurate measurement of body composition.[1] Conceptually, Heymsfield et al.[2] organized the human body into four different levels: atomic (e.g., oxygen, carbon, and hydrogen), molecular (i.e., water, lipid, protein, minerals, and glycogen), cellular (e.g., body cell mass and extracellular solids and fluids), and tissue (e.g., adipose tissue, skeletal muscle, bone, and visceral organs). Based on this framework, many multicompartment models have been developed to assess body composition. Methods based on these models have been facilitated by the advent of dual-energy x-ray absorptiometry (DXA).

More recently developed *high-tech* imaging options, such as computed tomography (CT) and magnetic resonance imaging (MRI), are being used with increasing frequency to measure body composition at tissue and organ levels. Although these methods offer excellent accuracy and reproducibility, several factors, including cost, technical complexity, and lack of portability, prohibit their routine use in large epidemiologic studies.[3] While DXA is becoming more widely available and accessible for use in relatively large field studies, CT and MRI are often used in small-scale studies that require a high degree of accuracy or as reference methods.

Despite technological advances in methods of body composition assessment, the simplicity and low cost of anthropometric measures, particularly of weight and height, make them the most commonly used variables in obesity epidemiologic research. Waist circumference (WC) as a measure of abdominal or central obesity has attracted particular attention because of its inclusion as a key criterion or prerequisite for the diagnosis of the metabolic syndrome.[4,5]

In this chapter, we first provide a brief overview of the "reference" body-composition methods, including underwater weighing, dilution methods, whole-body potassium counting, DXA, CT, and MRI. Next, we discuss bioelectrical impedance analysis (BIA), followed by a discussion of the validity of anthropometric measures, particularly self-reported height, weight, waist, and hip circumference in epidemiologic research. We also discuss ethnic differences in body composition and their implications for epidemiologic research. Finally, we examine statistical models and their interpretation in the analysis of various measures of adiposity in relation to morbidity and mortality. Table 5.1 provides a brief summary of the strengths and limitations of the different methods for measuring body composition.

Body Composition Reference Methods

In this section, we briefly describe body composition *reference* methods that are frequently used in small-scale studies to validate or calibrate anthropometric measures. For more detailed information refer to Heymsfield et al.[2]

Densitometry

Densitometry (also called underwater or hydrostatic weighing) is a classic technique for estimating body composition by measuring total body density. It is based on the principle that fat is less dense than water, and thus, the body density of an individual with more body fat will be lower than that of an individual with less body fat (fat is assumed to have a density of 0.9 g/cm^3 and FFM a density of 1.1 g/cm^3 at body temperature). Densitometry requires accurate recording of a subject's weight in air and underwater (submerged in a watertight tank), usually with a sensitive electronic scale. These measurements are used to estimate body volume (loss of weight in water, corrected for density of water), body density (body weight in air divided by the loss in weight in water), and percent body fat based on well-established formulas.[6,7] A critical methodological issue in the accuracy of densitometry is the need to measure and adjust for residual lung volume by standard techniques; inaccurate correction for residual lung volume is considered a major source of error.[1] Densitometry has long been the "gold standard" for measuring body composition because of its excellent precision and accuracy, and it will continue to be a useful criterion in validation studies of other body composition methods. However, the procedure is time-consuming, complicated, and requires active cooperation of the subject, which makes it unsuitable for younger children, the elderly, and morbidly obese patients.

A newer technique that uses air rather than water displacement for measuring body volume and density is more acceptable to participants, especially young children, the elderly, and other special populations. This method, called air-displacement plethysmography (ADP), measures raw body volume of subjects in minimal clothing (e.g., a swimsuit) as they sit in a testing chamber. Percent body fat is estimated using body volume and mass. As with densitometry, body volume needs to be corrected for the average amount of air in the lungs.[8] The BOD POD Body Composition System (Life Measurement Instruments, Concord, California) is now the most commonly used ADP method for assessing body volume and total body density.[9] Total body volume is estimated by applying the basic gas laws, using the differences in air pressure of the test chamber with and without the subject.

The system has an excellent between-day test-retest reliability ($r > .90$),[8] and validation studies have shown a good correlation between estimates of percent body fat by the BOD POD and densitometry ($R^2 = .78$ to $.94$). Although BOD POD tends to underestimate percent body fat, many studies have reported very good correlations between BOD POD

Table 5.1 A Comparison of Commonly Used Methods for Measuring Body Composition

Methods	Description	Strengths and Limitations
Reference methods		
Underwater weighing (densitometry)	This method is based on the principle that fat is less dense than water and that an individual with more body fat will thus have a lower body density. The technique involves measuring a subject's weight in air and underwater. Percent body fat is calculated with prediction equations based on the two-compartment model.	Densitometry has long been considered the "gold standard" for measuring body composition. However, the procedure is time-consuming and requires major active cooperation of the subjects. It is not suitable for children and older adults.
Air-displacement plethysmography (ADP)	ADP is a recently developed technique using air rather than water displacement for measuring body volume and density. The new BOD POD Body Composition System has been validated against densitometry.	The procedure is relatively quick, more comfortable, and does not require the subject to be submerged in water. It is an attractive alternative to the traditional densitometry method, especially for children.
Dilution method (hydrometry)	This method measures total body water using isotopes (deuterium is most commonly used) based on the principle that water exists in a relatively stable proportion to fat-free mass (≈ 0.73). Total body water is calculated with validated dilution equations.	The procedure is simple, safe, and relatively inexpensive. Measurements of total body water have high precision and accuracy. It can be used to measure body composition of morbidly obese patients. However, the assumption of a stable ratio of total body water to fat-free mass of 0.73 may not hold in patients who are ill, are in the early phase of weight loss, or have a different hydration status.
Dual-energy x-ray absorptiometry (DXA)	This technique is based on the principle that two x-ray beams of very low but different energy passing through the body are attenuated differentially by bone mineral tissue and soft tissue. It provides estimates for the three components of the whole body (fat-free mass, fat mass, and bone mineral density) for specific regions such as the arms, legs, and trunk.	The procedure has very high reproducibility and accuracy in measuring body fat and lean body mass and has gained increasing acceptance as a reference method for measuring body composition. Because x-ray exposure is extremely low, it is safe for children, but it is not suitable for pregnant women. The device is expensive and not portable. It cannot accurately distinguish visceral fat from subcutaneous fat.
Computed tomography (CT)/magnetic resonance imaging (MRI)	Both CT and MRI provide high-resolution cross-sectional scans of selected tissue or organs and are considered the most accurate methods for assessing body composition and regional fat distributions at tissue-organ levels.	Both methods accurately quantify percent body fat and visceral and subcutaneous fat. A major advantage of MRI over CT is the lack of radiation exposure. Both techniques are expensive and not readily available. They cannot usually accommodate morbidly obese people. *(continued)*

Table 5.1 continued

Methods	Description	Strengths and Limitations
Field methods		
Anthropometry BMI	BMI, defined as weight (kg)/height (m²), is the most widely used index of overall adiposity. The validity of BMI in predicting body fatness measured by a reference method is well-established in different age, sex, and racial groups. In numerous epidemiologic studies, BMI has been demonstrated to predict disease incidence and mortality.	BMI is simple and easy to calculate, and this measure is available in virtually all epidemiologic and clinical studies. Standardized cutoff points have been provided to define overweight and obesity in the general population. However, BMI is an indirect and imperfect measure of body fat because it does not distinguish fat mass and lean body mass components. BMI is a less valid predictor of body fat in elderly than in middle-aged adults. For a given BMI, Asians have a higher percent of body fat than do whites.
WC and waist-to-hip ratio (WHR)	WC and WHR are indirect measures of abdominal or central obesity. Both variables have been validated against measures of abdominal fat by DXA and CT scan and have been shown to predict disease incidence and mortality.	Measurements of waist and hip circumferences are relatively easy to obtain in large epidemiologic studies, although the measurement procedure is not entirely standardized. WC is now included as one of the key criteria for defining the metabolic syndrome. The interpretation of WHR is more complex, and the biological meaning of hip circumference is less clear.
Skinfold thicknesses	This method involves a special caliper to measure the thickness of a double layer of skin and the fat beneath it in predetermined sites, for example, triceps, biceps, subscapular, abdomen, and thighs. These measurements are commonly used as indirect assessments of body-fat distribution. They can be used to predict percent body fat based on prediction equations.	These measures are relatively simple to obtain in large epidemiologic studies and have been shown to predict total body fat and regional fat distribution, especially among children. However, interobserver errors are relatively large. The ability of skinfold thicknesses to predict morbidity and mortality is not well established.
Bioelectrical impedance analysis (BIA)	BIA is based on the principle that resistance to an applied alternating electrical current is a function of tissue composition: the more lean body mass or water a person has, the lower the resistance to the current. Calibrated prediction equations are used to calculate percent body fat, fat-free mass, and body water. Multifrequency BIA technology is increasingly replacing the traditional single-frequency BIA.	BIA equipment is relatively inexpensive, portable, and simple to operate. It can be used in relatively large field studies. However, the operation of the equipment and use of prediction equations need to be standardized. Because the method measures total body water, its accuracy can be affected by body structure, hydration status, and disease status.

estimates of percent fat and those provided by DXA (R^2 = .78 to .91).[10] Ginde et al.[11] demonstrated high accuracy in measuring body fat even in severely obese patients (body mass index, BMI ≥ 40). A high validity of BOD POD measurements of body fat has also been observed among children.[12] Because it has high validity and is less burdensome for participants, BOD POD has become an excellent alternative to traditional densitometry, especially in children, pregnant women, and morbidly obese persons.

Hydrometry

Hydrometry (or the dilution method) uses isotopes [deuterium (^2H_2O), tritium (^3H_2O), and oxygen-18-labeled water ($H_2^{18}O$)] to measure TBW.[13] Calculation of FFM is based on the dilution principle (the proportion of water to FFM is relatively stable: 0.73). This method is widely used as a reference method to estimate FFM and total body fat in vivo. Typically, an accurately weighed oral dose of isotope-labeled water is carefully administered to a subject after an overnight fast. Biological samples such as serum, urine, or saliva are collected before the dose is administered and at the end of equilibration, which usually takes 3 to 4 hours. TBW is calculated using validated dilution equations based on the degree of the dilution of the isotopes by total body fluid.[13] FFM is then calculated as TBW/0.73 and total body fat is calculated as the difference between body weight and FFM. The validity of this method relies on several reasonable assumptions: the presence of tracers in body water only; equal and rapid distribution of the tracer in all anatomical water compartments; and the absence of metabolism of both the tracer and body water during the course of equilibration after oral dosing.[13] The procedure is relatively straightforward, but achieving accurate and precise measurements requires careful attention to preparation of the subject, dosage, sample collection (urine, saliva, or blood), and isotopic analyses.[13]

Deuterium is the most widely used isotope because of its safety and relatively low cost. Oxygen-18-labeled water is also safe for children and pregnant women, but is more expensive than deuterium. The concentrations of both isotopes in biological samples are measured with high precision by a mass spectrometry technique. If the standard procedure is carefully followed, TBW measurements are highly accurate and precise, with technical errors in the range of 1% to 2%.[13] Overall, the use of hydrometry to estimate FFM and total body fat is simple and safe. It is one of the few methods that can be used to measure body composition in morbidly obese subjects; however, the assumption of a stable ratio of TBW to FFM of 0.73 may not be accurate in these subjects.[13] Disease, early phase of weight loss, or hydration status may also alter the ratio and affect the validity of estimates of FFM and body fat. Modified equations have been developed for estimating TBW and FFM in pregnant women according to different stages of pregnancy and the presence or absence of edema.[14]

Whole-Body Potassium Counting

Whole-body potassium counting is a classic reference method for estimating total body fat. It is based on the principle that the naturally occurring radioactive potassium isotope ^{40}K in human tissues represents total-body potassium (TBK); that ^{40}K accounts for 0.0118% of TBK; and that TBK is evenly distributed in intracellular components of FFM.[15] TBK can thus be quantified by using special equipment to detect γ-rays that emanate from ^{40}K. By assuming a constant proportion of FFM as potassium, one can estimate FFM by the following method:

$$FFM = TBK/63.3,$$

where 63.3 represents the TBK/FFM ratio in mmol/kg, reflecting the proportions of potassium for all FFM, including skeletal muscle mass in an average person.[1] Total body fat is then calculated as the difference between body weight and FFM. Because of the stable relationship between TBK and skeletal muscle in adults, TBK can be used to predict skeletal muscle mass.[16] Another major application of whole-body potassium counting is the measurement of total body cell mass, which consists of the cellular components of the body, including muscle, visceral organs, blood, and brain.[15]

The precision of the whole-body potassium counting technique is high (2% to 5% for adults).[15] The technique is also more accurate for measuring FFM and adiposity than densitometry, although its accuracy relies to some degree on the assumption of a constant TBK-FFM ratio. However, for different sex and ethnic groups, interpretation of results can be complicated because of substantial sex and ethnic differences in the rate of TBK change with age.[17] Although the method is relatively simple, safe, and accurate, it requires special and costly equipment that is not widely available. Thus, whole-body potassium counting has largely been replaced by DXA and imaging methods in measuring FFM and body fat. Nonetheless, it remains a useful means of assessing whole-body cell mass and skeletal muscle mass.

Imaging Methods

CT and MRI are considered the most accurate methods for assessing body composition and ascertaining fat distribution at the tissue-organ level.[18] Both CT and MRI provide high-resolution cross-sectional scans of selected tissues or organs and can be used to measure the volume and distribution of subcutaneous versus visceral fat, muscle mass, and organ composition. Unlike CT, MRI does not expose subjects to ionizing radiation. This makes it suitable for children and pregnant women. Multiple scans or whole-body scans can also be performed on the same person. Because both technologies are expensive and not readily accessible, they are not widely used in large field studies. However, they are the methods of choice for calibrating or validating simpler and less costly measurements of body fat distribution.

Both CT and MRI measurements of regional adipose tissue are highly reproducible and accurate by comparison with dissection in human cadavers.[18] Excellent correlations ($r = .89$ to .99) between cadaver and CT and MRI measures for lean skeletal muscle, visceral adipose tissue, and subcutaneous adipose tissue have been reported. Also, comparisons of CT and MRI measurements have shown very high agreement.[18] Skeletal muscle attenuation characteristics determined by CT have been shown to correlate well with muscle lipid content measured by biopsy.[19] In addition, both CT and MRI are useful and valid tools for measuring the composition of the liver and other organs.[18]

CT and MRI have been used in relatively small clinical and epidemiologic studies to measure total body adipose tissue mass, abdominal subcutaneous adipose tissue mass, visceral adipose tissue mass, and hepatic and intramuscular triglyceride content.[20,21] Several studies have found significant correlations between visceral adipose tissue mass (but not subcutaneous adipose tissue mass), insulin resistance, and metabolic and cardiovascular risk,[22] although results are not entirely consistent.[23] Weiss et al.[24] found that, in obese children and adolescents with impaired glucose tolerance, intramyocellular and intra-abdominal accumulation of lipids measured by MRI were closely correlated with the metabolic syndrome and severe peripheral insulin resistance.

Researchers in the Health Aging and Body Composition (Health ABC) Study of approximately 3000 elderly men and women used CT scans to measure visceral, subcutaneous abdominal, intramuscular, and subcutaneous thigh adipose tissue. Cross-sectional analyses suggested an association of higher amounts of intramuscular fat and visceral abdominal fat with increased prevalence of metabolic syndrome[25] as well as fasting insulin levels in normal-weight (BMI < 25 kg/m²) men ($r = .24$ for intramuscular fat, $r = .37$ for visceral abdominal fat) and women ($r = .20$ for intramuscular fat, $r = .40$ for visceral abdominal fat).[26] A significant association has also been noted between a high amount of subcutaneous thigh fat and decreased blood glucose (in men) and lipid (in both men and women) levels after accounting for abdominal fat depots.[27] A prospective analysis of the Health ABC Study found that visceral fat assessed by CT was a significant predictor of myocardial infarction (hazard ratio = 1.67, 95% CI: 1.28 to 2.17 per standard deviation increase) in women but not in men,[28] suggesting that the amount of adipose tissue stored in the intra-abdominal cavity is an important cardiovascular risk factor in elderly women.

Dual-Energy X-Ray Absorptiometry

DXA scanning was initially developed for measuring bone mineral density and diagnosing osteoporosis. It is now rapidly becoming one of the most frequently used methods for estimating human body composition in clinical studies.[29] It was used in NHANES 1999-2000,[30] and along with other imaging methods, in the Health ABC Study.[31] DXA can provide estimates of the three components of the whole body (FFM, FM, and bone mineral density) as well as specific regions, such as the arms, legs, and trunk. The procedure is relatively simple and quick. It is based on the principle that two x-ray beams of very low but differing energy passing through the body are attenuated differentially by bone mineral, soft tissue, fat tissue, and FFM. Because DXA provides highly reproducible and accurate measures of body fat and lean body mass (see below), it is becoming an accepted reference method for assessing body composition. DXA exposes subjects to extremely low levels of radiation, which makes it safe for use in a wide range of populations, including children. But it is not safe for pregnant women, and most currently available systems cannot accommodate morbidly obese subjects. The instrument itself is expensive and immobile—factors that preclude its widespread use in large epidemiologic studies of morbidity and mortality.

DXA produces very precise estimates of body composition. Kiebzak et al.[32] scanned 20 subjects once a day for four consecutive days with a Lunar DPX-L densitometer and manufacturer-supplied software. Coefficients of variation (CV%) were 0.62 for total body bone mineral density, 1.89 for total percentage fat, 0.63 for total body tissue mass, 2.0 for FM, 1.11 for lean mass, 1.10 for bone mineral content, and 1.09 for total bone calcium. Regional measurements (arm, leg, trunk, pelvis, and spine) were less precise than total body measurements, with CVs in the range of 1% to 5%. These data indicate that DXA produces highly precise short-term measurements of total and regional body composition. The long-term (3-month) reproducibility of DXA measurements (Hologic QDR 4500A absorptiometer) is also high.[33]

DXA estimates of body composition in humans have been validated extensively against criterion methods. Comparisons of body composition assessed by DXA and hydrodensitometry have generally provided highly consistent estimates of percent body fat.[29] However, differences in calibration between instruments from different manufacturers, as well as differences between various models and computer software from a single manufacturer, can lead to variability in DXA estimates.[34]

The accuracy of DXA has been further confirmed by small experiments in which exogenous fat was added to either central or peripheral body regions during the imaging process.[35] DXA estimates of total abdominal fat (TAF) and abdominal visceral fat (AVF) have been validated against a single-slice CT scan.[36] The DXA estimates of trunk and abdominal FM were strongly correlated with TAF ($r = .94$ to .97) and AVF ($r = .86$ to .90) as assessed by CT.

In the Health ABC Study of elderly men and women, Snijder et al.[31] compared the measurements of visceral fat from DXA and CT. Total body fat and trunk fat were measured by DXA with a Hologic QDR 1500. Visceral fat and TAF were measured with a 10 mm CT scan at the L4-L5 levels. The study showed a strong correlation between TAF measured by DXA (subregion) and CT (ranging from 0.87 in white men to 0.98 in black women). The DXA subregion underestimated TAF by 10% compared with the CT scan. This study supports the value of DXA as a good alternative to CT for predicting TAF in an elderly population. For the prediction of visceral fat, DXA was not superior to sagittal diameter (measured as the horizontal distance between the abdomen and the lower back).

Many studies have evaluated the relationship between DXA estimates of percent body fat and fat distribution and metabolic and cardiovascular risk factors.[29] In general, DXA estimates of body fatness correlate well with measures of insulin resistance, glucose intolerance, and blood lipids. However, the correlations between DXA measures and adverse cardiovascular risk factors in adults and children are no higher than those provided by simpler anthropometric measures, such as BMI, WC, and skinfold thicknesses.[37,38] Whether DXA estimates of body fat predict long-term risk of chronic disease or mortality has yet to be determined.

Body Composition Field Methods

Bioelectrical Impedance Analysis

BIA estimates body composition by measuring the impedance or resistance to a small electrical current (typically 800 μA, 50 kHz) passed across body tissues (i.e., between two detection electrodes attached to the right ankle and the right wrist of a subject). The method is based on the principle that resistance to an applied alternating electrical current is a function of tissue composition: the greater the lean body mass or water content of a person, the faster the current will pass through; the greater the fatty tissue, the greater the resistance to the current.[39]

Substantial technological advances in BIA have been developed over the past two to three decades, and many commercial BIA systems are now available to estimate body composition in children and adults. Simpler systems based on a single frequency have gradually been replaced by those based on multiple frequencies, with more complex methods for estimating body fat, FFM, skeletal muscle, body water, and water distribution. Numerous prediction equations have been developed to estimate percent body fat and FFM.[39] In developing these equations, researchers typically use TBW (measured by the reference method of isotope dilution) and FFM (measured by DXA or underwater weighing) as dependent variables, with measured resistance or closely related impedance as the predictor variables. The electrical measurements are usually adjusted for height. To improve statistical predictability, models typically include age, sex, race, weight, and other anthropometric measures. As with other prediction equations for body fat, those for BIA tend to be population specific.

In 1994, the National Institutes of Health organized a conference to assess the clinical and research applicability of BIA methods.[40] The consensus panel concluded that BIA, measured at a single frequency, provided a reliable estimate of TBW under most conditions. However, lack of a standardized methodology limited its clinical utility because estimates could be affected by numerous variables, including body position, hydration status, consumption of food and beverages, ambient air and skin temperature, recent physical activity, and conductance of the examining table. Since 1994, there have been two significant advances in BIA technology and modeling.[41] First, the original series resistance model has been replaced with a parallel resistance model that allows separate estimates of intracellular water (ICW) and extracellular water (ECW). Second, multifrequency and segmental BIA technologies were developed to provide more accurate measurement of body composition than single-frequency BIA.[42]

Recently, Sun et al.[43] compared multifrequency BIA and DXA estimates of percent body fat among 591 healthy subjects. They found correlations between BIA and DXA of 0.88 for the whole population, 0.78 for men and 0.85 for women. The mean percent body fat determined by BIA (32.89% ± 8.00%) was significantly lower than that measured by DXA (34.72% ± 8.66%). BIA overestimated percent body fat by 3.03% and 4.40% when the percent body fat was <15% in men and <25% in women, respectively; it underestimated it by 4.32% and 2.71% when the percent body fat was >25% in men and >33% in women, respectively. The study concluded that BIA is a good alternative for estimating percent body fat in subjects within a normal body fat range, but tends to overestimate it in lean subjects and underestimate it in obese subjects.

Use of standardized equipment, prediction equations, and body composition information are essential for clinical use of BIA.[44] Estimates of body fat in morbidly obese individuals should be considered with caution because BIA tends to underestimate percent body fat and overestimate FFM in this population.[45] Also, shape and size of various body parts are known to affect BIA measurements, with smaller cross-sectional areas (such as legs and arms) contributing the most to whole-body resistance. This could possibly affect measurements of percent body fat in different ethnic groups because of differences in body structure. Because BIA equipment is comparatively inexpensive, portable, and simple to operate, it can be used in relatively large epidemiologic studies. For example, NHANES III (1988-1994) included BIA measurements for 17,000 subjects aged 12 years or older.[46] However, a recent analysis showed that correlations between BIA-derived percent body fat and markers of cardiovascular disease (e.g., blood cholesterol, triglycerides, and blood pressure) were no stronger than those for BMI.[47]

Investigators from the Malmö Diet and Cancer Study[48] collected BIA data from a Swedish cohort of 10,902 men and 16,814 women aged 45 to 73 years. They found a somewhat stronger association between BIA-estimated percent of body fat at baseline and mortality than for BMI. However, WHR was an even stronger predictor of mortality independent of body fat, especially in women. Bigaard et al.[49] obtained BIA estimates of body fat and lean body mass from a Danish cohort of 27,178 men and 29,875 women 50 to 64 years old. Reliability and validity of the BIA method were referenced against a four-compartment model with whole-body potassium counting and the dilution method. Sex-specific equations developed in that study were used to estimate FFM.[50] The FFM index (FFMI) was calculated as FFM divided by height squared, and the BFM index (BFMI) was calculated as BMI minus FFMI. BMI was strongly correlated with both BFMI and FFMI, but the correlation was stronger for BFMI than for FFMI. The study found a U-shaped association between BMI and all-cause mortality, a slight J-shaped association between BFMI and mortality, and a reverse J-shaped association between

FFMI and mortality. These findings suggest that the U-shaped association between BMI and all-cause mortality observed in this cohort of older adults reflects the combination of opposite associations between BFMI and FFMI and mortality, and that high BFMI and low FFMI are both independent predictors of all-cause mortality. However, the high correlations between BMI and FFM make it difficult to tease out the independent effects of FM and FFM in most epidemiologic studies.

Anthropometry

Standardized methods are available to measure weight, height, and other anthropometric variables.[51] These approaches are especially important for national surveys that monitor obesity trends over time. The NHANES examination protocol and data collection methods are documented in the *NHANES Anthropometry Procedures Manual*.[52] The actual measurement techniques used in the survey are illustrated in the *NHANES III Anthropometric Procedures* video.[53] All NHANES body measurements are obtained by trained health technicians and routine calibration of the equipment is an important part of the study's quality-control plan. Body weight is measured in kilograms (to the second decimal place) using a self-zeroing digital scale; subjects wear foam slippers and a paper shirt and pants. Height is measured to the nearest millimeter with a stadiometer.

Among various anthropometric variables, weight and height are measured with the highest precision (reproducibility) and accuracy (little deviance from the true value), and the least amount of technical error.[54] Because measurements of waist and hip circumferences have greater between-technician variability, these measurements are best carried out by one person. Between-technician variability is even greater for skinfold measurements. Marks et al.[55] evaluated reliability for eight anthropometric measures in 95 male and 134 female subjects from NHANES II. Among the anthropometric measurements, the highest interobserver reliabilities were for weight, height, sitting height, and arm circumference ($R \geq .97$); the reliabilities for triceps and subscapular skinfolds, bitrochanteric breadth, and elbow breadth were lower but acceptable ($R = .81$ to $.95$).

Use of Height and Weight Variables in Epidemiologic Studies

Adult height is a complex variable determined primarily by genetics but also by nutritional factors, especially intakes of energy and protein during the preadult period.[56] Thus, adult height may serve as a marker of childhood or adolescent energy balance.[57] Consistent positive associations have been observed between adult height and increased risk of breast, prostate, and colorectal cancer.[58] In a pooled analysis of 337,819 postmenopausal women, the relative risk (RR) of breast cancer per height increment of 5 cm was 1.07 (95% CI: 1.03 to 1.12).[59] The association between adult height, which is influenced by both genetic and nutritional factors, and cancer risk may be mediated through hyperinsulinemia and increased IGF-1 levels associated with maximal growth in the preadult period.[60] In contrast to risk of cancer, shorter stature has been associated with increased cardiovascular mortality.[61]

Variables reflecting changes in body weight have been widely used in epidemiologic studies as both exposure and outcome variables, although their definitions differ substantially

Table 5.2 Definitions of Commonly Used Weight Variables in Epidemiologic Studies

Weight Variables	Definition	Comments
Attained weight	Current weight at a given time point.	It is not sufficient for use as an independent or dependent variable unless height or previous weight is adjusted for.
Weight gain	The amount of weight gained during a specified period of time (e.g., from adolescence to midlife).	Because height is constant in young and middle-aged adults, weight gain largely reflects an increase in body fat. When weight gain is used as a dependent variable, baseline weight needs to be controlled for.
Stable weight or weight maintenance	Gained or lost weight does not exceed a certain absolute amount (e.g., 4 kg) or percent of body weight (e.g., 5% of initial weight) within a specified period.	The group with stable weight is typically used as a reference in studies of health consequences associated with weight gain or loss. It can also be used as a dependent variable in studies on determinants of weight maintenance.
Intentional weight loss	Self-reported deliberate attempts to lose weight through diet/lifestyle changes or drugs.	Intentional weight loss has not been associated with adverse health outcomes. In some studies, it is associated with decreased mortality, but confounding by other health-conscious behaviors associated with attempted weight loss may explain the association.
Unintentional weight loss	Self-reported weight loss that is not voluntary.	Unintentional weight loss has been associated with increased mortality, but this association is largely explained by existing or undiagnosed illness. In older individuals, most weight loss is unintentional.
Weight cycling	Repeated loss and regain of body weight over time. Some definitions require that weight loss be intentional.	Such an analysis requires weight data across multiple time points. Weight cycling has been associated with greater weight gain and obesity but does not appear to be associated with adverse health outcomes if weight loss is intentional.
Body weight variability (BWV)	The root mean square error around the linear regression line of weight (or standard deviation divided by the average weight) across multiple time points.	BWV has been associated with mortality, but the association appears to be explained by unintentional weight loss associated with preexisting or undiagnosed illness in older individuals.

across studies (Table 5.2). In epidemiologic studies on determinants of obesity, weight gain is the most commonly used outcome variable. Changes in weight are typically defined as the difference in weight assessed between two time points (the interval ranging from several months to decades). A major weight gain has been defined as at least 25 kg over an extended period (e.g., 10-12 years).[62] Although this is an arbitrary definition, it is nevertheless useful to separate those with a substantial weight gain from those with moderate weight gain.

In epidemiologic studies on health consequences, weight gain during the period from late adolescence (18 to 20 years old) to middle age (30 to 55 years old) is of great interest. Many people gain the greatest amount of weight during this period, and for most, the added weight reflects increases in body fat. In the Nurses' Health Study (NHS), we calculated weight change between age 18 years and baseline (1976), and classified women into five categories according to the amount of weight gained (4 to 10 kg; 10.1 to 19.9 kg; 20 to 39.9 kg; ≥40 kg). There was a dose-response relationship between the amount of weight gained and risk of coronary heart disease (CHD)[63] and total mortality.[64] In these analyses, women with stable weight (gain or loss <4 kg) were used as the reference group. Note that the definition of stable weight or weight maintenance is arbitrary: some studies use the absolute weight change (e.g., gain or loss of ≤4 kg during a certain period), and others use percent weight change (e.g., ≤4% of change in body weight within a certain period).[65] Although it may seem easy to understand absolute weight change, the meaning of a 4 kg weight gain can differ depending on baseline weight and the time frame during which weight gain has occurred. Thus, epidemiologic analyses of weight change and health outcomes should adjust for baseline weight.

Although weight loss is a common exposure variable in epidemiologic studies, it is difficult to differentiate between intentional and unintentional weight loss. The distinction is important because unintentional weight loss rather than intentional weight loss has been associated with increased morbidity and mortality.[66] In the Iowa Women's Health Study,[67] unintentional weight loss was associated with higher total and cardiovascular mortality, but the finding was confined to women with prevalent disease, hypertension, or diabetes mellitus. Conversely, episodes of intentional weight loss of >9 kg during adulthood were not associated with increased total or cardiovascular mortality. Gregg et al.[68] found that self-reported unintentional weight loss was associated with significantly increased mortality rates, whereas intentional weight loss was associated with lower mortality rates. Similarly, Eilat-Adar et al.[69] found that intentional weight loss from a 6-month period of dieting predicted a lower incidence of CHD over 4 years of follow-up. These findings suggest an inverse association between intentional weight loss and CHD and mortality. However, such analyses can be easily confounded by other health-related behaviors associated with attempted weight loss.

In nonexperimental settings, weight loss, especially in older individuals, is often prompted by the presence of chronic conditions, such as diabetes, cancer, or chronic obstructive pulmonary disease (COPD). Although many studies exclude these participants, some predisposing conditions can be present for several years before clinical diagnosis in subjects who are not excluded. Weight loss or leanness caused by underlying disease rather than the contrary is called "reverse causation," a major source of bias in studies of obesity and mortality (see Chapter 11). Exclusion of deaths during the first few years of a study can reduce but not eliminate the impact of reverse causation, especially in studies of elderly populations. Because most weight loss in the elderly is unintentional, findings on weight loss and mortality from studies that include older individuals should be interpreted with caution.

Weight cycling, defined as the repeated loss and regain of body weight, is thought to be associated with adverse health outcomes, but epidemiologic data are limited. As with weight maintenance, there is no standard definition for weight cycling. Field et al.[70,71] classified women as weight cyclers if they reported an intentional loss of ≥20 lbs (≥9.1 kg) without maintaining the loss. Weight cyclers were further divided into severe (intentional weight loss of ≥20 lbs on at least three occasions) and mild weight cyclers (intentional weight loss of 10 to 19.9 lbs three or more times). Such definitions require the element of intentional weight loss. Therefore, it is not surprising that, in these analyses, weight cycling was not independently associated with hypertension[71] or diabetes.[70] In studies that did not distinguish between intentional and unintentional weight change, weight cycling or fluctuation (loss-gain or gain-loss across multiple time points) was associated with increased mortality.[66] However, the association disappeared when the analyses were restricted to healthy nonsmokers, suggesting that the observed association between weight cycling and mortality was confounded by unintentional weight loss caused by existing diseases.

Body weight variability (BWV) is another variable used to capture the effects of weight fluctuation over time. It is typically defined as the root mean square error of a regression fitted to each individual's weight or BMI values across multiple time points.[72] Whether BWV independently contributes to morbidity or mortality risk is uncertain. In the Chicago Western Electric Company Study, weight variability was not independently related to mortality after taking into account overall weight change.[73] In the Honolulu Heart Study, both weight loss and weight variability were associated with increased mortality.[74] However, these associations disappeared when the analyses were limited to healthy men who had never smoked, suggesting that the association between BWV and mortality was explained in part by confounding by smoking and the presence of preexisting disease. In the Framingham Study, BWV (calculated as the standard deviation of the nine BMI values of each subject divided by the average BMI for that subject) was significantly associated with subsequent mortality risk after adjusting for level and slope of BMI.[75] As with prior studies, this one did not take into account weight fluctuation caused by unintentional weight loss.

Adiposity Indexes Using Weight and Height

Although both height and weight are biologically meaningful variables in epidemiologic studies (discussed above), they do not represent body fatness. Nonetheless, the combination of these two variables can create useful, albeit not perfect, indexes of adiposity. Historically, insurance companies have developed, and periodically revised, height-weight tables based on associations with minimal mortality among insurees.[76] Relative weight is the ratio of an individual's observed weight to a standard or *ideal* weight according to age, sex, and height. The most widely used standard weights are the "desirable weights" of the Metropolitan Life Insurance Company.[77]

In earlier epidemiologic studies,[78,79] relative weight was examined prospectively in relation to subsequent mortality during follow-up. For example, in the Framingham Study,[79] overweight (weight >110%) nonsmoking men had 30-year mortality rates up to 3.9 times higher than those of men of desirable weight (weight 100% to 109%), according to the Metropolitan tables. Although relative weight is readily interpreted, it is often difficult to compare findings across studies if different standards were used.[57] Because of this limitation, the use of relative weight has become largely obsolete in epidemiologic studies.

Obesity indexes that use combinations of weight and height do not rely on a standard. The most commonly used obesity index is BMI. In 1835, Quetelet, a Belgian mathematician and astronomer, observed that in adults, body weight was proportional to the square of the height.[80] In 1972, Keys et al.[81] examined various weight-height indexes and found that BMI had the highest correlations with adiposity assessed by skinfold and body density measurements. Benn[82] advocated the use of an empirically fit value for the exponent of height (p) based on specific population studies to create an index uncorrelated with height. The validity of the Benn index (weight/height^p) has not been found to be superior to that of BMI (in which $P = 2$). For example, Revicki and Israel[83] examined the relationship between various adiposity indexes and hydrostatic measurements of body fat in 474 men aged 20 to 70 years. The weight-height ratio (W/H), Quetelet index or BMI (W/H^2), Khosla-Lowe index (W/H^3), and Benn index (W/H^p) were evaluated. The correlations among the various adiposity indexes were high, ranging from 0.91 to 0.99, and all were strongly correlated with weight ($r = .81$ to $.98$); while only W/H^2 ($r = -.03$) and W/H^p ($r = -.01$) had no correlation with height. The correlation of W/H^2 and W/H^p with hydrostatic measurement of adiposity were the strongest and similar (0.71 vs. 0.69).

Numerous studies have evaluated the validity of BMI in predicting body fatness measured by a *superior* method. Gallagher et al.[84] examined the relationship between BMI and total body fat in 504 white and 202 black men and women 20 to 94 years of age. The analysis was based on a four-compartment body composition model using the following equation:

$$\text{Fat mass} = 2.513 \times \text{BV} - 0.739 \times \text{TBW} + 0.947 \times \text{TBBM} - 1.79 \times \text{BW},$$

where BV is body volume as measured by hydrodensitometry, TBW is total body water as measured by tritium dilution, TBBM is total body bone mineral mass as measured by DXA, and BW is body weight.

BMI was strongly correlated with both absolute body fat and percent body fat (Table 5.3). The correlations were somewhat stronger for women than for men, and the correlations with absolute body fat were somewhat stronger than those for percent body fat. This study demonstrated that BMI is an excellent indicator of body fatness in different age, sex, and racial groups. Several other studies have shown a strong correlation between BMI and percent body fat assessed by DXA. Blew et al.[85] found a high correlation between the two variables ($r = .81$) in 317 postmenopausal women. Evans et al.[86] found similar high correlations between percent body fat and BMI in both black and white women, although race modified the prediction of percent body fat by BMI. Prediction equations have been developed to estimate percent of body fat based on BMI for both children and adults,[87,88] but these equations are not widely used.

Many studies have assessed the validity of BMI as a measure of body fatness to predict biochemical markers of obesity and cardiovascular risk. Circulating concentrations of adipocyte-secreted hormones, such as leptin and adiponectin, can be used as surrogate markers of body fat. Jurimae et al.[89] evaluated relationships between leptin levels and body fat assessed

Table 5.3 Correlation Coefficients for BMI and Body Composition Assessed Using a Four-Compartment Body Composition Model

	Women		Men	
	Black	*White*	*Black*	*White*
Height	−.07	−.19*	.02	−.04
Body weight	.89**	.87**	.85**	.84**
Body fat (%)	.75**	.72**	.63**	.58**
Body fat (kg)	.89**	.87**	.78**	.75**
Fat-free body mass (kg)	.42**	.33**	.48**	.44**

* $P < .01$; ** $P < .001$.
Adapted from Gallagher D, Visser M, Sepulveda D, Pierson RN, Harris T, Heymsfield SB. How useful is body mass index for comparison of body fatness across age, sex, and ethnic groups? *AM J Epidemiol.* 1996;143:228-239.[84]

by anthropometry and DXA. Among overweight and obese women (BMI > 27), BMI and percent body fat measured by DXA were similarly correlated with leptin concentrations (0.73 vs. 0.79). These correlations were much weaker among women with a BMI ≤ 27. In numerous studies, BMI has been inversely correlated with concentrations of adiponectin, a newly discovered adipocyte-derived hormone that is reduced in obese and diabetic subjects.[90]

The relationship between BMI and cardiovascular risk factors, such as blood pressure, high-density lipoprotein (HDL) cholesterol, fasting glucose, and triglycerides is well established. Spiegelman et al.[91] compared the associations of BMI, absolute FM, percent body fat, and regional fat distribution with fasting blood glucose and blood pressure in 1551 men and women between the ages of 15 and 79 years. Percent body fat and absolute FM were assessed by densitometry. In this study, BMI appeared to be more strongly correlated with absolute FM adjusted for height than with percent body fat. Also, overall and absolute FM were stronger predictors of blood pressure and blood glucose levels than was percent body fat (after adjustment for age, height, and current cigarette-smoking status). Correlations between body fat variables assessed by densitometry and blood pressure and blood glucose were not superior to those between BMI and these factors. These findings suggested that although BMI is a measure of both fat and lean body mass, the adverse effects of FM overrode the potential benefits of LBM in this young-adult and middle-aged population. This outcome may explain a strong association between BMI and cardiovascular morbidity and mortality observed in many epidemiologic studies (see Chapters 9 and 10).

Age and Sex Differences

Despite its established ability to predict body fat and health outcomes, BMI is an indirect and imperfect measure of adiposity. The components of BMI include both FM and lean body mass (LBM). Given the same BMI, the relative compositions of FM versus LBM appear to depend on age, sex, and ethnicity.[92] It is well known that for the same BMI, percent body fat is higher in women than in men.[84] The sex differences in body composition are established during adolescence and sexual maturation, when males develop more lean body mass, especially bone mass and skeletal muscle.[93] For children, BMI is a "moving target," in that normal changes with growth and maturation lead to greater increases in LBM than in FM.[94] Because it is inappropriate to use absolute values of BMI as a measure of fatness in children, national and international reference standards have been established to define childhood overweight and obesity using age and sex-specific distributions (see Chapter 20).

The validity of BMI as a marker of body fatness in older adults appears to be reduced due to changes in body composition associated with aging. According to NHANES data,[95] mean BMI gradually increases during young and middle-aged adult life, reaching peak values at 50 to 59 years of age, then declining slightly after age 60.[96] It is well established that aging is associated with a substantial loss in LBM and with some increase in FM.[84] For example, from 20 to 70 years of age, LBM, especially muscle, decreases by up to 40%.[96] Decreased muscle mass in the elderly is known as *sarcopenia*. Several studies have shown that the prevalence of sarcopenia increases rapidly at ages >60 years.[97,98]

Janssen et al.[99] observed a reduction in skeletal muscle mass starting during the third decade of life, with a more noticeable decrease in absolute skeletal muscle mass at the age of 45 (Fig. 5.1). This decrease was attributed primarily to a decrease in lower body skeletal muscle (e.g., thigh muscle). During 4 years of follow-up of the Health ABC cohort, Newman et al.[100] found that weight loss was strongly correlated with lean body mass loss in elderly men and women, especially in those whose weight loss occurred during hospitalization.

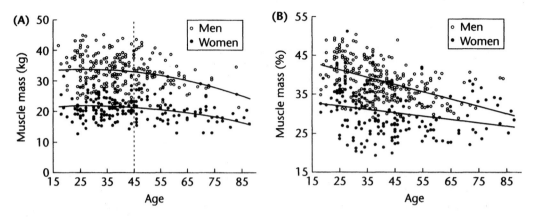

Figure 5.1 (A) Relationship between whole-body SM (skeletal muscle) mass and age in men and women. Solid lines, regression lines. Men: SM mass = −0.001 (age²) + 35.5; SE of estimate (SEE) = 5.1. Women: SM mass = −0.001 (age²) + 22.5; SEE = 3.6. (B) Relationship between relative SM mass (SM mass/body mass) and age in men and women. Solid lines, regression lines. Note that slope of regression line is greater ($P < .01$) in men than in women. Men: SM mass = −0.188 (age) + 46.0; SEE = 4.4. Women: SM mass = −0.084 (age) + 34.2; SEE = 5.4. Reproduced with permission from Janssen I, Heymsfield SB, Wang ZM, Ross R. Skeletal muscle mass and distribution in 468 men and women aged 18-88 yr. *J Appl Physiol.* 2000;89:81-88.[99]

Multiple factors may be responsible for the change in body composition with aging, including decreased testosterone levels and physical activity, and lower consumption of protein energy.[84] Because of age-related changes in body composition, between-person variations in BMI reflect, in part, variations in LBM, reducing the validity of BMI as a marker of body fat in the elderly.[57] Using data from NHANES I and NHANES II, Micozzi and Harris[101] found a stronger correlation between BMI and estimates of body fat in younger men and women than in older ones; in contrast, correlations between BMI and muscle mass were stronger in older individuals than in younger ones.

Aging is also associated with changes in body fat distribution. Hughes et al.[102] described 10-year changes in body composition and the metabolic and physical activity factors associated with these changes in 54 men and 75 women aged 60.4 ± 7.8 years at baseline. During the 10 years of follow-up, the amount of subcutaneous fat declined (−17.2%; $P < .001$), while total FM increased (7.2%; $P < .05$), primarily due to an increase in intra-abdominal fat. An increase in physical activity was associated with an attenuation of decline in FFM ($P < .007$). Other studies in the elderly have shown increased intramuscular and intrahepatic fat, which is associated with increased insulin resistance.[103]

The lower validity of BMI as a measure of adiposity in the elderly may explain why the relationship between BMI and mortality is less pronounced in older adults than in younger adults (see Chapter 11). In the elderly, a low BMI probably reflects low LBM rather than low FM.[104] A larger WC appears to be a better measure of adiposity, especially abdominal fatness, in older people. This may explain why, in some epidemiologic studies, WC is better than BMI as a predictor of mortality for the elderly.[105]

Ethnic Differences

The interpretation of BMI is complicated by well-recognized ethnic variations in body composition.[93] Wagner and Heyward[106] conducted a detailed comparative review on measures of body composition in blacks and whites. They noted that body mineral content, bone mineral density, and muscle mass as measured by DXA were greater in blacks than in whites, probably as a result of the relatively longer leg and arm lengths in blacks. Because of the difference in body structure, blacks tend to have lower adiposity and percent body fat than do whites for a given BMI. Several studies have shown that, although blacks tend to have higher BMI values than whites, the percent body fat as assessed by DXA is not significantly different in blacks and whites.[84,107]

There is consistent evidence that the percent body fat is higher in Asians than in whites with the same BMI.[108] Deurenberg et al.[109] found that the percent body fat in Asians was 3 to 5 percentage points higher than that in whites with the same BMI. Stated another way, for the same percent body fat, BMI was 3 to 4 units lower in Asians than in whites. The high body fat at low BMIs in Asians is probably related to their build, which is characterized by shorter legs and a smaller frame. Differences in muscularity may also be a contributing factor. Even among Asians, the relationship between BMI and percent body fat differs by subgroup. Deurenberg-Yap et al.[110] found that in a Singaporean population, Indians had higher percent body fat than did Chinese and Malaysians. A meta-analysis suggested that for the same level of body fat, age, and gender, the BMI of African Americans was 1.3 kg/m^2 higher than that of Caucasians, and that of Polynesians was 4.5 kg/m^2 higher than that of whites. In contrast, the BMIs of Chinese, Indonesians, and Thais were 1.9, 3.2, and 2.9 kg/m^2 lower, respectively, than those of whites[111] (Fig. 5.2). Available data also indicate that Asians tend to develop type 2 diabetes and cardiovascular disease at BMI levels lower than the current WHO cutoff point for overweight ($\geq$25 kg/m^2).[112] These data have been used as justifications by some to recommend lower cutoff values for overweight and obesity in Asian populations, but no clear BMI cutoff points for overweight and obesity have been established for different Asian groups.[112]

Validity of Self-reported Height and Weight

Many large epidemiologic studies use self-reported weight and height to calculate BMI.[57] Collection of self-reported measures is more feasible for large population samples. It is less burdensome for the study participants, and entails lower costs than the collection

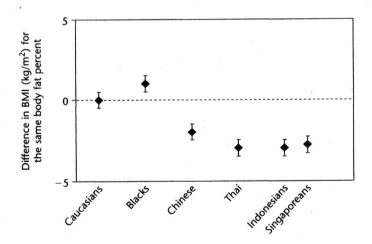

Figure 5.2 Adjustments to be made in BMI to reflect equal levels of percent body fat as compared with that in whites of the same age and sex. Reproduced with permission from Bray G, Bouchard C, James P, eds. *Handbook of Obesity*. New York: Dekker, 1998:81-92.[108]

of measured height and weight. Self-reported data, however, can lead to systematic bias in assessing BMI because heavy subjects are more likely to underreport their weight, while short individuals tend to overreport their height. Consequently, surveys using self-reported height and weight tend to underestimate prevalence of obesity. It is unclear whether self-reported BMIs are sufficiently accurate to be used in epidemiologic analyses of consequences or causes of obesity.

Almost three decades ago, Stunkard and Albaum[113] demonstrated that self-reported weights were highly accurate across different ages and sexes. That finding was confirmed by numerous subsequent studies. In the NHS, self-reported weight was first validated in a study subsample in 1980. There was a high correlation ($r = .97$) between self-reported and measured weights; the mean difference between measured and self-reported weights was 1.5 kg.[114] A similar correlation was observed for men in the Health Professionals' Follow-up Study (HPFS).[115] In addition, there was a high correlation between recalled weight at age 18 and measured weight from physical examination records [$r = .87$, mean difference (recalled − measured weight) = −1.4 kg] in a subsample of the NHS.[116]

We evaluated the validity of BMI based on self-reported data compared with technician-measured BMI as predictors of biomarkers of adiposity and cardiovascular disease among 10,639 NHANES III participants 20 years of age or older.[117] Mean BMI based on self-reported data (25.07 kg/m²) was lower than technician-measured BMI (25.52 kg/m²) due to underreporting of weight [−0.56 kg, 95% CI: −0.71 to −0.41] and overreporting of height [0.76 cm, 95% CI: 0.64 to 0.88]. The Bland-Altman plot in Figure 5.3 shows slightly more underreporting of BMI with increasing obesity levels. However, the correlations between self-reported and measured BMI values were high (0.95 for whites, 0.93 for blacks, and 0.90 for Mexican Americans). In terms of biomarkers, self-reported and measured BMI values were identically correlated with fasting blood glucose ($r = .43$), HDL cholesterol ($r = −.53$),

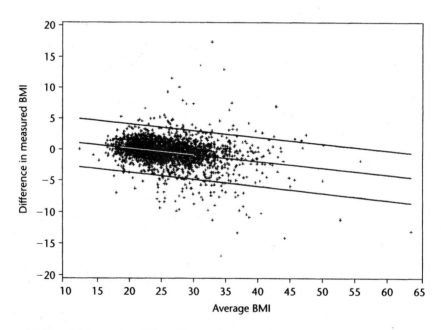

Figure 5.3 Bland-Altman plot of the difference between self-reported and measured BMI versus the average of these two measures of BMI. From McAdams MA, Van Dam RM, Hu FB. Comparison of self-reported and measured BMI as correlates of disease markers in US adults. *Obesity (Silver Spring)*. 2007;15:188-196.[117]

and systolic blood pressure ($r = .54$). Similar correlations were observed for both measures of BMI with plasma concentrations of triglycerides and leptin. These correlations did not differ by age, gender, ethnicity, or measured BMI. This study suggests that although use of self-reported BMI clearly leads to an underestimate of obesity prevalence, the accuracy of self-reported BMI is sufficient for epidemiologic studies using disease biomarkers.[118]

Waist and Hip Circumferences

There is increasing recognition that location of fat or body fat distribution contributes to obesity-related disease risk independent of overall adiposity.[119] The location of body fat has been used to delineate two body shapes: gynecoid (or "pear shape," with fat accumulated in the lower part of the body, such as the hips and thighs) versus android (or "apple shape," with fat accumulated in the upper part of the body, such as the abdomen). Consistent evidence indicates that android obesity is associated with more adverse metabolic and cardiovascular risk factors than is gynecoid obesity.[120]

WC and waist-to-hip ratio (WHR) are widely used as indirect measures of abdominal or central obesity in epidemiologic studies. WC is typically measured at the natural waist (midway between the lowest rib margin and the iliac crest), at the level of the umbilicus, or the narrowest WC.[121] Because a "natural waist" may be difficult to locate for obese subjects, the umbilicus site is preferred, although this may introduce substantial variations in defining the measurement site for very obese patients.[1] Hip circumference is typically measured as the maximal circumference over the buttocks.

There is some evidence that WC may be superior to WHR as a surrogate measure for central obesity. Clasey et al.[36] examined the utility of anthropometric measures and DXA to predict TAF and AVF measured by CT scan in 76 white adults 20 to 80 years of age. In both men and women, WC and abdominal sagittal diameter were strongly associated with TAF ($r = .87$ to $.93$) and AVF ($r = .84$ to $.93$). WHR was less predictive of TAF or AVF than WC. DXA estimates of trunk and abdominal FM were strongly associated with TAF ($r = .94$ to $.97$) and AVF ($r = .86$ to $.90$). This study demonstrates that WC is an excellent measure of both TAF and AVF, and that DXA does not offer a significant advantage over WC for estimation of AVF. In another study, Kamel et al.[122] found that in nonobese men, DXA, WC, and WHR predicted intra-abdominal fat measured by MRI equally well, while in nonobese women, DXA was superior to WC or WHR.

The WC-to-height ratio (WHtR) has been used as an alternative to the WHR as a measure of central adiposity. This index, which is adjusted for frame size (represented by height), is simple and conceptually appealing. However, there is no evidence that it is a better predictor of morbidity and mortality than WHR or WC.

Although WC is a well-accepted measure of abdominal fat, the biological meaning of hip circumference is less clear because a large hip may reflect more accumulation of subcutaneous fat, greater gluteal muscle mass, or larger bone structure (pelvic width).[57] Because WHR is the ratio of two complex variables, its interpretation is quite complicated. Increased WHR can reflect both increased visceral FM and/or reduced gluteofemoral muscle mass. Thus, a higher WHR, especially in the elderly, may be an indicator of visceral obesity combined with muscle loss.[123]

Several studies have suggested that waist and hip circumference may have opposite effects on metabolic and cardiovascular risk factors. In the Quebec Family Study, Seidell et al.[124] found that increased hip circumference was associated with decreased visceral fat and increased subcutaneous abdominal fat, especially in men. A large WC adjusted for BMI and hip circumference was significantly associated with low HDL-cholesterol concentrations ($P < .05$) and high fasting triglycerides, insulin, and glucose concentrations

($P < .01$). Hip circumference adjusted for BMI and WC was associated with these risk factors in the opposite direction. In a recent prospective analysis of participants in the HPFS, men whose WC had increased 14.6 cm or more after controlling for weight gain had 1.7 (95% CI: 1.0 to 2.8) times the risk of diabetes compared with men with a stable WC. In contrast, men who lost more than 4.1 cm in hip girth had 1.5 (95% CI: 1.0 to 2.3) times the risk of diabetes compared with men with a stable hip circumference.[125] These results suggest that increases or decreases in waist and hip circumferences reflect changes in different aspects of body composition, with varying implications for disease risk.

As previously discussed, differential loss of muscle associated with aging makes BMI a less valid measure of body fatness in older adults. However, WC has been shown to be a good predictor of adiposity, especially central obesity, in the elderly. In the HPFS, overall adiposity measured by BMI was a more important indicator of risk of CHD among men younger than 65 years of age, whereas central obesity measured by WC and WHR appeared to be a stronger predictor of risk than BMI among men older than 65 years.[126] These findings underscore the importance of measuring both overall adiposity and fat distribution in epidemiologic studies of obesity.

It remains controversial whether fat distribution should be routinely measured in clinical practice.[121] There is substantial evidence that fat distribution measurements have added value beyond BMI in predicting morbidity and mortality among patients who are of normal weight or moderately overweight (see Chapters 8 to 11). Thus fat distribution should provide additional value in risk assessment of obesity-related disease risk,[127] although such measurements may be unnecessary for morbidly obese patients (BMI $\geq$ 35 kg/m^2).

There are several rationales for the use of WC instead of WHR in practice. First, measuring WC is simpler than measuring WHR and has fewer measurement errors. Second, the association between WC and disease risk is easier to explain than is that for WHR (previously discussed). Third, several studies have suggested a stronger association between WC and the risk of developing health conditions, such as cardiovascular disease and type 2 diabetes, although the results are not entirely consistent.[128] A statement by the National Institutes of Health and the North American Association for the Study of Obesity concluded that WHR provides no advantage over WC alone.[129] Recommended WC cutoffs were 40 in. (102 cm) for men and 35 in. (88 cm) for women (corresponding cut-points for WHR of 0.95 for men and 0.88 for women). However, these cut-points are arbitrary, as the relationship between increased WC and elevated metabolic and cardiovascular risk appears to be linear. Also, the RR of chronic disease associated with central obesity varies across different age and ethnic groups. Nonetheless, these cutoff have been used in the National Cholesterol Education Program Adult Treatment Panel III (NCEP ATP III)[4] guidelines as a diagnostic criteria for metabolic syndrome. As with BMI, the risk of diabetes and cardiovascular disease appears to be higher at a lower WC in Asians than in whites.[130] Thus, the use of lower WC cutoff points has been proposed for Asians (e.g., >80 cm for women and >90 cm for men).[112] Recently, the International Diabetes Federation (IDF) proposed a new definition of metabolic syndrome that includes central obesity as a prerequisite for diagnosis along with gender- and ethnicity-specific cut-points for WC.[5] However, these varying cut-points, which remain controversial, complicate the definition and clinical diagnosis of metabolic syndrome in different populations.

Validity of Self-measured Waist and Hip Circumferences

In large epidemiologic surveys conducted by mail, participants are asked to measure and report body circumferences. Although participants (especially obese adults) tended to underreport WC, validation studies have generally found high correlations between self-reported and technician-measured WCs (0.7 to 0.9).[115,131-133]

In the NHS and HPFS cohorts, participants were mailed a specially designed paper tape measure and instructions on how to measure torso and hip circumferences. They were asked to make measurements to the nearest quarter of an inch while standing and to avoid measuring over bulky clothing. An illustration was provided as a guide to help standardize the location for proper waist and hip measurements. Participants were instructed to measure their waist at the umbilicus and their hips at the largest circumference between their waist and thighs. Rimm et al.[115] assessed the validity of circumference measurements obtained by self-report by analyzing data from 123 men aged 40 to 75 years and 140 women aged 41 to 65 years from the HPFS and NHS, respectively. Self-reported data were compared with standardized measurements taken approximately 6 months apart by technicians who visited participants at their homes. Pearson correlations between self-reported WC and the average of two technician-measured WCs were 0.95 for men and 0.89 for women. Correlations for hip measurements were 0.88 for men and 0.84 for women. For WHR, the correlations were 0.69 for men and 0.70 for women. Stratified analyses revealed no significant linear trends in accuracy of reported WC across quartiles of either age or BMI. The correlation coefficients between self-reported and measured WHR were somewhat lower, reflecting less between-person variation for the ratio than for the individual circumferences.

Bland-Altman plots were used to further examine the validity of self-reported waist measurements in the HPFS[134]. The differences between the self-reported WC and the average of the two technician-measured WCs were normally distributed, and the degree of bias was only 0.14 cm (95% CI: −0.40 to 0.69). These findings provide evidence to support the validity of self-measured WC data collected through standardized procedures.

Skinfolds

Skinfold thickness measurements are commonly used as an indirect assessment of body-fat distribution. A special caliper is used to measure the thickness of a double layer of skin and the fat beneath at in predetermined sites, such as triceps, biceps, the subscapular region, abdomen, and thigh.[135] Skinfolds must be measured at precise standard locations using standard techniques. Even so, skinfold measurements are more prone to interobserver variations and less reproducible than other anthropometric methods, such as weight, height, and body circumferences.[55,135] Skinfold thicknesses are particularly difficult to measure and have limited clinical value in morbidly obese patients.

Skinfold thicknesses are commonly used in prediction equations to assess total body FM and percent body fat in both adults and children. Two of the most widely used equations—those developed by Durnin and Womersley[136] and Jackson and Pollock[137]—are based on a two-compartment model. These equations have been shown to predict body fat reasonably well. Among a group of young and middle-aged women, the correlations between predicted and hydrostatically determined percent body fat exceeded 0.8.[138] With data from the Fels Longitudinal Study, Peterson et al.[139] developed new skinfold thickness equations using a four-compartment model as the reference. In both men and women, measures of percent body fat were more accurate compared with those calculated with the Durnin and Womersley and the Jackson and Pollock equations, both of which underestimated percent body fat. The improvement was attributed to use of the four-compartment model as the reference method, which is known to be more accurate than the two-compartment model in measuring percent body fat. More recent equations have combined skinfold thicknesses with circumferences and other anthropometric measures to predict percent body fat.[140] However, all prediction equations are population specific.

In epidemiologic studies, a variety of skinfold-related variables have been used to describe peripheral fat distribution (such as skinfold thickness in individual anatomical sites, mean values of skinfold thicknesses across several sites, and the ratio of the subscapular to triceps skinfolds). However, it is not yet fully established whether these measures independently predict disease risk. In the Northwick Park Heart Study, Kim et al.[141] showed that subscapular, forearm, and triceps skinfolds were predictive of fatal CHD and that subscapular skinfold was predictive of all-cause mortality in women. There was a significant association between BMI and CHD in both men and women, but none of the skinfold measures predicted risk of CHD or mortality in men. Tanne et al.[142] demonstrated that the ratio of subscapular to triceps skinfold thickness (as an indicator of trunk versus peripheral distribution of body fat) was more predictive of stroke mortality than was subscapular skinfold alone (as an indicator of trunk and overall adiposity). In several other studies, skinfold thicknesses did not appear to be independent predictors of CHD or mortality risk.[143,144] Several factors are probably responsible for the lack of consistent associations between skinfold thicknesses and morbidity and mortality. First, the measurement error is greater for skinfold thicknesses than for other anthropometric variables. Second, skinfold thicknesses are unreliable measurements of intra-abdominal fat or central adiposity. Finally, various skinfold sites are markers of different fat distributions despite high correlations among these sites.

Statistical Models of Anthropometric Variables and Disease Risk

Multivariate regression models are commonly used to evaluate the relationships between anthropometric variables and morbidity and mortality. These models should be carefully interpreted because of strong intercorrelations among the anthropometric variables and changes in the meaning of one variable after adjustments for another. In the simplest model, which includes height and weight as independent variables (model 1 in Table 5.4), the coefficient for weight can be interpreted as the effect of weight among individuals of identical height, which largely reflects overall adiposity across different individuals.[57] However, the interpretation of height adjusted for weight is uncertain. Conceptually, it is difficult to interpret variations in height among individuals of identical weight, which may largely reflect differences in lean body mass (body structure and muscle mass).

In model 2, interpretation of both variables is straightforward because there is little or no correlation between height and BMI. In this case, BMI represents the effects of overall adiposity, while height can be interpreted as an overall measure of body size or a surrogate measure of childhood and adolescent nutrition and energy balance (discussed earlier). An alternative method of obtaining weight—adjusted—for height is to calculate the residuals of weight by using a simple regression, with height as the independent variable and weight as the dependent variable. This procedure is analogous to that used for adjusting nutrient intake for total energy (see Chapter 6). The residuals of weight, by definition, are not correlated with height, and thus the same model (model 3) can be used to fully interpret weight adjusted for height (which represents overall adiposity) and height.

Researchers commonly include BMI and WC or WHR in the same model to *compare* the effects of overall adiposity and central or abdominal obesity (model 4). Although the meaning of WC or WHR is conceptually clear in such a model, the meaning of BMI is altered: instead of reflecting overall fatness, the model tends to reflect lean body mass to a greater degree because abdominal fatness is accounted

Table 5.4 Conceptual Meanings of Statistical Models Using Various Anthropometric Variables to Predict Disease Risk

Models	Interpretations
1. Y^* = Height + weight	Coefficient for weight can be interpreted as the association between overall body fatness and disease risk; the interpretation of height is unclear as, to some degree, it becomes a surrogate for lean body mass.
2. Y = Height + BMI	BMI and height are uncorrelated. BMI is measure of overall adiposity, while height can be interpreted as a surrogate of childhood and adolescent nutritional status.
3. Y = Height + weight adjusted for height	The correlation between height and weight adjusted for height (residuals) from a regression model is zero. Weight adjusted for height is a marker of overall adiposity, while height is a surrogate of childhood and adolescent nutritional status.
4. Y = BMI + WC (or WHR)	BMI and WC (or WHR) are highly correlated. While WC is a measure of central obesity, the interpretation of BMI (holding WC constant) is complicated, as it largely reflects the effects of muscularity rather than body fatness, especially in the elderly.
5. Y = BMI + WC adjusted for BMI	BMI and WC adjusted for BMI (residuals) in a regression model is zero. WC residuals represent the effects of central obesity adjusted for overall adiposity, while BMI represents the effects of overall adiposity.
6. Y = WC + hip circumference	Waist and hip circumferences are moderately correlated. While WC is a measure of central obesity or abdominal fat, hip circumference (holding WC constant) largely represents the effects of gluteal muscularity and bone structure.
7. Y = Baseline weight + current weight	After adjusting for baseline weight, current weight largely reflects the effects of change in body weight on disease risk.
8. Y = Change in weight + change in WC	Change in WC represents the effects of changes in body-fat distribution on disease risk, while change in weight (holding change in WC constant) largely reflects changes in lean body mass (e.g., in the elderly, weight loss is largely due to muscle loss).

Y^*: disease outcomes; BMI: body mass index; WC: waist circumference; WHR: waist-to-hip circumference ratio.

for by including WC in the model. Several studies show that when BMI and WC are included in the same model to predict disease risk, the effects of BMI are largely attenuated, and sometimes BMI becomes even inversely associated with disease or mortality risk.[123]

In such a model, however, WC may remain positively associated with disease risk, suggesting that fat distribution is an important predictor of disease risk independent of overall adiposity. This interpretation is biologically meaningful. The same regression method discussed earlier could be used to obtain residuals of WC after adjusting for BMI, with BMI and residuals of WC included in the same model to predict disease risk (model 5). This approach would maintain the biological meaning of BMI because BMI and residuals of WC (adjusted for BMI) are uncorrelated.

Another common practice is to include waist and hip circumferences in the same model to predict disease or mortality risk (model 6). Although WC clearly represents the effects of abdominal obesity, the meaning of hip circumference is more difficult to interpret because after WC is accounted for, a larger hip circumference largely reflects the effects of greater gluteal muscularity and bone structure. Therefore, hip circumference has been inversely associated with risk of chronic disease after adjusting for WC (see above).

Baseline and current weights are also commonly included in the same model to predict disease risk (model 7). When baseline weight is accounted for, current weight reflects the effects of weight change. In young and middle-aged people, weight change (mostly weight gain) largely reflects a gain in body fat. In the elderly, weight change (mostly weight loss) largely reflects loss in lean body mass, especially muscle, due to aging and chronic diseases. When both waist and weight changes are included in the same model (model 8), an increase in WC represents an increase in central or abdominal adiposity, while a change in weight is more difficult to interpret and may largely reflect a change in lean body mass (especially in the elderly who often lose weight but gain WC). Thus, in this situation, the changes in WC and weight may have opposite associations with disease risk.

Summary

Accurate measurement of the amount of and distribution of body fat is critical to obesity research. The past several decades have witnessed major advances in the field of body composition research. Compared to the traditional two-compartment body composition model, multicompartment models have improved the ability to accurately estimate body fatness. More recent *high-tech* imaging methods, such as CT and MRI, are able to produce high-resolution images of all major composition components at tissue-organ levels. DXA is rapidly becoming accessible and established as the reference body composition method and as an alternative to traditional methods, such as underwater weighing and hydrometry.

Despite these technological advances, anthropometric measures, particularly of weight and height, remain the least expensive and most widely used methods for assessing adiposity in epidemiologic studies. The validity of anthropometric measures in epidemiologic research, especially self-reported BMI and self-measured waist and hip circumference, has been extensively studied. Although self-reported measures tend to underestimate the prevalence of overweight and obesity, and are thus inappropriate for national surveys, numerous epidemiologic studies have demonstrated that self-reported BMI and WC are robust and strong predictors of biomarkers of adiposity, incidence of chronic disease, and premature mortality. However, we should bear in mind that these variables (whether measured or reported) are indirect measures of body fatness, and the validity of these measures, especially BMI, varies with age, sex, and ethnicity. Understanding biological meanings of these measures is essential to the interpretation of results from epidemiologic studies of body composition and disease incidence and mortality.

References

1. Heymsfield SB, Shen W, Wang J. Chapter 2. Evaluation of total and regional adiposity. In: Bray G, Bouchard C, James P, eds. *Handbook of Obesity*. New York: Dekker; 1998.
2. Heymsfield SB, Lohman TG, Wang Z, Going S, eds. *Human Body Composition*. 2nd ed. Champaign, IL: Human Kinetics; 2005.
3. Ellis KJ. Selected body composition methods can be used in field studies. *J Nutr.* 2001;131:1589S-1595S.
4. Expert Panel on Detection, Evaluation, and Treatment of High Blood Cholesterol in Adults. Executive summary of the Third Report of the National Cholesterol Education Program (NCEP) Expert Panel on Detection, Evaluation, and Treatment of High Blood Cholesterol in Adults (Adult Treatment Panel III). *JAMA*. 2001;285:2486-2497.
5. Zimmet P, Magliano D, Matsuzawa Y, Alberti G, Shaw J. The metabolic syndrome: a global public health problem and a new definition. *J Atheroscler Thromb.* 2005;12:295-300.
6. Siri W. Body composition from fluid spaces and density analysis of methods. In: Brozek J, Herschel A, eds. *Techniques for Measuring Body Composition*. Washington, DC: National Academies Press; 1961:223-244.
7. Brozek J, Grande F, Anderson J, Keys A. Densitometric analysis of body composition: revision of some quantitative assumptions. *Ann N Y Acad Sci.* 1963;110:113-140.
8. Going S. Chapter 2. Hydrodensitometry and air displacement plethysmography. In: Heymsfield SB, Lohman TG, Wang Z, Going S, eds. *Human Body Composition*. 2nd ed. Champaign, IL: Human Kinetics; 2005.
9. Dempster P, Aitkens S. A new air displacement method for the determination of human body composition. *Med Sci Sports Exerc.* 1995;27:1692-1697.
10. Fields DA, Goran MI, McCrory MA. Body-composition assessment via air-displacement plethysmography in adults and children: a review. *Am J Clin Nutr.* 2002;75:453-467.
11. Ginde SR, Geliebter A, Rubiano F, et al. Air displacement plethysmography: validation in overweight and obese subjects. *Obes Res.* 2005;13:1232-1237.
12. Fields DA, Higgins PB, Radley D. Air-displacement plethysmography: here to stay. *Curr Opin Clin Nutr Metab Care.* 2005;8:624-629.
13. Schoeller DA. Chapter 3. Hydrometry. In: Heymsfield SB, Lohman TG, Wang Z, Going S, eds. *Human Body Composition*. 2nd ed. Champaign, IL: Human Kinetics; 2005.
14. van Raaij JM, Peek ME, Vermaat-Miedema SH, Schonk CM, Hautvast JG. New equations for estimating body fat mass in pregnancy from body density or total body water. *Am J Clin Nutr.* 1988;48:24-29.
15. Ellis K. Whole-body counting and neutron activation analysis. In: Heymsfield SB, Lohman TG, Wang Z, Going SB, eds. *Human Body Composition*. 2nd ed. Champgaign, IL: Human Kinetics; 2005:51-62; Chapter 4.
16. Wang Z, Zhu S, Wang J, Pierson RN Jr, Heymsfield SB. Whole-body skeletal muscle mass: development and validation of total-body potassium prediction models. *Am J Clin Nutr.* 2003;77:76-82.
17. He Q, Heo M, Heshka S, et al. Total body potassium differs by sex and race across the adult age span. *Am J Clin Nutr.* 2003;78:72-77.
18. Ross R, Janssen I. Computer tomography and magnetic resonance imaging. In: Heymsfield SB, Lohman TG, Wang Z, Going S, eds. *Human Body Composition*. 2n ed. Champaign, IL: Human Kinetics; 2005:89-108; Chapter 7.
19. Goodpaster BH, Kelley DE, Thaete FL, He J, Ross R. Skeletal muscle attenuation determined by computed tomography is associated with skeletal muscle lipid content. *J Appl Physiol.* 2000;89:104-110.
20. Kvist H, Sjostrom L, Tylen U. Adipose tissue volume determinations in women by computed tomography: technical considerations. *Int J Obes.* 1986;10:53-67.

21. Abate N, Garg A, Peshock RM, Stray-Gundersen J, Grundy SM. Relationships of generalized and regional adiposity to insulin sensitivity in men. *J Clin Invest.* 1995;96:88-98.
22. Lebovitz HE, Banerji MA. Point: visceral adiposity is causally related to insulin resistance. *Diabetes Care.* 2005;28:2322-2325.
23. Miles JM, Jensen MD. Counterpoint: visceral adiposity is not causally related to insulin resistance. *Diabetes Care.* 2005;28:2326-2328.
24. Weiss R, Dufour S, Taksali SE, et al. Prediabetes in obese youth: a syndrome of impaired glucose tolerance, severe insulin resistance, and altered myocellular and abdominal fat partitioning. *Lancet.* 2003;362:951-957.
25. Goodpaster BH, Krishnaswami S, Harris TB, et al. Obesity, regional body fat distribution, and the metabolic syndrome in older men and women. *Arch Intern Med.* 2005;165:777-783.
26. Goodpaster BH, Krishnaswami S, Resnick H, et al. Association between regional adipose tissue distribution and both type 2 diabetes and impaired glucose tolerance in elderly men and women. *Diabetes Care.* 2003;26:372-379.
27. Snijder MB, Visser M, Dekker JM, et al. Low subcutaneous thigh fat is a risk factor for unfavourable glucose and lipid levels, independently of high abdominal fat. The Health ABC Study. *Diabetologia.* 2005;48:301-308.
28. Nicklas BJ, Penninx BW, Cesari M, et al. Association of visceral adipose tissue with incident myocardial infarction in older men and women: the Health, Aging and Body Composition Study. *Am J Epidemiol.* 2004;160:741-749.
29. Lohman TG, Chen Z. Dual-energy x-ray absorptiometry. In: Heymsfield SB, Lohman TG, Wang Z, Going S, eds. *Human Body Composition.* 2nd ed. Champaign, IL: Human Kinetics; 2005:63-78; Chapter 5.
30. Centers for Disease Control and Prevention. National Center for Health Statistics. NHANES 1999-2000 Public Data Release File Documentation.
31. Snijder MB, Visser M, Dekker JM, et al. The prediction of visceral fat by dual-energy x-ray absorptiometry in the elderly: a comparison with computed tomography and anthropometry. *Int J Obes Relat Metab Disord.* 2002;26:984-993.
32. Kiebzak GM, Leamy LJ, Pierson LM, Nord RH, Zhang ZY. Measurement precision of body composition variables using the lunar DPX-L densitometer. *J Clin Densitom.* 2000;3:35-41.
33. Cordero-MacIntyre ZR, Peters W, Libanati CR, et al. Reproducibility of DXA in obese women. *J Clin Densitom.* 2002;5:35-44.
34. Schoeller DA, Tylavsky FA, Baer DJ, et al. QDR 4500A dual-energy x-ray absorptiometer underestimates fat mass in comparison with criterion methods in adults. *Am J Clin Nutr.* 2005;81:1018-1025.
35. Madsen OR, Jensen JE, Sorensen OH. Validation of a dual energy x-ray absorptiometer: measurement of bone mass and soft tissue composition. *Eur J Appl Physiol Occup Physiol.* 1997;75:554-558.
36. Clasey JL, Bouchard C, Teates CD, et al. The use of anthropometric and dual-energy x-ray absorptiometry (DXA) measures to estimate total abdominal and abdominal visceral fat in men and women. *Obes Res.* 1999;7:256-264.
37. Sierra-Johnson J, Johnson BD, Bailey KR, Turner ST. Relationships between insulin sensitivity and measures of body fat in asymptomatic men and women. *Obes Res.* 2004;12:2070-2077.
38. Steinberger J, Jacobs DR, Raatz S, Moran A, Hong CP, Sinaiko AR. Comparison of body fatness measurements by BMI and skinfolds vs dual energy x-ray absorptiometry and their relation to cardiovascular risk factors in adolescents. *Int J Obes (Lond).* 2005;29:1346-1352.
39. Chumlea WC, Sun SS. Bioelectrical impedance analysis. In: Heymsfield SB, Lohman TG, Wang Z, Going S, eds. *Human Body Composition.* 2nd ed. Champaign, IL: Human Kinetics; 2005:79-88; Chapter 6.

40. NIH Consensus statement. Bioelectrical impedance analysis in body composition measurement. National Institutes of Health Technology Assessment Conference Statement. December 12-14, 1994. *Nutrition*. 1996;12:749-762.
41. Ellis KJ, Bell SJ, Chertow GM, et al. Bioelectrical impedance methods in clinical research: a follow-up to the NIH Technology Assessment Conference. *Nutrition*. 1999;15:874-880.
42. Kyle UG, Bosaeus I, De Lorenzo AD, et al. Bioelectrical impedance analysis-part II: utilization in clinical practice. *Clin Nutr*. 2004;23:1430-1453.
43. Sun G, French CR, Martin GR, et al. Comparison of multifrequency bioelectrical impedance analysis with dual-energy x-ray absorptiometry for assessment of percentage body fat in a large, healthy population. *Am J Clin Nutr*. 2005;81:74-78.
44. Kyle UG, Bosaeus I, De Lorenzo AD, et al. Bioelectrical impedance analysis—part I: review of principles and methods. *Clin Nutr*. 2004;23:1226-1243.
45. Coppini LZ, Waitzberg DL, Campos AC. Limitations and validation of bioelectrical impedance analysis in morbidly obese patients. *Curr Opin Clin Nutr Metab Care*. 2005;8:329-332.
46. Third National Health and Nutrition Examination Survey (NHANES III) Public-Use Data Files. U.S. Department of Health and Human Services, Centers for Disease Control and Prevention, National Center for Health Statistics.
47. Willett K, Jiang R, Lenart E, Spiegelman D, Willett W. Comparison of bioelectrical impedance and BMI in predicting obesity-related medical conditions. *Obesity (Silver Spring)*. 2006;14:480-490.
48. Lahmann PH, Lissner L, Gullberg B, Berglund G. A prospective study of adiposity and all-cause mortality: the Malmö Diet and Cancer Study. *Obes Res*. 2002;10:361-369.
49. Bigaard J, Frederiksen K, Tjonneland A, et al. Body fat and fat-free mass and all-cause mortality. *Obes Res*. 2004;12:1042-1049.
50. Heitmann BL. Prediction of body water and fat in adult Danes from measurement of electrical impedance. A validation study. *Int J Obes*. 1990;14:789-802.
51. Gibson RS. *Principles of Nutritional Assessment*. 2nd ed. New York: Oxford University Press; 2005.
52. Lohman TG, Roche AF, Martorell R. *Anthropometric Standardization Reference Manual*. Abridged edition. Champaign, IL: Human Kinetics Books; 1988.
53. U.S. Department of Health and Human Services. Centers for Disease Control and Prevention. NHANES III Anthropometric Procedures Video.
54. Ulijaszek SJ, Kerr DA. Anthropometric measurement error and the assessment of nutritional status. *Br J Nutr*. 1999;82:165-177.
55. Marks GC, Habicht JP, Mueller WH. Reliability, dependability, and precision of anthropometric measurements. The Second National Health and Nutrition Examination Survey 1976-1980. *Am J Epidemiol*. 1989;130:578-587.
56. Cole TJ. Secular trends in growth. *Proc Nutr Soc*. 2000;59:317-324.
57. Willett WC. *Nutritional Epidemiology*. 2nd ed. New York: Oxford University Press; 1998.
58. McCullough ML, Giovannucci EL. Diet and cancer prevention. *Oncogene*. 2004;23:6349-6364.
59. van den Brandt PA, Spiegelman D, Yaun SS, et al. Pooled analysis of prospective cohort studies on height, weight, and breast cancer risk. *Am J Epidemiol*. 2000;152:514-527.
60. Giovannucci E, Rimm EB, Liu Y, Willett WC. Height, predictors of C-peptide and cancer risk in men. *Int J Epidemiol*. 2004;33:217-225.
61. Smith GD, Greenwood R, Gunnell D, Sweetnam P, Yarnell J, Elwood P. Leg length, insulin resistance, and coronary heart disease risk: the Caerphilly Study. *J Epidemiol Community Health*. 2001;55:867-872.
62. Liu S, Willett WC, Manson JE, Hu FB, Rosner B, Colditz G. Relation between changes in intakes of dietary fiber and grain products and changes in weight and development of obesity among middle-aged women. *Am J Clin Nutr*. 2003;78:920-927.

63. Li TY, Rana JS, Manson JE, et al. Obesity as compared with physical activity in predicting risk of coronary heart disease in women. *Circulation*. 2006;113:499-506.

64. Hu FB, Willett WC, Li T, Stampfer MJ, Colditz GA, Manson JE. Adiposity as compared with physical activity in predicting mortality among women. *N Engl J Med*. 2004;351:2694-2703.

65. Wannamethee SG, Shaper AG, Walker M. Weight change, weight fluctuation, and mortality. *Arch Intern Med*. 2002;162:2575-2580.

66. Wannamethee SG, Shaper AG, Lennon L. Reasons for intentional weight loss, unintentional weight loss, and mortality in older men. *Arch Intern Med*. 2005;165:1035-1040.

67. French SA, Folsom AR, Jeffery RW, Williamson DF. Prospective study of intentionality of weight loss and mortality in older women: the Iowa Women's Health Study. *Am J Epidemiol*. 1999;149:504-514.

68. Gregg EW, Gerzoff RB, Thompson TJ, Williamson DF. Intentional weight loss and death in overweight and obese U.S. adults 35 years of age and older. *Ann Intern Med*. 2003;138:383-389.

69. Eilat-Adar S, Eldar M, Goldbourt U. Association of intentional changes in body weight with coronary heart disease event rates in overweight subjects who have an additional coronary risk factor. *Am J Epidemiol*. 2005;161:352-358.

70. Field AE, Manson JE, Laird N, Williamson DF, Willett WC, Colditz GA. Weight cycling and the risk of developing type 2 diabetes among adult women in the United States. *Obes Res*. 2004;12:267-274.

71. Field AE, Byers T, Hunter DJ, et al. Weight cycling, weight gain, and risk of hypertension in women. *Am J Epidemiol*. 1999;150:573-579.

72. French SA, Jeffery RW, Folsom AR, Williamson DF, Byers T. Relation of weight variability and intentionality of weight loss to disease history and health-related variables in a population-based sample of women aged 55-69 years. *Am J Epidemiol*. 1995;142:1306-1314.

73. Dyer AR, Stamler J, Greenland P. Associations of weight change and weight variability with cardiovascular and all-cause mortality in the Chicago Western Electric Company Study. *Am J Epidemiol*. 2000;152:324.

74. Iribarren C, Sharp DS, Burchfiel CM, Petrovitch H. Association of weight loss and weight fluctuation with mortality among Japanese American men. *N Engl J Med*. 1995;333:686-692.

75. Lissner L, Odell PM, D'Agostino RB, et al. Variability of body weight and health outcomes in the Framingham population. *N Engl J Med*. 1991;324:1839-1844.

76. Weigley ES. Average? Ideal? Desirable? A brief overview of height-weight tables in the United States. *J Am Diet Assoc*. 1884;84:417-423.

77. Metropolitan Life Insurance Company. New weight standards for men and women. *Stat Bull Metrop Insur Co*. 1959;40:1-5.

78. Lew EA, Garfinkel L. Variations in mortality by weight among 750,000 men and women. *J Chronic Dis*. 1979;32:563-576.

79. Garrison RJ, Castelli WP. Weight and thirty-year mortality of men in the Framingham Study. *Ann Intern Med*. 1985;103(6 pt 2):1006-1009.

80. Quetelet A. *Sur l'homme et le developpement de ses facultes, ou essai de phsyique sociale*. Paris: Bachelier; 1835.

81. Keys A, Fidanza F, Karvonen MJ, Kimura N, Taylor HL. Indices of relative weight and obesity. *J Chronic Dis*. 1972;25:329-343.

82. Benn RT. Some mathematical properties of weight-for-height indices used as measures of adiposity. *Br J Prev Soc Med*. 1971;25:42-50.

83. Revicki DA, Israel RG. Relationship between body mass indices and measures of body adiposity. *Am J Public Health*. 1986;76:992-994.

84. Gallagher D, Visser M, Sepulveda D, Pierson RN, Harris T, Heymsfield SB. How useful is body mass index for comparison of body fatness across age, sex, and ethnic groups? *Am J Epidemiol*. 1996;143:228-239.

85. Blew RM, Sardinha LB, Milliken LA, et al. Assessing the validity of body mass index standards in early postmenopausal women. *Obes Res.* 2002;10:799-808.
86. Evans EM, Rowe DA, Racette SB, Ross KM, McAuley E. Is the current BMI obesity classification appropriate for black and white postmenopausal women? *Int J Obes (Lond).* 2006:Epub ahead of print.
87. Deurenberg P, Weststrate JA, Seidell JC. Body mass index as a measure of body fatness: age- and sex-specific prediction formulas. *Br J Nutr.* 1991;65:105-114.
88. Pongchaiyakul C, Kosulwat V, Rojroongwasinkul N, et al. Prediction of percentage body fat in rural thai population using simple anthropometric measurements. *Obes Res.* 2005;13:729-738.
89. Jurimae T, Sudi K, Jurimae J, Payerl D, Ruutel K. Relationships between plasma leptin levels and body composition parameters measured by different methods in postmenopausal women. *Am J Hum Biol.* 2003;15:628-636.
90. Matsuzawa Y. Adiponectin: identification, physiology and clinical relevance in metabolic and vascular disease. *Atheroscler Suppl.* 2005;6:7-14.
91. Spiegelman D, Israel RG, Bouchard C, Willett WC. Absolute fat mass, percent body fat, and body-fat distribution: which is the real determinant of blood pressure and serum glucose? *Am J Clin Nutr.* 1992;55:1033-1044.
92. Garn SM, Leonard WR, Hawthorne VM. Three limitations of the body mass index. *Am J Clin Nutr.* 1986;44:996-997.
93. Malina RM. Variation in body composition associated with sex and ethnicity. In: Heymsfield SB, Lohman TG, Wang Z, Going S, eds. *Human Body Composition.* 2nd ed. Champaign, IL: Human Kinetics; 2005:271-298; Chapter 18.
94. Horlick M. Body mass index in childhood—measuring a moving target. *J Clin Endocrinol Metab.* 2001;86:4059-4060.
95. Flegal KM, Carroll MD, Ogden CL, Johnson CL. Prevalence and trends in obesity among US adults, 1999-2000. *JAMA.* 2002;288:1723-1727.
96. Villareal DT, Apovian CM, Kushner RF, et al. Obesity in older adults: technical review and position statement of the American Society for Nutrition and NAASO, The Obesity Society. *Obes Res.* 2005;13:1849-1863.
97. Baumgartner RN, Koehler KM, Gallagher D, et al. Epidemiology of sarcopenia among the elderly in New Mexico. *Am J Epidemiol.* 1998;147:755-763.
98. Janssen I, Heymsfield SB, Ross R. Low relative skeletal muscle mass (sarcopenia) in older persons is associated with functional impairment and physical disability. *J Am Geriatr Soc.* 2002;50:889-896.
99. Janssen I, Heymsfield SB, Wang ZM, Ross R. Skeletal muscle mass and distribution in 468 men and women aged 18-88 yr. *J Appl Physiol.* 2000;89:81-88.
100. Newman AB, Lee JS, Visser M, et al. Weight change and the conservation of lean mass in old age: the Health, Aging and Body Composition Study. *Am J Clin Nutr.* 2005;82:872-878.
101. Micozzi MS, Harris TM. Age variations in the relation of body mass indices to estimates of body fat and muscle mass. *Am J Phys Anthropol.* 1990;81:375-379.
102. Hughes VA, Roubenoff R, Wood M, Frontera WR, Evans WJ, Fiatarone Singh MA. Anthropometric assessment of 10-y changes in body composition in the elderly. *Am J Clin Nutr.* 2004;80:475-482.
103. Cree MG, Newcomer BR, Katsanos CS, et al. Intramuscular and liver triglycerides are increased in the elderly. *J Clin Endocrinol Metab.* 2004;89:3864-3871.
104. Seidell JC, Visscher TL. Body weight and weight change and their health implications for the elderly. *Eur J Clin Nutr.* 2000;54(Suppl 3):S33-S39.
105. Janssen I, Katzmarzyk PT, Ross R. Body mass index is inversely related to mortality in older people after adjustment for waist circumference. *J Am Geriatr Soc.* 2005;53:2112-2118.
106. Wagner DR, Heyward VH. Measures of body composition in blacks and whites: a comparative review. *Am J Clin Nutr.* 2000;71:1392-1402.

107. Kleerekoper M, Nelson DA, Peterson EL, Wilson PS, Jacobsen G, Longcope C. Body composition and gonadal steroids in older white and black women. *J Clin Endocrinol Metab.* 1994;79:775-779.

108. Deurenberg P, Deurenberg-Yap M. Ethnic and geographic influences on body composition. In: Bray G, Bouchard C, James P, eds. *Handbook of Obesity.* New York: Dekker, 1998:81-92; Chapter 3.

109. Deurenberg P, Deurenberg-Yap M, Guricci S. Asians are different from Caucasians and from each other in their body mass index/body fat per cent relationship. *Obes Rev.* 2002;3:141-146.

110. Deurenberg-Yap M, Schmidt G, van Staveren WA, Deurenberg P. The paradox of low body mass index and high body fat percentage among Chinese, Malays and Indians in Singapore. *Int J Obes Relat Metab Disord.* 2000;24:1011-1017.

111. Deurenberg P, Yap M, van Staveren WA. Body mass index and percent body fat: a meta analysis among different ethnic groups. *Int J Obes Relat Metab Disord.* 1998;22:1164-1171.

112. WHO Expert Consultation. Appropriate body-mass index for Asian populations and its implications for policy and intervention strategies. *Lancet.* 2004;363:157-163.

113. Stunkard AJ, Albaum JM. The accuracy of self-reported weights. *Am J Clin Nutr.* 1981;34:1593-1599.

114. Willett W, Stampfer MJ, Bain C, et al. Cigarette smoking, relative weight, and menopause. *Am J Epidemiol.* 1983;117:651-658.

115. Rimm EB, Stampfer MJ, Colditz GA, Chute CG, Litin LB, Willet TWC. Validity of self-reported waist and hip circumferences in men and women. *Epidemiology.* 1990;1:466-473.

116. Troy LM, Hunter DJ, Manson JE, Colditz GA, Stampfer MJ, Willett WC. The validity of recalled weight among younger women. *Int J Obes Relat Metab Disord.* 1995;19:570.

117. McAdams MA, Van Dam RM, Hu FB. Comparison of self-reported and measured BMI as correlates of disease markers in US adults. *Obesity (Silver Spring).* 2007;15:188-196.

118. Gillum RF, Sempos CT. Ethnic variation in validity of classification of overweight and obesity using self-reported weight and height in American women and men: the Third National Health and Nutrition Examination Survey. *Nutr J.* 2005;4:27.

119. Eckel RH, Grundy SM, Zimmet PZ. The metabolic syndrome. *Lancet.* 2005;365: 1415-1428.

120. Despres JP. Is visceral obesity the cause of the metabolic syndrome? *Ann Med.* 2006;38:52-63.

121. Klein S, Allison DB, Heymsfield SB, Kelley DE, Leibel RL, Nonas C. Waist Circumference and Cardiometabolic Risk. Diabetes Care 2007;30(6):1647-1652.

122. Kamel EG, McNeill G, Han TS, et al. Measurement of abdominal fat by magnetic resonance imaging, dual-energy x-ray absorptiometry and anthropometry in non-obese men and women. *Int J Obes Relat Metab Disord.* 1999;23:686-692.

123. Snijder MB, van Dam RM, Visser M, Seidell JC. What aspects of body fat are particularly hazardous and how do we measure them? *Int J Epidemiol.* 2006;35:83-92.

124. Seidell JC, Perusse L, Despres JP, Bouchard C. Waist and hip circumferences have independent and opposite effects on cardiovascular disease risk factors: the Quebec Family Study. *Am J Clin Nutr.* 2001;74:315-321.

125. Koh-Banerjee P, Wang Y, Hu FB, Spiegelman D, Willett WC, Rimm EB. Changes in body weight and body fat distribution as risk factors for clinical diabetes in US men. *Am J Epidemiol.* 2004;159:1150-1159.

126. Rimm EB, Stampfer MJ, Giovannucci E, et al. Body size and fat distribution as predictors of coronary heart disease among middle-aged and older US men. *Am J Epidemiol.* 1995;141:1117-1127.

127. Hu FB. Obesity and mortality: watch your waist, not just your weight. *Arch Int Med.* 2007;167(9):875-876.

128. Wang Y, Rimm EB, Stampfer MJ, Willett WC, Hu FB. Comparison of abdominal adiposity and overall obesity in predicting risk of type 2 diabetes among men. *Am J Clin Nutr.* 2005;81:555-563.

129. The practical guide: identification, evaluation, and treatment of overweight and obesity in adults. Bethesda, MD: National Institutes of Health, National Heart, Lung and Blood Institute, North American Association for the Study of Obesity, 2000.

130. Misra A, Wasir JS, Vikram NK. Waist circumference criteria for the diagnosis of abdominal obesity are not applicable uniformly to all populations and ethnic groups. *Nutrition.* 2005;21:969-976.

131. Kushi LH, Kaye SA, Folsom AR, Soler JT, Prineas RJ. Accuracy and reliability of self-measurement of body girths. *Am J Epidemiol.* 1988;128:740-748.

132. Freudenheim JL, Darrow SL. Accuracy of self-measurement of body fat distribution by waist, hip, and thigh circumferences. *Nutr Cancer.* 1991;15:179-186.

133. Bigaard J, Spanggaard I, Thomsen BL, Overvad K, Tjonneland A. Self-reported and technician-measured waist circumferences differ in middle-aged men and women. *J Nutr.* 2005;135:2263-2270.

134. Koh-Banerjee P, Chu NF, Spiegelman D, et al. Prospective study of the association of changes in dietary intake, physical activity, alcohol consumption, and smoking with 9-y gain in waist circumference among 16 587 US men. *Am J Clin Nutr.* 2003;78:719-727.

135. Lohman TG, Roche AF, Martorell R, eds. *Anthropometric Standardization Reference Manual.* Champaign, IL: Human Kinetics Books; 1998.

136. Durnin JV, Womersley J. Body fat assessed from total body density and its estimation from skinfold thickness: measurements on 481 men and women aged from 16 to 72 years. *Br J Nutr.* 1974;32:77-97.

137. Jackson AS, Pollock ML. Generalized equations for predicting body density of men. *Br J Nutr.* 1978;40:497-504.

138. Jackson AS, Pollock ML, Ward A. Generalized equations for predicting body density of women. *Med Sci Sports Exerc.* 1980;12:175-181.

139. Peterson MJ, Czerwinski SA, Siervogel RM. Development and validation of skinfold-thickness prediction equations with a 4-compartment model. *Am J Clin Nutr.* 2003;77:1186-1191.

140. Garcia AL, Wagner K, Hothorn T, Koebnick C, Zunft HJ, Trippo U. Improved prediction of body fat by measuring skinfold thickness, circumferences, and bone breadths. *Obes Res.* 2005;13:626-634.

141. Kim J, Meade T, Haines A. Skinfold thickness, body mass index, and fatal coronary heart disease: 30 year follow up of the Northwick Park heart study. *J Epidemiol Community Health.* 2006;60:275-279.

142. Tanne D, Medalie JH, Goldbourt U. Body fat distribution and long-term risk of stroke mortality. *Stroke.* 2005;36:1021-1025.

143. Spataro JA, Dyer AR, Stamler J, Shekelle RB, Greenlund K, Garside D. Measures of adiposity and coronary heart disease mortality in the Chicago Western Electric Company Study. *J Clin Epidemiol.* 1996;49:849-857.

144. Menottii A, Lanti M, Maiani G, Daan K. Forty-year mortality from cardiovascular diseases and their risk factors in men of the Italian rural areas of the Seven Countries Study. *Acta Cardiol.* 2005;60:521-531.

6

Dietary Assessment Methods

Frank B. Hu

For most people, significant weight gain results from a small but persistent positive energy balance over a long period of time, an imbalance that is too small to be detected by most instruments used in epidemiologic studies. This limitation notwithstanding, reasonably accurate methods are available to assess dietary composition and food patterns in free-living populations. Epidemiologic studies have demonstrated that many dietary factors have significant relationships with obesity and weight gain, either independently of, or mediated through, total energy intake (see Chapter 14). However, none of the dietary assessment approaches are perfect, and there are important methodological issues related to appropriate choices for specific research settings in obesity research.

In this chapter, we first discuss strengths and limitations of various dietary assessment methods—24-hour recall, food records, diet history, food-frequency questionnaires (FFQs), and biomarkers—and their validity and applications in obesity epidemiologic research. Next, we cover the assessment of, and adjustment for, total energy intake in epidemiologic research. We then discuss methods to correct for random and systematic measurement errors in nutritional epidemiologic studies. Finally, we review statistical approaches for assessing the impact of overall diet through dietary patterning analyses. The methods discussed in this chapter are not unique to obesity epidemiologic studies, but are relevant to virtually all areas of epidemiology involving dietary exposures.[1]

Dietary Assessment Methods in Obesity Epidemiologic Studies

Several methods are available to assess individual intakes of foods, nutrients, and total energy; these include single 24-hour recalls, FFQs, diet histories, food or diet records, and biomarkers. Each approach has its strengths and limitations. In the following section, we briefly discuss the application of these methods to assess dietary intake in epidemiologic research. For more detailed information, please refer to texts in nutritional epidemiology[1] and dietary assessments.[2]

24-Hour Recalls

The 24-hour dietary recall involves the collection of detailed information on all foods and beverages consumed by a subject in the previous day or past 24 hours. This method is most widely used by national nutritional surveys (e.g., the National Health and Nutrition Examination Survey (NHANES), USDA Nationwide Food Consumption Surveys, and the Continuing Surveys of Food Intakes by Individuals) to estimate average intakes of populations. The recall method, especially the unannounced recall (see below), is frequently used in dietary intervention trials to monitor adherence. A single 24-hour dietary recall can be useful for estimating mean intakes of a population in national surveys, but it alone cannot be used to estimate usual intakes of individuals, or provide correct distributions for the population because of large within-person variations in dietary intakes.[3]

The 24-hour recall is usually conducted by a trained or certified interviewer. The interview is often face to face, but can also be done by telephone. In the face-to-face interview, visual aids, such as food models or shapes, can be used to obtain more accurate information on quantities of foods. To help with portion size estimation in telephone-administered interviews, two-dimensional food portion visual aids or photographs are sometimes mailed to the respondents' homes beforehand.[4] To avoid changes in participants' eating habits, 24-hour recalls are best administered *unannounced*, that is, not scheduled on a specific day. The *surprise* aspect of the unannounced telephone interview is especially important for monitoring compliance in dietary intervention studies.[5]

Traditional paper-and-pencil or computerized systems can be used to collect data from 24-hour recalls. The Minnesota Nutrient Data System (NDS) has been specifically designed for conducting real-time interactive interviews[6] and a computer program, EPIC-SOFT, has been developed to standardize interview-based 24-hour recalls in the European Prospective Investigation into Cancer and Nutrition (EPIC) study.[7]

The multiple-pass 24-hour recall is a method in which interviewers use several (3 or 5) distinct *passes* or steps (with multiple cues and opportunities for participants) to collect information about a subject's food intake over the preceding 24 hours.[8] The USDA 5-pass method involves five steps.[9,10] The first pass is a *quick list* of all foods or beverages the participant consumed in the previous day. The second pass (termed *forgotten list*) involves a probe of possible forgotten foods, for example, snacks, sweets, and soft drinks. The third pass (*time and occasion*) asks the subject to describe the time and situation in which the foods were eaten. The fourth step (the *detailed pass*) involves probing for detailed information on preparation, ingredients, and portion sizes (use of two-dimensional food models can help subjects estimate portion sizes). The last step (the *final review pass*) involves reviewing the recalled information and probing for information on any additional food items. The multiple-pass 24-hour recall method has led to improvement in food recalls.[9,11] However, the approach is still prone to underreporting that typically occurs with self-reported methods, a problem that involves memory lapses and difficulties in estimating portion sizes.

It is well known that a single 24-hour recall does not represent usual intake or reliably rank subjects according to nutrient intakes because of large day-to-day variations. Multiple recalls are required to estimate an individual's usual diet, however, the optimal number of recalls depends on the nutrients or foods of interest; those with large day-to-day variations will require more recalls than those with smaller day-to-day variations. In large cohort studies, the cost of collecting and processing dietary data from multiple 24-hour recalls is often prohibitive. However, it is possible to do so in a subset of the cohort for validation purposes.

Food or Dietary Records

With the food record or food diary method, the subject (or observer) records in detail all foods and beverages consumed on one or more days.[3] In most studies, participants are asked to enter information on a standardized hard copy form, but new methods have been developed to collect tape-recorded or bar-coded food consumption information. Whereas weighed food records involve weighing all food and beverages consumed on a small scale, estimated food records require participants to estimate the portion sizes of all foods consumed using household measures or aids (e.g., food models or photographs). Participants should be trained in advance in methods for weighing and recording foods. Ideally, they should weigh and record each portion of food before eating it so that the food records do not depend on memory, although this is not feasible in many situations. In some situations (such as a population with low literacy rates), an observer or field worker is needed to weigh the raw ingredients and cooked dishes to estimate household and individual dietary intakes.[3]

Food records are typically collected for 3 to 7 days, but multiple 7-day records across different seasons are often required to reflect long-term diet. Multiple 7-day records are often used as the "gold standard" for validating other methods, such as the FFQ. Weighted diet records, if done correctly, have a clear advantage of not relying on a subject's memory, and of allowing direct and accurate quantification of food intakes. Drawbacks include the need for literate, trained, and highly motivated subjects. Food records place a high burden on participants,[8] and the quality of recording declines as the number of days increase. The process itself tends to modify eating habits, with some participants even losing weight. Due to day-to-day variations in diet, short-term (e.g., 3 days) records can misrepresent usual intake, a problem remedied by repeated recording over different time periods and seasons. Food records, as with other self-reported dietary assessment methods, are prone to underreporting bias (see below), especially among the obese.

Food records are most commonly used as a reference method for validating FFQs, however, the cost of collecting and processing the data in large cohort studies has been prohibitive. Nonetheless, some newer cohort studies (e.g., the European Prospective Investigation of Cancer (EPIC) in Norfolk) have simultaneously collected 7-day diet records and FFQ data.[12] Diet records can be a cost-effective approach in nested case-control studies for assessment of exposure or for validation purposes. However, it is unclear whether single 7-day diet records can adequately reflect long-term dietary intake.

Food-Frequency Questionnaires

Short-term diet and recall methods fail to represent usual intake, are inappropriate for assessment of past diet, and are costly. Because of these limitations, alternative methods have been developed to measure long-term dietary intake. Among these methods, the FFQ has emerged as the preferred approach. FFQs are easy for participants to complete, can be processed by computer, and are inexpensive—features that make them feasible for use in large prospective studies.

The FFQ is based on two principles—that average long-term diet is conceptually more important than short-term diet, and that relative ranking of individual intakes is more important than absolute intakes in predicting chronic disease risk.[1] (Absolute intakes are difficult, if not impossible, to measure precisely in large epidemiologic studies.) The foundation for this framework dates back to the dietary history interview developed in 1947 by Burke (discussed below).[13] In the past several decades, the food-frequency method has become the main dietary assessment tool in large nutritional epidemiologic studies, and numerous versions of FFQs have been developed for applications in various populations and contexts.

The FFQ asks respondents to report their usual frequency of consumption of each food from a list of foods during a specific period (typically from a few months to a year). The questionnaire consists of a structured listing of individual foods and beverages. For each food item, participants are asked to indicate their average frequency of consumption in terms of a specified serving size by checking one of multiple frequency categories (ranging, for example, from "almost never" to "six or more times a day"). The selected frequency category for each food item can be converted to a daily intake; for example, a response of "two to four per week" converts to 0.43 servings per day (or three times per week). The number or types of food items may vary by study purpose and population. Comprehensive FFQs used in most epidemiologic studies generally include 60 to 180 food items. The questionnaires can be administered by trained personnel in face-to-face interviews, by telephone, or through self-administered postal surveys. FFQs can be optically scanned, which improves the accuracy and efficiency of data entry and makes them suitable for use in large epidemiologic studies.

Collection of portion size information varies according to types of FFQs. In nonquantitative FFQs, portion size information is not collected. Such questionnaires, which cannot provide estimates of nutrient intakes, are typically used for screening purposes. In semiquantitative FFQs, portion sizes are specified as standardized portions or choices. For example, in the FFQ developed by Willett,[14] portion size information is included as part of the food item rather than as a separate question. Other questionnaires (such as the Block FFQ) ask respondents to indicate usual portion sizes for each food (e.g., small, medium, or large) (using food models as a unit of reference).[15] The NCI Diet History Questionnaire (DHQ) includes an additional question about portion size for each food.[16,17]

Whether adding portion size information to FFQs improves estimation of nutrients is still a matter of debate. In that most of the variation in food intakes is explained by frequency of intake rather than differences in portion sizes,[1] available evidence suggests only marginal improvement in the validity of FFQs that include portion size data compared with those that do not. In a Danish study, the mean correlations between food-frequency data, with and without individually estimated portion sizes, and weighed diet records were similar, suggesting that little extra information was obtained by adding questions about portion size.[18] Conversely, Subar et al. suggested that portion size information could improve estimates of absolute macronutrient intake,[16] but not necessarily the validity of energy-adjusted nutrients.

Carefully developed FFQs offer a conceptual advantage over short-term 24-hour recalls or food records in assessing average long-term diet. They are also relatively inexpensive and impose a low burden on participants, factors that make them feasible for use in large epidemiologic studies. However, FFQs have significant limitations. Because they lack the detail and specificity of diet records or recalls they may not provide accurate estimates of absolute nutrient intakes. Constant changes in food supplies and compositions require that items in the FFQ and nutrient database be updated in a timely manner. In addition, the completion of FFQs involves memory, recall, and cognitive estimation skills. As a result, FFQs, as with other self-reported dietary assessment instruments, are subject to both random and systematic errors (see below).

FFQs need to be specific to individual cultures and populations. In some populations, low education levels may restrict the usefulness of self-administered surveys. These limitations need to be balanced against the strengths of FFQs. As the least expensive and most efficient dietary assessment tool, they have become the method of choice in large epidemiologic studies. However, questions on the validity of nutrient estimates by FFQs in epidemiologic studies of obesity and chronic diseases continue to be raised. Later in this chapter, we will discuss the validity and reproducibility of FFQs.

Diet History Method

As discussed earlier, the diet history method was originally described by Burke in 1947.[13] It consists of three parts: a detailed face-to-face interview; a cross-check food-frequency list; and a 3-day diet record. The food-frequency list and 3-day records were used by Burke to check the internal consistency of the interview. The purpose of the diet history method is to obtain usual food consumption patterns. The interview typically starts with a 24-hour recall prompted by careful probing of current and past food consumption patterns. Interviews, often lasting 1 to 2 hours, require substantial cooperation from the participants.

Several medium-sized prospective studies and clinical trials have used the diet history method. For example, in the Western Electric Study,[19] nutritionists conducted an initial examination followed by a second interview 1 year later. Using standardized interviews and questionnaires, they collected data on usual eating patterns, special diets, and changes in eating habits. To gauge the internal consistency of the interview, they used a 195-item cross-check food-frequency list. Estimates of portion sizes were based on wax models of commonly consumed foods and dishes. Participants' wives, using mailed questionnaires, provided further information on food preparation, as did neighborhood restaurants and bakeries.

The CARDIA diet history was modeled after the Western Electric dietary history method,[20] but the list of foods was expanded from 150 items to approximately 700 to accommodate various populations and ethnic groups. Liu et al.[20] reported on the reliability and validity of the CARDIA Diet History in 128 young adults. The reproducibility correlations for the log-transformed nutrient values and calorie-adjusted nutrient values from the two diet histories were generally in the range of 0.50 to 0.80 for Caucasians. For African Americans, the correlations were lower, with a majority in the range of 0.30 to 0.70. The validity correlations between mean daily nutrient intakes from the CARDIA diet history and means from 7 randomly scheduled 24-hour recalls were generally above 0.50.

The Diabetes Control and Complications Trial (DCCT) also used a modified Burke type diet history method. Trained dietitians interviewed participants for approximately 1.5 to 2 hours to collect quantitative and qualitative information on a usual week of dietary intake over the previous year. Schmidt et al.[21] found that 1-year reproducibility correlation coefficients ranged from 0.51 for dietary fiber to 0.72 for dietary cholesterol.

Conceptually, the diet history method has advantages over 24-hour recalls and FFQs because it collects more accurate quantitative data on long-term consumption patterns. However, the method is time consuming, expensive, and hard to standardize. Thus, it is not often feasible for use in large epidemiologic studies involving tens of thousands of people. Similar to other dietary assessment methods described earlier, the diet history method is prone to recall bias caused by faulty memory or problems in estimating intake frequencies. It can also be affected by interviewer bias.

Biomarkers

In that the dietary assessment methods discussed earlier are imprecise and subject to bias, the use of biomarkers to assess nutrient intake has been of great interest to the nutritional epidemiology community. Biomarkers offer the advantages of increased reliability and objectivity (they do not depend on memory). Although they are not immune to measurement errors, these are not correlated with measurement errors in self-reported dietary assessments. Still, useful biomarkers are not available for all nutrients, and there are no satisfactory and specific biomarkers for intakes of most foods and food groups. The most important requirement for a biomarker is sensitivity to intake, which typically means a dose-response relationship between the biomarker and nutrient intake.[22] However, in many situations, there is a threshold effect at very low levels of intake and a plateau effect at very high levels. Another criterion for a useful biomarker is time integration. Because long-term dietary exposure is the main interest of chronic disease epidemiology, a valid biomarker should reflect the cumulative effect of diet over an extended period of time rather than short-term fluctuations. Thus, tissues with longer half-lives (e.g., adipose tissue, erythrocytes, and toenails) can be used to reflect dietary intake over the previous months or years. Below, we describe several key biomarkers that are commonly used in laboratory and field studies.

Doubly Labeled Water

The doubly labeled water (DLW) method is an objective and accurate measure of energy expenditure in free-living subjects.[23] Its use as a measure of energy intake is based on the principle that energy expenditure should be equal to energy intake for individuals in energy balance. This method involves the oral administration of a carefully weighed dose of water containing enriched quantities of the stable isotopes deuterium (^2H_2O) and oxygen-18 ($H_2^{18}O$) and collection of several urine or plasma samples over the next 15 days. The oxygen-18 is eliminated from the body in the form of both carbon dioxide ($C^{18}O_2$) and water ($H_2^{18}O$), whereas the deuterium is eliminated in water (^2H_2O) only. Therefore, the difference in disappearance rate between these two isotopes from the body water pool is a measure of carbon dioxide production from which total energy expenditure can be calculated using standard equations for indirect calorimetry.[24] The DLW method has been shown to have high accuracy and precision,[25] but because the method is expensive and analysis requires specialized and sophisticated laboratory equipment, it cannot be used in large epidemiologic studies. However, the approach has been widely used in dietary validation studies of total energy intake (see below).

Total energy expenditure consists of three components: the resting metabolic rate (RMR), the thermic effect of food, and energy expended in physical activity.[26] Thus, an alternate way to estimate total energy intake is to measure energy expended in physical activity and RMR, which together comprises approximately 90% of the total daily energy expenditure of sedentary persons. RMR can be measured by calorimetry and physical activity energy expenditure can be measured by accelerometers (see Chapter 7). Because the thermic effect of food accounts for approximately 10% of total energy expenditure, the estimated total energy expenditure can be calculated as (RMR + energy expended in physical activity) $\times$ 1.10.

Similar to the DLW method, indirect calorimetry is often infeasible in large epidemiologic studies. Several prediction equations have been developed to estimate RMR based on age, sex, height, and weight.[27,28] These equations provide a rough estimate of minimal energy intake required for an individual's survival. To estimate total energy expenditure, the RMR is multiplied by an activity factor according to different physical activity levels.[29,30] The estimated energy expenditure can then be compared with reported energy expenditure by a dietary instrument, which can be used to identify underreporters. For example, a nominal factor of 1.35 (the ratio of estimated to reported total energy intake) has been used to estimate the lowest physiological limit for someone with minimal physical activity.[29,30]

24-Hour Urinary Nitrogen

Urinary nitrogen is commonly used as a biomarker for protein intake. Because most nitrogen intake (>80%) is excreted in the urine and 16% of protein is nitrogen, urinary nitrogen can provide an unbiased marker of protein intake.[31,32] Bingham and Cummings[31] investigated the value of 24-hour urine nitrogen (N) excretion as a way of validating dietary methods of measuring protein intake in four men and four women living in a metabolic ward. Daily N intake and excretion were measured for 28 days. The completeness of the 24-hour urine collections was verified by the use of PABA (p-aminobenzoic acid) taken by the patients with meals. The within-person coefficient of variation (CV%) in dietary intake of protein ranged from 14% to 26%, whereas CV% for urinary N varied from 11% to 18% within individuals. The correlation between 28 days urinary N and 28 days of protein intake was 0.99 with a CV% of 2% for urinary N; the correlation between 8 days urinary N and 28 days diet was 0.95 with a CV% of 5% for urinary N; the correlation between a single-day diet and urinary N was 0.47 with a CV% of 24% for urinary N. This study suggests that multiple-day (at least eight 24-hour collections) urinary nitrogen measurements are needed to provide stable estimates of nitrogen intake. Subsequent studies have found that partial 24-hour urine collection (even repeated overnight) cannot replace full 24-hour urine collection in measuring urea N.[33] The collection of multiple 24-hour urine samples poses a major challenge for large epidemiologic studies.

24-Hour Urine Sodium and Potassium

In healthy individuals, blood levels of sodium and potassium do not reflect dietary intakes because of tight homeostatic control. Urine is the major route of excretion of these electrolytes, and thus 24-hour urinary sodium and potassium can serve as valid biomarkers of dietary intake of these nutrients.[34] Large day-to-day variations of sodium and potassium intake make it necessary to conduct multiple 24-hour urine collections to obtain stable estimates of these electrolytes, and as with urine N, even repeat overnight collections cannot replace full 24-hour collections.[35] Because 77% of dietary potassium is excreted in the urine,[36] the (dietary potassium × 0.77)/urinary potassium ratio has been used to identify under- and overreporting of potassium intake assessed by other dietary assessment instruments.[37]

Total Fat and Dietary Fatty Acids

Dietary fat is probably the most commonly studied dietary exposure variable, yet there is no specific biomarker for total fat intake. This limits the ability to objectively evaluate the validity of total fat intake assessed by dietary instruments. However, it is well established in controlled metabolic studies[38] that plasma fasting triglyceride levels are reduced with higher fat intake, and can thus serve as a nonspecific biomarker for fat intake. Willett et al.[39] examined the relationship between total fat intake assessed by FFQs and plasma lipid levels among 185 women in the Nurses' Health Study (NHS) and 269 men in the Health Professionals Follow-up Study (HPFS). In a multiple regression analysis adjusted for age, smoking, alcohol consumption, physical activity, body mass index (BMI), and intakes of protein, dietary fiber, and total energy, total fat intake was inversely associated with fasting triglycerides (a fat increase of 1% of energy, lowered triglyceride levels by 2.5% [95% CI: −3.7 to −1.3%, $P = .0002$]). For reported fat intake of 20% or less of energy, the geometric mean fasting triglyceride level was 179, and for more than 40% of energy it was 102 mg/dL (Fig. 6.1). This relationship was actually stronger than what

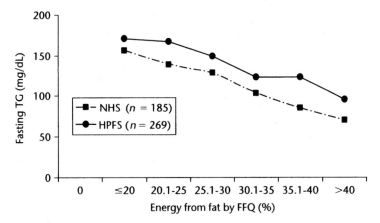

Figure 6.1 Adjusted geometric mean fasting triglyceride (TG) levels by category of total fat intake among men in the Health Professionals' Follow-Up Study (HPFS) (1994) and women in the Nurses' Health Study (NHS) (1990). Values for men were adjusted for age in 1994, smoking, alcohol consumption, physical activity, BMI, total energy intake, and total protein intake. Values for women were adjusted for age; age at menarche; age at menopause; smoking status; BMI at age 18 years; intakes of total energy, fiber, protein, and alcohol; physical activity; history of breast cancer; history of benign breast disease; parity age at first birth; laboratory batch; and time of day of phlebotomy. Reproduced with permission from Willett W, Stampfer M, Chu NF, Spiegelman D, Holmes M, Rimm E. Assessment of questionnaire validity for measuring total fat intake using plasma lipid levels as criteria. *Am J Epidemiol.* 2001;154: 1107-1112.[39]

would be predicted by the equations derived from metabolic studies,[38] probably because the participants in the cohorts were middle-aged and older, and thus had greater body fat and insulin resistance than subjects typically enrolled in metabolic studies. These findings indicate that biomarkers sensitive to (but not necessarily specific for) the dietary factor being evaluated are of value for assessing the validity of dietary questionnaires or evaluation of compliance in intervention studies.

Concentrations of fatty acids in tissue can be used as biomarkers for the intake of different types of fatty acids. These tissues include plasma, erythrocytes, platelets, adipose tissue, various lipoprotein subfractions, and others.[40] Useful fatty acid biomarkers are those that cannot be endogenously synthesized, such as polyunsaturated fatty acids (n-3 and n-6), trans fatty acids, and odd-numbered saturated fatty acids (e.g., 15:0, 17:0). Endogenously synthesized saturated (lauric, myristic, palmitic, and stearic acids) and monounsaturated fatty acids in tissue are not considered good biomarkers of intake. For saturated and monounsaturated fat intake, however, changes in nonspecific biomarkers (e.g., serum cholesterol and triglycerides) can be used as markers of intake. Controlled metabolic trials have shown that substituting saturated fat for carbohydrates significantly increases low-density lipoprotein (LDL) and high-density lipoprotein (HDL) cholesterol and decreases triglycerides, whereas substituting mono- or polyunsaturated fat for carbohydrates significantly decreases LDL cholesterol and triglycerides and increases HDL cholesterol.[38] These effects can be predicted by well-established equations derived from metabolic studies.[38,41,42]

There has been considerable interest in using plasma levels of fatty acids as biomarkers of intake. Baylin and Campos[40] summarized the quantitative effect of fatty acid substitution in the diet on changes in fatty acid composition in plasma cholesterol esters

(CEs), plasma triglycerides, and phospholipids from dietary metabolic trials. There was a clear dose-response relationship between increasing dietary linoleic acid intake and observed changes in serum CE or triglyceride linoleic acid concentrations. However, the dose-response relationship between serum phospholipids and dietary linoleic acid was much weaker, suggesting that more tightly regulated tissues (in particular, phospholipids of membranes) may not adequately reflect long-term intake.

Sun et al.[43] compared fatty acid content of erythrocytes to that of plasma with respect to their abilities to reflect usual dietary fatty acid intake as measured by a FFQ. Docosahexaenoic acid (DHA, 22:6n-3) in plasma and erythrocytes provided the strongest correlations with its dietary intake, but erythrocytes ($r = .56$) were better than plasma ($r = .48$) as a biomarker. Similarly, total trans fatty acids ($r = .43$) and total 18:1 trans isomers ($r = .42$) in erythrocytes were more strongly correlated with dietary intake than plasma markers ($r = .30$ and $r = .29$, respectively). In addition, use of repeated measures of diet further improved these correlation coefficients.

Baylin et al.[44] evaluated whole blood as a biomarker of intake. The diet-whole blood correlations were 0.43 for linoleic acid, 0.38 for alpha-linolenic acid, and 0.26 for 18:2 trans fatty acids. These results show that whole blood was a reasonable alternative for plasma for the assessment of fatty acid intake.

Adipose tissue is considered the best choice to assess long-term fatty acid intake because of its slow turnover rate. In a secondary prevention trial of coronary disease by substituting unsaturated fat for saturated fat, Dayton et al.[45] observed that adipose tissue linoleic acid increased from 11% in the first year to 32% in year 5, suggesting excellent compliance with the intervention. In epidemiologic studies, intakes of linoleic and trans fatty acids estimated by FFQs are reasonably correlated with corresponding lipids in adipose tissue (with correlations in the range of 0.40 to 0.50).[22] However, these correlations are only modestly higher than those for plasma markers.[46]

Adipose tissue levels of pentadecanoic acid (15:0) (PDA) and heptadecanoic acid (17:0) (HAD) can be used to reflect average long-term dairy fat consumption in free-living subjects. In a study of 81 healthy women aged 30 to 77 years in Sweden, Wolk et al.[47] found a Pearson correlation coefficient of 0.63 between the 15:0 content in adipose tissue and intake from dairy foods from diet records, with a somewhat lower correlation for 17:0 ($r = .42$). Baylin et al.[48] reported a correlation of 0.31 between adipose tissue content of 15:0 (also 17:0) and dairy product intake in Costa Rican men and women. Sun et al.[49] reported correlation coefficients between 15:0 content and average dairy fat intake in 1986-1990 were 0.36 for plasma and 0.30 for erythrocytes. Trans 16:1n-7 in plasma ($r = .30$) and erythrocytes ($r = .32$) were also correlated with dairy fat intake.

Because of their high cost, laboratory measurements of fatty acids are most suitable for use in nested case-control or case-cohort studies, or as a reference method in validation studies. In addition, because they are usually expressed as a percentage of total fatty acids, they only reflect relative intake, with no measure of absolute fatty acid intake.[40] Thus, changes in one fatty acid affect the distributions of the others.

Carbohydrates and Quality of Carbohydrates

As with total fat, there is no specific biomarker for total carbohydrate intake. However, plasma triglycerides rise in response to increasing carbohydrate intake (and decreasing fat intake),[38] and can be used as a sensitive but nonspecific marker of carbohydrate intake. Because both the amount and quality of carbohydrates are important determinants of fasting plasma triacylglycerol concentrations, glycemic load has been used as a measure that incorporates the quantity as well as the quality of dietary carbohydrates consumed.[50]

The glycemic load of a specific food—calculated as the product of that food's carbohydrate content and its glycemic index value—has direct physiologic meaning in that each unit can be interpreted as the equivalent of 1 g of carbohydrate from white bread (or glucose depending on the reference used in determining the glycemic index). Liu et al.[50] found a positive relationship between serum fasting triglycerides and total carbohydrate intake, the overall dietary glycemic index, and the dietary glycemic load among postmenopausal women, with the strongest relationship for glycemic load. The association between triglycerides and glycemic load appears to be stronger for overweight women than those who are not overweight, implying a biological interaction between underlying insulin resistance and carbohydrate metabolism.

Biomarkers of One-Carbon (Methyl) Metabolism

Folate, B_{12}, B_6, B_2, choline, methionine, and betaine play key roles in one-carbon metabolism that involve transfer and utilization of one-carbon groups from one compound to another.[51,52] One of folate's main biological functions is remethylation of homocysteine to methionine. Folate status can be measured in serum (or plasma) and red cells. Serum folate reflects short-term folate status (within the past few days), while a concentration of red cell folate represents longer term and integrated folate intake because the half-life of red cells is approximately 4 months.[53] Thus, red cell folate more closely reflects tissue folate status. Vitamin B_{12} status is measured by the serum cobalamin assay, and vitamin B_6 status is indicated by the circulating concentration of pyridoxial-5'-phosphate (PLP). Elevated serum or plasma homocysteine is a sensitive and nonspecific marker of both folate and vitamin B_{12} deficiency, but it is not a reliable indicator of vitamin B_6 status.[53] In a recent study, Cho et al.[54] demonstrated a significant association between dietary intake of choline plus betaine (assessed by FFQ in the Framingham Offspring Study) and lower homocysteine concentrations. Main sources of choline in the diet included red meat, poultry, milk, eggs, and fish, while main sources of betaine included spinach, pasta, white bread, cold breakfast cereal, and English muffins, bagels, or rolls.

Dietary folate assessed by FFQ is well correlated with biomarkers of folate status, including serum or plasma folate: $r = .56$ among 385 participants in the Framingham Heart Study,[55] and $r = .63$ among 139 Boston-area participants.[56] For red cell folate, the r was .42.[57] The measurement of genomic DNA methylation in blood mononuclear cells may also serve as a useful biomarker for dietary folate intake.[53]

Biomarkers of Isoflavones and Lignans

Isoflavones and lignans are naturally occurring plant-derived phytoestrogens that may have biologically active properties.[58] Lignans are present in grains, beans, green vegetables, fruits, nuts, and grasses, whereas isoflavones are concentrated in soybeans and soy foods. Common dietary isoflavonoids and metabolites include genistein, daidzein, dihydrodaidzein, O-desmethylangolensin, and equol; common lignans and metabolites include enterolactone, enterodiol, matairesinol, and secoisolariciresinol. In a typical Western diet, the daily intake of phytoestrogens is very low (<1 mg/day).[59]

Biochemical indicators of isoflavones and lignans can be measured in urine and blood specimens. However, these measurements often reflect only short-term intake, that is, several to 24 hours before a blood draw.[22,60,61] Isoflavone excretion is substantial in the urine of Asian populations, which have high soy intake.[61] Populations that consume a typical Western diet have very low blood concentrations or urinary excretion of isoflavone, and large within-person variations.[62]

Urinary or plasma isoflavone and lignan concentrations can be used as measures of adherence for dietary intervention trials of soy or isoflavone supplementation.[62] Cross-sectional studies have demonstrated good correlations between dietary intakes of soy and urinary concentrations of isoflavone in several Asian populations.[63,64] Because these biomarkers reflect short-term intake, their usefulness in predicting long-term disease risk, especially in populations consuming a Western diet, is unclear.

Biomarkers of Trace Minerals

Hambidge[65] provided a comprehensive review of biomarkers of trace mineral intake and status. Although there are no reliable biomarkers of iron intake, plasma ferritin is considered the best marker of body iron stores in the absence of acute inflammation. A higher ferritin concentration has been associated with increased consumption of heme iron and iron supplementation assessed by a FFQ.[66] However, serum ferritin is also influenced by nondietary determinants, such as age, postmenopausal hormone use, obesity, physical activity, aspirin use, gastrointestinal ulcer, and genetic polymorphisms. Thus, ferritin is a nonspecific marker of iron stores. Plasma soluble transferrin receptor concentration (sTfR) is considered a sensitive and specific marker of early iron deficiency.

Selenium can be measured in plasma, red cells, and toenails. Selenium intake calculated from duplicate meals correlated well with serum ($r = .63$), whole blood ($r = .62$), and toenail ($r = .59$) selenium concentrations.[67] Plasma selenium levels appear to be sensitive to short-term changes in dietary intake of selenium, whereas erythrocyte selenium can reflect relatively long-term exposure (e.g., several months). Toenail selenium levels are considered the best time-integrated biomarker of long-term selenium intake because toenails have a slow turnover rate. Hunter et al.[68] showed a dose-response relationship between selenium supplementation and toenail selenium levels in free-living women. Longnecker et al.[69] conducted an intervention study in which 12 males were fed high-dose (4.91 μmol Se/d), medium-dose (2.61 μmol Se/d), or control (0.41 μmol Se/d) whole wheat bread for 1 year, with the concentration of selenium measured in toenail clippings collected every 12 weeks for 2 years. Toenail selenium concentration was unaffected by dietary intake in the first 3 months and appeared to provide a time-integrated measure of intake over a period of 26-52 weeks. Thus, toenail concentration of selenium is a useful marker of long-term average intake. This is important because highly variable selenium concentrations in different samples of the same food make it difficult to calculate dietary selenium intake accurately. Other trace elements (e.g., chromium, magnesium, zinc, and copper) can also be measured in toenails using the same procedure as that used to measure selenium (instrumental neutron-activation analysis).[70] Whether these biomarkers reflect long-term dietary intakes needs to be studied further.

Use of Biomarkers in Obesity Epidemiologic Studies

Nutritional biomarkers are used in several important ways in obesity epidemiologic studies. Because measurement errors of biomarkers are essentially uncorrelated with errors in any dietary assessment methods, they can be used as a reference method for validating self-reported dietary instruments. DLW, considered the gold standard for measuring energy intake (in the absence of weight change), is now widely used in validation studies of total energy intake measured by self-reported methods (see below). Similarly, urinary nitrogen has been used as a reference marker of dietary protein intake. Sensitive but nonspecific biomarkers, such as HDL cholesterol and triglycerides, can be used to validate long-term intakes of dietary fat and carbohydrates. These biomarkers are also useful in monitoring dietary compliance in weight loss trials.

Some biomarkers can serve as surrogate indicators of long-term dietary intake in studies on dietary predictors of obesity. For example, essential fatty acid composition in adipose tissue can be used to predict long-term weight gain and obesity risk. In nutritional epidemiologic studies, the relationship between biomarkers of nutritional intake and status and risk of chronic disease incidence and mortality are typically investigated in a nested case-control design. The same design can be used to study the associations between nutrient biomarkers and onset of obesity. Hunter[22] provided a comprehensive list of biochemical markers that are used in epidemiologic studies along with representative values of their reproducibility and validity.

Sufficiently valid biomarkers for intakes of food and food groups can also be useful in dietary intervention trials or in studies of dietary determinants of obesity and obesity-related chronic diseases. For example, plasma carotenoids are known to be useful biomarkers of vegetable and fruit intake.[71] As discussed earlier, urinary or plasma concentrations of isoflavones can reflect soy-rich diets and adipose tissue levels of 15:0 and 17:0 are reasonable markers of dairy fat. However, biomarkers cannot substitute for self-reported dietary assessment methods for several reasons. First, not all nutrients have sensitive biomarkers that are practical to measure, and most foods and food groups have no useful biomarkers. Second, many biomarkers reflect short-term intake rather than usual diet. This limits their usefulness in validation studies of usual diet, and in investigations of the relationship between diet and long-term risk of obesity and obesity-related conditions.

Biochemical indicators are not influenced by dietary intake alone because individuals generally differ to some degree in the absorption and metabolism of most nutrients. Other sources of physiologic or genetic variations, such as levels of binding proteins or diurnal or menstrual cycles, may also influence the biochemical levels of nutrients and their metabolites.[22] Finally, measurements of biomarkers are prone to many sources of laboratory errors. Thus, careful attention to specimen collection, storage, and assays, and sound epidemiologic design are critical in studies involving biomarkers.

Validation of Dietary Assessment Methods

Validation studies are designed to evaluate the reproducibility and validity of dietary measurements against one or more "reference methods." Reproducibility refers to "consistency of questionnaire measurements on more than one administration to the same person at different times"; validity refers to "the degree to which the questionnaire actually measures the aspect of diet that it was designed to measure."[14] A *precise* reproducible instrument shows good agreement in repeated administrations, while a valid instrument is *accurate* in measuring unbiased *true intake* (typically the usual diet over a period of time). Ideally, an instrument should be precise as well as accurate. However, random and systematic errors can lead to inaccuracy and imprecision (Fig. 6.2).[72]

In validation studies, the choice of the reference method is a critical issue. One dilemma facing nutritional epidemiologists is the lack of a true gold standard against which to assess habitual dietary intakes. Nelson[73] discussed limitations of reference methods that are commonly used in validation studies of test instruments (Table 6.1). For example, repeat 24-hour recalls and multiple diet records can provide a quantitative assessment of food consumption, but the number of recalls or records required to reflect usual diet is large (depending on the magnitude of the intraindividual variations of the nutrients). Underreporting of energy intake is common for both instruments. *Objective* methods (e.g., DLW, urinary nitrogen excretion, adipose tissue fatty acid composition, and

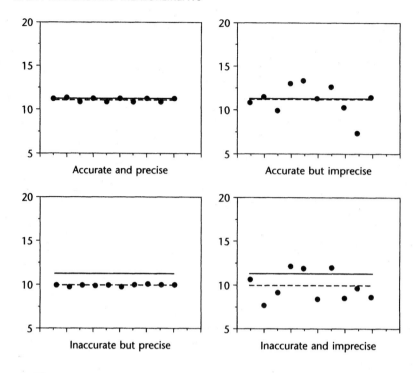

Figure 6.2 Visual representation of accuracy (validity) and precision (repeatability). True average (*solid lines*), repeat measurements (*filled circle*) and measured average (*dashed lines*). Reproduced with permission from Livingstone MB, Black AE. Markers of the validity of reported energy intake. *J Nutr.* 2003;133(Suppl 3):895S-920S.[72]

toenail concentrations of trace minerals) have the advantage of measurement errors that are independent of test instrument errors. However, these methods can be used to validate only one or a few nutrients at a time, and some methods, such as DLW and urinary nitrogen excretion, may not be sufficient to reflect long-term energy and protein intake unless multiple assessments are done over a prolonged period of time.

Because of drawbacks associated with reference methods, validation studies of nutrient intake often rely on *alloyed* standards. Diet records are the standard that is most commonly used to evaluate test methods, especially FFQs. A major advantage of diet records is that they do not depend on memory; similarly, weighed records do not depend on perceptions of portion size or amount of foods consumed. Diet records should be kept for a sufficient number of days over a prolonged period of time (e.g., 1 year) to represent long-term average intake. Multiple 24-hour recalls are also a popular choice as a reference method. Unlike diet records, repeat 24-hour recalls do not alter participants' regular eating habits. In the past two decades, numerous validation studies have been conducted to examine the validity of FFQs developed for different populations and cultures. Since Willett's summary of validation studies published through 1997,[1] the literature on the validity of FFQs has continued to grow.

The validity of FFQs can vary considerably across different populations or cultures. However, average correlations between nutrients assessed by FFQs and reference methods (e.g., one- or multiple-week diet records or repeat 24-hour recalls), when adjusted for total energy intake, are generally in the range of 0.4 to 0.7.[14] For example, in a validation study of the 136-item Willett questionnaire in the NHS,

Table 6.1 Limitations of Reference Methods Appropriate for Validation of Dietary Assessment Measures

Reference Method	Limitations
Doubly labeled water	• Energy only • Assumptions of model regarding water partitioning may not apply in cases of gross obesity or high alcohol intake • Very expensive
Urinary nitrogen (completeness of samples confirmed using PABA)	• Protein only • Requires multiple 24-h urine collections • PABA analysis affected by paracetamol and related products
Urinary nitrogen only	• Protein only • Danger of incomplete samples
Weighed records or household measures	• Underreporting • Not representative of *usual* diet due to insufficient number of days • Distortion of food habits due to recording process
Diet history	• Interviewer bias • Inaccuracy of portion size reporting due to conceptualization and memory errors • Errors in reporting of frequency, especially overreporting of related foods listed separately (e.g., individual fruits and vegetables) • Requires regular eating habits
Repeat 24-h recalls	• Under- or overreporting of foods due to reporting process (e.g., alcohol and fruit) • Not representative of *usual* diet due to insufficient number of days • Inaccuracy of portion size reporting due to conceptualization and memory errors
Biochemical measurements of nutrients in blood or other tissues	• Complex relationship with intake mediated by digestion, absorption, uptake, utilization, metabolism, excretion, and homeostatic mechanisms • Cost and precision of assays • Invasive • Sensitive biomarkers do not exist for many nutrients

Adapted from Nelson M. The validation of dietary assessment. In: Margetts BM, Nelson MC, eds. *Design Concepts in Nutritional Epidemiology.* 2nd ed. New York: Oxford University Press;1997;241-272;Chapter 8.[73]

the mean deattenuated correlation coefficient for nutrient intakes (corrected for within-person variation) between FFQs and diet records was 0.62. A similar FFQ was also evaluated in a sample of 127 male participants in the HPFS.[74] During a 1-year interval, men completed two 1-week diet records spaced approximately 6 months apart. Intraclass correlation coefficients for nutrient intakes assessed by questionnaires 1 year apart ranged from 0.47 for vitamin E without supplements to 0.80 for vitamin C with supplements. Correlation coefficients between the energy-adjusted nutrient intakes measured by diet records and the second questionnaire (which asked about diet during the year encompassing the diet records) ranged from 0.28 for iron without supplements to 0.86 for vitamin C with supplements (mean $r = .59$). These correlations were higher after adjusting for week-to-week variation in diet record intakes (mean $r = .65$). Food-based analyses reported an average correlation coefficient of >0.60 comparing the FFQ and dietary record for foods in dietary questionnaires after correcting for within-person variation in both men[75] and women.[76] These data indicate that the FFQ provides a useful measure of intake for many nutrients and foods over a 1-year period.

In a validation study of FFQs against repeated 24-hour recalls in the European Prospective Investigation into Cancer and Nutrition (EPIC), Kroke et al.[77] also obtained energy-adjusted correlation coefficents ranging from 0.54 for dietary fiber to 0.86 for alcohol. Similarly, in a validation study of the FFQ used in the Shanghai Women's Health Study,[78] nutrient and food intake assessed by the FFQ and the multiple 24-hour dietary recall were reasonably correlated, with the energy-adjusted correlation coefficients ranging from 0.59 to 0.66 for macronutrients, from 0.41 to 0.59 for micronutrients, and from 0.41 to 0.66 for major food groups.

Several studies have compared different versions of FFQs commonly used in nutritional epidemiologic studies. Caan et al.[79] compared the performance of the Block and Willett FFQs with a longer, interviewer-administered diet history in two separate subsamples of participants. Although both questionnaires generally provided lower absolute intake estimates than the diet history, the ability to rank or classify individuals was very similar, and comparable to that of the diet history. In a comparison of the Block and Willett FFQs against multiple 24-hour recalls, Wirfalt et al.[80] found different performance characteristics for the two FFQs with respect to categorizing of individuals according to different nutrients. Subar and colleagues conducted a detailed study to compare the validity of the Block, Willett, and NCI DHQs against four 24-hour recalls completed over a 1-year period.[16] They found that the crude validity correlation coefficients tended to be lower for the Willett FFQ, but the energy-adjusted correlation coefficients were similar across the different questionnaires.

Numerous validation studies have employed biomarkers as the reference method. As discussed earlier, sensitive and specific biomarkers that represent long-term dietary intake are only available for a limited number of nutrients, and no specific biomarkers exist for most nutrients and foods. However, sensitive though nonspecific biomarkers can still be useful in evaluating the validity of nutrient measures. For example, because plasma triglycerides are responsive to an increase in carbohydrates, they can serve as an indirect biomarker for changes in fat and carbohydrate composition in the diet. Plasma HDL cholesterol level, another nonspecific biomarker, is not only responsive to changes in dietary fat and carbohydrates, but is also influenced by habitual alcohol consumption.[81] For this reason, HDL cholesterol has been used as a biomarker to validate long-term alcohol consumption assessed by FFQs or other dietary assessment instruments.[82] The urinary excretion of 5-hydroxytryptophol (5-HTOL):5-hydroxyindole-3-acetic acid (5-HIAA) ratio has been shown to be a sensitive marker of recent alcohol intake based on a single 24-hour recall.[83]

For most nutrients, correlations with biomarkers are in the range of 0.3 to 0.5. These moderate correlations result from imperfections in dietary assessment instruments as well as technical errors in measurement of biomarkers. In many situations, they are also due to homeostatic control of biomarker metabolism and nondietary determinants of biomarkers. Nonetheless, these correlations provide useful and objective evidence for the validity of nutrient intake assessed by a dietary instrument.

Method of Triads

Biomarkers and a reference dietary method (e.g., repeat 24-hour recalls or food records) provide complementary information on the validity of a FFQ. These measures can also be used to estimate the correlation between FFQs and the *true* measure of long-term diet by using the method of triads.[84] Kabagambe et al.[85] employed this method to assess the validity of a FFQ used in a Hispanic population. Seven 24-hour dietary recalls and two FFQ interviews (12 months apart) were conducted to estimate dietary intake during the past year. Plasma and adipose tissue samples were collected from all subjects. The validity coefficient (VC) was estimated from three pair wise correlations between the FFQ, the reference method, and the biomarker (Fig. 6.3). Suppose Q, R, and M are the measurements from the FFQ, the reference method, and the biomarker, respectively, VCs for the reference method and the biomarker can be estimated as follows:

and
$$\text{VC}_{QT} = \sqrt{\left(\left(r_{QR} \times r_{QM}\right)/r_{RM}\right)}, \ \text{VC}_{RT} = \sqrt{\left(\left(r_{QR} \times r_{RM}\right)/r_{QM}\right)}$$

$$\text{VC}_{MT} = \sqrt{\left(\left(r_{QM} \times r_{RM}\right)/r_{QR}\right)},$$

where r is the correlation corrected for within-subject variation and T is a latent variable representing the *true* but unknown long-term dietary intake.

Kabagambe et al.[85] found that the median VCs for tocopherols and carotenoids estimated by repeat 24-hour recalls, the average of the two FFQs, and plasma were 0.71, 0.60, and 0.52, respectively. Plasma measures were better biomarkers for carotenoids and tocopherols than adipose tissue. However, adipose tissue appeared to be a better biomarker for polyunsaturated fatty acids (VC, 0.45 to 1.00) and lycopene (VC, 0.51). In general, the biomarkers did not perform better than the FFQs, and thus, the authors concluded that biomarkers should be used to complement the FFQ rather than substitute for it.

The method of triads has also been used in several other studies.[86-88] Though useful, it requires the assumption that the errors between the methods are independent. This method has an important drawback. In some situations, VCs are inestimable, or >1, a condition referred to as Heywood case.[84]

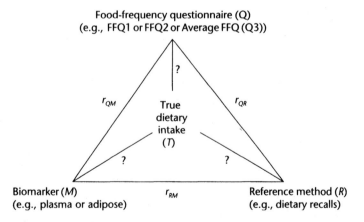

Figure 6.3 Diagrammatic representation of the method of triads used to estimate the correlation between true long-term nutrient intake and intake estimated using dietary assessment methods. Reproduced with permission from Kabagambe EK, Baylin A, Allan DA, Siles X, Spiegelman D, Campos H. Application of the method of triads to evaluate the performance of food-frequency questionnaires and biomarkers as indicators of long-term dietary intake. *Am J Epidemiol.* 2001;154:1126-1135.[85]

Improving the Validity of FFQs through Repeated Measures

As discussed earlier, in most validation studies the correlations between nutrients assessed by FFQs and diet records or repeat 24-hour recalls range from 0.4 to 0.7. This *ceiling effect* results not only from the inability of FFQs to capture the complexity of diets fully but also from lack of a true gold standard for comparison.[89] Use of repeated measures from FFQs in prospective studies can potentially improve the validity of dietary measures by reducing random errors. Repeated measures are also more likely to represent long-term dietary intake.

As part of the evaluation of the expanded FFQ used in the NHS in 1986, we included participants from a similar study done 6 years earlier (in 1980). The series of diet records from the same women after a 6-year interval allowed us to assess the ability of repeated measurement of intakes by FFQs to represent long-term diet. In the validation study of the original FFQ in 1980, participants were asked to complete four 1-week diet records over a 1-year period. In the validation study of the expanded FFQ, participants were asked to complete two 7-day diet records approximately 6 months apart. To capture seasonal changes in diet, the first set of records was completed in the winter or spring, and the second set in the summer or fall of 1987 (Fig. 6.4).

To assess the ability of FFQs to reflect long-term diet, we compared the averages of nutrient intakes from the 1980 and 1986 diet record means with nutrient intakes assessed by FFQs in 1980, 1984, and 1986, separately, and the average intakes from the 1980, 1984, and 1986 FFQs. In both the 1980 and 1986 validation studies, FFQs were administered twice, before and after completing the diet records. We used the second FFQ for this analysis because it covered the time period in which the diet records were completed. Rather than using only one set of diet records, we used two sets (i.e., 1980 and 1986) as the comparison method. To compensate for attenuation of correlation coefficients, we used the within- and between-person components of variation in diet records (treating the two sets of diet records as two random units of observation) to deattenuate correlation coefficients for intakes of macronutrients (see below). This approach provided an estimate of the correlation that would have been observed had we collected diet records for each year during the 6-year period.

Pearson correlations between nutrient intakes from the 1980 and 1986 diet records ranged from 0.42 for saturated fat to 0.74 for carbohydrates (mean = 0.55). For the FFQs, the mean reproducibility coefficients were 0.37 between 1980 and 1984, 0.53 between 1984 and 1986, and 0.34 between 1980 and 1986. When the averages of nutrients from the 1980 and 1986 diet records were compared with the questionnaires (Table 6.2), the mean correlations for the above macronutrients (after correction for within-person variability in diet records) were 0.57 for the 1980 questionnaire, 0.65

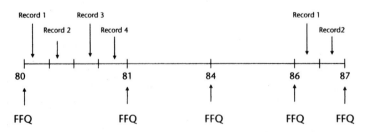

Figure 6.4 An outline of the time frame for the 1980 and 1986 FFQ validation studies in the Nurses' Health Study.

Table 6.2 Pearson Correlation Coefficients (Deattenuated) for Energy-Adjusted Macronutrient Intakes Assessed by FFQs and the Average Intakes Assessed by 1980 and 1986 Diet Records

	1980 FFQ vs. Average Diet Records	1984 FFQ vs. Average Diet Records	1986 FFQ vs. Average Diet Records	Average of 1980, 1984, 1986 FFQs vs. Average Diet Records
Total fat	0.44	0.47	0.62	0.64
	(0.57)	(0.61)	(0.81)	(0.83)
Saturated fat	0.50	0.49	0.64	0.68
	(0.70)	(0.68)	(0.90)	(0.95)
Cholesterol	0.52	0.61	0.58	0.67
	(0.69)	(0.82)	(0.78)	(0.90)
Protein	0.39	0.38	0.50	0.56
	(0.48)	(0.46)	(0.61)	(0.68)
Carbohydrates	0.37	0.59	0.69	0.68
	(0.43)	(0.68)	(0.79)	(0.78)
Mean	0.44	0.51	0.61	0.65
	(0.57)	(0.65)	(0.78)	(0.83)

for the 1984 questionnaire, and 0.78 for the 1986 questionnaire. The mean correlation increased to 0.83 when the averages of nutrients from the three questionnaires were compared with the averages from the 1980 and 1986 diet records. This correlation was appreciably greater than the average correlations derived from evaluations of single comprehensive FFQs, which range from 0.40 to 0.70. These data indicate that repeated measures of diet by FFQs provide useful measures of long-term average dietary intakes over a 6-year period. This finding is critically important in studies of chronic diseases that develop over a period of many years, such as cancers or atherosclerosis. Consistent with these findings, we found in a previous analysis that use of the cumulative average of dietary intakes of fatty acids was more predictive of coronary heart disease (CHD) risk than use of only baseline diet.[90]

Underreporting and Adjustment for Total Energy Intake

Underreporting of total energy intake by dietary instruments is widely recognized. Livingstone and Black[72] conducted a comprehensive review of studies in which energy intake (EI) was reported and energy expenditure (EE) was measured using the DLW method. Under the condition of stable weight, EI should equal EE. Under- and overreporters were identified by using EI:EE <0.82 or >1.18. Figure 6.5 shows EI:EE from 43 studies of adults (73 subgroups), with a mean $\pm$ SD EI:EE of 0.83 $\pm$ 0.14. In 29% of subgroups, EI and EE agreed to within $\pm$10%, but 69% of the subgroups had a reported mean EI >10% below the mean EE, whereas less than 3% had a mean EI >10% above the mean EE. There were no significant differences between different dietary assessment methods (Table 6.3). However, in the Observing Protein and Energy Nutrition (OPEN) Study, Subar et al.[91] found a greater degree of underreporting with FFQs than with 24-hour recalls. The likelihood of underreporting appears to be strongly related to participants' weight status. In most of the studies, underreporting is more common in the obese than in normal weight subjects.

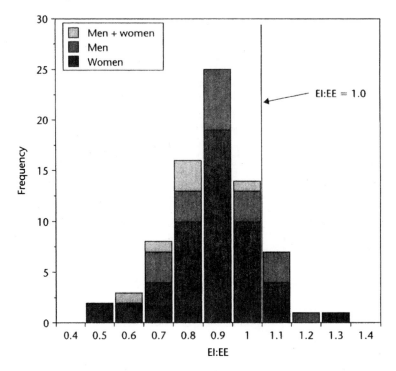

Figure 6.5 Frequency distribution of the ratio of energy intake to energy expenditure (EI:EE) by sex in 43 doubly labeled water (DLW) energy expenditure (DLW-EE) studies of adults comprising 77 subgroups (men and women separately). Reproduced with permission from Livingstone MB, Black AE. Markers of the validity of reported energy intake. *J Nutr.* 2003;133(Suppl 3):895S-920S.[72]

Table 6.3 Comparison of Reported Energy Intake by Dietary Assessment Method with Energy Expenditure Measured by Doubly Labeled Water

Dietary Method	N (# Studies)	Mean (EI/ EE Ratio)	SD
Observation	5	1.06	0.09
Weighed records*	22	0.84	0.11
Estimated records*	25	0.84	0.10
Diet history	4	0.84	0.14
Twenty-four-hour recall (single or multiple)	6	0.84	0.08
Food-frequency questionnaire	6	0.87	0.12
All	68	0.86	0.13

* Excluding studies on subjects recruited as obese or as large or small eaters.
Reproduced with permission from Livingstone MB, Black AE. Markers of the validity of reported energy intake. *J Nutr.* 2003;133(Suppl 3):895S-920S.[72]

The impact of underreporting energy intake on the analysis and interpretation of diet and disease relationships is uncertain. The main interest in nutritional epidemiology is the composition of the diet, as represented by energy-adjusted nutrient intakes (see below), rather than simply increasing or decreasing energy-bearing nutrient intakes.[1] In addition, in epidemiologic studies, factors that may be related to underreporting of energy intakes, such as age, sex, and BMI, are often adjusted for in the analyses. Total energy intake is seldom used as an exposure or outcome variable because it is difficult to measure and interpret. In free-living populations, between-person variations in total energy intake are primarily determined by individual differences in physical activity, body size, and metabolic efficiency; energy balance over a period of time is primarily reflected in body weight change. After controlling for total or lean body mass, the variation in total energy intake appears to be primarily determined by physical activity levels. The substantial contribution of physical activity to between-person variations in total energy intake may explain a positive association between total energy intake and physical activity levels observed in some epidemiologic studies.[92] Although there are individual differences in metabolic efficiency, it is infeasible to measure them in epidemiologic studies.

The best way to deal with underreporting in analyses is unclear. Some studies exclude underreporters from the data set. This approach not only reduces power, but may also introduce selection bias because subjects with high BMI levels are more likely to be excluded.[72] Nonetheless, this approach can be used in sensitivity or secondary analyses. For example, in the analysis of the relationship between dietary fat and CHD, we calculated the ratio of reported caloric intake to predicted caloric intake for each participant using their age and weight. Excluding women with the greatest likelihood for underreporting (the lowest quintile of the ratio) did not change the associations.[90] It is possible that simultaneous adjustment for BMI and total energy in the overall analyses may have already taken care of potential biases caused by underreporting.

These analyses demonstrate the importance of measuring and adjusting for total energy intake in epidemiologic studies. Adjustment for total energy intake in data analyses has several conceptual and practical advantages.[14] First, control for total energy in epidemiologic studies mimics *isocaloric* substitution of one macronutrient (e.g., fat) for another (e.g., carbohydrates) in controlled experimental studies. In most situations, dietary composition rather than absolute intake is the primary interest in nutritional epidemiologic studies. Absolute increase or decrease in nutrient or food intakes can often lead to changes in total energy intake. Unless physical activity levels are also changed, the changes in food intake will, theoretically, lead to weight gain or loss that make it difficult to interpret the nutrient-disease association. Second, because measurement errors for energy and nutrient intakes are correlated, they tend to *cancel* each other in energy-adjusted nutrients. The correlated errors between nutrients and energy typically result from overreporting or underreporting of specific foods. In many validation studies, the correlation coefficients between nutrient intakes calculated by the FFQs and reference methods improve after adjusting for energy intake,[1] which can be largely attributed to reduced measurement errors. Third, energy adjustment also removes "extraneous variation" that results from the differences in energy requirements among individuals of different body sizes and physical activity levels. It should be noted that because energy adjustment leads to a reduction in between-person variations in nutrient intakes, it can sometimes reduce the correlations between energy-adjusted nutrient intakes calculated by the FFQ and diet records.

Another reason to adjust for total energy intake is to control for confounding in cases where total energy is associated with disease risk, and a spurious association between nutrient intake and disease may occur because of confounding by total energy intake. Using an energy-adjusted nutrient instead of absolute intake should eliminate such confounding because this variable is, by definition, not correlated with total energy intake.

The most commonly used method to adjust for total energy is to calculate nutrient density (i.e., percentage of calories contributed by a macronutrient). Public health recommendations are generally expressed in these units. For nonenergy contributing nutrients, density can be expressed as absolute intake per 1,000 cal. The major limitation of using nutrient densities in epidemiologic studies is that it does not control adequately for confounding by total energy intake. An alternative method proposed by Willett and Stampfer[93] is to calculate nutrient residuals. In this method, energy-adjusted nutrient intakes are computed as the residuals from a regression model, with total energy intake as the independent variable and absolute nutrient intake as the dependent variable (Fig. 6.6). Thus, the nutrient residuals, by definition, provide a measure of nutrient intake uncorrelated with total energy. Because the residuals have a mean of zero and include negative values, a constant is added to make them more interpretable. Typically, the predicted nutrient intake for the mean energy intake of the study population is added to the residuals. In multivariate analyses of nutrient-disease relationships, several statistical models are available for energy adjustments (Table 6.4): (a) the standard multivariate model; (b) the nutrient residual model; (c) the energy-partition model; and (d) the multivariate nutrient density model. The standard multivariate model includes total energy along with absolute intake of the nutrient of interest. The nutrient residual model includes the nutrient residuals obtained by regressing

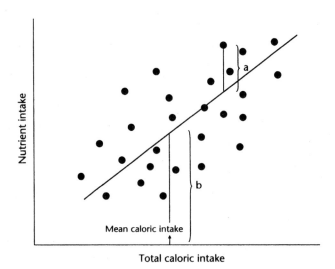

Figure 6.6 Calorie-adjusted intake = a + b, where a = residual for subject from regression model with nutrient intake as the dependent variable and total caloric intake as the independent variable and b = the expected nutrient intake for a person with mean caloric intake. Reproduced with permission from Willett W, Stampfer MJ. Total energy intake: implications for epidemiologic analyses. *Am J Epidemiol.* 1986;124:17-27.[93]

Table 6.4 Statistical Models for Adjusting for Total Energy Intake in Epidemiologic Analyses

Model	Relation Expressed
Model 1A (standard multivariate)	Disease risk = β_1 nutrient + α (total energy)
Model 1B (residual nutrient)	Disease risk = β_1 nutrient residual* + β_2 total energy
Model 1C (energy partition)	Disease risk = $(\alpha + \beta_1)$ nutrient + α (energy from nonnutrient sources)
Model 2 (multivariate nutrient density)	Disease risk = β_3 nutrient/total energy + β_4 total energy

* "Nutrient residual" is the residual from the regression of a specific nutrient on energy.
From Willett WC. *Nutritional Epidemiology.* 2nd ed. New York: Oxford University Press; 1998.[1]

nutrient intake as an independent variable on total energy intake (see above); total energy intake is also included as a covariate. In the energy-partition model, total energy is partitioned into contributions by different energy sources. The coefficient for one type of energy source (e.g., fat) represents the effect of increasing absolute intake of this nutrient while holding other energy sources (i.e., protein and carbohydrates) constant. Therefore, it represents the effect of *adding fat*, which includes both its energy and nonenergy effect. This would be analogous to conducting a trial holding protein or carbohydrate constant, while varying the amount of fat as well as total calories. The multivariate nutrient density model includes the nutrient densities (percentages of energy) from the macronutrients of interest (e.g., fat) as exposure variables with total energy included as a covariate. The coefficients from this model also have an *isocaloric* interpretation. It represents the substitution of fat for an equal amount of energy from carbohydrate (if percentage of energy from protein is included in the model), but in units of the percentage of energy.

Although the first three methods are mathematically equivalent when the nutrients are in their continuous form,[94] the interpretation of the coefficients varies. For the standard, residual, and nutrient density models, the estimated associations all have the "isocaloric substitution" interpretation. However, interpretations of the associations for total energy are different. In the standard model, the associations should be interpreted as the effect of the sources of energy that are not included in the model, whereas the meaning of total energy intake is retained in the residual and nutrient density models. In the energy-partition model, total energy is not held constant. Therefore, an increase in absolute intake of one macronutrient will lead to an increase in total energy intake. As discussed earlier, the consequence of altered energy intake on body weight can complicate the interpretation of the nutrient-disease association.

In many circumstances, dietary variables are categorized according to quartiles or quintiles to avoid incorrect specification of the model, and to reduce the influence of outliers. Unfortunately, statistical equivalence among the standard, residual, and energy-partition models ceases to exist once a nutrient has been categorized. In a comparison of the standard multivariate and residual methods, Brown et al.[94] found the latter more powerful for detecting linear trends in associations, and more robust to residual confounding when the adjustment variable was categorized. We have also reported that when dietary exposures were categorized into quantiles, the residual and nutrient density models yielded stronger associations and narrower 95% confidence intervals for the associations between polyunsaturated and trans fats and risk of CHD than did the standard multivariate and energy-partition models.[95]

Adjusting for Total Energy Intake in Obesity Epidemiologic Studies

Because weight gain results from positive energy balance, total energy intake can be interpreted as an intermediate end point between higher consumption of energy-bearing nutrients, foods, or beverages and subsequent weight gain. Thus, in studies on determinants of obesity and weight gain, total energy intake should be treated as a mediator rather than a confounder. For example, in analyzing the relationship between macronutrient intake (e.g., dietary fat) and weight gain, it is best to use percentage of calories from fat as the exposure variable. Not controlling for total calories in the multivariate model allows testing of the hypothesis that higher consumption of dietary fat may lead to obesity through passive overconsumption of calories. In an alternative analysis, total calories can be added to the model to see whether the association between the macronutrient and weight gain is mediated through excess energy intake.

Schulze et al.[96] examined the relationship between sugar-sweetened soft drink consumption, calorie intake, and weight gain in a large cohort of younger and middle-aged women. Women who increased their sugar-sweetened soft drink consumption between 1991 and

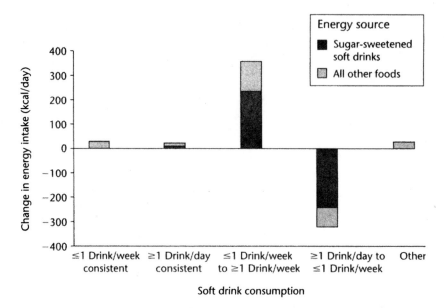

Figure 6.7 Mean change in energy consumption according to time trends in sugar-sweetened soft drink consumption between 1991 and 1995 in 51,603 women in the Nurses' Health Study II. Reproduced with permission from Schulze MB, Manson JE, Ludwig DS, et al. Sugar-sweetened beverages, weight gain, and incidence of type 2 diabetes in young and middle-aged women. *JAMA.* 2004;292:927-34.[96]

1995 from low (≤1 per week) to high (≥1 per day) significantly increased their reported total energy intake by an average of 358 kcal/day (Fig. 6.7), whereas women who reduced their sugar-sweetened soft drink consumption between 1991 and 1995 also reduced their total energy consumption by a mean of 319 kcal/day. Changes in energy intake from food sources other than sugar-sweetened soft drinks accounted for about one third of the changes in total energy intake. These findings suggest that intake of sugar-sweetened beverages is an important source of excess calories, thereby resulting in a positive caloric balance and development of obesity. In this situation, to estimate the association between soft drink consumption and weight gain, the increase in total calories should be treated as an intermediate variable.

Measurement Error Corrections

All dietary assessment methods inevitably lead to measurement errors, which include random errors due to day-to-day variations in food intakes and systematic errors arising from inaccurate assessments of food intake frequency and portion sizes, errors in food composition tables, and selective underreporting or overreporting of consumption of certain foods.[1] In epidemiologic research, daily variations in intakes of specific nutrients have been studied extensively using the analysis of variance technique.[97-99] Beaton et al.[98] observed that ratios of the within-person and between-person components of variance differed tremendously across nutrients, ranging from 1.0 for calories to >100 for vitamin A in men, and 1.4 for calories to 47.6 for vitamin A in women. Similarly, Willett reported that the ratios ranged from 1.9 for calories to 11.7 for vitamin A among

173 women.[1] In that total energy intake is quite well regulated by physiologic mechanisms, there is relatively low day-to-day variation for total calories. In contrast, the concentration of vitamin A and other micronutrients in certain foods can cause intake to vary considerably from day to day, depending on food choices and seasonable availability of foodstuffs.

Because of day-to-day variations in diet, a single 24-hour recall provides a poor estimate of a person's usual diet. However, repeated measures can be used to improve the estimate. In validation studies, repeated measures of the reference method are commonly used to correct for within-person variations in dietary intakes. For example, deattenuated correlation coefficients for the nutrient of interest between a FFQ and weighed diet records were corrected for week-to-week variation in diet records by using the following formula.[99]

$$r_t = r_0 \sqrt{(1 + \gamma/k)} \tag{6.1}$$

where r_t is the corrected correlation between the dietary pattern scores derived from the FFQ and diet records, r_0 is the observed correlation, γ is the ratio of estimated within-person and between-person variation in nutrient intakes derived from the two 1-week diet records, and k is the number of repeated observations of diet records. Conceptually, these corrected correlations provide an estimate of the correlations between the FFQ and *true* intake whereby each person's intake was measured by a very large number of diet records. Rosner and Willett[100] provided an estimate of the standard error for the corrected or deattenuated correlation coefficient and an associated $100\% \times (1 - \alpha)$ confidence interval.

In epidemiologic studies of diet and disease risk, the regression calibration approach can be used to correct for both random and systematic errors, but this approach requires a validation study in a subsample of the cohort. Rosner et al.[101] developed a method to correct odds ratio estimates from logistic regression models for measurement errors in continuous exposures within cohort studies; these errors could be systematic or due to random within-person variation. Let X denote true dietary intake by a reference method and Z denote surrogate exposure by a FFQ. Ignoring measurement error, the logistic regression model for regressing a dichotomous disease variable D on Z,

$$\log[D/(1 - D)] = \alpha + \beta z \tag{6.2}$$

True intake (X) is estimated as a function of observed surrogate intake (Z) from a regression derived from validation study data ($X = \alpha' + \lambda Z + \varepsilon$). The corrected β^* is obtained by

$$\beta^* = \beta/\lambda \tag{6.3}$$

where β is the uncorrected logistic regression coefficient of D on Z from the main study (from equation 6.2), and λ is the estimated regression slope of X on Z from the validation study.

Koh-Banerjee et al.[102] extended the regression calibration method to estimate regression coefficients adjusted for measurement error in an analysis of the relationship between changes in diet and 9-year gain in waist circumference. Such an analysis requires validation studies conducted at two separate time points.

Let: X_1 represent true dietary intake (diet record) in time 1; X_2 represent true dietary intake (diet record) in time 2.
Z_1 represent dietary intake measured by a surrogate (FFQ) in time 1.
Z_2 represent dietary intake measured by a surrogate (FFQ) in time 2.

Using the same regression calibration approach discussed earlier, the change in true dietary intakes $(X_2 - X_1)$ is estimated as a function of the change in surrogate intakes $(Z_2 - Z_1)$ derived from the validation study data:

$$(X_2 - X_1) = \alpha + (\gamma)(Z_2 - Z_1) + \varepsilon \qquad (6.4)$$

In a linear regression with the amount of weight or waist change as the outcome, the corrected point estimate for the exposure measure (i.e., difference in observed dietary intake over time) is:

$$\beta^* = \beta/\gamma$$

where β is the estimated (or uncorrected) linear regression coefficient from the main study, and γ is the estimated regression slope of changes in X on changes in Z from the validation studies.

Using this method, Koh-Banerjee et al.[102] estimated that after error correction, the substitution of trans fats as 2% of energy for polyunsaturated fats was associated with a 2.7 cm increase in waist circumference over 9 years ($P < .001$) (as compared with a 0.77 cm waist gain, uncorrected). An increase of 12 g fiber/day ($r = .68$ between FFQs and diet records) was associated with a 2.21 cm reduction in waist circumference after error correction ($P < .001$) (0.63 cm waist gain, uncorrected). The same method was employed by Liu et al.[103] to correct for measurement error in the analyses of changes in dietary fiber intake and weight gain during 12 years of follow-up in the NHS. After further correction for measurement errors in changes in dietary fiber intake, they estimated that an increase of 12 g in dietary fiber intake was associated with ≈3.5 kg (8 lb) less weight gain in 12 years.

Dietary Pattern Analyses

A growing interest in the study of overall dietary patterns in relation to obesity and chronic diseases[104] has been spurred, in part, by several conceptual and methodological challenges associated with the traditional approach of examining individual nutrients and foods. These include high levels of intercorrelations among nutrients and foods, lack of consideration of synergistic or cumulative effects of multiple nutrients, multiple comparison problems, and confounding by other dietary components. Patterns are characterized based on similarity of habitual food use, which minimizes confounding by other foods or nutrient. Thus, in dietary pattern analysis, the collinearity of nutrients and foods can be used to advantage. Classifying individuals according to their overall eating pattern (i.e., by considering how foods and nutrients are consumed in combination) can yield a larger contrast between exposure groups than analyses based on single nutrients. Because overall patterns of dietary intake might be easy for the public to interpret or translate into diets, research on dietary patterns could have important public health implications.

Several methods have been commonly used to characterize dietary patterns using collected dietary information, including factor analysis, cluster analysis, and dietary indices. Factor analysis, as a generic term, includes both principal component analysis (PCA) and common factor analysis. PCA is commonly used to define dietary patterns because the principal components are expressed by certain mathematical functions of the observed consumption of food items.[105] The method aggregates specific food items or food groups based on the degree to which food items in the data set are correlated with one another. A summary score for each pattern is then derived and can be used in either correlation or regression analysis to examine relationships between various eating patterns and outcomes of interest, such as weight gain[106] and chronic diseases.[107,108] In a validation study, we found that two major patterns (the prudent and Western patterns) identified through PCA of food consumption data assessed by FFQs were reproducible over time and correlated reasonably well with the patterns identified from two 1-week diet records.[109]

Cluster analysis is another multivariate method for characterizing dietary patterns. In contrast to factor analysis, cluster analysis aggregates individuals into relatively homogeneous subgroups (clusters) with similar diets. Individuals have been clustered on the basis of the frequency of food consumed; the percentage of energy contributed by each food or food group, the average grams of food intakes, or standardized nutrient intakes.[110-112] When the cluster procedure is completed, further analyses (e.g., comparing dietary profiles across clusters) are necessary to interpret the identified patterns.[113] Earlier studies have examined the relationships between dietary patterns identified by cluster analysis and weight gain.[114]

A variety of dietary indices have been proposed to assess overall diet quality.[115,116] These are typically constructed on the basis of dietary recommendations or existing dietary patterns. Commonly used dietary indices include the diet quality index-revised (DQI),[117] the USDA Healthy Eating Index (HEI),[118] the Recommended Food Score (RFS),[119] and the Mediterranean Diet Index (MDI).[120,121] We have created an alternate HEI (AHEI) by incorporating components regarding trans fat, polyunsaturated to saturated fat ratio, moderate alcohol use, and multivitamin use.[122] Several studies have examined the relationships between various dietary indices and risk of obesity and weight gain.[123]

Both factor and cluster analyses are considered a posteriori because the eating patterns are derived through statistical modeling of dietary data at hand.[124] The dietary index approach, in contrast, is a priori, because the indices are created based on previous knowledge of a *healthy* diet. Because the factor and cluster analysis approaches generate patterns based on available empirical data without a priori hypotheses, they do not necessarily represent optimal patterns for disease prevention. On the other hand, the dietary index approach is limited by current knowledge and understanding of diet-disease relationships, and can also be fraught with uncertainties in selecting individual components of the score and subjectivity in defining cutoff points. Typically, dietary indices are constructed on the basis of prevailing dietary recommendations, some of which may not represent the best available evidence.[104]

A newly developed approach that bridges the gap between the two major dietary pattern approaches is Reduced Rank Regression (RRR).[125-127] The RRR method takes into account the biological pathways from diet to outcome by identifying dietary patterns associated with biomarkers of a specific disease, then uses the identified patterns to predict disease occurrence. Unlike analyses using PCA, which derives dietary patterns based on observed covariance among food groups, the RRR method utilizes information on biomarkers to derive dietary patterns (Fig. 6.8). Thus, this approach is considered a combination of a priori and a posteriori methods.

Because RRR patterns are derived based on biological pathways rather than patterns of eating behavior, they could be more predictive of disease risk. The method has been applied to studies of CHD[128] and type 2 diabetes.[129] The RRR approach requires response (biomarker) information. However, such data may not be available in many studies. Also, the biomarker information available in a study may not reflect the current status of knowledge. Nonetheless, the hypothesis-driven nature of the RRR method is considered complementary to the traditional factor analysis approach.

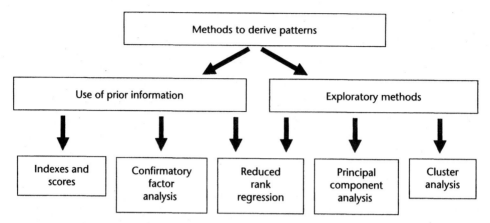

Figure 6.8 Approaches to define dietary patterns in epidemiologic studies. Adapted from Schulze MB, Hoffmann K. Methodological approaches to study dietary patterns in relation to risk of coronary heart disease and stroke. *Br J Nutr.* 2006 May;95:860-869.[127]

Summary

Despite many advances in dietary assessment methodologies in the past two decades, it remains a major challenge in epidemiologic studies to accurately quantify dietary intakes in free-living populations. Sufficiently valid dietary assessment is particularly important for studying dietary determinants of obesity. However, such studies are made exceedingly complex by combinations of large day-to-day variations in nutrient and food intakes, biased reports associated with obesity status, and difficulties in controlling for confounding variables. The same methodological problems also apply to nutritional epidemiologic studies on dietary determinants of chronic disease risk. These require careful choice of the most appropriate dietary assessment methods, and rigorous validation studies and statistical analyses and interpretation.

Because there is no perfect dietary assessment method, choice of a dietary instrument has to balance strengths and limitations of various methods in specific research settings. FFQs offer low cost and the ability to assess usual diet, the main interest in most epidemiologic studies of obesity and related chronic diseases. In the past two decades, the FFQ has become the method of choice for large epidemiologic studies involving hundreds and thousands of people. However, the validity of a FFQ is population- and culture specific; it is crucial to consider population characteristics, such as age, sex, education/literacy, and cultural characteristics when developing a FFQ.

One emerging trend in nutritional epidemiologic studies is to assess overall dietary patterns in relation to obesity and chronic diseases. Such analyses take advantage of a FFQ's ability to assess habitual diet and examine cumulative effects of overall diet. Dietary pattern analysis will certainly not replace nutrient or food analysis, but instead, be complementary to more traditional analysis. Evidence is enhanced when the results from multiple lines of research (i.e., biomarkers of nutrient intake, nutrients, foods, and dietary patterns) are consistent.

Another emerging trend in large epidemiologic studies is to collect repeated measures of diet during follow-up. These can be used to reduce measurement error and best represent long-term diet. They can be useful in correcting for both random and systematic measurement errors in analyses of changes in diet, body weight, or waist circumference over time.

A recent development in large epidemiologic studies is to combine different types of dietary assessment methods. For example, NHANES III added a FFQ to its 24-hour recall.[130] In the EPIC-Norfolk study, 7-day diet records and FFQ data were collected simultaneously from subjects who were willing to provide food records.[131] Although the combined approach may provide a more complete picture on the complexity of diet, different data from the various methods may create a dilemma in the interpretation of the findings. In addition, the cost of collecting food record data from hundreds of thousands of people is often prohibitive for most cohort studies, especially if repeated measures of diet are considered.

There is a general consensus that adjusting for total energy intake when estimating individual nutrient intake from FFQs can reduce correlated errors and improve estimates in validation studies. Thus, in most situations, nutrient density (percentage of calories from specific macronutrients) or nutrient residuals should be used as the primary exposure variable in studying dietary determinants of obesity or chronic diseases. Total energy is typically adjusted in multivariate analyses of diet and incidence of chronic diseases (e.g., heart disease or cancer) to simulate isocaloric substitution of one macronutrient (e.g., fat) for another (e.g., carbohydrates). Whether such adjustment should be done in studies on dietary determinants of obesity and weight gain is more complicated because total energy is considered an intermediate biological variable between macronutrient intake and body weight. If the main interest is weight gain in relation to changes in dietary composition (without change in energy intake), then total energy intake should be adjusted in the model. On the other hand, if one hypothesizes that increased consumption of a particular nutrient or food may lead to an increase in subsequent energy intake, then total energy should not be controlled for in the model.

It has become critically important for large cohort studies of obesity and chronic diseases to collect and store biological samples such as plasma, red blood cells, toenails, and DNA for biomarker analyses. Effective biomarkers of nutrient intake and status can provide valuable data on the validity of dietary assessment methods, and also serve as an objective and time-integrated dietary exposure for some nutrients that are difficult to assess through self-reports. However, biomarkers are a complement to, rather than a replacement for, dietary assessment methods in epidemiologic studies. The combination of repeated measures of FFQs and biomarker data is likely to provide reasonably accurate measures of long-term diet in large cohort studies of obesity and chronic diseases.

References

1. Willett WC. *Nutritional Epidemiology.* 2nd ed. New York: Oxford University Press; 1998.
2. Gibson RS. *Principles of Nutritional Assessment.* 2nd ed. New York: Oxford University Press; 2005.
3. Buzzard M. 24-hour dietary recall and food record methods. In: Willet WC, ed. *Nutritional Epidemiology.* 2nd ed. New York: Oxford University Press; 1998;50-73.
4. Posner BM, Borman CL, Morgan JL, Borden WS, Ohls JC. The validity of a telephone-administered 24-hour dietary recall methodology. *Am J Clin Nutr.* 1982;36:546-553.
5. Buzzard IM, Faucett CL, Jeffery RW, et al. Monitoring dietary change in a low-fat diet intervention study: advantages of using 24-hour dietary recalls vs food records. *J Am Diet Assoc.* 1996;96:574-579.
6. Feskanich D, Sielaff BH, Chong K, Buzzard IM. Computerized collection and analysis of dietary intake information. *Comput Methods Programs Biomed.* 1989;30:47-57.
7. Slimani N, Ferrari P, Ocke M, et al. Standardization of the 24-hour diet recall calibration method used in the European prospective investigation into cancer and nutrition (EPIC): general concepts and preliminary results. *Eur J Clin Nutr.* 2000;54:900-917.

8. Johnson RK. Dietary intake—how do we measure what people are really eating? *Obes Res.* 2002;10(Suppl 1):63S-68S.

9. Conway JM, Ingwersen LA, Moshfegh AJ. Accuracy of dietary recall using the USDA five-step multiple-pass method in men: an observational validation study. *J Am Diet Assoc.* 2004;104:595-603.

10. Conway JM, Ingwersen LA, Vinyard BT, Moshfegh AJ. Effectiveness of the US Department of Agriculture 5-step multiple-pass method in assessing food intake in obese and nonobese women. *Am J Clin Nutr.* 2003;77:1171-1178.

11. Johnson RK, Driscoll P, Goran MI. Comparison of multiple-pass 24-hour recall estimates of energy intake with total energy expenditure determined by the doubly labeled water method in young children. *J Am Diet Assoc.* 1996;96:1140-1144.

12. Bingham SA, Welch AA, McTaggart A, et al. Nutritional methods in the European Prospective Investigation of Cancer in Norfolk. *Public Health Nutr.* 2001;4:847-858.

13. Burke BS. The dietary history as a tool in research. *J Am Diet Assoc.* 1947;23: 1041-1046.

14. Willett WC. *Food-Frequency Methods. Nutritional Epidemiology.* 2nd ed. New York: Oxford University Press; 1998;74-100.

15. Block G, Thompson FE, Hartman AM, Larkin FA, Guire KE. Comparison of two dietary questionnaires validated against multiple dietary records collected during a 1-year period. *J Am Diet Assoc.* 1992;92:686-693.

16. Subar AF, Thompson FE, Kipnis V, et al. Comparative validation of the Block, Willett, and National Cancer Institute food-frequency questionnaires: the Eating at America's Table Study. *Am J Epidemiol.* 2001;154:1089-1099.

17. Subar AF. Developing dietary assessment tools. *J Am Diet Assoc.* 2004;104:769-770.

18. Tjonneland A, Haraldsdottir J, Overvad K, Stripp C, Ewertz M, Jensen OM. Influence of individually estimated portion size data on the validity of a semiquantitative food-frequency questionnaire. *Int J Epidemiol.* 1992;21:770-777.

19. Orencia AJ, Daviglus ML, Dyer AR, Shekelle RB, Stamler J. Fish consumption and stroke in men. 30-year findings of the Chicago Western Electric Study. *Stroke.* 1996;27:204-209.

20. Liu K, Slattery M, Jacobs D Jr, et al. A study of the reliability and comparative validity of the cardia dietary history. *Ethn Dis.* 1994;4:15-27.

21. Schmidt LE, Cox MS, Buzzard IM, Cleary PA. Reproducibility of a comprehensive diet history in the Diabetes Control and Complications Trial. The DCCT Research Group. *J Am Diet Assoc.* 1994;94:1392-1397.

22. Hunter D. Biochemical indicators of dietary intake. In: Willet WC, ed. *Nutritional Epidemiology.* 2nd ed. New York: Oxford University Press; 1998.

23. Speakman JR. *Doubly Labeled Water: Theory and Practice.* London: Chapman & Hall; 1997.

24. Trabulsi J, Schoeller DA. Evaluation of dietary assessment instruments against doubly labeled water, a biomarker of habitual energy intake. *Am J Physiol Endocrinol Metab.* 2001;281:E891-E899.

25. Schoeller DA, Schoeller DA. Validation of habitual energy intake. *Public Health Nutr.* 2002;5:883-888.

26. Horton ES. Introduction: an overview of the assessment and regulation of energy balance in humans. *Am J Clin Nutr.* 1983;38:972-977.

27. Schofield WN. Predicting basal metabolic rate, new standards and review of previous work. *Hum Nutr Clin Nutr.* 1985;39(Suppl 1):5-41.

28. Mifflin MD, St Jeor ST, Hill LA, Scott BJ, Daugherty SA, Koh YO. A new predictive equation for resting energy expenditure in healthy individuals. *Am J Clin Nutr.* 1990;51:241-247.

29. Goldberg GR, Black AE, Jebb SA, et al. Critical evaluation of energy intake data using fundamental principles of energy physiology: 1. Derivation of cut-off limits to identify under-recording. *Eur J Clin Nutr.* 1991;45:569-581.

30. Black AE. Critical evaluation of energy intake using the Goldberg cut-off for energy intake: basal metabolic rate. A practical guide to its calculation, use and limitations. *Int J Obes Relat Metab Disord.* 2000;24:1119-1130.

31. Bingham SA, Cummings JH. Urine nitrogen as an independent validatory measure of dietary intake: a study of nitrogen balance in individuals consuming their normal diet. *Am J Clin Nutr.* 1985;42:1276-1289.

32. Matthews DE. Proteins and amino acids. In: Shils ME, Olson JA, Shike M, et al., eds. *Modern Nutrition in Health and Disease.* 9th ed. Baltimore, MD: Williams & Wilkins Company; 1999:11-48.

33. Margetts BM, Nelson M. *Design Concepts in Nutritional Epidemiology.* 2nd ed. New York: Oxford University Press; 1997.

34. Kesteloot H, Joossens JV. The relationship between dietary intake and urinary excretion of sodium, potassium, calcium, and magnesium: Belgian Interuniversity Research on Nutrition and Health. *J Hum Hypertens.* 1990;4:527-533.

35. Liu K, Stamler J. Assessment of sodium intake in epidemiological studies on blood pressure. *Ann Clin Res.* 1984;16(Suppl):49-54.

36. Holbrook JT, Patterson KY, Bodner JE, et al. Sodium and potassium intake and balance in adults consuming self-selected diets. *Am J Clin Nutr.* 1984;40:786-793.

37. Zhang J, Temme EH, Sasaki S, Kesteloot H. Under- and overreporting of energy intake using urinary cations as biomarkers: relation to body mass index. *Am J Epidemiol.* 2000;152:453-462.

38. Mensink RP, Katan MB. Effect of dietary fatty acids on serum lipids and lipoproteins. A meta-analysis of 27 trials. *Arterioscler Thromb.* 1992;12:911-919.

39. Willett W, Stampfer M, Chu NF, Spiegelman D, Holmes M, Rimm E. Assessment of questionnaire validity for measuring total fat intake using plasma lipid levels as criteria. *Am J Epidemiol.* 2001;154:1107-1112.

40. Baylin A, Campos H. The use of fatty acid biomarkers to reflect dietary intake. *Curr Opin Lipidol.* 2006;17:22-27.

41. Keys A. Serum cholesterol response to dietary cholesterol. *Am J Clin Nutr.* 1984;40:351-359.

42. Hegsted DM, Ausman LM, Johnson JA, Dallal GE. Dietary fat and serum lipids: an evaluation of the experimental data. *Am J Clin Nutr.* 1993;57:875-883.

43. Sun Q, Ma J, Campos H, Hankinson SE, Hu FB. Comparison between plasma and erythrocyte fatty acid content as biomarkers of fatty acid intake in U.S. women. *Am J Clin Nutr.* 2007;86(1):74-81.

44. Baylin A, Kim MK, Donovan-Palmer A, et al. Fasting whole blood as a biomarker of essential fatty acid intake in epidemiologic studies: comparison with adipose tissue and plasma. *Am J Epidemiol.* 2005;162:373-381.

45. Dayton S, Hashimoto S, Dixon W, Pearce ML. Composition of lipids in human serum and adipose tissue during prolonged feeding of a diet high in unsaturated fat. *J Lipid Res.* 1966;7:103-111.

46. Ma J, Folsom AR, Shahar E, Eckfeldt JH. Plasma fatty acid composition as an indicator of habitual dietary fat intake in middle-aged adults. The Atherosclerosis Risk in Communities (ARIC) Study Investigators. *Am J Clin Nutr.* 1995;62:564-571.

47. Wolk A, Vessby B, Ljung H, Barrefors P. Evaluation of a biological marker of dairy fat intake. *Am J Clin Nutr.* 1998;68:291-295.

48. Baylin A, Kabagambe EK, Siles X, Campos H. Adipose tissue biomarkers of fatty acid intake. *Am J Clin Nutr.* 2002;76:750-757.

49. Sun Q, Ma J, Campos H, Hankinson S, Hu FB. Plasma and erythrocyte biomarkers of dairy fat intake and risk of coronary heart disease. *Am J Clin Nutr.* 2007;86:929-937.

50. Liu S, Manson JE, Stampfer MJ, et al. Dietary glycemic load assessed by food-frequency questionnaire in relation to plasma high-density-lipoprotein cholesterol and fasting plasma triacylglycerols in postmenopausal women. *Am J Clin Nutr.* 2001; 73:560-566.

51. Selhub J. Folate, vitamin B12 and vitamin B6 and one carbon metabolism. *J Nutr Health Aging.* 2002;6:39-42.
52. Stanger O. Physiology of folic acid in health and disease. *Curr Drug Metab.* 2002;3:211-223.
53. Mason JB. Biomarkers of nutrient exposure and status in one-carbon (methyl) metabolism. *J Nutr.* 2003;133:941S-947S.
54. Cho E, Zeisel SH, Jacques P, et al. Dietary choline and betaine assessed by food-frequency questionnaire in relation to plasma total homocysteine concentration in the Framingham Offspring Study. *Am J Clin Nutr.* 2006;83:905-911.
55. Selhub J, Jacques PF, Wilson PW, Rush D, Rosenberg IH. Vitamin status and intake as primary determinants of homocysteinemia in an elderly population. *JAMA.* 1993;270:2693-2698.
56. Jacques PF, Sulsky SI, Sadowski JA, Phillips JC, Rush D, Willett WC. Comparison of micronutrient intake measured by a dietary questionnaire and biochemical indicators of micronutrient status. *Am J Clin Nutr.* 1993;57:182-189.
57. Green TJ, Allen OB, O'Connor DL. A three-day weighed food record and a semiquantitative food-frequency questionnaire are valid measures for assessing the folate and vitamin B-12 intakes of women aged 16 to 19 years. *J Nutr.* 1998; 128:1665-1671.
58. van der Schouw YT, de Kleijn MJ, Peeters PH, Grobbee DE. Phyto-oestrogens and cardiovascular disease risk. *Nutr Metab Cardiovasc Dis.* 2000;10:154-167.
59. de Kleijn MJ, van der Schouw YT, Wilson PW, et al. Intake of dietary phytoestrogens is low in postmenopausal women in the United States: the Framingham study(1-4). *J Nutr.* 2001;131:1826-1832.
60. Karr SC, Lampe JW, Hutchins AM, Slavin JL. Urinary isoflavonoid excretion in humans is dose dependent at low to moderate levels of soy-protein consumption. *Am J Clin Nutr.* 1997;66:46-51.
61. Adlercreutz H, Fotsis T, Lampe J, et al. Quantitative determination of lignans and isoflavonoids in plasma of omnivorous and vegetarian women by isotope dilution gas chromatography-mass spectrometry. *Scand J Clin Lab Invest Suppl.* 1993;215:5-18.
62. Lampe JW. Isoflavonoid and lignan phytoestrogens as dietary biomarkers. *J Nutr.* 2003;133(Suppl 3):956S-964S.
63. Seow A, Shi CY, Franke AA, Hankin JH, Lee HP, Yu MC. Isoflavonoid levels in spot urine are associated with frequency of dietary soy intake in a population-based sample of middle-aged and older Chinese in Singapore. *Cancer Epidemiol Biomarkers Prev.* 1998;7:135-140.
64. Chen Z, Zheng W, Custer LJ, et al. Usual dietary consumption of soy foods and its correlation with the excretion rate of isoflavonoids in overnight urine samples among Chinese women in Shanghai. *Nutr Cancer.* 1999;33:82-87.
65. Hambidge M. Biomarkers of trace mineral intake and status. *J Nutr.* 2003;133(Suppl 3):948S-955S.
66. Liu JM, Hankinson SE, Stampfer MJ, Rifai N, Willett WC, Ma J. Body iron stores and their determinants in healthy postmenopausal US women. *Am J Clin Nutr.* 2003;78:1160-1167.
67. Swanson CA, Longnecker MP, Veillon C, et al. Selenium intake, age, gender, and smoking in relation to indices of selenium status of adults residing in a seleniferous area. *Am J Clin Nutr.* 1990;52:858-862.
68. Hunter DJ, Morris JS, Chute CG, et al. Predictors of selenium concentration in human toenails. *Am J Epidemiol.* 1990;132:114-122.
69. Longnecker MP, Stampfer MJ, Morris JS, et al. A 1-y trial of the effect of high-selenium bread on selenium concentrations in blood and toenails. *Am J Clin Nutr.* 1993;57:408-413.
70. Garland M, Morris JS, Colditz GA, et al. Toenail trace element levels and breast cancer: a prospective study. *Am J Epidemiol.* 1996;144:653-660.

71. Martini MC, Campbell DR, Gross MD, Grandits GA, Potter JD, Slavin JL. Plasma carotenoids as biomarkers of vegetable intake: the University of Minnesota Cancer Prevention Research Unit Feeding Studies. *Cancer Epidemiol Biomarkers Prev.* 1995;4:491-496.

72. Livingstone MB, Black AE. Markers of the validity of reported energy intake. *J Nutr.* 2003;133(Suppl 3):895S-920S.

73. Nelson M. The validation of dietary assessment. In: Margetts BM, Nelson MC, eds. *Design Concepts in Nutritional Epidemiology.* 2nd ed. New York: Oxford University Press; 1997;241-272;Chapter 8.

74. Rimm EB, Giovannucci EL, Stampfer MJ, Colditz GA, Litin LB, Willett WC. Reproducibility and validity of an expanded self-administered semiquantitative food-frequency questionnaire among male health professionals. *Am J Epidemiol.* 1992;135:1114.

75. Feskanich D, Rimm EB, Giovannucci EL, et al. Reproducibility and validity of food intake measurements from a semiquantitative food-frequency questionnaire. *J Am Diet Assoc.* 1993;93:790-796.

76. Salvini S, Hunter DJ, Sampson L, et al. Food-based validation of a dietary questionnaire: the effects of week-to-week variation in food consumption. *Int J Epidemiol.* 1989;18:858-867.

77. Kroke A, Klipstein-Grobusch K, Voss S, et al. Validation of a self-administered food-frequency questionnaire administered in the European Prospective Investigation into Cancer and Nutrition (EPIC) Study: comparison of energy, protein, and macronutrient intakes estimated with the doubly labeled water, urinary nitrogen, and repeated 24-h dietary recall methods. *Am J Clin Nutr.* 1999;70:439-447.

78. Shu XO, Yang G, Jin F, et al. Validity and reproducibility of the food-frequency questionnaire used in the Shanghai Women's Health Study. *Eur J Clin Nutr.* 2004; 58:17-23.

79. Caan BJ, Slattery ML, Potter J, Quesenberry CP Jr, Coates AO, Schaffer DM. Comparison of the Block and the Willett self-administered semiquantitative food-frequency questionnaires with an interviewer-administered dietary history. *Am J Epidemiol.* 1998;148:1137-1147.

80. Wirfalt AK, Jeffery RW, Elmer PJ. Comparison of food-frequency questionnaires: the reduced Block and Willett questionnaires differ in ranking on nutrient intakes. *Am J Epidemiol.* 1998;148:1148-1156.

81. Rimm EB, Klatsky A, Grobbee D, Stampfer MJ. Review of moderate alcohol consumption and reduced risk of coronary heart disease: is the effect due to beer, wine, or spirits. *BMJ.* 1996;312:731-736.

82. Giovannucci E, Colditz G, Stampfer MJ, et al. The assessment of alcohol consumption by a simple self-administered questionnaire. *Am J Epidemiol.* 1991;133:810-817.

83. Kroke A, Klipstein-Grobusch K, Hoffmann K, Terbeck I, Boeing H, Helander A. Comparison of self-reported alcohol intake with the urinary excretion of 5-hydroxytryptophol:5-hydroxyindole-3-acetic acid, a biomarker of recent alcohol intake. *Br J Nutr.* 2001;85:621-627.

84. Kaaks RJ. Biochemical markers as additional measurements in studies of the accuracy of dietary questionnaire measurements: conceptual issues. *Am J Clin Nutr.* 1997;65(4 Suppl):1232S-1239S.

85. Kabagambe EK, Baylin A, Allan DA, Siles X, Spiegelman D, Campos H. Application of the method of triads to evaluate the performance of food-frequency questionnaires and biomarkers as indicators of long-term dietary intake. *Am J Epidemiol.* 2001;154:1126-1135.

86. Ocke MC, Kaaks RJ. Biochemical markers as additional measurements in dietary validity studies: application of the method of triads with examples from the European Prospective Investigation into Cancer and Nutrition. *Am J Clin Nutr.* 1997;65(4 Suppl):1240S-1245S.

87. Bhakta D, dos Santos Silva I, Higgins C, et al. A semiquantitative food-frequency questionnaire is a valid indicator of the usual intake of phytoestrogens by south Asian women in the UK relative to multiple 24-h dietary recalls and multiple plasma samples. *J Nutr.* 2005;135:116-123.

88. McNaughton SA, Marks GC, Gaffney P, Williams G, Green A. Validation of a food-frequency questionnaire assessment of carotenoid and vitamin E intake using weighed food records and plasma biomarkers: the method of triads model. *Eur J Clin Nutr.* 2005;59:211-218.

89. Willett W. Invited commentary: a further look at dietary questionnaire validation. *Am J Epidemiol.* 2001;154:1100.

90. Hu FB, Stampfer MJ, Manson JE, et al. Dietary fat intake and the risk of coronary heart disease in women. *N Engl J Med.* 1997;337:1491-1499.

91. Subar AF, Kipnis V, Troiano RP, et al. Using intake biomarkers to evaluate the extent of dietary misreporting in a large sample of adults: the OPEN study. *Am J Epidemiol.* 2003;158:1-13.

92. Saltzman E, Roberts SB. The role of energy expenditure in energy regulation: findings from a decade of research. *Nutr Rev.* 1995;53:209-220.

93. Willett W, Stampfer MJ. Total energy intake: implications for epidemiologic analyses. *Am J Epidemiol.* 1986;124:17-27.

94. Brown CC, Kipnis V, Freedman LS, Hartman AM, Schatzkin A, Wacholder S. Energy adjustment methods for nutritional epidemiology: the effect of categorization. *Am J Epidemiol.* 1994;139:323-338.

95. Hu FB, Stampfer MJ, Rimm E, et al. Dietary fat and coronary heart disease: a comparison of approaches for adjusting for total energy intake and modeling repeated dietary measurements. *Am J Epidemiol.* 1999;149:531-540.

96. Schulze MB, Manson JE, Ludwig DS, et al. Sugar-sweetened beverages, weight gain, and incidence of type 2 diabetes in young and middle-aged women. *JAMA.* 2004;292:927-934.

97. Beaton GH, Milner J, Corey P, et al. Sources of variance in 24-hour dietary recall data: implications for nutrition study design and interpretation. *Am J Clin Nutr.* 1979;32:2546-2559.

98. Beaton GH, Milner J, McGuire V, Feather TE, Little JA. Source of variance in 24-hour dietary recall data: implications for nutrition study design and interpretation. Carbohydrate sources, vitamins, and minerals. *Am J Clin Nutr.* 1983;37:986-995.

99. Liu K, Stamler J, Dyer A, McKeever J, McKeever P. Statistical methods to assess and minimize the role of intra-individual variability in obscuring the relationship between dietary lipids and serum cholesterol. *J Chronic Dis.* 1978;31:399-418.

100. Rosner B, Willett WC. Interval estimates for correlation coefficients corrected for within-person variation: implications for study design and hypothesis testing. *Am J Epidemiol.* 1988;127:377-386.

101. Rosner B, Willett WC, Spiegelman D. Correction of logistic regression relative risk estimates and confidence intervals for systematic within-person measurement error. *Stat Med.* 1989;8:1051-1069.

102. Koh-Banerjee P, Chu NF, Spiegelman D, et al. Prospective study of the association of changes in dietary intake, physical activity, alcohol consumption, and smoking with 9-y gain in waist circumference among 16 587 US men. *Am J Clin Nutr.* 2003;78:719-727.

103. Liu S, Willett WC, Manson JE, Hu FB, Rosner B, Colditz G. Relation between changes in intakes of dietary fiber and grain products and changes in weight and development of obesity among middle-aged women. *Am J Clin Nutr.* 2003;78:920-927.

104. Hu FB. Dietary pattern analysis: a new direction in nutritional epidemiology. *Curr Opin Lipidol.* 2002;13:3-9.

105. Kleinbaum DG, Kupper LL, Muller KE. Chapter 24. Variable reduction and factor analysis. *Applied Regression Analysis and Other Multivariate Methods.* Boston: PWS-KENT Publishing Company; 1988:595-640.

106. Newby PK, Muller D, Hallfrisch J, Andres R, Tucker KL. Food patterns measured by factor analysis and anthropometric changes in adults. *Am J Clin Nutr.* 2004;80:504-513.
107. van Dam RM, Rimm EB, Willett WC, Stampfer MJ, Hu FB. Dietary patterns and risk for type 2 diabetes mellitus in U.S. men. *Ann Intern Med.* 2002;136:201-209.
108. Fung TT, Hu FB, Holmes MD, et al. Dietary patterns and the risk of postmenopausal breast cancer. *Int J Cancer.* 2005;116:116-121.
109. Hu FB, Rimm E, Smith-Warner SA, et al. Reproducibility and validity of dietary patterns assessed with a food-frequency questionnaire. *Am J Clin Nutr.* 1999;69: 243-249.
110. Millen BE, Quatromoni PA, Copenhafer DL, Demissie S, O'Horo CE, D'Agostino RB. Validation of a dietary pattern approach for evaluating nutritional risk: the Framingham Nutrition Studies. *J Am Diet Assoc.* 2001;101:187-194.
111. Tucker KL, Dallal GE, Rush D. Dietary patterns of elderly Boston-area residents defined by cluster analysis. *J Am Diet Assoc.* 1992;92:1487-1491.
112. Wirfalt AK, Jeffery RW. Using cluster analysis to examine dietary patterns: nutrient intakes, gender, and weight status differ across food pattern clusters. *J Am Diet Assoc.* 1997;97:272-279.
113. Newby PK, Tucker KL. Empirically derived eating patterns using factor or cluster analysis: a review. *Nutr Rev.* 2004;62:177-203.
114. Newby PK, Muller D, Hallfrisch J, Qiao N, Andres R, Tucker KL. Dietary patterns and changes in body mass index and waist circumference in adults. *Am J Clin Nutr.* 2003;77:1417-1425.
115. Fung TT, McCullough ML, Newby PK, et al. Diet-quality scores and plasma concentrations of markers of inflammation and endothelial dysfunction. *Am J Clin Nutr.* 2005;82:163-173.
116. Kant AK. Dietary patterns and health outcomes. *J Am Diet Assoc.* 2004;104:615-635.
117. Newby PK, Hu FB, Rimm EB, et al. Reproducibility and validity of the Diet Quality Index Revised as assessed by use of a food-frequency questionnaire. *Am J Clin Nutr.* 2003;78:941-949.
118. Kennedy ET, Ohls J, Carlson S, Fleming K. The Healthy Eating Index: design and applications. *J Am Diet Assoc.* 1995;95:1103-1108.
119. Kant AK, Schatzkin A, Graubard BI, Schairer C. A prospective study of diet quality and mortality in women. *JAMA.* 2000;283:2109-2115.
120. Martinez-Gonzalez MA, Fernandez-Jarne E, Serrano-Martinez M, Marti A, Martinez JA, Martin-Moreno JM. Mediterranean diet and reduction in the risk of a first acute myocardial infarction: an operational healthy dietary score. *Eur J Nutr.* 2002;41:153-160.
121. Trichopoulou A. Traditional Mediterranean diet and longevity in the elderly: a review. *Public Health Nutr.* 2004;7:943-947.
122. McCullough ML, Feskanich D, Stampfer MJ, et al. Diet quality and major chronic disease risk in men and women: moving toward improved dietary guidance. *Am J Clin Nutr.* 2002;76:1261-1271.
123. Kennedy E. Dietary diversity, diet quality, and body weight regulation. *Nutr Rev.* 2004;62(7 Pt 2):S78-S81.
124. Trichopoulos D, Lagiou P. Dietary patterns and mortality. *Br J Nutr.* 2001;85:133-134.
125. Hoffmann K, Schulze MB, Schienkiewitz A, Nothlings U, Boeing H. Application of a new statistical method to derive dietary patterns in nutritional epidemiology. *Am J Epidemiol.* 2004;159:935-944.
126. Hoffmann K, Zyriax BC, Boeing H, Windler E. A dietary pattern derived to explain biomarker variation is strongly associated with the risk of coronary artery disease. *Am J Clin Nutr.* 2004;80:633-640.
127. Schulze MB, Hoffmann K. Methodological approaches to study dietary patterns in relation to risk of coronary heart disease and stroke. *Br J Nutr.* 2006;95: 860-869.

128. Weikert C, Hoffmann K, Dierkes J, et al. A homocysteine metabolism-related dietary pattern and the risk of coronary heart disease in two independent German study populations. *J Nutr.* 2005;135:1981-1988.

129. Schulze MB, Hoffmann K, Manson JE, et al. Dietary pattern, inflammation, and incidence of type 2 diabetes in women. *Am J Clin Nutr.* 2005;82:675-684.

130. Third National Health and Nutrition Examination Survey (NHANES III) Public-Use Data Files. U.S. Department of Health and Human Services, Centers for Disease Control and Prevention, National Center for Health Statistics, 2004.

131. Bingham SA, Luben R, Welch A, Wareham N, Khaw KT, Day N. Are imprecise methods obscuring a relation between fat and breast cancer? *Lancet.* 2003;362:212-214.

7

Physical Activity Measurements

Frank B. Hu

Physical activity is a major determinant of between-person differences in total energy expenditure (see Chapter 6). To understand more fully the causes of obesity and to design effective prevention and intervention strategies, it is important to accurately quantify physical activity levels. However, the effects of physical activity on health go far beyond energy balance. Much evidence indicates that type and intensity of activity have many health benefits independent of adiposity. The purpose of physical activity measures is not only to obtain accurate assessments of energy expenditure but also to capture complex dimensions of physical activity, including type, duration, frequency, and intensity. From this perspective, strong parallels exist between assessment of dietary composition and physical activity measurements. Both variables represent complex behaviors with large day-to-day variations. In both cases, the primary focus of epidemiologic studies is to measure long-term, habitual patterns.

As with dietary assessment tools, measures of physical activity are prone to errors from day-to-day variations, inaccurate memory and estimation, and biased recalls associated with obesity status. To some degree, it is more challenging to measure different dimensions of physical activity—especially moderate activities that are part of routine daily life—than it is to measure dietary variables. Despite these challenges, epidemiologic studies have produced strong evidence, even with crude instruments, for the benefits of physical activity on a wide range of health outcomes, including body weight (see Chapter 15). Perhaps more refined instruments and automated technology will enable researchers to identify more subtle effects of physical activity on health outcomes.

In this chapter, we begin by discussing conceptual definitions and the multidimensional aspects of physical activity and exercise. Next, we describe self-reported methods and monitoring devices for measuring physical activity that are commonly used in epidemiologic studies. Then we discuss validation studies of physical activity questionnaires and methods used to correct for measurement errors in analyses of physical activity and obesity and weight change.

Conceptual Definitions

The terms *physical activity, exercise,* and *physical fitness* have been defined in a variety of ways and sometimes used interchangeably. However, these terms have clear and distinct definitions with important implications for measurements. Physical activity is "any bodily movement produced by skeletal muscles that results in calorie expenditure."[1] This definition "incorporates all forms of movement as physical activity and operationalizes these movements as contributors to overall energy expenditure."[2] Exercise is a subset of physical activity, defined as "physical activity that is planned or structured. It involves repetitive bodily movement done to improve or maintain one or more of the components of physical fitness—cardiorespiratory endurance (aerobic fitness), muscular strength, muscular endurance, flexibility, and body composition." Physical fitness, in turn, is defined as "a set of attributes that people have or achieve that relates to the ability to perform physical activity."[3] Thus, while physical activity is a behavior, physical fitness is a functional attribute that can be influenced by physical activity.

Physical activity can be characterized by type and intensity. Broad categories of physical activities include occupational, transportation, household, and leisure-time. Occupational physical activities are performed regularly as part of one's job (e.g., walking, hauling, lifting, pushing, carpentry work, shoveling, and packing boxes).[3] Leisure-time physical activities consist of exercise, sports, recreation, or hobbies that are not associated with regular job-, household-, or transportation-related activities. Metabolically, exercise can be classified as aerobic (with oxygen) or anaerobic (without oxygen). Examples of aerobic exercise include walking or hiking, running, jogging, cycling, cross-country skiing, rowing, stair climbing, aerobic dancing, swimming, and skating. Resistance training, such as weight lifting, is anaerobic exercise used to increase muscular size, strength, and endurance. Stretching exercises increase muscle flexibility. The type of physical activity directly affects its intensity, energy expenditure, and health outcomes.

Intensity can be defined in absolute or relative terms.[4] Absolute intensity is usually expressed in metabolic equivalent tasks (METs), which estimate the amount of oxygen consumed or rate of energy expenditure. One MET (the energy expended by sitting quietly) is equivalent to 3.5 mL of oxygen uptake per kilogram of body weight per minute or 1 kcal/kg of body weight per hour. For example, 1 hour of running is equivalent to 7 METs and 1 hour of brisk walking is equivalent to 4 METs. Ainsworth et al.[5,6] published an extensive compendium of MET values for different types of physical activities. They considered light-intensity activities to be those that require less than 3 METs; moderate intensity, 3 to 6 METs; and vigorous activity >6 METs. However, these cutoff points are arbitrary, and the associated percents of maximal capacity may vary with age and physical fitness. The cutoff value of 6 METs for vigorous activity is considered too low for adults who are younger or more fit but too high for those who are older or less fit.[2] Also, MET values, which are derived from nonobese individuals, may be less accurate for obese subjects.[7] MET values for obese subjects are likely to be overestimated during nonweight-bearing activities but underestimated during weight-bearing activities.[7] Also, metabolic costs associated with individual physical activities are typically based on data for young adults, and thus, tend to overestimate energy expenditure in older people.[8,9] Spadano et al.[10] observed that body weight strongly influenced energy costs of activity in 12-year-old girls; that use of average MET values to estimate energy costs of walking would lead to underestimation in heavier girls and overestimation in thinner ones.

Relative intensity refers to "the relative percentage of maximal aerobic power that is maintained during exercise."[4] It can be expressed as percentage of maximal oxygen uptake ($VO_{2 max}$), percentage of maximum heart rate (HR max), or Borg Rating of Perceived Exertion (RPE). $VO_{2 max}$ is the maximum amount of oxygen uptake in milliliters (in 1 minute/kg of body weight) during exercise. There is a linear relationship between increase in oxygen uptake and increase in heart rate. Borg[11] developed the RPE, which is based on a scale from 6 to 20, to describe a person's perception of exertion during exercise. Activities that are 40% to 60% of $VO_{2\,max}$ are generally considered moderate intensity, which corresponds to absolute intensity of 4.0 to 6.0 METs for middle-aged persons and 2.0 to 3.0 METs for those older than 80 years of age (Table 7.1).

Inactivity and Sedentary Behaviors

Inactivity is defined as "not engaging in any regular pattern of physical activity beyond daily functioning" or "a state in which bodily movement is minimal."[3] Physical inactivity is closely related to sedentary behaviors; that is, those that expend little energy beyond resting metabolic rate (RMR), such as watching television (TV), reading, working on a computer, and passive commuting (e.g., riding in a car).[6] Among these behaviors, TV watching is the most common sedentary behavior in both adults and children. Although leisure-time physical activity is generally low in the United States, there is no evidence that it has declined in recent decades.[12] However, sedentary lifestyles have become more prevalent, a trend reflected by increasing time spent watching TV and using computers. Growth in sedentary behaviors, especially TV watching, may be contributing to the obesity epidemic in the United States.

In epidemiologic studies, the correlation between sedentary behaviors and physical activity is minimal,[13] suggesting that sedentary behaviors are not simply the opposite of physical activity. TV watching is frequently associated with increased caloric intake and unhealthy eating patterns, probably owing to constant exposure to food advertisements.[14] It is now well established that independent of physical activity, prolonged TV watching is associated with obesity in both children[15,16] and adults.[13,17]

Nonexercise Activity Thermogenesis

Levine et al.[18] devised the concept of nonexercise activity thermogenesis (NEAT) to aggregate "the energy expenditure of all physical activities other than volitional sporting-like exercise." NEAT ranges from energy expended walking to that used in fidgeting, and includes daily activities such as typing, yard work, occupational activities, household chores, and shopping. NEAT is determined by both genetic and environmental factors.[18] In that exercise-related energy expenditure is typically very low, NEAT explains the majority of between-person variations in total daily energy expenditure. As such, it plays an important role in weight gain and obesity.

However, measurements of NEAT are difficult to obtain because virtually all NEAT activities in modern societies are of light to moderate intensity, and many are incorporated into daily routines. In addition, it is almost impossible to measure energy expenditure due to fidgeting in free-living populations. However, because total energy expenditure is the sum of RMR, the thermic effect of food (TEF), energy expenditure due to exercise, and NEAT, an alternative approach can be used to estimate total NEAT: subtraction of RMR (measured by indirect calorimetry), energy expenditure due to exercise, and TEF (estimated as 10% of total energy expenditure) from total daily energy expenditure (which can be measured by doubly labeled water [DLW], see below). This approach, however, is expensive, time consuming, and burdensome for participants, and is therefore not feasible for large epidemiologic studies. In addition, a representative assessment of NEAT probably requires multiple-day measurements across different seasons to offset large day-to-day variability. In sum, despite the conceptual appeal of NEAT, quantifying it is not practical in large epidemiological studies.

Table 7.1 Classification of Physical Activity Intensity*

| Intensity | Relative Intensity | | | Endurance-Type Activity | | | | Strength-Type Exercise/Relative Intensity* |
| | | | | Absolute Intensity in Healthy Adults (Age), METs | | | | |
	$VO_{2\,max}$ %	Maximum Heart Rate, %	RPE†	Young (20-39)	Middle-aged (40-64)	Old (65-79)	Very Old (80+)	Maximum Voluntary Contraction, %
Very light	<20	<35	<10	<2.4	<2.0	<1.6	<1.0	<30
Light	20-39	35-54	10-11	2.4-4.7	2.0-3.9	1.6-3.1	1.1-1.9	30-49
Moderate	40-59	55-69	12-13	4.8-7.1	4.0-5.9	3.2-4.7	2.0-2.9	50-69
Hard	60-84	70-89	14-16	7.2-10.1	6.0-8.4	4.8-6.7	3.0-4.25	70-84
Very hard	≥85	≥90	17-19	≥10.2	≥8.5	≥6.8	≥4.24	≥85
Maximum‡	100	100	20	12.0	10.0	8.0	5.0	100

* Based on 8 to 12 repetitions for persons <50 to 60 y old and 10 to 15 repetitions for persons aged >60 y.

† Borg rating of Relative Perceived Exertion (RPE), 6 to 20 scale.

‡ Maximum values are mean values achieved during maximum exercise by healthy adults. Absolute intensity values are approximate mean values for men. Mean values for women are −1 to 2 METs lower than those for men.

Reproduced with permission from Fletcher GF, Balady GJ, Amsterdam EA, et al. Exercise standards for testing and training: a statement for healthcare professionals from the American Heart Association. Circulation. 2001;104:1694-1740.[4]

Measuring Physical Activity

Physical activity is a complex and multifaceted behavior that is challenging to measure. Many approaches have been used to assess this variable in epidemiologic studies; each has its advantages and disadvantages. Several comprehensive reviews have discussed methods for measuring physical activity.[6,12,19,20] These methods have been broadly categorized as self-reported (e.g., physical diaries, logs, recalls, and questionnaires) or objective (e.g., activity monitors, DLW, indirect calorimetry, pedometers, and heart rate monitors). Table 7.2 lists advantages and disadvantages for each method.[21]

Various methods do not necessarily measure the same dimension of physical activity. Lamonte and Ainsworth[19] emphasized the conceptual distinction between physical activity and energy expenditure. Physical activity is a behavior that can be directly measured by motion detectors and physical activity records, while energy expenditure reflects the energy costs of behaviors that can be directly measured by DLW and indirectly by physiological parameters, such as heart rate and oxygen uptake (Fig. 7.1). Therefore, the two terms should not be used interchangeably. Although DLW is often used to validate self-reported measures, it reflects total energy expenditure due in part to physical activity but is not a direct measure of the behavior itself.

Objective Methods

Doubly Labeled Water

As discussed in Chapter 6, DLW is an objective and accurate measure of total energy expenditure in free-living subjects.[22] This method involves the oral administration of a carefully weighed dose of water containing enriched quantities of the stable isotopes deuterium (^2H) and oxygen-18 (^{18}O) to subjects who are required to provide several urine samples over days or weeks. The difference in disappearance rates between these two isotopes from the body water pool is a measure of carbon dioxide production from which total energy expenditure can be calculated.[23] This technique measures all volitional and nonvolitional activities with high accuracy and is thus widely used as the reference method for validating dietary and physical activity assessment instruments. However, it is expensive, time consuming, and cannot be used to determine the type, intensity, frequency, or duration of activities.[24]

Indirect Calorimetry

In contrast to direct calorimetry, which directly measures heat production by the body, indirect calorimetry calculates energy expenditure from a measurement of oxygen uptake and carbon dioxide production using established equations.[25] Advances in gas exchange measurement have made this technique practical, safer, and easier to use in free-living populations. In short-term studies, subjects wear a mouthpiece, face mask, or canopy during exercise; longer-term studies usually require confinement to a metabolic chamber for an extended period of time (i.e., 24 hours to assess RMR). RMR, which accounts for largest fraction of daily energy expenditure, is primarily determined by lean body mass, but it is also affected by age, sex, race, and physical fitness. RMR measured by indirect calorimetry, coupled with total daily energy expenditure measured by the DLW technique, can be used to estimate physical activity energy expenditure, assuming that

Table 7.2 Advantages and Disadvantages of Various Physical Activity Methods

Measure	Units of Measurement	Advantages	Disadvantages
Self-report (physical activity diaries or records)	Bouts of physical activity	• Captures quantitative and qualitative information • Detailed information on type, duration, frequency, and intensity of activities • Minimal recall bias • Information available to estimate energy expenditure from daily living (i.e., Compendium of Physical Activities)	• Expensive, time consuming • High participant burden • Multiple-day records for different seasons are needed to measure long-term physical activity pattern • May alter participants' physical activity behaviors
Self-report (physical activity questionnaire)	Bouts of physical activity	• Captures quantitative and qualitative information • Inexpensive, allowing large sample size • Usually low participant burden • Can be administered quickly • Information available to estimate energy expenditure from daily living (i.e., Compendium of Physical Activities)	• Reliability and validity problems associated with recall of activity • Potential content validity problems associated with misinterpretation of physical activity in different populations
Accelerometers	Movement counts	• Objective indicator of body movement (acceleration) • Useful in laboratory and field settings • Provides indicator of intensity, frequency, duration, and energy expenditure based on calibration equations • Noninvasive • Ease of data collection and analyses • Provides minute-by-minute information • Allows for extended periods of recording (weeks)	• Financial cost may prohibit assessment of large numbers of participants • Inaccurate assessment of a large range of activities (e.g., upper-body movement, incline walking, water-based activities) • Lack of field-based equations to accurately estimate energy expenditure in specific populations • Cannot guarantee accurate monitor placement on participants during long, unobserved periods of data collection
Heart rate monitor	Beats (per min)	• Physiological parameter • Good association with energy expenditure • Valid in laboratory and field settings • Low participant burden for limited recording periods (30 min to 6 h)	• Financial cost may prohibit assessment of large numbers of participants • Some discomfort for participants, especially over extended recording periods • Useful only for aerobic activities

Method	Measure	Advantages	Disadvantages
		• Describes intensity, frequency, and duration well (adults); energy expenditure estimates are based on calibration equations • Easy and quick for data collection and analyses	• Heart rate (HR) characteristics and the training state affect HR-VO_{2max} relation • Some uncertainty as to the best way of using HR data to predict energy expenditure
Pedometers	Step counts	• Inexpensive, noninvasive • Potential for use in a variety of settings, including workplaces and schools • Easy to administer to large groups • Potential to promote behavior change • Objective measure of common activity behavior (i.e., walking)	• Reduced accuracy when used to assess jogging or running • Possibility of participant tampering • Are specifically designed to assess walking only
Direct observation	Activity rating	• Provide excellent quantitative and qualitative information • Physical activity categories established a priori, allowing specific targeting of physical activity behaviors • Software programs now available to enhance data collection and recording	• Time-intensive training needed to establish between-observer and within-observer agreement • Labor- and time-intensive data collection, which limits the number of study participants • Observer presence may artificially alter normal physical activity patterns • Limited research reporting on validation of direct observation coding systems against physiological criteria
Indirect calorimetry	O_2 consumption, CO_2 production	• Precision of measure • Light portable devices have been developed	• High participant burden • High cost
Doubly labeled water (DLW)	Total energy expenditure by measuring disappearing rate of stable isotopes in urine	• Highly accurate • Gold standard for measuring total energy expenditure	• High participant burden • Not possible to differentiate different types of activity • High cost

Adapted from Dale D, Welk GJ, Matthews CE. Chapter 1. Methods for assessing physical activity and challenges for research. In: Welk GJ, ed. *Physical Activity Assessments for Health-Related Research.* Champaign, Illinois: Human Kinetics, Inc.; 2002:19-34.[21]

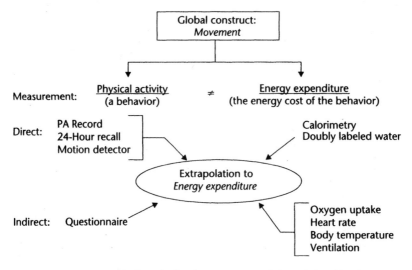

Figure 7.1 A conceptual model of methods of assessment and the relationships between movement, physical activity, and energy expenditure. Adapted from Lamonte MJ, Ainsworth BE. Quantifying energy expenditure and physical activity in the context of dose response. *Med Sci Sports Exerc.* 2001;33(6 Suppl):S370-S378.[19]

thermogenic effects of food account for 10% of total daily energy expenditure.[24] The formula is as follows:

$$\text{Physical activity energy expenditure (kcal/day)}$$
$$= (\text{total daily energy expenditure} \times 0.90) - \text{RMR}$$

Recently, Manini et al.[26] used the above method to calculate daily activity energy expenditure for 302 older adults in the Health ABC study. The estimated daily activity energy expenditure was 672 kcal/day (SD = 287). The authors found a significant inverse association between this variable and mortality risk during 6 years of follow-up. As exercise was minimal in this population, most of daily activity energy expenditure was NEAT.

Physical activity level (PAL) index is calculated as the ratio of total daily energy expenditure to RMR. As RMR is primarily determined by body size, PAL is *automatically* corrected for body weight. Typical PAL index ranges from 1.2 for completely resting, to 1.5 for sedentary work, 1.8 for moderately active individuals, and >2.0 for those who are highly active.[24]

The indirect calorimetry approach is relatively expensive and burdensome for participants. Thus, it is not feasible for large epidemiologic studies. However, because of its high accuracy, indirect calorimetry is widely used as a reference method for validating other physical activity assessment methods. The new generation of portable handheld devices for measuring RMR is likely to improve its acceptability and increase its use in field studies.[27]

Direct Observation

Direct observation of free-living physical activity behaviors can provide detailed and objective information on type, intensity, duration, and contexts of physical activity.[28] This method is particularly useful for assessing physical activity among young children, who have difficulty with self-reported methods. Several computer programs are now available to assist data collection and analyses. Although this method provides excellent quantitative and qualitative information on physical activity, it is time consuming and labor intensive, and may alter participants' usual physical activity patterns.

Pedometers

The pedometer is a device that measures steps in walking or running. Over the past few decades, many brands of pedometers have become commercially available.[29] Their reliability and validity vary with different models. Bassett et al.[30] compared the accuracy of five electronic pedometers (Freestyle, Pacer, Eddie Bauer, Yamax, and Accusplit) for measuring distance walked and found significant differences. The Yamax, Pacer, and Accusplit models demonstrated high accuracy. The Yamax Digi-Walker SW-200 (YX200) appeared to be more accurate than the Pacer and Eddie Bauer at slow-to-moderate speeds ($p < .05$), though no significant differences were seen at the fastest speed. Schneider et al.[31] compared the accuracy of 13 models of pedometers over a 24-hour period among 10 middle-aged males and females. The criterion pedometer, the Yamax, was worn on the left side of the body, with a comparison pedometer on the right. Measurements from the different pedometers ranged from underestimates of 25% to overestimates of 45%. The authors concluded that only four of the 13 brands were reasonably accurate for research purposes.

A review by Tudor-Locke et al.[32] found a strong correlation (median $r = .86$) between steps measured by pedometers and different brands of accelerometers (see below). There was a strong correlation ($r = .82$) between pedometers and time in observed activity of the subjects, and a negative correlation (median $r = -.44$) between pedometer outputs and time in observed inactivity. The correlation between pedometer output and observed steps appeared to depend on walking speed. Ambulatory activity (i.e., running and walking) or sitting produced the highest agreement. Conversely, the lowest level of accuracy was seen with slow walking. A subsequent study[33] showed an inverse correlation between pedometer output and prevalence of overweight (median $r = -.27$); a positive correlation between pedometer output and various fitness measures, for example, the 6-minute walk test (median $r = .69$) and the timed treadmill test (median $r = .41$); and a positive correlation with estimated maximum oxygen uptake (median $r = .22$). The magnitude of correlations varied with the different models of pedometers.

Since they are simple to use and inexpensive, pedometers are useful in physical activity intervention research and epidemiologic studies. However, they have important limitations, including an inability to store data, distinguish different intensities of walking and running, or capture data for activities other than walking. Different models of pedometers also vary widely in reliability and validity.

Tudor-Locke and Bassett[34] have proposed the following categories to classify pedometer-determined physical activity in healthy adults: sedentary (<5,000 steps/day); low active (5,000-7,499 steps per day); somewhat active (7,500-9,999 steps per day); and active (≥10,000 steps per day). Individuals who take >12,500 steps per day are classified as highly active. Such classifications, albeit arbitrary, can help monitor adherence to exercise programs and motivate participation in walking and other moderate intensity activities.

Accelerometers

Accelerometers are motion sensors that provide real-time monitoring of the frequency, duration, and intensity of all activities in free-living individuals. Over the years, advances in accelerometry-based technology have made motion sensing the most popular way to obtain objective assessments of physical activity in relatively small epidemiologic and clinical studies. (Several detailed reviews on this topic have recently been published.[35-38])

Accelerometers have clear practical advantages; they are portable, lightweight, noninvasive, and allow for extended periods of recording. Thus, they have been used to track physical activity, evaluate intervention programs, and monitor adherence. As their measurement errors are not correlated with those of self-reported methods, accelerometers are particularly useful for validating physical activity questionnaires and other self-reported instruments. As technology advances and costs continue to fall, the potential for use of accelerometers in relatively large-scale epidemiologic studies will increase. The Caltrac Personal Activity Monitor (Muscle Dynamics, Torrance, California) ushered in the first generation of devices for research purposes. Today several other monitors have become commercially available, including Tritrac-R3D, ActiGraph, Actical, BioTrainer, Actiwatch, and ActiTrac. ActiGraph (Actigraph, LLC, Fort Walton Beach, FL) has recently been used in the NHANES to monitor physical activity patterns in the U.S. population.[39]

The reliability and validity of accelerometry-based activity monitors have been extensively studied. In general, reports indicate relatively high interinstrument and within-individual reliability coefficients (intraclass correlation coefficients >0.90). Reliability appears to be higher for dynamic activities, such as walking and running, than for other activities (e.g., stepping, sliding, or cycling).[40] Laboratory-based validation studies in both adults[41] and children[42] have shown that raw movement counts derived from accelerators are strongly correlated with *criterion* measures, such as DWL and oxygen uptake ($VO_{2\,max}$). The correlations are weaker in field-based validation studies, where the validity of the accelerometers may vary with population characteristics and the activity being studied.[41]

For example, it is more difficult to use accelerometers to capture light activity or motion in older adults with limited mobility. Campell et al.[43] found that compared with portable indirect calorimetry, the Tritrac overestimated the energy expenditure of walking and jogging, and underestimated that of stair climbing and stationary cycling in middle-aged women. Similarly, Welk et al.[44] reported that various accelerometers consistently underestimated the energy costs of both indoor chores (i.e., sweeping, stacking, and vacuuming) and outdoor ones (i.e., shoveling, mowing grass, and raking leaves) by 38% to 48% compared with energy expenditure measured by indirect calorimetry. Accelerometers cannot usually capture energy expenditure from aquatic activities, such as swimming, and tend to substantially underestimate energy expenditure from static activities, such as cycling and weight lifting.[41]

Bassett et al.[45] tested the validity of four motion sensors for measuring energy expenditure during physical activities of moderate intensity in field and laboratory settings against energy expenditure measured using a portable indirect calorimeter. Participants wore three accelerometers (Computer Science and Applications [CSA], Inc. model 7164; Caloric; and Kens Select 2) and one pedometer (Amax SW-701). The mean error scores (calculated as indirect calorimetry minus device) across all activities ranged from 0.05 MET for CSA to 1.12 MET for Amax. The correlation coefficients ranged from 0.33 to 0.62 between indirect calorimetry and various motion sensors. Motion sensors tended to overestimate energy expenditure during walking but underestimate energy costs of light to moderate activities related to upper body movements. Similarly, a field study by Hendelman et al.[46] found that accelerometers substantially underestimated the metabolic costs of golf and household activities by 30% to 60%.

A literature review by Trost et al.[38] on methodological issues related to accelerometer-based assessments of physical activity in free-living individuals found no convincing evidence of greater validity or reliability for one make or model of accelerometer over another. Thus, they suggested that accelerometer selection be based on cost, technical support, and comparability with other studies. They also noted that the use of multiple accelerometers to estimate energy expenditure produced only marginal improvements in prediction power compared with estimates from a single accelerometer. In addition, there was no clear evidence that multiaxial accelerometers (detecting accelerations in multiple dimensions) are better for detecting physical activity than uniaxial devices (detecting motion in one plane, usually vertical). However, multiaxial accelerometers are more sensitive to light activities (e.g., slow walking), and provide more accurate measurements of static trunk movement in activities like cycling and rowing.[37] A newly developed accelerometer (Intelligent Device for Energy Expenditure and Activity [IDEEA]) has shown promising results in measuring type, duration, and intensity of physical activity and improving energy expenditure estimation in laboratory-based settings,[47,48] but field-based validation studies are needed.

Standardized placement of accelerometers on the body (typically mounted to the waist) can help to reduce extraneous variations in measurements, although evidence is lacking regarding the superiority of one position versus another.[36] Output of measurements can be expressed in multiple ways including total movement counts, energy expenditure calculated by prediction equations, or time spent performing individual activities. The estimated energy expenditure largely depend on the accuracy of prediction equations derived from various calibration studies,[49] which appear to be population-specific and can yield different activity cut points for defining various intensities of physical activity.[50] How to enhance the comparability of different calibration studies remains a challenge in the field.

To account for day-to-day variations and reliably estimate habitual physical activity in adults, Mathews et al.[51] suggested 3 to 5 days of monitoring (optimally 7 days, including 1 weekend day). Trost[52] recommended 4 to 9 days of monitoring for children and adolescents. In a subsequent study, Trost et al.[38] found that repeated measures across different seasons might be required to estimate long-term physical activity.

Accelerometer-based devices are an attractive way to measure physical activity in children.[53] In laboratory conditions with structured activities, accelerometer activity counts among children were found to be strongly correlated with energy expenditure measured by DLW and indirect calorimetry.[54,55] As in adult studies, accelerometer validity has been found to vary by type and intensity of activities.[56] Lopez-Alarcon et al.[57] reported that accelerometry had limited value in measuring free-living energy expenditure among very young children. An 8-day field test of Actiwatch activity monitors in children 4 to 6 years old showed that activity counts did not reflect total energy expenditure assessed by DLW and were not correlated with percentage fat mass.

Heart Rate Monitoring

Because of the linear relationship between heart rate increases and oxygen consumption of contracting skeletal muscles during moderate to vigorous physical activity, heart rate monitoring can provide a continuous record of physical activity energy expenditure in free-living populations.[58] Currently available heart rate monitors are lightweight, small, and have large data-storage capability. Heart rate data are used to predict energy expenditure by calibrating heart rate against the maximum volume of oxygen consumed ($VO_{2\,max}$). There are several approaches for estimating energy expenditure, including the flex heart rate (Flex HR) method,[59] percent heart rate reserve (% HRR), or % $VO_{2\,max}$ reserve.[60] In general, validation studies have demonstrated a moderate to high degree of accuracy of both Flex HR and % HRR methods in estimating energy expenditure measured by DLW and indirect calorimetry ($r = .54$ to $.98$).[58]

After correcting for age and fitness level, Strath et al.[60] reported a strong correlation between heart rate and energy expenditure ($r = .87$) measured by indirect calorimetry during field- and laboratory-based moderate intensity activities. However, the reliability and validity of heart rate monitors for measuring low-intensity physical activity are known to be considerably lower because of nonlinearity of heart rate and $VO_{2\,max}$ during resting and light activity.[58] Thus, heart rate monitors have been combined with accelerometry-based technology to assess sedentary and light activity. In addition, other factors (e.g., psychological stress or changes in body temperature) can influence heart rate. Extended periods of monitoring can cause skin irritation and discomfort, considering that multiple-day monitoring (including both weekdays and weekends) is required to reflect usual activity patterns.

There is some evidence that combining heart rate monitors with movement sensors can improve the precision and accuracy of physical activity measurements. Strath et al.[61] showed a higher accuracy of energy expenditure estimated by the simultaneous heart rate-motion sensor technique (CSA accelerometers and Yamax pedometer) than that estimated by heart rate and motion sensors used independently among 16 men and 14 women. The combined technique also provided more accurate estimates of energy expenditure at different intensities of activity.[62]

Physical Fitness

Although physical fitness and physical activity are closely related concepts, they are not synonymous and should not be used interchangeably. As already mentioned, physical fitness is a functional construct, while physical activity consists of behaviors. Bouchard and Shephard[63] refined the concept of health-related fitness by dividing it into four major components: cardiorespiratory endurance (or fitness), body composition, muscular strength, and flexibility. Among these components, cardiorespiratory fitness is the most extensively studied in clinical and epidemiologic settings.

Cardiorespiratory fitness, also termed aerobic fitness or endurance, is defined as "a health-related component of physical fitness that relates to the ability of the circulatory and respiratory systems to supply oxygen during sustained physical activity."[3] Habitual physical activity status is one of the major modifiable determinants of cardiorespiratory fitness. Other influencing factors include age, sex, genetics, and medical conditions.[64] In epidemiologic studies, assessments of cardiorespiratory fitness have been used as objective and surrogate measures of physical activity to validate self-reported physical activity questionnaires.

$VO_{2\,max}$, the gold standard or criterion measure of cardiorespiratory fitness and exercise capacity,[4] is the maximum volume of oxygen that muscles can use while performing dynamic exercises, such as walking, running, or cycling. It is commonly expressed as multiples of METs. $VO_{2\,max}$ is typically estimated according to a protocol that involves the performance of an activity, usually running or cycling, until exhaustion. The test can be performed on a treadmill or bicycle ergometer, and oxygen uptake can be accurately estimated from the rate of work (speed, grade, and resistance).[64] Cardiorespiratory fitness measures have been obtained in several relatively large epidemiologic studies, notably the Aerobics Center Longitudinal Study (ACLS),[65] Lipid Research Clinics Mortality

Follow-up Study (LRC),[66] and the Coronary Artery Risk Development in Young Adults (CARDIA) study.[67] Somewhat different maximal treadmill test protocols have been used in various studies. For example, ACLS used the Balke procedure,[68] whereas LRC used the Bruce protocol.[69] Despite these differences, these studies found a strong inverse association between cardiorespiratory fitness measures and cardiovascular disease incidence or mortality.[65,66]

In the NHANES 1999-2002, a submaximal treadmill exercise protocol was used to gather information on cardiorespiratory fitness levels based on age- and sex-specific cut points of estimated $VO_{2\,max}$.[70,71] The initial goal of the submaximal test was to achieve 75% of the age-predicted maximum heart rate (220–age); it was later modified to allow adolescents and adults to achieve up to 90% and 85%, respectively, of their age-predicted maximum heart rate. $VO_{2\,max}$ was extrapolated from submaximal heart rate response by assuming a linear relationship between oxygen uptake and heart rate. Because it relies on prediction equations, the submaximal treadmill test provides a less accurate measure of cardiorespiratory fitness than the maximal exercise test. Nonetheless, low fitness assessed by submaximal tests has been strongly associated with increased risk for overweight, obesity, and metabolic disorders in both adolescents and adults.[71]

Various field-testing procedures are also available for rapid assessments of cardiorespiratory fitness in large populations. These include Cooper's 12-minute run, the Canadian Home Fitness Test, the 2 km walk test, and the 20-minute shuttle run.[72] Fitchett[73] found significant positive correlations between the predicted $VO_{2\,max}$ for the submaximal tests and the measured $VO_{2\,max}$, although $VO_{2\,max}$ predicted by submaximal cycle ergometry and bench-stepping procedures significantly underestimated measured $VO_{2\,max}$. Similarly, Montgomery et al.[74] found a good correlation between predicted $VO_{2\,max}$ by the step and shuttle run tests and the maximal treadmill test.

Self-reported Methods

Self-reported methods include physical activity records and diaries, logs, recalls, and questionnaires. Physical activity questionnaires are the most commonly used method in large epidemiologic studies because they are practical, inexpensive, and put a low burden on participants.

Physical Activity Records or Diaries

Subjects using physical activity or diary methods are instructed to provide a detailed record of virtually all physical activity performed in a day. As with food records, accurate recall is facilitated by the recording of activities shortly after completion. Because detailed information is collected on type, duration, and intensity of activities, multiple-day physical activity records have been used as a *reference* method to calibrate physical activity questionnaires. However, several weeks of records over different seasons of the year are often required to represent long-term physical activity patterns. Therefore, this method puts a considerable burden on participants and may even influence their physical activity behavior. It has been reported that recording physical activity leads to increased physical activity (a phenomenon called "reactivity").[75] The recent development of handheld electronic diary systems may reduce the burden on participants and improve compliance. It can also facilitate automation of data entry and scoring of physical activity.

Physical Activity Logs

Logs differ from diaries in that participants record broad categories of activities (e.g., walking, running, sitting, and standing) rather than individual bouts of each activity during the day. A preexisting form is typically used. Similar to diaries, physical activity logs require substantial efforts from motivated participants. A digital activity log developed by the U.S. Department of Agriculture allows subjects to record duration and intensity of physical activity in a handheld computer.[76] This can potentially reduce subject burden and improve data quality.

Short-term Recalls

Physical activity short-term recalls are analogous to 24-hour diet recalls, although their time frames have ranged from 24 hours to 1 month. The Stanford Seven-Day Physical Activity Recall is a survey that collects information on moderate and vigorous exercise, work-related activity, walking, and gardening over the preceding 7 days.[77] Because of daily and weekly variations in physical activity, a large number of recalls may be required to capture long-term physical activity patterns. As with 24-hour diet recalls, unannounced telephone-administered interviews are used to ask participants to recall the amount of time spent during the past 24 hours in activities of various intensities for household, occupational, and leisure-time activities.[78] If a sufficient number of 24-hour recalls are obtained, this method can provide reasonably accurate data on long-term physical activity. However, it is time-consuming, expensive, and requires participants' cooperation and cognitive ability to recall and estimate.

Habitual Physical Activity Questionnaires

Physical activity questionnaires are the most commonly used tool to assess habitual physical activity patterns in large epidemiologic studies. They are analogous to FFQs in objectives (measurement of long-term patterns), formats (semiquantitative response categories), and time frames (the past several months to 1 year),[20] although habitual physical activity questionnaires are typically much shorter than FFQs. Items in physical activity questionnaires range from simple global questions (e.g., active vs nonactive) to comprehensive lists of activities. Questionnaires are designed to elicit information on multiple dimensions of physical activities, including types, average frequency, duration, and intensity.[20]

Typically, such questionnaires are relatively simple and can be self-administered with little burden on respondents. Participants are asked to report the average weekly time spent at a number of specified activities (e.g., walking or hiking outdoors, jogging, running, bicycling, swimming, tennis, squash or racquetball, calisthenics, or rowing, weight lifting, and heavy outdoor work). Some questionnaires also ask about time spent on sedentary behaviors, such as watching TV, or sitting at home, work or in transit. The response categories range from none to ≥40 hours/week. Other information requested includes the average daily number of flights of stairs climbed and walking pace.

Over the past two to three decades, more than 30 physical activity questionnaires have been developed. Detailed descriptions of some of the questionnaires and information on their reproducibility and validity can be found in several excellent reviews.[79,80] Specific questionnaires on occupational physical activity have also been developed.[80] There are questionnaires for specific populations, such as children[53] and the elderly.[81] Questionnaires have also been developed to assess lifetime physical activity.[82] In addition, an International Physical Activity Questionnaire has been used to collect physical activity information across nations in a standardized way.[83] Among the many physical activity questionnaires, the most commonly used ones include the Minnesota Leisure-Time Physical Activity Questionnaire,[84] the College Alumni Questionnaire,[85,86] the Lipid Research Clinics Questionnaire,[87] the Baecke Physical Activity Questionnaire,[88] the Nurses' Health Study Questionnaire,[89] the Godin Questionnaire,[90] and the Stanford Usual Activity Questionnaire.[77]

Total energy expenditure from physical activity can be derived from questionnaire data. Usually, time spent at each activity in hours per week is multiplied by typical energy expenditure expressed in METs, which are then summed over all activities to yield a MET-hour score. As discussed earlier, 1 MET is equivalent to RMR; an activity with 7 METs (e.g., running) expends seven times the energy as RMR. Thus, MET values represent relative physical activity energy expenditure. Since 1 MET is equivalent to 3.5 mL/kg/min of oxygen consumption or roughly 1 kcal/kg/min, RMR is approximately 60 kcal/hour for a subject weighing 60 kg. Thus, absolute physical activity energy expenditure can be calculated by multiplying MET-hour by RMR (Fig. 7.2).[75] Such estimates are based on the average value of physical activity energy cost for the population and average RMR estimates proportional to body mass; they cannot readily account for between-individual differences in energy costs and RMR.

Physical activity questionnaires have the conceptual advantage of assessing average long-term activity patterns. They are also relatively inexpensive and impose a low burden on participants. As such, they are practical for use in large epidemiologic studies. However, they also have well-recognized limitations.[91] Self-reporting of such complex behavior as physical activity through questionnaires is a cognitive challenge for many people, especially children and the elderly. Thus, questionnaire data are prone to both random and systematic errors. In general, subjects tend to overreport physical activity and underreport sedentary behaviors that are influenced by cultural and social desirability factors.[91] In the subsequent sections, we will discuss the reproducibility and validity of physical activity questionnaires and methods for correcting measurement errors.

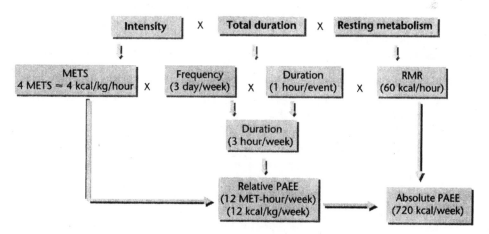

Figure 7.2 Computation of physical activity energy expenditure summary measures. PAEE, physical activity energy expenditure; RMR, resting metabolic rate. Adapted and reproduced with permission from Matthews CE. Use of self-report instruments to assess physical acitvity. In: Welk GJ, ed. *Physical Activity Assessments for Health-Related Research.* Champaign, IL: Human Kinetics, Inc., 2002; Chapter 7.[75]

Validation Studies of Physical Activity Questionnaires

Because of feasibility and cost considerations, large epidemiological studies rely primarily on physical activity questionnaires. Numerous such questionnaires have been developed and tested for their reproducibility (or test-retest reliability) and criterion-related validity. The major obstacle in physical activity questionnaire validation is lack of a true gold standard. In the literature, a variety of reference methods have been used in validation studies, including DLW, indirect calorimetry, accelerometry, fitness measures (maximal heart rate, $VO_{2\ max}$), and physical activity diary/records. These methods are considered more objective than questionnaires, but none can capture all dimensions of physical activity. Validity coefficients vary widely depending on the reference method used. Nevertheless, because measurement errors in the reference method are unlikely to be correlated with questionnaire-associated errors, carefully conducted validation studies can still provide useful information on the validity of questionnaires to measure long-term patterns of physical activity.

In a comprehensive review of available physical activity questionnaires, Pereira et al.[80] noted that most questionnaires had relatively high test-retest reliability correlation coefficients (0.5 to 0.8 for total and vigorous activity). However, validity coefficients were relatively low, especially for light to moderate intensity physical activity (typically less than 0.5). Most questionnaires focused on recreational physical activity because it is easier to recall than occupational, transportation, and household physical activity. In the general population, however, recreational physical activity accounts for only a small part of total physical activity.

Jacobs et al.[92] conducted one of the most detailed validation studies of 10 commonly used physical activity questionnaires among 78 men and women 20 to 59 years of age. Multiple reference methods were used, including treadmill exercise performance, vital capacity, body fatness, the average of 14 four-week physical activity histories, and the average of 14 two-day accelerometer readings. One-year reliability was high for all questionnaires measuring long-term physical activity (0.62 to 0.93). In fact, these coefficients were comparable to those for the reference measures (e.g., Caltrac accelerometer, body fatness, and treadmill tests). The validity of the questionnaires, however, varied with the types of activities and was generally low. Correlations were typically higher for total and vigorous or heavy activities than for light and household chores. In general, questionnaires had higher correlations with $VO_{2\ max}$ (in the range of 0.4 to 0.5) than with accelerometry-based measures (in the range of 0.2 to 0.3). It is possible that physical fitness is a better measure of long-term physical activity patterns than accelerometer data (even with 24 readings in a 1-year period). Only the household chores measured by the Minnesota Leisure-Time Physical Activity Questionnaire were correlated with those assessed by 4-week physical activity histories. Despite relatively high test-retest reliability, occupational activity measured by these questionnaires was not correlated with the criterion measures. A subsequent analysis of occupational data revealed that 93% of total occupational energy expenditure was attributable to light-intensity activities including sitting, standing, and walking.[93] This study underscores the difficulty of measuring light to moderate physical activity.

Wareham et al.[94] assessed the validity of a comprehensive questionnaire designed to measure total physical activity in the European Prospective Investigation into Cancer Study-Norfolk cohort (EPIC-Norfolk). They randomly selected 173 individuals from the cohort. Energy expenditure was assessed by four separate episodes of 4-day heart rate monitoring over a 1-year period. As with other studies, the repeatability of the sum of recreational and occupational reported activity was high ($r = .73$). However, energy expenditure in recreation and at work, as estimated by the questionnaire, was only modestly correlated with daytime energy expenditure measured by heart rate monitoring after adjusting for age and sex ($r = .28$, $P < .001$). The correlation was slightly higher in men than in women (.30 vs. .23). These validity correlation coefficients are similar to other studies using accelerometers as the reference method (from 0.14 to 0.53).[95] A recent validation study[96] of the Spanish version of the physical activity questionnaire used in the Nurses' Health Study found a relatively high correlation ($r = .51$) between the questionnaire and a triaxial accelerometer (RT3 Triaxial Research Tracker).

Using the DLW method as the criterion, Philippaerts et al.[97] evaluated the validity of the Baecke Questionnaire, the Five City Project Questionnaire, and the Tecumseh Community Health Study Questionnaire in 19 Flemish males. Physical activity indices estimated by all three questionnaires showed high correlations with the DLW method (from 0.57 to 0.69). Other studies, however, found much weaker correlations of physical activity questionnaires with the DLW method. Bonnefoy et al.[81] simultaneously validated 10 physical activity questionnaires against the DLW method in 19 healthy older men (aged 73.4 ± 4.1 years). Correlation coefficients between the questionnaires and total energy expenditure estimated by the DLW ranged from 0.11 for the Yale Physical Activity Survey (YPAS) total index to 0.63 for the Stanford Usual Activity Questionnaire (average $r = .32$).

Physical activity diaries or records are also commonly used as a reference method to validate habitual physical activity questionnaires. Assuming that physical activity is recorded more or less at the same time the activity is performed, diaries offer the advantage of not being subject to recall bias. Thus, diary-related measurement errors can be considered reasonably independent of the recall and estimation errors associated with questionnaires. Another advantage is that diaries record actual behaviors, thereby providing detailed information on multiple dimensions of physical activity (e.g., type, frequency, duration, and intensity). However, physical activity diaries have a major disadvantage; because the recording process may alter subjects' behaviors, data may not represent usual activity patterns. Physical activity diaries are also subject to reporting biases, and like diet records, put a high burden on participants. In addition, many days of recording (typically at least one week of recording in each season) are required to represent long-term physical activity patterns.

Wolf et al.[89] evaluated the reproducibility and validity of self-administered questionnaires on physical activity and inactivity in a random sample of the Nurses' Health Study cohort. Past-week activity recalls and 7-day activity diaries—the reference methods—were sent to participants four times over a 1-year period. Correlations between activity reported in diaries and those reported on questionnaires were 0.62 and 0.59 for whites and African American women, respectively. Similar or somewhat lower correlation coefficients were found for other physical activity questionnaires when validated against physical diaries or logs.[92,98,99] In most studies, higher validity correlation coefficients were found for vigorous activities (typically greater than 0.50) than for light to moderate ones (typically lower than 0.40).

Taken together, validation studies indicate that carefully developed physical activity questionnaires are reasonably accurate in measuring vigorous activity. However, most questionnaires have low to moderate validity coefficients, reflecting the imperfections of physical activity questionnaires; on the other hand, they underscore the complexity of physical activity as a behavior that contains multiple underlying and biologically meaningful constructs, including total energy expenditure, aerobic intensity, and weight bearing.[100] Unfortunately, neither questionnaires nor criterion methods (e.g., motion sensors) can capture all the dimensions of physical activity. One obvious reason is that most physical activity is of light to moderate intensity, a difficult category to capture with any methods. In addition, physical activity questionnaires and criterion methods often reflect different dimensions as well as time frames of exposure. For example, DLW and indirect calorimetry typically measure the energy cost of all daily activity within a few days, whereas physical activity questionnaires assess frequency, intensity, and duration of habitual physical activity behaviors in the past few months or one year. Because these methods measure different conceptual variables, and all are prone to errors, the correlations between the physical activity questionnaire and the reference methods will generally underestimate the validity of the questionnaires.

Validity of Physical Activity Questionnaire by Obesity Status

There is some evidence that the validity of physical activity questionnaires may vary with obesity status. Norman et al.[101] compared a physical activity questionnaire with two 7-day activity records performed 6 months apart in 111 men 44 to 78 years of age. The Spearman correlation coefficient between total daily activity scores estimated from the questionnaire and the records was 0.56. Significantly higher correlations were observed in men with BMI < 26 kg/m^2 compared with heavier men ($r = .73$ vs. $r = .39$). Compared with overweight women, Schmidt et al.[102] also reported higher validity coefficients between physical activity questionnaires and accelerometer estimates in leaner women.

There are several potential explanations for these findings. First, overweight individuals are more likely to overreport their physical activity than people of normal weight, thereby lowering the validity of their physical activity questionnaires. Second, as discussed above, individual physical activity MET values used to calculate total energy expenditure are derived from people of normal weight, and are therefore less accurate for obese subjects. Finally, overweight and obese subjects are less likely to engage in vigorous physical activity, a factor that could decrease between-subject variability in the overall estimate of physical activity, and lead to a lower validity coefficient.

Measurement Error Correction

Whether subjective or objective, measurement error is inevitable in physical activity assessments. As with dietary measurement errors, those associated with physical activity instruments can be either random or systematic. Random measurement errors resulting from within-person variability tend to underestimate the strength of the association between physical activity and obesity or other health outcomes (regression dilution bias). Systematic errors result from underreporting or overreporting of physical activity, instrument tampering and defects, and recall bias; they can lead to underestimation as well as overestimation of associations.

As with many dietary factors, within-subject variation of physical activity is considerably greater than between-subject variation. Matthews et al.[103] conducted a detailed analysis of the sources of variance in physical activity among 580 participants in the Seasonal Variation of Blood Cholesterol Study. Fifteen unannounced 24-hour physical activity recalls of total, occupational, and nonoccupational activity were collected over 12 months. Variance components for subject, season, day of the week, and residual error were estimated using a random effects model. The largest contributor to variance in total and nonoccupational activity was within-subject variance (50% to 60%), followed by between-subject variance (20% to 30% of the overall variance in total activity); seasonal and day-of-the-week effects accounted for 6% and 15%, respectively (Table 7.3). The authors estimated that for total activity 7 to 10 days of assessment in men and 14 to 21 days of assessment in women were required to achieve 80% reliability. Within-subject variation in accelerometer-based physical activity measures were found to be lower, although reliable measures of physical activity required at least 7 days of monitoring.[51]

The same measurement error correction methods for dietary instruments (see Chapter 6) can be used in physical activity studies. For example, Matthews et al.[51] used three repeated measures of 24-hour recalls in the Seasonal Variation of Blood Cholesterol Study to calculate deattenuated correlation coefficients between 24-hour physical activity recalls and the Baecke Questionnaire. The correlation coefficients for total and leisure-time physical activity in men increased from 0.29 to 0.34 and from 0.49 to 0.68, respectively; for women they increased from 0.41 to 0.60 and from 0.47 to 0.68, respectively.

Using multiple measurements of physical activity and physical fitness over a 1-year period, Franks et al.[104] corrected for random within-individual variability in analyses of the association between physical activity and the metabolic syndrome. Although the procedure had little effect on estimates of cardiovascular fitness ($VO_{2\,max}$) measured by heart rate monitors, it substantially improved estimates for physical activity energy expenditure. A similar measurement error correction method was used in an analysis of the relationship between physical activity and changes in body composition.[105]

As with dietary assessments, cumulatively averaged physical activity measurements from repeatedly administered questionnaires during follow-up can reduce random measurement error. In a subsample of the Health Professionals' Follow-up Study (HPFS), Fung et al.[106] found that average activity levels over 8 years had a stronger association with high-density lipoprotein (HDL) cholesterol than did a single, cross-sectional measure. Repeated measurements over time are known to reduce measurement error due to within-person variation; in turn, composite scores based on them may be more reliable, and can be considered stable measurements of long-term physical activity.

As discussed earlier, a validation study in a subsample of the cohort is required to correct systematic errors. Rosner et al.[107] provided a method to correct relative risk estimates from logistic regression models for systematic or within-person measurement errors in continuous dietary exposures within cohort studies (see Chapter 6). This method can also be applied to physical activity studies. In a study of physical activity and risk of coronary heart disease (CHD) in the HPFS, Tanasescu et al.[108] applied the measurement error method where the correction factor λ is derived by regressing observed physical activity on *true* physical activity measured by multiple 7-day activity records from the validation study. When physical activity was modeled as a continuous variable, every 50 MET-hours/week increase of baseline physical activity was associated with a 21% reduction in risk of CHD (multivariate relative risk = 0.77, 95% CI: 0.67 to 0.89). The association was strengthened considerably after correction for measurement error (corrected relative risk = 0.49, 95% CI: 0.30 to 0.81).

In an analysis of the relationship between changes in diet and physical activity and 9-year gain in waist circumference in the HPFS, Koh-Banerjee et al.[109] extended the regression calibration method to estimate regression coefficients corrected for random and systematic measurement errors in the measure of physical activity changes over time. Because the changes in physical activity were not assessed in the validation study, they assumed that levels of error in the assessments of changes in vigorous physical activity and in dietary exposure were comparable, and thus, applied the same correction factor for dietary fats to the analyses of vigorous activity. After correction for measurement error, an increase of 25 MET-hours/week of vigorous activity was associated with

Table 7.3 Variance Components for Total, Occupational, and Nonoccupational Physical Activity in Men and Women, Seasonal Variation of Blood Cholesterol Study, Worcester, Massachusetts, 1994-1998

| | Type of Activity* | | | | | | | | |
| | Total | | | Occupational | | | Nonoccupational | | |
	Variance	95% CI[†]	Total Percentage[‡]	Variance	95% CI	Total Percentage	Variance	95% CI	Total Percentage
Men (n = 300)									
Subject	39.3	32.2-49.0	31	37.9	31.2-46.9	35	8.7	6.6-12.0	14
Season	7.1	4.8-11.5	6	3.0	1.8-6.2	3	6.1	4.4-8.9	10
Day	19.3	15.8-24.1	15	28.3	24.8-32.5	26	8.9	6.9-11.8	14
Residual	60.7	56.7-65.1	48	38.3	35.7-41.2	36	39.9	37.3-42.7	63
Total	126.4			107.5			63.5		
Women (n = 280)									
Subject	10.4	8.2-13.6	19	9.6	7.8-12.1	29	5.5	4.1-7.7	13
Season	3.6	2.5-6.0	7	1.0	0.5-2.5	3	3.3	2.4-5.1	8
Day	6.5	5.0-8.9	12	6.7	5.6-8.2	20	7.4	6.0-9.3	18
Residual	32.9	30.7-35.3	62	15.7	14.5-16.9	48	24.9	23.2-36.7	61
Total	53.5			32.9			41.1		

* Units for physical activity variables were metabolic equivalent-hours/day.
[†] CI, confidence interval.
[‡] Percentage of total variance attributable to a given source.

Reproduced with permission from Matthews CE, Hebert JR, Freedson PS, et al. Sources of variance in daily physical activity levels in the seasonal variation of blood cholesterol study. *Am J Epidemiol.* 2001;153:987-995.[103]

a 1.33 cm decrease in waist circumference ($P < .001$) compared with an uncorrected 0.38 cm waist gain.

Summary

Accurate quantification of physical activity remains a major challenge in epidemiologic studies. Similar to diet, physical activity is a complex human behavior with large day-to-day variations. Because the type, intensity, frequency, and duration of physical activity can exert independent effects on health outcomes, including obesity, its benefits go beyond energy expenditure. Structured exercise or sports participation is relatively easy to assess by standardized questionnaires. However, physical activities of light to moderate intensity, which are often incorporated into daily routines (e.g., transportation, occupation, and household chores), are more difficult to measure. In this chapter we reviewed two types of methods for measuring physical activity: objective (e.g., activity monitors, DLW/indirect calorimetry, pedometers, and heart rate monitors) and self-reported (e.g., physical diaries, logs, recalls, and questionnaires). Each method has strengths and limitations. Recent advances in accelerometry-based devices enable participants to provide real-time monitoring of the frequency, duration, and intensity of all activities in free-living populations. Accelerometry has the potential to improve the accuracy and precision of physical activity measurements in intervention and epidemiologic studies, although use of this approach to measure long-term physical activity patterns probably needs at least 1 week of recording for each season of the year. This may not be feasible in large epidemiologic studies with extended follow-up.

Among various self-reported methods, physical activity diaries or records are considered most accurate because they can provide detailed information on activity context, type (e.g., aerobic, weight lifting), frequency, intensity, and duration. Similar to diet records, activity diaries require substantial efforts from participants and are therefore not feasible in large epidemiologic studies involving hundreds and thousands of participants. Thus, validated questionnaires remain the mainstay of physical activity measurement method in large epidemiologic studies. Despite many refinements and improvements, the validity coefficients of most habitual physical activities from questionnaires are modest ($r = .3$ to $.5$) relative to other direct or indirect measures of physical activity and energy expenditure. The low validity coefficients reflect both the complexity of physical activity behavior and the lack of a true gold standard in measuring long-term physical activity.

It is clear that both sides of the energy balance equation are difficult to measure. However, even with relatively crude measurements of the various sources of energy intake and expenditure, epidemiologic studies have demonstrated the important roles of diet and physical activity in the development of obesity and chronic diseases. Continued advances in diet and activity measurements will depend on further refinements in questionnaire-based and objective methods (e.g., biomarkers, and motion sensors). In most situations, the use of a validated physical activity questionnaire in the overall cohort, combined with objective measurements by either accelerometers or cardiorespiratory fitness tests in a subsample, will provide sufficiently valid data on physical activity in large epidemiologic studies. Moreover, improvements in epidemiologic study design and analytic strategies, such as periodic updating of diet and physical activity information during follow-up and measurement error correction, will enhance our ability to detect and understand important relationships between factors related to energy balance and obesity in free-living populations.

References

1. Caspersen CJ, Powell KE, Christenson GM. Physical activity, exercise, and physical fitness: definitions and distinctions for health-related research. *Public Health Rep.* 1985;100:126-131.
2. Welk GJ, Morrow JRJ, Falls HB, eds. *Fitnessgram Reference Guide.* Dallas, TX: The Cooper Institute; 2002.
3. U.S. Department of Health and Human Services. Physical activity and health: a report of the Surgeon General. Atlanta: U.S. Department of Health and Human Services, Centers for Disease Control and Prevention, National Center for Chronic Disease Prevention and Health Promotion; 1996.
4. Fletcher GF, Balady GJ, Amsterdam EA, et al. Exercise standards for testing and training: a statement for healthcare professionals from the American Heart Association. *Circulation.* 2001;104:1694-1740.
5. Ainsworth BE, Haskell WL, Leon AS, et al. Compendium of physical activities: classification of energy costs of human physical activities. *Med Sci Sports Exerc.* 1993;25(1):71-80.
6. Ainsworth BE, Haskell WL, Whitt MC, et al. Compendium of physical activities: an update of activity codes and MET intensities. *Med Sci Sports Exerc.* 2000;32 (9 Suppl):S498-S504.
7. Saris WH, Blair SN, van Baak MA, et al. How much physical activity is enough to prevent unhealthy weight gain? Outcome of the IASO 1st Stock Conference and consensus statement. *Obes Rev.* 2003;4:101-114.
8. Harada ND, Chiu V, King AC, Stewart AL. An evaluation of three self-report physical activity instruments for older adults. *Med Sci Sports Exerc.* 2001;33:962-970.
9. Rikli RE. Reliability, validity, and methodological issues in assessing physical activity in older adults. *Res Q Exerc Sport.* 2000;71(2 Suppl):S89-S96.
10. Spadano JL, Must A, Bandini LG, Dallal GE, Dietz WH. Energy cost of physical activities in 12-y-old girls: MET values and the influence of body weight. *Int J Obes Relat Metab Disord.* 2003;27:1528-1533.
11. Borg G. *Borg's Perceived Exertion and Pain Scales.* Champaign, IL: Human Kinetics; 1998.
12. Dishman RK, Washburn RA, Heath GW. *Physical Activity Epidemiology.* Champaign, IL: Human Kinetics, Inc.; 2004.
13. Hu FB, Li TY, Colditz GA, Willett WC, Manson JE. Television watching and other sedentary behaviors in relation to risk of obesity and type 2 diabetes mellitus in women. *JAMA.* 2003;289:1785-1791.
14. Wiecha JL, Peterson KE, Ludwig DS, Kim J, Sobol A, Gortmaker SL. When children eat what they watch: impact of television viewing on dietary intake in youth. *Arch Pediatr Adolesc Med.* 2006;160:436-442.
15. Gortmaker SL, Must A, Sobol AM, Peterson K, Colditz GA, Dietz WH. Television viewing as a cause of increasing obesity among children in the United States, 1986-1990. *Arch Pediatr Adolesc Med.* 1996;150:356-362.
16. Andersen RE, Crespo CJ, Bartlett SJ, Cheskin LJ, Pratt M. Relationship of physical activity and television watching with body weight and level of fatness among children: results from the Third National Health and Nutrition Examination Surve. *JAMA.* 1998;279:938-942.
17. Hu FB, Leitzmann MF, Stampfer MJ, Colditz GA, Willett WC, Rimm EB. Physical activity and television watching in relation to risk for type 2 diabetes mellitus in men. *Arch Intern Med.* 2001;161:1542-1548.
18. Levine JA, Vander Weg MW, Hill JO, Klesges RC. Non-exercise activity thermogenesis: the crouching tiger hidden dragon of societal weight gain. *Arterioscler Thromb Vasc Biol.* 2006;26:729-736.
19. Lamonte MJ, Ainsworth BE. Quantifying energy expenditure and physical activity in the context of dose response. *Med Sci Sports Exerc.* 2001;33(6 Suppl):S370-S378.

20. Welk GJ, ed. *Physical Activity Assessments for Health-Related Research*. Champaign, IL: Human Kinetics, Inc.; 2002.
21. Dale D, Welk GJ, Matthews CE. Chapter 1. Methods for assessing physical activity and challenges for research. In: Welk GJ, ed. *Physical Activity Assessments for Health-Related Research*. Champaign, IL: Human Kinetics, Inc.; 2002;19-34.
22. Speakman JR. *Doubly Labelled Water. Theory and Practice*. London: Chapman and Hall; 1997.
23. Trabulsi J, Schoeller DA. Evaluation of dietary assessment instruments against doubly labeled water, a biomarker of habitual energy intake. *Am J Physiol Endocrinol Metab*. 2001;281:E891-E899.
24. Starling RD. Chapter 12. Use of doubly labeled water and indirect calorimetry to assess physical activity. In: Welk GJ, ed. *Physical Activity Assessments for Health-Related Research*. Champaign, IL: Human Kinetics, Inc.; 2002.
25. da Rocha EE, Alves VG, da Fonseca RB. Indirect calorimetry: methodology, instruments and clinical application. *Curr Opin Clin Nutr Metab Care*. 2006;9:247-256.
26. Manini TM, Everhart JE, Patel KV, et al. Daily activity energy expenditure and mortality among older adults. *JAMA*. 2006;296:171-179.
27. Nieman DC, Austin MD, Chilcote SM, Benezra L. Validation of a new handheld device for measuring resting metabolic rate and oxygen consumption in children. *Int J Sport Nutr Exerc Metab*. 2005;15:186-194.
28. McKenzie TL. Chapter 13. Use of direct observation to assess physical activity In: Welk GJ, ed. *Physical Activity Assessments for Health-Related Research*. Champaign, IL: Human Kinetics, Inc.; 2002;213-226.
29. Bassett DR Jr, Strath SJ. Chapter 10. Use of pedometers to assess physical activity. In: Welk GJ, ed. *Physical Activity Assessments for Health-Related Research*. Champaign, IL: Human Kinetics, Inc.; 2002;164-178.
30. Bassett DR Jr, Ainsworth BE, Leggett SR, et al. Accuracy of five electronic pedometers for measuring distance walked. *Med Sci Sports Exerc*. 1996;28:1071-1077.
31. Schneider PL, Crouter SE, Bassett DR. Pedometer measures of free-living physical activity: comparison of 13 models. *Med Sci Sports Exerc*. 2004;36:331-335.
32. Tudor-Locke C, Williams JE, Reis JP, Pluto D. Utility of pedometers for assessing physical activity: convergent validity. *Sports Med*. 2002;32:795-808.
33. Tudor-Locke C, Williams JE, Reis JP, Pluto D. Utility of pedometers for assessing physical activity: construct validity. *Sports Med*. 2004;34:281-291.
34. Tudor-Locke C, Bassett DR Jr. How many steps/day are enough? Preliminary pedometer indices for public health. *Sports Med*. 2004;34:1-8.
35. Chen KY, Bassett DR Jr. The technology of accelerometry-based activity monitors: current and future. *Med Sci Sports Exerc*. 2005;37(11 Suppl):S490-S500.
36. Welk GJ. Principles of design and analyses for the calibration of accelerometry-based activity monitors. *Med Sci Sports Exerc*. 2005;37(11 Suppl):S501-S511.
37. Steele BG, Belza B, Cain K, Warms C, Coppersmith J, Howard J. Bodies in motion: monitoring daily activity and exercise with motion sensors in people with chronic pulmonary disease. *J Rehabil Res Dev*. 2003;40(5 Suppl):45-58.
38. Trost SG, McIver KL, Pate RR. Conducting accelerometer-based activity assessments in field-based research. *Med Sci Sports Exerc*. 2005;37(11 Suppl):S531-S543.
39. NHANES 2003-2004. U.S. Department of Health and Human Services Available at: http://0-www.cdc.gov.mill1.sjlibrary.org/nchs/about/major/nhanes/nhanes2003-2004/nhanes03_04.htm. Accessed November 1, 2007.
40. Jakicic JM, Winters C, Lagally K, Ho J, Robertson RJ, Wing RR. The accuracy of the TriTrac-R3D accelerometer to estimate energy expenditure. *Med Sci Sports Exerc*. 1999;31:747-754.
41. Matthews CE. Calibration of accelerometer output for adults. *Med Sci Sports Exerc*. 2005;37(11 Suppl):S512-S522.

42. Freedson P, Pober D, Janz KF. Calibration of accelerometer output for children. *Med Sci Sports Exerc.* 2005;37(11 Suppl):S523-S530.

43. Campbell KL, Crocker PR, McKenzie DC. Field evaluation of energy expenditure in women using Tritrac accelerometers. *Med Sci Sports Exerc.* 2002;34:1667-1674.

44. Welk GJ, Blair SN, Wood K, Jones S, Thompson RW. A comparative evaluation of three accelerometry-based physical activity monitors. *Med Sci Sports Exerc.* 2000;32(9 Suppl):S489-S497.

45. Bassett DR Jr, Ainsworth BE, Swartz AM, Strath SJ, O'Brien WL, King GA. Validity of four motion sensors in measuring moderate intensity physical activity. *Med Sci Sports Exerc.* 2000;32(9 Suppl):S471-S480.

46. Hendelman D, Miller K, Baggett C, Debold E, Freedson P. Validity of accelerometry for the assessment of moderate intensity physical activity in the field. *Med Sci Sports Exerc.* 2000;32(9 Suppl):S442-S449.

47. Zhang K, Werner P, Sun M, Pi-Sunyer FX, Boozer CN. Measurement of human daily physical activity. *Obes Res.* 2003;11:33-40.

48. Zhang K, Pi-Sunyer FX, Boozer CN. Improving energy expenditure estimation for physical activity. *Med Sci Sports Exerc.* 2004;36:883-889.

49. Welk GJ. Chapter 8. Use of accelerometry-based activity monitors to assess physical activity In: Welk GJ, ed. *Physical Activity Assessments for Health-Related Research.* Champaign, IL: Human Kinetics, Inc.; 2002.

50. Matthew CE. Calibration of accelerometer output for adults. *Med Sci Sports Exerc.* 2005;37:S512-S522.

51. Matthews CE, Ainsworth BE, Thompson RW, Bassett DR Jr. Sources of variance in daily physical activity levels as measured by an accelerometer. *Med Sci Sports Exerc.* 2002;34:1376-1381.

52. Trost SG. Objective measurement of physical activity in youth: current issues, future directions. *Exerc Sport Sci Rev.* 2001;29:32-36.

53. Goran MI. Measurement issues related to studies of childhood obesity: assessment of body composition, body fat distribution, physical activity, and food intake. *Pediatrics.* 1998;101(3 Pt 2):505-518.

54. Freedson PS. Electronic motion sensors and heart rate as measures of physical activity in children. *J Sch Health.* 1991;61:220-223.

55. Puyau MR, Adolph AL, Vohra FA, Butte NF. Validation and calibration of physical activity monitors in children. *Obes Res.* 2002;10:150-157.

56. Eisenmann JC, Strath SJ, Shadrick D, Rigsby P, Hirsch N, Jacobson L. Validity of uniaxial accelerometry during activities of daily living in children. *Eur J Appl Physiol.* 2004;91:259-263.

57. Lopez-Alarcon M, Merrifield J, Fields DA, et al. Ability of the actiwatch accelerometer to predict free-living energy expenditure in young children. *Obes Res.* 2004;12:1859-1865.

58. Janz KF. Chapter 9. Use of heart rate monitors to assess physical activity. In: Welk GJ, ed. *Physical Activity Assessments for Health-Related Research.* Champaign, IL: Human Kinetics, Inc.; 2002.

59. Wareham NJ, Hennings SJ, Prentice AM, Day NE. Feasibility of heart-rate monitoring to estimate total level and pattern of energy expenditure in a population-based epidemiological study: the Ely Young Cohort Feasibility Study 1994-5. *Br J Nutr.* 1997;78:889-900.

60. Strath SJ, Swartz AM, Bassett DR Jr, O'Brien WL, King GA, Ainsworth BE. Evaluation of heart rate as a method for assessing moderate intensity physical activity. *Med Sci Sports Exerc.* 2000;32(9 Suppl):S465-S470.

61. Strath SJ, Bassett DR Jr, Swartz AM, Thompson DL. Simultaneous heart rate-motion sensor technique to estimate energy expenditure. *Med Sci Sports Exerc.* 2001;33:2118-2123.

62. Strath SJ, Bassett DR Jr, Thompson DL, Swartz AM. Validity of the simultaneous heart rate-motion sensor technique for measuring energy expenditure. *Med Sci Sports Exerc.* 2002;34:888-894.

63. Bouchard C, Shephard RJ. Physical activity, fitness and health: the model and key concepts. In: Bouchard C, Shepard RJ, Stephens T, eds. *Physical Activity, Fitness and Health, International Proceedings and Consensus Statement.* Champaign, IL: Human Kinetics, Inc.; 1994:77-88.

64. Haskell WL, Kiernan M. Methodologic issues in measuring physical activity and physical fitness when evaluating the role of dietary supplements for physically active people. *Am J Clin Nutr.* 2000;72(2 Suppl):541S-550S.

65. Blair SN, Kohl HW III, Paffenbarger RS Jr, Clark DG, Cooper KH, Gibbons LW. Physical fitness and all-cause mortality. A prospective study of healthy men and women. *JAMA.* 1989;262:2395-2401.

66. Stevens J, Cai J, Evenson KR, Thomas R. Fitness and fatness as predictors of mortality from all causes and from cardiovascular disease in men and women in the lipid research clinics study. *Am J Epidemiol.* 2002;156:832-841.

67. Carnethon MR, Gidding SS, Nehgme R, Sidney S, Jacobs DR Jr, Liu K. Cardiorespiratory fitness in young adulthood and the development of cardiovascular disease risk factors. *JAMA.* 2003;290:3092-3100.

68. Balke B, Ware RW. An experimental study of physical fitness of Air Force personnel. *U S Armed Forces Med J.* 1959;10:875-888.

69. Bruce RA, Fisher LD, Cooper MN, Gey GO. Separation of effects of cardiovascular disease and age on ventricular function with maximal exercise. *Am J Cardiol.* 1974;34:757-763.

70. Duncan GE, Li SM, Zhou XH. Cardiovascular fitness among U.S. adults: NHANES 1999-2000 and 2001-2002. *Med Sci Sports Exerc.* 2005;37:1324-1328.

71. Carnethon MR, Gulat IM, Greenland P. Prevalence and cardiovascular disease correlates of low cardiorespiratory fitness in adolescents and adults. *JAMA.* 2005; 294:2981-2988.

72. Shephard RJ. Tests of maximum oxygen intake. A critical review. *Sports Med.* 1984;1:99-124.

73. Fitchett MA. Predictability of VO2 max from submaximal cycle ergometer and bench stepping tests. *Br J Sports Med.* 1985;19:85-88.

74. Montgomery DL, Reid G, Koziris LP. Reliability and validity of three fitness tests for adults with mental handicaps. *Can J Sport Sci.* 1992;17:309-315.

75. Matthews CE. Chapter 7. Use of self-report instruments to assess physical acitvity. In: Welk GJ, ed. *Physical Activity Assessments for Health-Related Research.* Champaign, IL: Human Kinetics, Inc.; 2002.

76. Keim NL, Blanton CA, Kretsch MJ. America's obesity epidemic: measuring physical activity to promote an active lifestyle. *J Am Diet Assoc.* 2004;104:1398-1409.

77. Sallis JF, Haskell WL, Wood PD, et al. Physical activity assessment methodology in the Five-City Project. *Am J Epidemiol.* 1985;121:91-106.

78. Matthews CE, Freedson PS, Hebert JR, Stanek EJ III, Merriam PA, Ockene IS. Comparing physical activity assessment methods in the Seasonal Variation of Blood Cholesterol Study. *Med Sci Sports Exerc.* 2000;32:976-984.

79. Washburn RA, Montoye HJ. The assessment of physical activity by questionnaire. *Am J Epidemiol.* 1986;123:563-576.

80. Pereira MA, FitzerGerald SJ, Gregg EW, et al. A collection of Physical Activity Questionnaires for health-related research. *Med Sci Sports Exerc.* 1997;29(6 Suppl): S1-S205.

81. Bonnefoy M, Normand S, Pachiaudi C, Lacour JR, Laville M, Kostka T. Simultaneous validation of ten physical activity questionnaires in older men: a doubly labeled water study. *J Am Geriatr Soc.* 2001;49:28-35.

82. Friedenreich CM, Courneya KS, Bryant HE. The lifetime total physical activity questionnaire: development and reliability. *Med Sci Sports Exerc.* 1998;30:266-274.

83. Craig CL, Marshall AL, Sjostrom M, et al. International physical activity questionnaire: 12-country reliability and validity. *Med Sci Sports Exerc.* 2003;35:1381-1395.

84. Leon AS, Connett J, Jacobs DR Jr, Rauramaa R. Leisure-time physical activity levels and risk of coronary heart disease and death. The Multiple Risk Factor Intervention Trial. *JAMA*. 1987;258:2388-2395.

85. Paffe nbarger RS Jr, Hyde RT, Wing AL, Lee IM, Jung DL, Kampert JB. The association of changes in physical-activity level and other lifestyle characteristics with mortality among men. *N Engl J Med*. 1993;328:538-545.

86. Lee IM, Hsieh CC, Paffenbarger RS Jr. Exercise intensity and longevity in men. The Harvard Alumni Health Study. *JAMA*. 1995;273:1179-1184.

87. Siscovick DS, Ekelund LG, Hyde JS, Johnson JL, Gordon DJ, LaRosa JC. Physical activity and coronary heart disease among asymptomatic hypercholesterolemic men (the Lipid Research Clinics Coronary Primary Prevention Trial). *Am J Public Health*. 1988;78:1428-1431.

88. Baecke JA, Burema J, Frijters JE. A short questionnaire for the measurement of habitual physical activity in epidemiological studies. *Am J Clin Nutr*. 1982;36:936-942.

89. Wolf AM, Hunter DJ, Colditz GA, et al. Reproducibility and validity of a self-administered physical activity questionnaire. *Int J Epidemiol*. 1994;23:991-999.

90. Godin G, Shephard RJ. A simple method to assess exercise behavior in the community. *Can J Appl Sport Sci*. 1985;10:141-146.

91. Shephard RJ. Limits to the measurement of habitual physical activity by questionnaires. *Br J Sports Med*. 2003;37:197-206.

92. Jacobs DR Jr, Ainsworth BE, Hartman TJ, Leon AS. A simultaneous evaluation of 10 commonly used physical activity questionnaires. *Med Sci Sports Exerc*. 1993;25:81-91.

93. Ainsworth BE, Jacobs DR Jr, Leon AS, Richardson MT, Montoye HJ. Assessment of the accuracy of physical activity questionnaire occupational data. *J Occup Med*. 1993;35:1017-1027.

94. Wareham NJ, Jakes RW, Rennie KL, Mitchell J, Hennings S, Day NE. Validity and repeatability of the EPIC-Norfolk Physical Activity Questionnaire. *Int J Epidemiol*. 2002;31:168-174.

95. Sallis JF, Saelens BE. Assessment of physical activity by self-report: status, limitations, and future directions. *Res Q Exerc Sport*. 2000;7(2 Suppl):S1-S14.

96. Martinez-Gonzalez MA, Lopez-Fontana C, Varo JJ, Sanchez-Villegas A, Martinez JA. Validation of the Spanish version of the physical activity questionnaire used in the Nurses' Health Study and the Health Professionals' Follow-up Study. *Public Health Nutr*. 2005;8:920-927.

97. Philippaerts RM, Westerterp KR, Lefevre J. Doubly labeled water validation of three physical activity questionnaires. *Int J Sports Med*. 1999;20:284-289.

98. Richardson MT, Ainsworth BE, Wu HC, Jacobs DR Jr, Leon AS. Ability of the Atherosclerosis Risk in Communities (ARIC)/Baecke Questionnaire to assess leisure-time physical activity. *Int J Epidemiol*. 1995;24:685-693.

99. Matthews CE, Shu XO, Yang G, et al. Reproducibility and validity of the Shanghai Women's Health Study physical activity questionnaire. *Am J Epidemiol*. 2003;158:1114-1122.

100. Rennie KL, Wareham NJ. The validation of physical activity instruments for measuring energy expenditure: problems and pitfalls. *Public Health Nutr*. 1998;1:265-271.

101. Norman A, Bellocco R, Bergstrom A, Wolk A. Validity and reproducibility of self-reported total physical activity—differences by relative weight. *Int J Obes Relat Metab Disord*. 2001;25:682-688.

102. Schmidt MD, Freedson PS, Chasan-Taber L. Estimating physical activity using the CSA accelerometer and a physical activity log. *Med Sci Sports Exerc*. 2003;35:1605-1611.

103. Matthews CE, Hebert JR, Freedson PS, et al. Sources of variance in daily physical activity levels in the seasonal variation of blood cholesterol study. *Am J Epidemiol*. 2001;153:987-995.

104. Franks PW, Ekelund U, Brage S, Wong MY, Wareham NJ. Does the association of habitual physical activity with the metabolic syndrome differ by level of cardiorespiratory fitness? *Diabetes Care.* 2004;27:1187-1193.
105. Ekelund U, Brage S, Franks PW, et al. Physical activity energy expenditure predicts changes in body composition in middle-aged healthy whites: effect modification by age. *Am J Clin Nutr.* 2005;81:964-969.
106. Fung TT, Hu FB, Yu J, et al. Leisure-time physical activity, television watching, and plasma biomarkers of obesity and cardiovascular disease risk. *Am J Epidemiol.* 2000;152:1171-1178.
107. Rosner B, Willett WC, Spiegelman D. Correction of logistic regression relative risk estimates and confidence intervals for systematic within-person measurement error. *Stat Med.* 1989;8:1051-1069.
108. Tanasescu M, Leitzmann MF, E.B. R, Willett WC, Stampfer MJ, Hu FB. Exercise type and intensity in relation to coronary heart disease in men. *JAMA.* 2002;288:1994-2000.
109. Koh-Banerjee P, Chu NF, Spiegelman D, et al. Prospective study of the association of changes in dietary intake, physical activity, alcohol consumption, and smoking with 9-y gain in waist circumference among 16 587 US men. *Am J Clin Nutr.* 2003;78:719-727.

Part II

Epidemiologic Studies of Consequences of Obesity

8

Metabolic Consequences of Obesity

Frank B. Hu

Obesity triggers a plethora of metabolic disturbances, including insulin resistance, hypertension, hyperglycemia, hypertriglyceridemia, and reduced levels of high-density lipoprotein (HDL) cholesterol, together referred to as the metabolic syndrome.[1] While excess body weight is a well-established risk factor for the development of these metabolic conditions, mounting evidence also supports independent effects of body fat distribution. In addition, increasing evidence suggests ethnic differences with respect to the effects of obesity on risk of metabolic diseases, especially type 2 diabetes. Another area of growing interest is the impact of obesity on complications or "fellow travelers" of the metabolic syndrome, including gallstones, gout, polycystic ovary syndrome (PCOS), chronic kidney disease (CKD), and sleep apnea.

In this chapter, we review links between obesity and individual components of the metabolic syndrome as well as underlying biological mechanisms, for example, insulin resistance, systemic inflammation, and endothelial dysfunction. We will discuss recent epidemiologic studies on risk of diabetes in relation to changes in fat distribution, the role of overall adiposity versus abdominal obesity, and the relative importance of fatness versus fitness. We also briefly examine epidemiologic literature related to "fellow travelers" of the metabolic syndrome. Figure 8.1 depicts the biological pathways through which overall adiposity and central obesity influence metabolic disorders and related conditions.

Defining the Metabolic Syndrome

In his Banting Award Lecture in 1988,[2] Gerald Reaven used the term "Syndrome X" to describe the close interrelationships among obesity, hyperinsulinemia, glucose intolerance, and dyslipidemia. In 1989, Kaplan[3] used the term "deadly quartet" to describe the clustering of upper body obesity, hypertriglyceridemia, glucose intolerance, and hypertension. In 1998, the World Health Organization (WHO) coined the phrase "metabolic syndrome" and defined it as insulin resistance and/or impaired glucose regulation with at least two of the following conditions: dyslipidemia (elevated triglycerides or low HDL); high blood pressure; obesity (high waist-to-hip ratio [WHR] or body mass index [BMI]); or microalbuminuria.[4] In 2001, the Third Report of the Expert Panel on Detection, Evaluation, and Treatment of High Blood Cholesterol in Adults (Adult Treatment

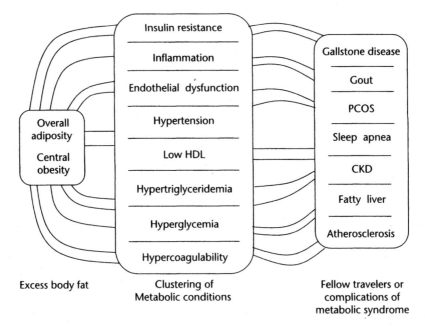

Figure 8.1 Pathways through which overall adiposity and central obesity influence metabolic disorders and related conditions. PCOS denotes polycystic ovary syndrome and CKD denotes chronic kidney disease.

Panel III [ATP III])[5] defined the metabolic syndrome as three or more of the following (Table 8.1): abdominal obesity (waist circumference >102 cm in men and >88 cm in women); hypertriglyceridemia (≥150 mg/dL or 1.69 mmol/L); low HDL cholesterol (<40 mg/dL or 1.04 mmol/L in men and <50 mg/dL or 1.29 mmol/L in women); high blood pressure (≥130/85 mm Hg); and high fasting glucose (≥110 mg/dL or 6.1 mmol/L). Using data from NHANES III, Ford et al.[6] estimated that approximately one quarter of U.S. adults (or 47 million people) have the metabolic syndrome.

In 2005, the International Diabetes Federation (IDF) proposed another definition of metabolic syndrome—central obesity plus any two of the following conditions: hypertension, hypertriglyceridemia, reduced HDL cholesterol, or impaired fasting glucose.[7] The IDF definition included gender- and ethnic-specific cutpoints for central obesity measured by waist circumference, but justifications for these cutpoints remain controversial.

Although the various descriptions of metabolic syndrome differ somewhat, they all include a similar cluster of metabolic disorders and central obesity. Most notably, all conclude that the co-occurrence of obesity, hypertension, high cholesterol, and insulin resistance is not due to chance alone, but rather, to a common underlying process.[8] Still, there is vigorous debate over competing definitions of metabolic syndrome. Issues include the validity of the *syndrome* classification, the criteria for diagnosis, the appropriate cutpoints for individual components, and the underlying causes of risk factor clustering. Other points of contention include the degree to which the metabolic syndrome is more than the sum of its parts in predicting cardiovascular disease (CVD) incidence and mortality, and whether diagnosis of the syndrome improves treatment over traditional approaches.[9-11] Despite difficulties in resolving these issues, prospective epidemiologic studies have consistently found that the metabolic syndrome, regardless of varying diagnostic criteria,

Table 8.1 Diagnostic Criteria according to WHO, ATP III, and IDF Definitions

WHO 1999	*ATPIII 2001*	*IDF 2005*
Diabetes or impaired glucose tolerance or insulin resistance*		Central Obesity Waist circumference[†]- ethnicity specific
Plus two or more of the following:	Three or more of the following:	Plus any two of the following:
1. Obesity: BMI > 30 kg/m² or WHR > 0.9 (Male) or 0.85 (Female)	1. Central obesity: Waist circumference > 102 cm (Male), >88 cm (Female)	1. Raised triglycerides: ≥150 mg/dL (1.7 mmol/L) or specific treatment for this lipid abnormality
2. Dyslipidemia: Triglycerides ≥ 150 mg/dL (1.7 mmol/L) or HDL cholesterol < 35 mg/dL (0.9 mmol/L) (Male) < 39 mg/dL (Female) (1.0 mmol/L)	2. Hypertriglyceridemia: Triglycerides ≥ 150 mg/dL (1.7 mmol/L)	2. Reduced HDL cholesterol: < 40 mg/dL (1.03 mmol/L) in males, <50 mg/dL (1.29 mmol/L) in females or specific treatment for this lipid abnormality
3. Hypertension: Blood pressure ≥ 140/90 mm Hg or medication	3. Low HDL cholesterol: < 40 mg/dL (1.03 mmol/L) (Male), <50 mg/dL (1.29 mmol/L) (Female)	3. Raised blood pressure: *systolic*: ≥130 mm Hg or *diastolic*: ≥ 85 mm Hg or treatment of previously diagnosed hypertension
4. Microalbuminuria: Albumin excretion ≥20 µg/min or albumin: creatinine ratio ≥ 30 mg/g	4. Hypertension: Blood pressure ≥130/85 mm Hg or medication	4. Raised fasting plasma glucose[‡] Fasting plasma glucose ≥ 100 mg/dL (5.6 mmol/L) or previously diagnosed type 2 diabetes. If above 5.6 mmol/L or 100 mg/dL, OGTT is strongly recommended but is not necessary to define presence of the syndrome
	5. Fasting plasma glucose ≥ 110 mg/dL (6.1 mmol/L)	

* Defined as the top quartile of fasting insulin in the nondiabetic population.
† If BMI is > 30 kg/m² then central obesity can be assumed, and waist circumference does not need to be measured.
‡ In clinical practice, IGT is also acceptable, but all reports of the prevalence of the metabolic syndrome should use only the fasting plasma glucose and presence of previously diagnosed diabetes to assess this criterion. Prevalences also incorporating the 2-h glucose results can be added as supplementary findings.

strongly predicts future risk of CVD.[12,13] Below, we will discuss the role of adipose tissue cytokines in the etiology of the metabolic syndrome and examine the links between various metabolic disorders and the amount and distribution of body fat.

Adipose Tissue as an Endocrine Organ

The metabolic syndrome has provided a useful theoretical framework for studying the biological basis for the clustering of obesity and multiple metabolic disorders. Insulin resistance is often considered the common link between obesity and metabolic risk factors.[2] However, there is a recent recognition that chronic inflammation induced by adipocyte-secreted cytokines may be the underlying pathophysiology in the development of insulin resistance and the metabolic syndrome. For this reason, the metabolic syndrome has also been called "the inflammatory syndrome."[14]

Excess adiposity, especially abdominal obesity, is recognized as the primary driving force behind the current epidemic of the metabolic syndrome. Although mechanisms linking obesity to elevated risk of individual components of the syndrome are not yet fully understood, evidence suggests that specific hormones, cytokines, and free fatty acids (FFAs) secreted by adipose tissue play crucial roles. Demonstration of crosstalk between adipose tissue and other insulin target tissues (e.g., skeletal muscle and liver) has greatly advanced our understanding of the link between obesity and insulin resistance.[15,16] Such crosstalk is mediated through molecules released by adipocytes, including leptin, tumor necrosis factor-alpha (TNF-α), interleukin-6 (IL-6), resistin, and adiponectin[17] (Fig. 8.2). Acting in concert, these cytokines or *adipokines* play critical roles in energy metabolism and insulin sensitivity.[16] Epidemiologic studies have consistently demonstrated positive associations between overall and central adiposity and increased plasma concentrations of leptin, TNF-α, and IL-6. Subjects with obesity, insulin resistance, and type 2 diabetes have lower plasma levels of adiponectin.[18] Resistin's relationship to obesity and insulin resistance is not as clear.[19] Recent data suggest that retinol-binding protein 4 (RBP4), another protein secreted by adipocytes, is linked to insulin resistance and type 2 diabetes.[20]

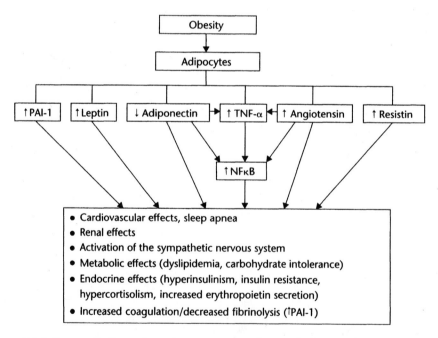

Figure 8.2 Influence of adipose tissue hormones or proteins on obesity-associated organic and metabolic abnormalities. Angiotensin and adiponectin are active both *via* the NFκB pathway or directly by other pathways. $\uparrow$, increased in obesity; $\downarrow$, decreased in obesity; NFκB, nuclear factor-kappa B. PAI-1 denotes plasminogen activator inhibitor-1. Adapted from Wiecek A, Kokot F, Chudek J, Adamczak M. The adipose tissue—a novel endocrine organ of interest to the nephrologist. *Nephrol Dial Transplant.* 2002;17:191-195.[17]

FFAs, the primary oxidative fuel for several tissues including liver and resting skeletal muscle, also play an important role in insulin resistance.[21,22] Excess body fat can lead to fatty acid *spillover* from adipose to nonadipose tissue, causing peripheral insulin resistance and abnormal glucose metabolism.[15,16,21]

Obesity and Systemic Inflammation

As adipose tissue is a major secretory organ for proinflammatory cytokines, obesity is considered to be a state of low-level inflammation. The relationship between obesity and inflammation is, in part, reflected by its close relationship with plasma concentrations of C-reactive protein (CRP), a sensitive marker for acute-phase systemic inflammation. Studies show that elevated serum high-sensitivity CRP (hsCRP) concentrations are a significant predictor for incidence of the metabolic syndrome[23] and type 2 diabetes.[24-26] In many prospective cohort studies, hsCRP has also been linked with coronary heart disease,[27] although the causal implication of the association is still a matter of debate.

The relationship between obesity and CRP is well-established. In an analysis of data from 16 616 men and women from NHANES III, Visser et al.[28] found a strong association between obesity and hsCRP levels, especially in women. After adjustment for potential confounders, the odds ratio (OR) for elevated CRP (>1 mg/dL) was 6.21 (95% CI: 4.94 to 7.81) for obese women and 2.13 (95% CI: 1.56 to 2.91) for obese men.

In general, BMI and waist circumference (or WHR) have similar correlations with hsCRP levels (0.2 to 0.4 in men and 0.3-0.5 in women).[29] In a Japanese study, Saijo et al.[30] found that visceral fat accumulation measured by CT scan was more strongly correlated with hsCRP than total or subcutaneous fat. On the other hand, Lemieux et al.[31] reported stronger correlations of hsCRP levels with body fat mass ($r = .41$) and waist girth ($r = .37$) than with visceral adipose tissue (VAT) accumulation measured by CT scan at L4 to L5 ($r = .28$).

Obesity and Insulin Resistance

Insulin resistance refers to reduced insulin-mediated glucose uptake in insulin-sensitive tissues, specifically skeletal muscle and the liver.[32] In obese individuals, in particular, insulin resistance is both common and closely related to the amount of fat in the central abdominal region. Thus, insulin resistance is often considered the common mechanism underlying the clustering of multiple metabolic disorders related to obesity[33] as well as the defining pathophysiological defect in the metabolic syndrome.[34] However, not all insulin-resistant subjects meet the diagnostic criteria for metabolic syndrome, and recent evidence suggests that insulin resistance and the metabolic syndrome are independent predictors of atherosclerosis.[35]

VAT, which is closely associated with insulin resistance and the metabolic syndrome,[36] consists mainly of mesenteric and omental fat masses and can be precisely measured with imaging methods such as CT scans and MRI (see Chapter 5). VAT accounts for a relatively small proportion of total body fat mass, approximately 10%, but for 25% to 50% of total abdominal fat mass, which is largely subcutaneous.[37] Nonetheless, many investigators believe that VAT, with its higher lipolysis rates than subcutaneous fat tissue (SAT) and its close proximity to the portal circulation, is a major contributor to insulin resistance. Lebovitz and Banerji[38] cited several lines of evidence supporting a causal relationship between the amount of VAT and insulin resistance.

The first line of evidence, albeit inconsistent, suggests that in diverse populations, VAT is more strongly associated with insulin resistance than total or subcutaneous fat masses.[39,40] Second, Lemieux et al.[41] found that increases in VAT, but not total fat mass, predicted changes in glucose tolerance and insulin secretion in a cohort of women followed for 7 years. Third, Klein and colleagues reported that liposuction of abdominal subcutaneous adipose tissue did not appear to improve insulin action and cardiovascular risk factors in obese subjects.[42] Lastly, treatment with peroxisome proliferator-activated receptor (PPAR) agonists (e.g., pioglitazone and rosiglitazone) led to a shift of fat distribution from visceral to subcutaneous adipose depots, and that this shift was associated with improvements in hepatic and peripheral tissue sensitivity to insulin.[43]

Conversely, several lines of evidence argue against the causal relationship between VAT and insulin resistance. Miles and Jensen[37] noted that differences in the amount of SAT account for most of the between-person variability in abdominal fat, while the relative content of VAT is similar between lean and obese individuals. In addition, some studies have shown similar correlations between SAT and VAT and insulin resistance.[44] Moreover, Goodpaster et al.[44] found that FFAs released by VAT were correlated with visceral fat mass, but relative amounts of FFAs derived from VAT lipolysis were much lower than those derived from SAT. Visceral lipolysis accounts for only 5% to 10% of portal vein FFAs in lean individuals and 20% to 25% of portal vein FFAs in obese individuals.

Martin and Jensen,[45] for example, reported that upper body nonvisceral fat lipolysis contributes most to systemic FFAs availability in obese men and women. When Kelley et al.[46] subdivided abdominal SAT into deep and superficial compartments, they found that deep SAT and VAT were similarly correlated with insulin-stimulated glucose utilization measured by euglycemic clamp ($r \approx -.60$). Conversely, there was no significant association between superficial SAT and insulin sensitivity.

Together, current evidence suggests that both VAT and SAT contribute to insulin resistance. Theoretically, VAT is more relevant to the development of insulin resistance, but the data on the relative importance of SAT and VAT are conflicting. In epidemiologic studies, waist circumference as a measure of abdominal or upper body obesity reflects the effects of both SAT and VAT. Thus, in practice, distinction between these two fat locations may not be easy or essential.

Obesity and Vascular Endothelial Dysfunction

The vascular endothelium was traditionally considered a static monolayer of cells, serving as a semipermeable barrier between the bloodstream and tissue.[47] It is now well established that the endothelium is an active and dynamic tissue that plays an essential role in cell adhesion and migration, thrombosis, and fibrinolysis. Proinflammatory stimuli can activate the vascular endothelium to increase production and expression of soluble adhesion molecules, such as intercellular adhesion molecule-1 (ICAM-1), vascular cell adhesion molecule-1 (VCAM-1), and e-selectin and p-selectin.[48] In several prospective studies, elevated levels of ICAM-1 and e-selectin were significant predictors of future risk of CVD[49] and type 2 diabetes.[50] In addition, microalbuminuria, a marker of diffuse endothelial dysfunction, has been associated with type 2 diabetes and CVD.[51] These results suggest that endothelial dysfunction is a common precursor of multiple metabolic disorders associated with obesity.

Several epidemiologic studies have examined the relationship between overall adiposity, fat distribution, and endothelial function. In a cohort of healthy women, Wexler et al.[52] found similar correlations between plasma concentrations of e-selectin with both BMI and waist circumference ($r \approx .3$). Adhesion molecules were significantly elevated in women with central adiposity but low BMI, and markers of endothelial dysfunction appeared to largely mediate the relationship between central body fat, insulin resistance, and incident diabetes.

Brachial artery flow-mediated dilation (FMD) is a direct measure of endothelial vasodilator function in humans. Endothelial dysfunction, reflected by decreased FMD, is correlated with inflammation, metabolic disorders, and cardiovascular events.[53] In the Framingham Heart Study, BMI was an independent predictor of reduced FMD.[54] In addition, Brook et al.[55] found that abdominal obesity, reflected by a higher WHR, was a significant predictor of endothelial function assessed by FMD of the brachial artery. Similarly, Arcaro et al.[56] reported a significant correlation between degree of vascular dysfunction and body fat distribution independent of BMI. These data indicate that endothelial dysfunction may be a common cellular mechanism linking obesity to the metabolic syndrome and CVD. Thus, vascular endothelial dysfunction can be considered a unifying factor for the diabetogenic effects of excess adiposity, low-grade inflammation, and the metabolic syndrome.

Obesity and Hypertension

The relationship between obesity and hypertension is well established. Even within lean populations in developing countries, individuals with greater body mass have substantially elevated blood pressure and higher rates of hypertension.[57,58] Overweight and obesity are the most important modifiable risk factors for hypertension, accounting for more than 66% of the risk in some populations.[59] In the Nurses' Health Study (NHS), multivariate analyses showed that BMI values at 18 years of age and midlife were both significantly associated with hypertension.[60] There was a significant association between long-term weight loss after 18 years of age and decreased risk of hypertension, while weight gain after 18 years dramatically increased the risk; multivariate relative risks (RRs) were 0.85 for a loss of 5.0 to 9.9 kg; 0.74 for a loss of 10 kg or more; 1.74 for a gain of 5.0 to 9.9 kg; and 5.21 for a gain of 25.0 kg or more. The association remained significant after adjusting for current BMI, suggesting that both attained BMI and history of weight change are independent predictors of hypertension. In the Framingham Study, Moore et al.[61] reported that a modest weight loss, particularly when sustained, was associated with 22% to 26% lower risk of hypertension during 38 years of follow-up.

Several studies have suggested that waist circumference or WHR significantly predicts risk of hypertension independent of BMI.[62-64] In a cohort of Japanese Americans, visceral adiposity measured by CT was a better predictor of incident hypertension than BMI or waist circumference.[65] There was no significant association between subcutaneous fat and hypertension.

Multiple mechanisms have been proposed to explain the relationship between obesity and hypertension. Overweight and obesity are known to cause renal structural changes that lead to tubular reabsorption and sodium retention.[66,67] Increased arterial pressure further damages nephron function, creating the vicious cycle of obesity, hypertension, and renal injury.[67] For these reasons, obesity and the metabolic syndrome have been commonly associated with microalbuminuria and CKD.[68,69] Another mechanism is related to enhanced sympathetic nervous system (SNS) activity in obese individuals. In subjects who lost weight and then regained it, plasma norepinephrine levels were significantly higher than they were in subjects who maintained weight loss.[70] Activation of SNS activity has been linked to increased plasma insulin levels and insulin resistance, elevated FFAs, angiotensin II and leptin levels, and decreased baroreflex sensitivity.[67]

The relationship between hyperinsulinemia and hypertension has received a great deal of attention. More than 40 years ago, Welborn et al.[71] observed that nondiabetic patients with essential hypertension had significantly higher plasma insulin concentrations than normotensive individuals. Several longitudinal studies have since confirmed this positive relationship, but results have not been entirely consistent.[72] In some studies, the association between hyperinsulinemia and incident hypertension disappeared after adjustment for BMI, suggesting that the association might be confounded by adiposity.[73]

In the past decade, the concept of adipose tissue as an endocrine organ has provided a new paradigm for explaining the relationship between obesity and hypertension. As discussed already, adipose tissue secretes a number of cytokines that have proinflammatory or anti-inflammatory properties. Some of these adipokines have both direct and indirect effects on blood pressure control. For example, angiotensinogen (AGT) secreted by adipocytes is the precursor of vasoactive angiotensin II, a molecule in the renin-angiotensin system (RAS) that plays an important role in the regulation of blood pressure.[74,75] In addition, higher CRP levels have been associated with increased risk of developing hypertension.[76]

Leptin is mainly secreted and expressed in SAT.[77] The role of leptin in activation of the SNS has been studied extensively in animal experiments.[67] In humans, however, there is little evidence that plasma leptin levels significantly predict incident hypertension independent of BMI. As discussed already, plasma adiponectin levels, which are associated with improved insulin sensitivity, are decreased in obese individuals. Studies show that PPAR-gamma agonists or thiazolidinediones (TZDs), which lead to increased adiponectin levels, produce a modest reduction in blood pressure.[78,79] Whether the relationship between adiponectin levels and blood pressure is causal is unclear.

Obesity and Dyslipidemia

Dyslipidemia is one of the most common metabolic disorders associated with obesity. In many studies, indices of body size and adiposity—including BMI, WHR, subscapular skinfolds, and percent body fat—are strongly correlated with hypertriglyceridemia, hypercholesterolemia, and low HDL cholesterol. Low HDL cholesterol, high TG, and small dense LDL are among the most common features of dyslipidemia related to the metabolic syndrome.[80,81]

The link between overweight and dyslipidemia is complex and not well understood. However, evidence suggests that insulin resistance may be the underlying mechanism.[80] Under normal physiological conditions, insulin suppresses the release of fatty acids from adipose tissue and the production of very-low-density lipoprotein (VLDL). Conversely, insulin resistance diminishes this inhibitory effect. Thus, in obese subjects, increased flux of FFAs from the blood to the liver stimulates hepatic TG synthesis and overproduction of TG containing VLDL and also increases production of ApoB by the liver. Consequently, hypertriglyceridemia in metabolic syndrome results from both increased production and impaired clearance. In overweight individuals, one of the best biomarkers of insulin resistance appears to be hypertriglyceridemia or the TG-to-HDL ratio.[82]

In the metabolic syndrome, low HDL cholesterol is considered a direct consequence of elevated TG. Large amounts of TG-rich lipoproteins with prolonged residence time in circulation increase the exchange between esterified cholesterol in HDL and TG in TG-rich lipoproteins.[80] The faster catabolic rate of TG-enriched and cholesterol-depleted HDL (compared with normal HDL) increases HDL clearance from the circulation. In addition, hypertriglyceridemia increases the clearance of ApoA, the main protein of HDL, and causes a shift from large buoyant LDL to small dense LDL enriched with ApoB. Small dense LDL has frequently been associated with insulin resistance and the metabolic syndrome.[83]

Obesity and Thrombogenic Factors

Plasma thrombogenic factors (e.g., fibrinogen, factor VII, and plasminogen activator inhibitor-1 [PAI-1]) are elevated in subjects with the metabolic syndrome and may contribute to increased cardiovascular risk.[84] Ditschuneit et al.[85] found that fibrinogen correlated with BMI, waist circumference, and WHR, and that weight loss substantially lowered fibrinogen levels. Avellone et al.[86] reported that PAI-1 concentrations were positively associated with VAT and upper-body fat distribution in women.

Ferguson et al.[87] demonstrated that even in early childhood, adiposity was associated with unfavorable homeostatic factors, for example, increased fibrinogen and PAI-1 levels. Strong correlations between fasting insulin levels and levels of fibrinogen and PAI-1 have also been found. The Cardiovascular Health Study reported positive correlations between factor VII concentrations and several cardiovascular risk factors including obesity, dyslipidemia, and fasting insulin levels.[88] In the Framingham Offspring Study, significant associations were observed between hyperinsulinemia and levels of PAI-1 and tissue-plasminogen activator (t-PA).[89]

Obesity and Type 2 Diabetes

Among all lifestyle risk factors for type 2 diabetes, overweight and obesity are the most important. In the NHS,[90] the RRs were 20.1 for 30.0 to 34.9 kg/m^2 and 38.8 for $\geq$35 kg/m^2 (compared with <23 kg/m^2). Even a BMI within a normal range (23 to 24.9 kg/m^2) was associated with substantially elevated risk for type 2 diabetes (RR, 2.67; 95% CI: 2.13 to 3.34). In this cohort, 61% (95% CI: 58% to 64%) of diabetes cases could be attributed to overweight and obesity (using 25 kg/m^2 as a cutpoint). Abdominal obesity assessed by waist circumference or WHR predicted risk of diabetes independent of BMI.[91] After controlling for BMI and other potential confounding factors, the RR for the 90th percentile of WHR (WHR = 0.86) versus the 10th percentile (WHR = 0.70) was 3.1 (95% CI: 2.3 to 4.1). The RR for the 90th percentile of waist circumference (36.2 in or 92 cm) versus the 10th percentile (26.2 in or 67 cm) was 5.1 (95% CI: 2.9 to 8.9).

Weight gain during adulthood, even at modest levels (e.g., $\leq$10 kg), has been associated with increased risk of diabetes. In the NHS,[92] compared with those whose weight remained stable (a gain or loss of $\leq$5 kg between the age of 18 and baseline in 1976), the RRs for diabetes were: 1.9 (95% CI: 1.5 to 2.3) for women with a weight gain of 5.0 to 7.9 kg; 2.7 (95% CI: 2.1 to 3.3) for a weight gain of 8.0 to 10.9 kg; and 12.3 (95% CI: 10.9 to 13.8) for an increase of 20.0 kg or more. In contrast, women who lost more than 5.0 kg reduced their risk for diabetes by 50% or more.

We recently compared the accuracy of BMI, waist circumference, and WHR in predicting type 2 diabetes among 27,270 men in the Health Professionals' Follow-up Study (HPFS).[93] The risk of diabetes, already significant at the second decile for BMI, waist

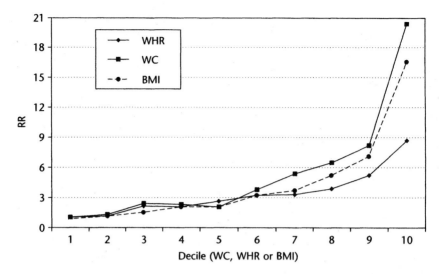

Figure 8.3 Age-adjusted RR of type 2 diabetes by baseline waist circumference (WC), waist-to-hip ratio (WHR), and body mass index (BMI) deciles. Reproduced with permission from Wang Y, Rimm EB, Stampfer MJ, Willett WC, Hu FB. Comparison of abdominal adiposity and overall obesity in predicting risk of type 2 diabetes among men. *Am J Clin Nutr.* 2005;81:555-563.[93]

circumference, and WHR, increased more dramatically between the 9th and 10th deciles. A high (upper decile) waist circumference was a powerful risk factor for type 2 diabetes (RR, 20.4; 95% CI: 12.3 to 33.8), stronger than WHR (RR, 8.7; 95% CI: 5.8 to 13.0) or BMI (RR, 16.5; 95% CI: 10.4 to 26.3) (Fig. 8.3). Joint analyses showed that BMI and waist circumference were independent predictors of diabetes.

Koh-Banerjee et al.[94] examined relationships between changes in body weight and body fat distribution (1986-1996) and subsequent risk of diabetes (1996-2000) among participants in the HPFS cohort. Weight gain was monotonically related to risk, and for every kilogram of weight gained, risk increased by approximately 7%. In this cohort, the correlation of 0.51 between changes in body weight and waist was smaller than that between BMI and waist at baseline ($r = .77$). This suggests that changes in body weight alone does not adequately capture changes in body fat in older individuals, who may be losing muscle mass and gaining adiposity (see Chapter 5).

In multivariate analyses, men who lost more than 2.6 cm of waist girth had an RR of 0.8 (95% CI: 0.5 to 1.1) for developing diabetes compared with men whose waist size remained stable (±2.5 cm).[94] In contrast, men whose waist circumference increased by 2.6 to 6.4 cm had a multivariate RR of 1.3 (95% CI: 1.0 to 1.7), while those with the greatest waist gain (≥14.6 cm) had 2.4 (95% CI: 1.5 to 3.7) times the risk of diabetes. Men who lost more than 4.1 cm in hip girth had 1.5 (95% CI: 1.0 to 2.3) times the risk of diabetes compared with men with stable hip circumference. The increased risk with loss in hip girth may reflect the effect of a loss of muscle mass on insulin sensitivity and diabetes risk.

In the Hoorn Study, large hip girth was associated with a lower risk of type 2 diabetes after adjusting for age, BMI, and waist circumference.[95] Evidence from cross-sectional studies suggests that leg fat depot, unlike truncal fat depot, may confer protection against metabolic disturbances.[96] However, this observation needs to be confirmed in additional prospective studies, and the mechanisms for the divergent effects of different fat depots need to be elucidated.

Ethnic Differences in Risk of Metabolic Syndrome and Diabetes

Data from NHANES III show that minority groups have a disproportionately higher prevalence of the metabolic syndrome than whites.[6] Mexican Americans have the highest age-adjusted prevalence of the metabolic syndrome (31.9% versus 23.7% in the overall population). Abdominal obesity is one of the most common components of the syndrome. The prevalence of abdominal obesity is higher in African Americans (44.6%) and Mexican Americans (45.7%) than in whites (37.2%). The prevalence is particularly high in minority women, exceeding 60% in both African American and Mexican American women compared with 40% in white women. Among other components of the metabolic syndrome, Mexican Americans have the highest prevalence of impaired fasting glucose or diabetes (20%) and hypertriglyceridemia (37.7%), while African Americans have the highest prevalence of hypertension (46.3%).

There is substantial evidence that East Asians (e.g., Chinese, Japanese, and Korean individuals) develop the metabolic syndrome at much lower BMI levels than whites, and that the slopes between BMI and individual components of the metabolic syndrome are steeper than those observed for whites.[97,98] As discussed in Chapter 5, ethnic variations in metabolic risk may be attributed to different fat distribution and percent body fat among different ethnic groups. At the same BMI, percentage of body fat in Asians is 3%-5% higher than in Caucasians with the same BMI.[99]

Few prospective cohort studies have examined ethnic differences in risk of developing diabetes while taking dietary and lifestyle factors into account. In a prospective study of ethnic differences in type 2 diabetes risk among 78,419 healthy middle-aged women in the NHS,[100] we repeatedly collected detailed information on diet and lifestyle factors during 20 years of follow-up. Compared with whites, the age and BMI-adjusted RRs were 2.26 (1.70 to 2.99) for Asians; 1.86 (1.40 to 2.47) for Hispanics; and 1.34 (1.12 to 1.61) for blacks. These RRs did not change appreciably after further adjustment for dietary and lifestyle risk factors. For each five-unit increment in BMI, the multivariate RR of diabetes was 2.36 (1.83 to 3.04) for Asians; 2.21 (1.75 to 2.79) for Hispanics; 1.96 (1.93 to 2.00) for whites; and 1.55 (1.36 to 1.77) for blacks. For each 5 kg weight gain between the ages of 18 and baseline, risk of diabetes increased by 84% for Asians; 44% for Hispanics; 37% for whites; and 38% for blacks.

This study indicates that the risk of developing diabetes is significantly higher among Asians, Hispanics, and blacks than among whites after accounting for BMI and other diabetes risk factors. The association between increasing BMI and greater weight gain and risk of diabetes was most pronounced among Asian women. The biological basis for the ethnic differences has not been fully elucidated. A metabolic study by Dickinson et al.[101] found markedly higher postprandial glucose in Asians compared with whites. Among lean, healthy subjects matched for age, BMI, waist circumference, birth weight, and current diet, Asians (particularly those of Southeast Asian descent) had significantly higher postprandial glycemia and lower insulin sensitivity compared with whites in response to a 75 g carbohydrate load. In several epidemiologic studies,[102-104] minority populations including blacks, Asians, and Mexican Americans had reduced insulin sensitivity than non-Hispanic whites after adjusting for obesity. These findings suggest that reduced insulin sensitivity, which may be caused by both genetic and environmental factors, underlies the increased risk of type 2 diabetes in U.S. minorities, particularly Asians.[100]

Relative Effects of Adiposity and Physical Activity on Diabetes

Both obesity and physical inactivity are well-known risk factors for development of type 2 diabetes. It has been suggested that higher levels of physical activity and fitness can mitigate the impact of overweight and obesity on morbidity and mortality; in other words, obesity may not be detrimental to those who are physically active or fit.[105] However, a recent study indicated a much greater magnitude of association of type 2 diabetes with BMI than with physical inactivity, and physical activity appeared to be less predictive of diabetes in overweight and obese individuals than in those who were lean.[106]

We recently examined the relative impact of adiposity and physical activity on incident diabetes in the NHS.[107] Using a reference group of physically active (exercise at least 21.8 MET hours/week) women at healthy weight (BMI < 25 kg/m²), the RRs of type 2 diabetes were 16.8 (95% CI: 14.0 to 20.0) for women who were obese (BMI ≥ 30 kg/m²) and sedentary (exercise < 2.1 MET hours/week); 10.7 (95% CI: 8.7 to 13.2) for those who were active but obese; and 2.08 (95% CI: 1.66 to 2.61) for women who were lean but inactive. In this study, obesity and physical inactivity independently contributed to the development of type 2 diabetes, with the magnitude of risk conferred by obesity being much greater than that conferred by lack of physical activity. Although increasing physical activity was beneficial for diabetes prevention in both obese and nonobese individuals, being physically active was not sufficient to counteract the adverse effects of obesity on diabetes. Given the utmost importance of adiposity in the development of type 2 diabetes, maintenance of healthy body weight should be emphasized as an eventual goal to prevent the onset of type 2 diabetes.[107]

Obesity and "Fellow Travelers" of the Metabolic Syndrome

Gallstone Disease

Gallstone disease or cholelithiasis is commonly associated with the metabolic syndrome. The majority of gallstones develop from cholesterol;[108] their formation results primarily from the hypersecretion of cholesterol into the biliary tree. Obesity has long been a recognized risk factor for gallstones, especially in women.[108] Mounting evidence indicates that gallstone disease is associated with all the individual components of the metabolic syndrome, for example, low HDL, high TG, high blood pressure, insulin resistance, and impaired glucose tolerance or type 2 diabetes.[109,110] Recent data suggest that prevalence of gallstone disease is significantly elevated among subjects with the metabolic syndrome, increased insulin resistance, or fatty liver (even after taking BMI into account).[111,112] Prevalence of CVD is also two to three times higher among subjects with gallstone disease than among those without it.[112] Given these findings, gallstone disease has been dubbed as a "fellow traveler" of the metabolic syndrome.[113]

Recent evidence indicates a strong and independent association between abdominal adiposity and risk of gallstone disease in both men and women. Tsai et al.[114] examined the association of abdominal circumference and WHR with risk of symptomatic gallstone disease in a cohort of 29,847 men in the HPFS; all were free of previous gallstone disease. After adjustment for BMI and other risk factors for gallstones, RRs across quintiles of height-adjusted waist circumference were 1.0, 1.22, 1.30, 1.41, 1.80, and 2.29 (P for trend < .001). The corresponding RRs across quintiles of WHR were 1.0, 1.22, 1.48, 1.73, and 1.78 (P for trend < .001). BMI was also strongly associated with increased risk of gallstone disease, but the association became nonsignificant after controlling for height-adjusted waist circumference. These results suggest that central fat distribution in men may be a more important risk factor for gallstone development than overall obesity. However, as described in Chapter 5, including BMI and waist circumference in the same model alters the meaning of BMI; controlling for abdominal obesity essentially accounts for the fat mass component of BMI, changing it, for the most part, into a surrogate for lean body mass.

Rapid weight loss in obese patients through very-low-calorie diets or bariatric surgery has been associated with gallstone disease.[115] Syngal et al.,[116] in a study of long-term weight patterns relative to risk of cholecystectomy in a cohort of women, found that 54.9% of the women reported weight cycling, with at least one episode of intentional weight loss associated with weight regain. Overall, 20.1% of the women were light cyclers (5 to 9 lb of weight loss and gain), 18.8% were moderate cyclers (10 to 19 lb), and 16.0% were severe cyclers ($\geq$20 lb of weight loss and gain). Only 11.1% of the cohort maintained weight within 5 lb over the 16-year period (weight maintainers). Compared with weight maintainers, the RR for cholecystectomy among light cyclers (adjusted for BMI, age, alcohol intake, fat intake, and smoking) was 1.20 (95% CI: 0.96 to 1.50); 1.31 (95% CI: 1.05 to 1.64) among moderate cyclers; and 1.68 (95% CI: 1.34 to 2.10) among severe cyclers. These results suggest that weight cycling resulting from intentional attempts to lose weight is a significant risk factor for gallstone formation independent of attained BMI. Thus, preventing weight gain and maintaining a healthy body weight during adulthood are critical for reducing risk of gallstone disease.

Gout

Gout, an inflammatory arthritis characterized by deposits of uric acid crystals within the joints, is a metabolic disorder caused by chronic hyperuricemia.[117] Hyperinsulinemia, insulin resistance, and the metabolic syndrome together are highly common in patients suffering from gout.[118] Hyperuricemia is strongly associated with individual components of the metabolic syndrome (e.g., obesity, hypertension, dyslipidemia, and hyperglycemia/diabetes mellitus)[119] as well as diet (e.g., meats and seafood), alcohol use, renal failure, and intake of certain drugs.[117] Hyperuricemia has been associated with increased cardiovascular and total mortality in several prospective cohort studies.[120,121] However, the associations have been relatively small, and the causality is uncertain.[122] Lee et al.[123] found that obesity may increase hyperuricemia through increased urate production and decreased renal clearance, and that renal excretion of urate is also reduced in the presence of insulin resistance. In light of hyperuricemia's close relationships with lipid, glucose, and insulin metabolism, Zavaroni et al.[124] suggested that hyperuricemia be added to the cluster of metabolic or insulin resistance syndrome risk factors.

Although many cross-sectional and case-control studies have found a close relationship between obesity and gout, prospective data are limited. In the Johns Hopkins Precursors Study, Roubenoff et al.[125] found that BMI at age 35, weight gain, and hypertension were independent predictors of gout. Choi et al.[126] prospectively examined the relationships between BMI and incident gout in 47,150 male participants during 12 years of follow-up. Compared with men with a BMI of 21 to 22.9, the multivariate RRs of gout were 1.95 (95% CI: 1.44 to 2.65) for men with a BMI of 25 to 29.9; 2.33 (1.62 to 3.36) for those with a BMI of 30 to 34.9; and 2.97 (1.73 to 5.10) for men with a BMI of 35 or greater (P for trend <.001). BMI at age 21 was significantly associated with increased risk of gout, although the association was weaker than that for current BMI.

Abdominal obesity, reflected by increasing WHR, was also independently associated with incident gout in men.[126] In addition, weight gain since age 21 was associated with increased risk of gout, whereas weight loss was associated with a lower risk. Hypertension was significantly associated with increased risk of gout even after adjusting for BMI.

Polycystic Ovary Syndrome

PCOS, characterized by ovulatory dysfunction and hyperandrogenism, is strongly related to obesity; over half of women with PCOS are overweight or obese, and most have abdominal obesity.[127] The majority of women with PCOS have various components of the metabolic syndrome and insulin resistance.[128,129] In cross-sectional analyses, metabolic syndrome was highly prevalent in women with PCOS, even at the relatively young age of approximately 30 years.[130] Thus, the term "syndrome XX" has been used to refer to PCOS, with the implication that it is a "female-specific form of the metabolic syndrome."[131] Cross-sectional data suggest increased rates of atherosclerosis and CHD among women with PCOS.[132] In prospective studies, highly irregular menstrual cycles, a common feature of PCOS, have been associated with incident type 2 diabetes[133] and CVD.[132]

Insulin resistance is thought to play an important role in the development of PCOS. Among women with PCOS, insulin-mediated glucose disposal is significantly reduced, and the degree of insulin resistance is similar to that in patients with type 2 diabetes.[134] The reduction in insulin sensitivity is also evident among nonobese women with PCOS, suggesting that defective insulin action in PCOS is not completely caused by obesity. In addition to insulin resistance, both obese and nonobese women with PCOS have significantly decreased beta-cell function.[135] The fundamental causes of insulin resistance in PCOS are not completely understood, but abdominal obesity, hyperandrogenism, and genetic defects all appear to play a role in its development.[128]

Sleep Apnea

Sleep apnea is a common clinical manifestation of the metabolic syndrome and insulin resistance.[136] Obstructive sleep apnea (OSA), defined as a lack of airflow despite continued respiratory efforts, is strongly correlated with age, obesity, weight gain, male gender, and smoking.[137] Heavy snoring is a cardinal symptom of sleep apnea, and epidemiologic data have indicated a strong association between obesity and regular snoring.[138]

There is growing evidence that sleep apnea is independently associated with insulin resistance. In a cross-sectional study, Ip et al.[139] found that those with OSA (defined as an apnea-hypopnea index or AHI of $\geq$ 5) had significantly higher levels of fasting serum insulin ($P = .001$) and homeostasis model assessment of insulin resistance (HOMA-IR) ($P < .001$). This association was seen in obese as well as nonobese subjects. Similarly, Punjabi et al.[140] found an association between sleep-disordered breathing and increased risk of impaired glucose tolerance (odds ratio, 2.15; 95% CI: 1.05 to 4.38) after adjusting for BMI and percentage body fat. There was a dose-response relationship between the severity of oxygen desaturation and the impairment in glucose tolerance. A positive association between sleep-disordered breathing with glucose intolerance and insulin resistance was also found among community-dwelling subjects ($n = 2,656$) in the Sleep Heart Health Study.[141]

The cross-sectional nature of these analyses makes it difficult to know whether sleep apnea is the cause or consequence of insulin resistance. However, increasing evidence suggests that sleep disorders (e.g., reduced sleep hours) may increase risk of weight gain and obesity (see Chapter 16). Also, prospective studies have found that sleep apnea or regular snoring significantly predict future risk of hypertension,[142] type 2 diabetes,[143,144] and CVD in healthy individuals.[145,146]

Sleep apnea has been associated with increased concentrations of proinflammatory cytokines (e.g., IL-6 and TNF-α) that are thought to mediate the relationship between sleep apnea and CVD.[136] It has also been associated with other cardiovascular risk factors, for example, vascular endothelial dysfunction, increased oxidative stress, inflammation, and increased platelet aggregation.[147] Because of the close relationship between sleep disorders and metabolic and cardiovascular risk factors, the term *Syndrome Z* has been used to describe the addition of sleep apnea to the cluster of risk factors in the metabolic syndrome.[148]

Chronic Kidney Disease

Chronic kidney disease (CKD is another "fellow traveler" of the metabolic syndrome. Because the kidney plays an important role in the development of hypertension and hyperuricemia, Reaven considered it "an unwilling accomplice in Syndrome X." [149] Data suggest a strong relationship between the metabolic syndrome and CKD. Chen et al.[150] demonstrated that subjects with the metabolic syndrome had a significantly higher odds ratio of CKD (defined as a glomerular filtration rate [GFR] of less than 60 mL/min per 1.73 m^2) and microalbuminuria (defined as a urinary albumin-creatinine ratio of 30 to 300 mg/g) compared with subjects without the metabolic syndrome; adjusted odds ratios were 2.60 (95% CI: 1.68 to 4.03) for CKD and 1.89 (95% CI: 1.34 to 2.67) for microalbuminuria.

These cross-sectional relationships were confirmed by a prospective cohort analysis from the Atherosclerosis Risk in Communities study.[151] This analysis included 10 096 nondiabetic participants with normal kidney function at baseline. Compared with participants with no traits of the metabolic syndrome, those with one, two, three, four, or five traits had respective RRs of CKD of 1.13, 1.53, 1.75, 1.84, and 2.45 (*P* for trend <.001).

Several recent studies have reported an independent association between obesity and renal disease. In the Framingham Study, Fox et al.[152] found that higher BMI was associated with an increased risk of developing CKD, defined by a GFR in the fifth or lower percentile (≤59.25 mL/min per 1.73 m^2 in women and ≤64.25 mL/min per 1.73 m^2 in men) after adjusting for hypertension, diabetes, and other cardiovascular risk factors (RR, 1.23 per 1 standard deviation; 95% CI: 1.08 to 1.41). Hsu et al.[153] examined whether excess weight was an independent risk factor for end-stage renal disease (ESRD). Using multivariable models that adjusted for age, sex, race, education level, smoking status, history of myocardial infarction, serum cholesterol level, urinalysis proteinuria, urinalysis hematuria, and serum creatinine level (Fig. 8.4), they found a significant association

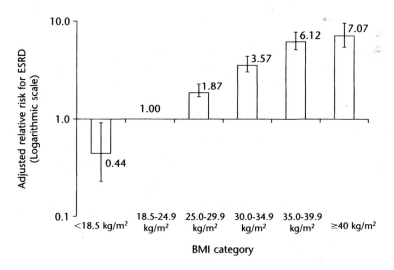

Figure 8.4 Adjusted RR for end-stage renal disease (ESRD) by body mass index (BMI). Model adjusted for multiphasic health checkup period, age, sex, race, education level, smoking status, history of myocardial infarction, serum cholesterol level, proteinuria, hematuria, and serum creatinine level. Error bars represent 95% CIs. Reproduced with permission from Hsu CY, McCulloch CE, Iribarren C, Darbinian J, Go AS. Body mass index and risk for end-stage renal disease. *Ann Intern Med.* 2006;144:21-28.[153]

between increasing BMI and increasing risk of developing ESRD in a cohort of 320,252 adult members of Kaiser Permanente who volunteered for screening health checkups between 1964 and 1985. This association remained significant even after additional adjustments for baseline blood pressure level and the presence or absence of diabetes mellitus.

These analyses indicate that the adverse effects of obesity on kidney disease are not completely mediated through hypertension or diabetes. Insulin resistance and compensatory hyperinsulinemia, both associated with reduced GFR,[154] may directly contribute to renal cell damage by causing renal vasodilation and glomerular hyperfiltration.[69,155] Proinflammatory cytokines secreted by adipose tissue, such as IL-6, TNF-α, and leptin, may also mediate the relationship between obesity and renal disease pathophysiology.[156]

Nonalcoholic Fatty Liver Disease

Nonalcoholic fatty liver disease (NAFLD), or fatty liver, results from an accumulation of fat within the liver and frequently coexists with various components of the metabolic syndrome.[157] Both overall adiposity and abdominal obesity are associated with substantially increased risk of fatty liver. In a study of elderly men and women in Japan, Akahoshi et al.[158] found that the prevalence of fatty liver increased from 3.3% in males with BMI less than 26 kg/m^2 to 21.6% in those with BMI of 26 kg/m^2 or greater; the respective prevalence among women was 3.8% and 18.8%.

In a cross-sectional study of 83 obese men and women with type 2 diabetes, Kelley et al.[159] found that a majority (63%) of subjects with type 2 diabetes met CT scan criteria for fatty liver, compared with 20% of obese individuals without type 2 diabetes, and none of the lean, nondiabetic volunteers. NAFLD appeared to be more strongly correlated with VAT than BMI or subcutaneous fat. Subjects with fatty liver also had significantly elevated concentrations of proinflammatory cytokines (e.g., CRP, IL-6, and TNF-α). Even among nonobese individuals, fatty liver has been associated with increased waist circumference, insulin resistance, and iron overload reflected by serum ferritin levels.[160]

In nonobese and nondiabetic Koreans, the presence of fatty liver was significantly associated with increased waist circumference, TG levels, and insulin resistance.[161] Marchesini et al.[162] reported a nearly 50% reduction in glucose disposal during the euglycemic clamp in patients with fatty liver assessed by biopsy. Insulin-mediated suppression of lipolysis was also significantly reduced in patients with fatty liver. Garg[163] noted that fatty liver was common in subjects with lipodystrophies; that such patients, with virtually no adipose tissue, had metabolic abnormalities similar to those in obesity-induced metabolic syndrome (e.g., insulin resistance, diabetes mellitus, and hypertriglyceridemia).

In a cross-sectional study conducted in Shanghai, Fan et al.[164] observed a strong correlation between fatty liver diagnosed by ultrasonography and the metabolic syndrome defined by ATP III criteria. Subjects with the metabolic syndrome had nearly 40-fold higher odds of being diagnosed with fatty liver than those without the syndrome. Hamaguchi et al.[165] conducted a prospective study in healthy Japanese men and women 21 to 80 years of age with a mean BMI of 22.6 kg/m^2. Men with the metabolic syndrome (according to ATP III criteria) at baseline were four times (95% CI: 2.63 to 6.08) more likely to develop fatty liver during follow-up. In women, the corresponding RR was substantially higher (RR of 11.20; CI: 4.85 to 25.87). Cross-sectional and case-control studies also suggest that fatty liver disease is associated with increased atherosclerosis.[166,167] Whether this association is independent of insulin resistance or individual components of the metabolic syndrome is unclear.

Summary

Although the clustering of obesity-related abnormalities has long been recognized, clinical definitions of the metabolic syndrome have only recently been formalized. Despite controversies regarding the precise definition of the syndrome, there is a consensus that excess adiposity, especially central obesity, is the driving force behind the metabolic syndrome. Insulin resistance is widely considered the unifying mechanism for obesity-related metabolic disorders, but proinflammatory cytokines secreted by adipose tissue also appear to play an important role in causing insulin resistance and inducing a cascade of metabolic disturbances. Studies suggest that these cytokines exert an endocrine effect conducive to the development of insulin resistance in liver, skeletal muscle, and vascular endothelial tissue; changes that ultimately lead to the clinical expression of type 2 diabetes, CVD, and other complications of the metabolic syndrome (e.g., gallbladder disease, gout, PCOS, fatty liver, sleep apnea, and CKD).

Excess adiposity is the single most important factor in the development of various metabolic disorders, in particular, hypertension and type 2 diabetes. Numerous epidemiologic studies have shown that BMI and fat distribution independently predict various metabolic disorders. Weight gain has also been identified as a powerful predictor of virtually all metabolic conditions, and there is solid evidence that some ethnic groups, especially Asians, are more susceptible to the adverse effects of excess adiposity. Recent evidence also suggests that increasing waist circumference during adulthood is a risk factor for incident diabetes independent of weight gain. Therefore, it is important to monitor measures of both overall and regional adiposity, such as body weight and waist circumference, in assessing metabolic risks associated with obesity.

References

1. Eckel RH, Grundy SM, Zimmet PZ. The metabolic syndrome. *Lancet*. 2005;365: 1415-1428.
2. Reaven GM. Banting lecture 1988. Role of insulin resistance in human disease. *Diabetes*. 1988;37:1595-1607.
3. Kaplan NM. The deadly quartet. Upper-body obesity, glucose intolerance, hypertriglyceridemia, and hypertension. *Arch Intern Med*. 1989;149:1514-1520.
4. Alberti KG, Zimmet PZ. Definition, diagnosis and classification of diabetes mellitus and its complications. Part 1: diagnosis and classification of diabetes mellitus provisional report of a WHO consultation. *Diabet Med*. 1998;15:539-553.
5. Executive Summary of the Third Report of the National Cholesterol Education Program (NCEP) Expert Panel on Detection, Evaluation, and Treatment of High Blood Cholesterol In Adults (Adult Treatment Panel III). *JAMA*. 2001;285:2496-2497.
6. Ford ES, Giles WH, Dietz WH. Prevalence of the metabolic syndrome among US adults: findings from the third National Health and Nutrition Examination Survey. *JAMA*. 2002;287:356-359.
7. Alberti KG, Zimmet P, Shaw. J; IDF Epidemiology Task Force Consensus Group. The metabolic syndrome—a new worldwide definition. *Lancet*. 2005;366:1059-1062.
8. Liese AD, Mayer-Davis EJ, Haffner SM. Development of the multiple metabolic syndrome: an epidemiologic perspective. *Epidemiol Rev*. 1998;20:157-172.
9. Kahn R, Buse J, Ferrannini E, Stern M. American Diabetes Association, European Association for the Study of Diabetes. The metabolic syndrome: time for a critical appraisal: joint statement from the American Diabetes Association and the European Association for the Study of Diabetes. *Diabetes Care*. 2005;28:2289-2304.
10. Reaven GM. The metabolic syndrome: requiescat in pace. *Clin Chem*. 2005;51:931-938.

11. Grundy SM. Metabolic syndrome: connecting and reconciling cardiovascular and diabetes worlds. *J Am Coll Cardiol.* 2006;47:1093-1100.

12. Ford ES. Risks for all-cause mortality, cardiovascular disease, and diabetes associated with the metabolic syndrome: a summary of the evidence. *Diabetes Care.* 2005;28:1769-1778.

13. Dekker JM, Girman C, Rhodes T, et al. Metabolic syndrome and 10-year cardiovascular disease risk in the Hoorn Study. *Circulation.* 2005;112:666-673.

14. Wisse BE. The inflammatory syndrome: the role of adipose tissue cytokines in metabolic disorders linked to obesity. *J Am Soc Nephrol.* 2004:2792-2800.

15. Abel ED, Peroni O, Kim JK, et al. Adipose-selective targeting of the GLUT4 gene impairs insulin action in muscle and liver. *Nature.* 2001;409:729-733.

16. Saltiel AR. You are what you secrete. *Nat Med.* 2001;7:887-888.

17. Wiecek A, Kokot F, Chudek J, Adamczak M. The adipose tissue—a novel endocrine organ of interest to the nephrologist. *Nephrol Dial Transplant.* 2002;17:191-195.

18. Havel PJ. Control of energy homeostasis and insulin action by adipocyte hormones: leptin, acylation stimulating protein, and adiponectin. *Curr Opin Lipidol.* 2002;13:51-59.

19. Lee JH, Bullen JW, Jr., Stoyneva VL, Mantzoros CS. Circulating resistin in lean, obese, and insulin-resistant mouse models: lack of association with insulinemia and glycemia. *Am J Physiol Endocrinol Metab.* 2005;288:E625-E632.

20. Graham TE, Yang Q, Bluher M, et al. Retinol-binding protein 4 and insulin resistance in lean, obese, and diabetic subjects. *N Engl J Med.* 2006;354:2552-2563.

21. Lewis GF, Carpentier A, Adeli K, Giacca A. Disordered fat storage and mobilization in the pathogenesis of insulin resistance and type 2 diabetes. *Endocr Rev.* 2002;23:201-229.

22. Daval M, Foufelle F, Ferre P. Functions of AMP-activated protein kinase in adipose tissue. *J Physiol.* 2006;1;574(Pt 1):55-62.

23. Han TS, Sattar N, Williams K, Gonzalez-Villalpando C, Lean ME, Haffner SM. Prospective study of C-reactive protein in relation to the development of diabetes and metabolic syndrome in the Mexico City Diabetes Study. *Diabetes Care.* 2002; 25:2016-2021.

24. Pradhan AD, Manson JE, Rifai N, Buring JE, Ridker PM. C-reactive protein, interleukin 6, and risk of developing type 2 diabetes mellitus. *JAMA.* 2001;286:327-334.

25. Spranger J, Kroke A, Mohlig M, et al. Inflammatory cytokines and the risk to develop type 2 diabetes: results of the prospective population-based European Prospective Investigation into Cancer and Nutrition (EPIC)-Potsdam Study. *Diabetes.* 2003;52: 812-817.

26. Hu FB, Meigs JB, Li TY, Rifai N, Manson JE. Inflammatory markers and risk of developing type 2 diabetes in women. *Diabetes.* 2004;53:693-700.

27. Willerson JT, Ridker PM. Inflammation as a cardiovascular risk factor. *Circulation.* 2004;109(21 Suppl 1):II2-II10.

28. Visser M, Bouter LM, McQuillan GM, Wener MH, Harris TB. Elevated C-reactive protein levels in overweight and obese adults. *JAMA.* 1999;282:2131-2135.

29. Erlinger TP, Selvin E. Chapter 14. Effects of adiposity and weight loss on C-reactive protein. In: Ridker PM, Rifai N, eds. C-reactive protein and cardiovascular disease: MediEdition, 2006;199-212.

30. Saijo Y, Kiyota N, Kawasaki Y, et al. Relationship between C-reactive protein and visceral adipose tissue in healthy Japanese subjects. *Diabetes Obes Metab.* 2004;6: 249-258.

31. Lemieux I, Pascot A, Prud'homme D, et al. Elevated C-reactive protein: another component of the atherothrombotic profile of abdominal obesity. *Arterioscler Thromb Vasc Biol.* 2001;21:961-967.

32. DeFronzo RA, Ferrannini E. Insulin resistance. A multifaceted syndrome responsible for NIDDM, obesity, hypertension, dyslipidemia, and atherosclerotic cardiovascular disease. *Diabetes Care.* 1991;14:173-194.

33. Golay A, Ybarra J. Link between obesity and type 2 diabetes. *Best Pract Res Clin Endocrinol Metab.* 2005;19:649-663.
34. de Luca C, Olefsky JM. Stressed out about obesity and insulin resistance. *Nat Med.* 2006;12:41-42.
35. Reilly MP, Wolfe ML, Rhodes T, Girman C, Mehta N, Rader DJ. Measures of insulin resistance add incremental value to the clinical diagnosis of metabolic syndrome in association with coronary atherosclerosis. *Circulation.* 2004;110:803-809.
36. Despres JP. Is visceral obesity the cause of the metabolic syndrome? *Ann Med.* 2006;38:52-63.
37. Miles JM, Jensen MD. Counterpoint: visceral adiposity is not causally related to insulin resistance. *Diabetes Care.* 2005;28:2326-2328.
38. Lebovitz HE, Banerji MA. Point: visceral adiposity is causally related to insulin resistance. *Diabetes Care.* 2005;28:2322-2325.
39. Miyazaki Y, Glass L, Triplitt C, Wajcberg E, Mandarino LJ, DeFronzo RA. Abdominal fat distribution and peripheral and hepatic insulin resistance in type 2 diabetes mellitus. *Am J Physiol Endocrinol Metab.* 2002;283:E1135-E1143.
40. Banerji MA, Faridi N, Atluri R, Chaiken RL, Lebovitz HE. Body composition, visceral fat, leptin, and insulin resistance in Asian Indian men. *J Clin Endocrinol Metab.* 1999;84:137-144.
41. Lemieux S, Prud'homme D, Nadeau A, Tremblay A, Bouchard C, Despres JP. Seven-year changes in body fat and visceral adipose tissue in women. Association with indexes of plasma glucose-insulin homeostasis. *Diabetes Care.* 1996 September;19:983-991.
42. Klein S, Fontana L, Young VL, et al. Absence of an effect of liposuction on insulin action and risk factors for coronary heart disease. *N Engl J Med.* 2004;350:2549-2557.
43. Miyazaki Y, Mahankali A, Matsuda M, et al. Effect of pioglitazone on abdominal fat distribution and insulin sensitivity in type 2 diabetic patients. *J Clin Endocrinol Metab.* 2002;87:2784-2791.
44. Goodpaster BH, Thaete FL, Simoneau JA, Kelley DE. Subcutaneous abdominal fat and thigh muscle composition predict insulin sensitivity independently of visceral fat. *Diabetes.* 1997;46:1579-1585.
45. Martin ML, Jensen MD. Effects of body fat distribution on regional lipolysis in obesity. *J Clin Invest.* 1991;88:609-613.
46. Kelley DE, Thaete FL, Troost F, Huwe T, Goodpaster BH. Subdivisions of subcutaneous abdominal adipose tissue and insulin resistance. *Am J Physiol Endocrinol Metab.* 2000;278:E941-E948.
47. Hu FB, Stampfer MJ. Is type 2 diabetes mellitus a vascular condition? *Arterioscler Thromb Vasc Biol.* 2003;23:1715-1716.
48. Davies MJ, Gordon JL, Gearing AJ, et al. The expression of the adhesion molecules ICAM-1, VCAM-1, PECAM, and E-selectin in human atherosclerosis. *J Pathol.* 1993;171:223.
49. Pradhan AD, Rifai N, Ridker PM. Soluble intercellular adhesion molecule-1, soluble vascular adhesion molecule-1, and the development of symptomatic peripheral arterial disease in men. *Circulation.* 2002;106:820-825.
50. Meigs JB, Hu FB, Rifai N, Manson JE. Biomarkers of endothelial dysfunction and risk of type 2 diabetes mellitus. *JAMA.* 2004;291:1978-1986.
51. Meigs JB, D'Agostino RB, Sr., Nathan DM, Rifai N, Wilson PW, Framingham Offspring Study. Longitudinal association of glycemia and microalbuminuria: the Framingham Offspring Study. *Diabetes Care.* 2002;25:977-983.
52. Wexler DJ, Hu FB, Manson JE, Rifai N, Meigs JB. Mediating effects of inflammatory biomarkers on insulin resistance associated with obesity. *Obes Res.* 2005;13:1772-1783.
53. Vita JA, Keaney JF, Jr. Endothelial function: a barometer for cardiovascular risk? *Circulation.* 2002;106:640-642.

54. Benjamin EJ, Larson MG, Keyes MJ, et al. Clinical correlates and heritability of flow-mediated dilation in the community: the Framingham Heart Study. *Circulation.* 2004;109:613-619.

55. Brook RD, Bard RL, Rubenfire M, Ridker PM, Rajagopalan S. Usefulness of visceral obesity (waist/hip ratio) in predicting vascular endothelial function in healthy overweight adults. *Am J Cardiol.* 2001;88:1264-1269.

56. Arcaro G, Zamboni M, Rossi L, et al. Body fat distribution predicts the degree of endothelial dysfunction in uncomplicated obesity. *Int J Obes Relat Metab Disord.* 1999;23:936-942.

57. Long AE, Prewitt TE, Kaufman JS, Rotimi CN, Cooper RS, McGee DL. Weight-height relationships among eight populations of West African origin: the case against constant BMI standards. *Int J Obes Relat Metab Disord.* 1998;22:842-846.

58. Hu FB, Wang B, Chen C, et al. Body mass index and cardiovascular risk factors in a rural Chinese population. *Am J Epidemiol.* 2000;151:88-97.

59. Garrison RJ, Kannel WB, Stokes J III, Castelli WP. Incidence and precursors of hypertension in young adults: the Framingham Offspring Study. *Prev Med.* 1987;16:235-251.

60. Huang Z, Willett WC, Manson JE, et al. Body weight, weight change, and risk for hypertension in women. *Ann Intern Med.* 1998;128:81-88.

61. Moore LL, Visioni AJ, Qureshi MM, Bradlee ML, Ellison RC, D'Agostino R. Weight loss in overweight adults and the long-term risk of hypertension: the Framingham study. *Arch Intern Med.* 2005;165:1298-1303.

62. Dyer AR, Liu K, Walsh M, Kiefe C, Jacobs DR, Jr., Bild DE. Ten-year incidence of elevated blood pressure and its predictors: the CARDIA study. Coronary Artery Risk Development in (Young) Adults. *J Hum Hypertens.* 1999;13:13-21.

63. Guagnano MT, Ballone E, Colagrande V, et al. Large waist circumference and risk of hypertension. *Int J Obes Relat Metab Disord.* 2001;25:1360-1364.

64. Zhu S, Wang Z, Heshka S, Heo M, Faith MS, Heymsfield SB. Waist circumference and obesity-associated risk factors among whites in the third National Health and Nutrition Examination Survey: clinical action thresholds. *Am J Clin Nutr.* 2002;76:743-749.

65. Hayashi T, Boyko EJ, Leonetti DL, et al. Visceral adiposity is an independent predictor of incident hypertension in Japanese Americans. *Ann Intern Med.* 2004;140:992-1000.

66. Davy KP, Hall JE. Obesity and hypertension: two epidemics or one? *Am J Physiol Regul Integr Comp Physiol.* 2004;286:R803-R813.

67. Aneja A, El-Atat F, McFarlane SI, Sowers JR. Hypertension and obesity. *Recent Prog Horm Res.* 2004;59:169-205.

68. Hall JE. The kidney, hypertension, and obesity. *Hypertension.* 2003;41(3 Pt 2):625-633.

69. Bagby SP. Obesity-initiated metabolic syndrome and the kidney: a recipe for chronic kidney disease? *J Am Soc Nephrol.* 2004;15:2775-2791.

70. Masuo K, Katsuya T, Kawaguchi H, et al. Rebound weight gain as associated with high plasma norepinephrine levels that are mediated through polymorphisms in the beta2-adrenoceptor. *Am J Hypertens.* 2005;18:1508-1516.

71. Welborn TA, Breckenridge A, Rubinstein AH, Dollery CT, Fraser TR. Serum-insulin in essential hypertension and in peripheral vascular disease. *Lancet.* 1966;1:1336-1337.

72. Arnlov J, Pencina MJ, Nam BH, et al. Relations of insulin sensitivity to longitudinal blood pressure tracking: variations with baseline age, body mass index, and blood pressure. *Circulation.* 2005;112:1719-1727.

73. Hu FB, Stampfer MJ. Insulin resistance and hypertension: the chicken-egg question revisited. *Circulation.* 2005;112:1678-1680.

74. Prat-Larquemin L, Oppert JM, Clement K, et al. Adipose angiotensinogen secretion, blood pressure, and AGT M235T polymorphism in obese patients. *Obes Res.* 2004;12:556-561.

75. Engeli S, Schling P, Gorzelniak K, et al. The adipose-tissue renin-angiotensin-aldosterone system: role in the metabolic syndrome? *Int J Biochem Cell Biol.* 2003;35:807-825.

76. Sesso HD, Buring JE, Rifai N, Blake GJ, Gaziano JM, Ridker PM. C-reactive protein and the risk of developing hypertension. *JAMA.* 2003;290:2945-2951.

77. Russell CD, Petersen RN, Rao SP, et al. Leptin expression in adipose tissue from obese humans: depot-specific regulation by insulin and dexamethasone. *Am J Physiol.* 1998;275(3 Pt 1):E507-E515.

78. Raji A, Seely EW, Bekins SA, Williams GH, Simonson DC. Rosiglitazone improves insulin sensitivity and lowers blood pressure in hypertensive patients. *Diabetes Care.* 2003;26:172-178.

79. Sarafidis PA, Lasaridis AN, Nilsson PM, et al. Ambulatory blood pressure reduction after rosiglitazone treatment in patients with type 2 diabetes and hypertension correlates with insulin sensitivity increase. *J Hypertens.* 2004;22:1769-1777.

80. Ginsberg HN, Zhang YL, Hernandez-Ono A. Metabolic syndrome: focus on dyslipidemia. *Obesity.* 2006;14(Suppl 1):41S-49S.

81. Kolovou GD, Anagnostopoulou KK, Cokkinos DV. Pathophysiology of dyslipidaemia in the metabolic syndrome. *Postgrad Med J.* 2005;81:358-366.

82. McLaughlin T, Abbasi F, Cheal K, Chu J, Lamendola C, Reaven G. Use of metabolic markers to identify overweight individuals who are insulin resistant. *Ann Intern Med.* 2003;139:802-809.

83. Garvey WT, Kwon S, Zheng D, et al. Effects of insulin resistance and type 2 diabetes on lipoprotein subclass particle size and concentration determined by nuclear magnetic resonance. *Diabetes.* 2003;52:453-462.

84. Skurk T, Hauner H. Obesity and impaired fibrinolysis: role of adipose production of plasminogen activator inhibitor-1. *Int J Obes Relat Metab Disord.* 2004;28: 1357-1364.

85. Ditschuneit HH, Flechtner-Mors M, Adler G. Fibrinogen in obesity before and after weight reduction. *Obes Res.* 1995;3:43-48.

86. Avellone G, Di Garbo V, Cordova R, Raneli G, De Simone R, Bompiani G. Coagulation, fibrinolysis and haemorheology in premenopausal obese women with different body fat distribution. *Thromb Res.* 1994;75:223-231.

87. Ferguson MA, Gutin B, Owens S, Litaker M, Tracy RP, Allison J. Fat distribution and hemostatic measures in obese children. *Am J Clin Nutr.* 1998;67:1136-1140.

88. Cushman M, Yanez D, Psaty BM, et al. Association of fibrinogen and coagulation factors VII and VIII with cardiovascular risk factors in the elderly: the Cardiovascular Health Study. Cardiovascular Health Study Investigators. *Am J Epidemiol.* 1996;143: 665-676.

89. Meigs JB, Mittleman MA, Nathan DM, et al. Hyperinsulinemia, hyperglycemia, and impaired hemostasis: the Framingham Offspring Study. *JAMA.* 2000;283:221-228.

90. Hu FB, Manson JE, Stampfer MJ, et al. Diet, lifestyle, and the risk of type 2 diabetes mellitus in women. *N Engl J Med.* 2001;345:790-797.

91. Carey VJ, Walters EE, Colditz GA, et al. Body fat distribution and risk of non-insulin-dependent diabetes mellitus in women. The Nurses' Health Study. *Am J Epidemiol.* 1997;145:614-619.

92. Colditz GA, Willett WC, Rotnitzky A, Manson JE. Weight gain as a risk factor for clinical diabetes mellitus in women. *Ann Intern Med.* 1995;122:481-486.

93. Wang Y, Rimm EB, Stampfer MJ, Willett WC, Hu FB. Comparison of abdominal adiposity and overall obesity in predicting risk of type 2 diabetes among men. *Am J Clin Nutr.* 2005;81:555-563.

94. Koh-Banerjee P, Wang Y, Hu FB, Spiegelman D, Willett WC, Rimm EB. Changes in body weight and body fat distribution as risk factors for clinical diabetes in US men. *Am J Epidemiol.* 2004;159:1150-1159.

95. Snijder MB, Dekker JM, Visser M, et al. Associations of hip and thigh circumferences independent of waist circumference with the incidence of type 2 diabetes: the Hoorn Study. *Am J Clin Nutr.* 2003;77:1192-1197.

96. Van Pelt RE, Evans EM, Schechtman KB, Ehsani AA, Kohrt WM. Contributions of total and regional fat mass to risk for cardiovascular disease in older women. *Am J Physiol Endocrinol Metab.* 2002;282:E1038-E1038.

97. Colin Bell A, Adair LS, Popkin BM. Ethnic differences in the association between body mass index and hypertension. *Am J Epidemiol.* 2002;155:346-353.

98. Pan WH, Flegal KM, Chang HY, Yeh WT, Yeh CJ, Lee WC. Body mass index and obesity-related metabolic disorders in Taiwanese and US whites and blacks: implications for definitions of overweight and obesity for Asians. *Am J Clin Nutr.* 2004;79:31-39.

99. Deurenberg P, Deurenberg-Yap M. Chapter 3. Ethnic and geographic influences on body composition. In: Bray G, Bouchard C, James P, eds. *Handbook of Obesity.* New York: Dekker, 1998:81-92.

100. Shai I, Jiang R, Manson JE, et al. Ethnicity, obesity, and risk of type 2 diabetes in women: a 20-year follow-up study. *Diabetes Care.* 2006;29:1585-1590.

101. Dickinson S, Colagiuri S, Faramus E, Petocz P, Brand-Miller JC. Postprandial hyperglycemia and insulin sensitivity differ among lean young adults of different ethnicities. *J Nutr.* 2002;132:2574-2579.

102. Torrens JI, Skurnick J, Davidow AL, et al. Ethnic differences in insulin sensitivity and beta-cell function in premenopausal or early perimenopausal women without diabetes: the Study of Women's Health Across the Nation (SWAN). *Diabetes Care.* 2004;27:354-361.

103. Chiu KC, Chuang LM, Yoon C. Comparison of measured and estimated indices of insulin sensitivity and beta cell function: impact of ethnicity on insulin sensitivity and beta cell function in glucose-tolerant and normotensive subjects. *J Clin Endocrinol Metab.* 2001;86:1620-1625.

104. Haffner SM, D'Agostino R, Saad MF, et al. Increased insulin resistance and insulin secretion in nondiabetic African-Americans and Hispanics compared with non-Hispanic whites. The Insulin Resistance Atherosclerosis Study. *Diabetes.* 1996;45:742-748.

105. Blair SN, Brodney S. Effects of physical inactivity and obesity on morbidity and mortality: current evidence and research issues. *Med Sci Sports Exerc.* 1999;31 (11 Suppl):S646-S662.

106. Weinstein AR, Sesso HD, Lee IM, et al. Relationship of physical activity vs body mass index with type 2 diabetes in women. *JAMA.* 2004;292:1188-1194.

107. Rana JS, Li TY, Manson JE, Hu FB. Adiposity compared with physical inactivity and risk of type 2 diabetes in women. *Diabetes Care.* 2007;30:53-58.

108. Diehl AK. Epidemiology and natural history of gallstone disease. *Gastroenterol Clin North Am.* 1991;20:1-19.

109. Ruhl CE, Everhart JE. Association of diabetes, serum insulin, and C-peptide with gallbladder disease. *Hepatology.* 2000;31:299-303.

110. Dubrac S, Parquet M, Blouquit Y, et al. Insulin injections enhance cholesterol gallstone incidence by changing the biliary cholesterol saturation index and apo A-I concentration in hamsters fed a lithogenic diet. *J Hepatol.* 2001;35:550-557.

111. Nervi F, Miquel JF, Alvarez M, et al. Gallbladder disease is associated with insulin resistance in a high risk Hispanic population. *J Hepatol.* 2006;Feb 17:Epub ahead of print.

112. Mendez-Sanchez N, Chavez-Tapia NC, Motola-Kuba D, et al. Metabolic syndrome as a risk factor for gallstone disease. *World J Gastroenterol.* 2005;11:1653-1657.

113. Grundy SM. Cholesterol gallstones: a fellow traveler with metabolic syndrome? *Am J Clin Nutr.* 2004;80:1-2.

114. Tsai CJ, Leitzmann MF, Willett WC, Giovannucci EL. Prospective study of abdominal adiposity and gallstone disease in US men. *Am J Clin Nutr.* 2004;80:38-44.

115. Yang H, Petersen GM, Roth MP, Schoenfield LJ, Marks JW. Risk factors for gallstone formation during rapid loss of weight. *Dig Dis Sci.* 1992;37:912-918.

116. Syngal S, Coakley EH, Willett WC, Byers T, Williamson DF, Colditz GA. Long-term weight patterns and risk for cholecystectomy in women. *Ann Intern Med.* 1999;130:471-477.

117. Choi HK, Mount DB, Reginato AM, American College of Physicians, American Physiological Society. Pathogenesis of gout. *Ann Intern Med.* 2005;143:499-516.

118. Fam AG. Gout, diet, and the insulin resistance syndrome. *J Rheumatol.* 2002;29:1350.

119. Vazquez-Mellado J, Alvarez Hernandez E, Burgos-Vargas R. Primary prevention in rheumatology: the importance of hyperuricemia. *Best Pract Res Clin Rheumatol.* 2004;18:111-124.

120. Fang J, Alderman MH. Serum uric acid and cardiovascular mortality the NHANES I epidemiologic follow-up study, 1971-1992. National Health and Nutrition Examination Survey. *JAMA.* 2000;283:2404-2410.

121. Niskanen LK, Laaksonen DE, Nyyssonen K, et al. Uric acid level as a risk factor for cardiovascular and all-cause mortality in middle-aged men: a prospective cohort study. *Arch Intern Med.* 2004;164:1546-1551.

122. Baker JF, Krishnan E, Chen L, Schumacher HR. Serum uric acid and cardiovascular disease: recent developments, and where do they leave us? *Am J Med.* 2005;118:816-826.

123. Lee J, Sparrow D, Vokonas PS, Landsberg L, Weiss ST. Uric acid and coronary heart disease risk: evidence for a role of uric acid in the obesity-insulin resistance syndrome. The Normative Aging Study. *Am J Epidemiol.* 1995;142:288-294.

124. Zavaroni I, Mazza S, Fantuzzi M, et al. Changes in insulin and lipid metabolism in males with asymptomatic hyperuricaemia. *J Intern Med.* 1993;234:25-30.

125. Roubenoff R, Klag MJ, Mead LA, Liang KY, Seidler AJ, Hochberg MC. Incidence and risk factors for gout in white men. *JAMA.* 1991;266:3004-3007.

126. Choi HK, Atkinson K, Karlson EW, Curhan G. Obesity, weight change, hypertension, diuretic use, and risk of gout in men: the health professionals follow-up study. *Arch Intern Med.* 2005;165:742-748.

127. Gambineri A, Pelusi C, Vicennati V, Pagotto U, Pasquali R. Obesity and the polycystic ovary syndrome. *Int J Obes Relat Metab Disord.* 2002;26:883-896.

128. Dunaif A. Insulin resistance and the polycystic ovary syndrome: mechanism and implications for pathogenesis. *Endocr Rev.* 1997;18:774-800.

129. Ehrmann DA. Polycystic ovary syndrome. *N Engl J Med.* 2005;352:1223-1236.

130. Ehrmann DA, Liljenquist DR, Kasza K, et al. Prevalence and predictors of the metabolic syndrome in women with polycystic ovary syndrome. *J Clin Endocrinol Metab.* 2006;91:48-53.

131. Sam S, Dunaif A. Polycystic ovary syndrome: syndrome XX? *Trends Endocrinol Metab.* 2003;14:365-370.

132. Birdsall MA, Farquhar CM, White HD. Association between polycystic ovaries and extent of coronary artery disease in women having cardiac catheterization. *Ann Intern Med.* 1997;126:32-35.

133. Solomon CG, Hu FB, Dunaif A, et al. Long or highly irregular menstrual cycles as a marker for risk of type 2 diabetes mellitus. *JAMA.* 2001;286:2421-2426.

134. Dunaif A, Segal KR, Futterweit W, Dobrjansky A. Profound peripheral insulin resistance, independent of obesity, in polycystic ovary syndrome. *Diabetes.* 1989;38:1165-1174.

135. Dunaif A, Finegood DT. Beta-cell dysfunction independent of obesity and glucose intolerance in the polycystic ovary syndrome. *J Clin Endocrinol Metab.* 1996;81:942-947.

136. Vgontzas AN, Bixler EO, Chrousos GP. Sleep apnea is a manifestation of the metabolic syndrome. *Sleep Med Rev.* 2005;9:211-224.

137. Vgontzas AN, Bixler EO, Chrousos GP. Metabolic disturbances in obesity versus sleep apnoea: the importance of visceral obesity and insulin resistance. *J Intern Med.* 2003;254:32-44.

138. Hu FB, Willett WC, Colditz GA, et al. Prospective study of snoring and risk of hypertension in women. *Am J Epidemiol*. 1999;150:806-816.

139. Ip MS, Lam B, Ng MM, Lam WK, Tsang KW, Lam KS. Obstructive sleep apnea is independently associated with insulin resistance. *Am J Respir Crit Care Med*. 2002;165:670-676.

140. Punjabi NM, Sorkin JD, Katzel LI, Goldberg AP, Schwartz AR, Smith PL. Sleep-disordered breathing and insulin resistance in middle-aged and overweight men. *Am J Respir Crit Care Med*. 2002;165:677-682.

141. Punjabi NM, Shahar E, Redline S, et al. Sleep-disordered breathing, glucose intolerance, and insulin resistance: the Sleep Heart Health Study. *Am J Epidemiol*. 2004;160:521-530.

142. Young T, Finn L, Hla KM, Morgan B, Palta M. Snoring as part of a dose-response relationship between sleep-disordered breathing and blood pressure. *Sleep*. 1996;19(10 Suppl):S202-S205.

143. Al-Delaimy WK, Manson JE, Willett WC, Stampfer MJ, Hu FB. Snoring as a risk factor for type II diabetes mellitus: a prospective study. *Am J Epidemiol*. 2002;155:387-393.

144. Mallon L, Broman JE, Hetta J. High incidence of diabetes in men with sleep complaints or short sleep duration: a 12-year follow-up study of a middle-aged population. *Diabetes Care*. 2005;28:2762-2767.

145. Elwood P, Hack M, Pickering J, Hughes J, Gallacher J. Sleep disturbance, stroke, and heart disease events: evidence from the Caerphilly cohort. *J Epidemiol Community Health*. 2006;60:69-73.

146. Hu FB, Willett WC, Manson JE, et al. Snoring and risk of cardiovascular disease in women. *J Am Coll Cardiol*. 2000;35:308-313.

147. Shamsuzzaman AS, Gersh BJ, Somers VK. Obstructive sleep apnea: implications for cardiac and vascular disease. *JAMA*. 2003;290:1906-1914.

148. Wilcox I, McNamara SG, Collins FL, Grunstein RR, Sullivan CE. "Syndrome Z": the interaction of sleep apnoea, vascular risk factors and heart disease. *Thorax*. 1998;53(Suppl 3):S25-S28.

149. Reaven GM. The kidney: an unwilling accomplice in syndrome X. *Am J Kidney Dis*. 1997;30:928-931.

150. Chen J, Muntner P, Hamm LL, et al. The metabolic syndrome and chronic kidney disease in U.S. adults. *Ann Intern Med*. 2004;140:167-174.

151. Kurella M, Lo JC, Chertow GM. Metabolic syndrome and the risk for chronic kidney disease among nondiabetic adults. *J Am Soc Nephrol*. 2005;16:2134-2140.

152. Fox CS, Larson MG, Leip EP, Culleton B, Wilson PW, Levy D. Predictors of new-onset kidney disease in a community-based population. *JAMA*. 2004;291:844-850.

153. Hsu CY, McCulloch CE, Iribarren C, Darbinian J, Go AS. Body mass index and risk for end-stage renal disease. *Ann Intern Med*. 2006;144:21-28.

154. De Cosmo S, Trevisan R, Minenna A, et al. Insulin resistance and the cluster of abnormalities related to the metabolic syndrome are associated with reduced glomerular filtration rate in patients with type 2 diabetes. *Diabetes Care*. 2006;29:432-434.

155. Hall JE, Henegar JR, Dwyer TM, et al. Is obesity a major cause of chronic kidney disease? *Adv Ren Replace*. 2004;11:41-54.

156. Wolf G, Chen S, Han DC, Ziyadeh FN. Leptin and renal disease. *Am J Kidney Dis*. 2002;39:1-11.

157. Angulo P. Nonalcoholic fatty liver disease. *N Engl J Med*. 2002;346:1221-1231.

158. Akahoshi M, Amasaki Y, Soda M, et al. Correlation between fatty liver and coronary risk factors: a population study of elderly men and women in Nagasaki, Japan. *Hypertens Res*. 2001;24:337-343.

159. Kelley DE, McKolanis TM, Hegazi RA, Kuller LH, Kalhan SC. Fatty liver in type 2 diabetes mellitus: relation to regional adiposity, fatty acids, and insulin resistance. *Am J Physiol Endocrinol Metab*. 2003;285:E906-E916.

160. Hsiao TJ, Chen JC, Wang JD. Insulin resistance and ferritin as major determinants of nonalcoholic fatty liver disease in apparently healthy obese patients. *Int J Obes Relat Metab Disord.* 2004;28:167-172.
161. Kim HJ, Kim HJ, Lee KE, et al. Metabolic significance of nonalcoholic fatty liver disease in nonobese, nondiabetic adults. *Arch Intern Med.* 2004;164:2169-2175.
162. Marchesini G, Brizi M, Bianchi G, et al. Nonalcoholic fatty liver disease: a feature of the metabolic syndrome. *Diabetes.* 2001;50:1844-1850.
163. Garg A. Lipodystrophies. *Am J Med.* 2000;108:143-152.
164. Fan JG, Zhu J, Li XJ, et al. Fatty liver and the metabolic syndrome among Shanghai adults. *J Gastroenterol Hepatol.* 2005;20:1825-1832.
165. Hamaguchi M, Kojima T, Takeda N, et al. The metabolic syndrome as a predictor of nonalcoholic fatty liver disease. *Ann Intern Med.* 2005;143:722-728.
166. Brea A, Mosquera D, Martin E, Arizti A, Cordero JL, Ros E. Nonalcoholic fatty liver disease is associated with carotid atherosclerosis: a case-control study. *Arterioscler Thromb Vasc Biol.* 2005;25:1045-1050.
167. Targher G, Bertolini L, Padovani R, et al. Non-alcoholic fatty liver disease is associated with carotid artery wall thickness in diet-controlled type 2 diabetic patients. *J Endocrinol Invest.* 2006;29:55-60.

9

Obesity and Cardiovascular Disease

Frank B. Hu

A strong relationship between obesity and cardiovascular disease (CVD) has been documented in numerous prospective studies, yet several issues remain unsettled. For example, the relative importance of overall adiposity versus body fat distribution in predicting risk of coronary heart disease (CHD) and stroke is still a matter of debate. Another unresolved issue is whether obesity should be included in global CHD risk assessment tools. Although obesity is a recognized coronary risk factor, it has not yet been incorporated into the Framingham score because it is believed that the effects of obesity are entirely mediated through established risk factors such as hypertension, dyslipidemia, and diabetes. However, recent studies have suggested that the association between overall adiposity or central obesity and CHD risk is not completely explained by traditional risk factors, and there is increasing evidence that markers of inflammation, endothelial dysfunction, and thrombogenic factors also play a role in mediating the relationship between excess adiposity and CVD risk (Fig. 9.1). In addition, although weight gain during adulthood is known to raise CHD risk, the health consequences of weight loss are controversial, and until recently, most epidemiologic studies did not distinguish intentional from unintentional weight loss. Another controversial issue is related to the phenomenon called "obesity paradox"—increasing body mass index (BMI) has been associated with improved survival among patients with congestive heart failure (CHF) or other advanced diseases.

In this chapter, we first review current evidence on the relationship between obesity and CHD, paying special attention to the effects of moderate overweight, body fat distribution, weight change, and the relative importance of excess adiposity and physical activity. We then review evidence regarding obesity and other cardiovascular conditions including CHF, atrial fibrillation (AF), and sudden cardiac death (SCD). In addition, we discuss methodological issues related to "obesity paradox."

BMI and Risk of CHD

Over the past several decades, there have been more than 100 prospective cohort studies on the relationship between adiposity and risk of CHD in various populations. Three meta-analyses—including 92 prospective studies, with virtually no overlap, and more than 1.1 million participants worldwide—have summarized the association between

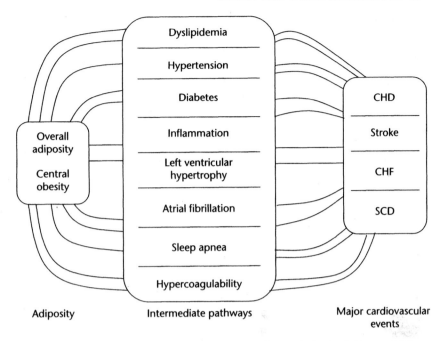

Figure 9.1 Pathways through which overall adiposity and central obesity influence cardiovascular diseases. CHD, coronary heart disease; CHF, congestive heart failure; and SCD, sudden cardiac death.

BMI and CHD incidence and mortality. Table 9.1 summarizes the key characteristics and main results from these meta-analyses. The Asian Pacific Cohort Studies Collaboration analyzed 33 cohort studies from Asian and Pacific countries (12 from Japan, 11 from mainland China, 2 from Singapore, 2 from Taiwan, 1 from Hong Kong, 1 from South Korea, 1 from New Zealand, and 3 from Australia).[1] In total, 310,283 participants contributed more than 2.1 million person-years of follow-up (average 6.9 years). As expected, the Asian cohorts were very lean (average BMI 22.9 kg/m²) compared with those from Australia and New Zealand (average BMI 26.4 kg/m²).

There were 2073 cases of incident CHD (849 nonfatal and 1224 fatal) during follow-up. After adjustment for age, sex, and smoking status, the relationship between increasing BMI and risk of CHD was linear. Each two-unit increment in BMI was associated with an 11% (95% CI: 9% to 13%) increased risk of CHD. The association was similar for men at 12% (10% to 15%) and women at 10% (6% to 13%). Adjustment for systolic blood pressure attenuated the overall association by approximately one-third to 8% (6% to 10%). The association was similar between the Asian and Australia/New Zealand cohorts. This meta-analysis clearly demonstrated a dose-response relationship between increasing BMI and risk of CHD, with elevated risk starting well below the cutpoint for normal BMI (25 kg/m²). There was a similar association for stroke (results summarized in the following sections), which is more common than CHD in Asian populations.

The second meta-analysis, the Diverse Populations Collaboration,[2] used person-level data from 26 cohort studies with 388,622 individuals. The main end point was total mortality (see summary of results in Chapter 11); secondary end points included CHD ($n = 17,708$) and CVD mortality ($n = 27,099$). Males and females were analyzed separately, with adjustments for age and smoking status. The summary relative risks (RRs) of CHD mortality for overweight women compared with normal-weight women was

Table 9.1 A Summary of Three Meta-analyses on Obesity and CVD

First Author	Cohort	Participants	End Points	Main Findings	Comments
Asian Pacific Cohort studies collaboration[1]	33 (cohort studies from Korea, China, Japan, Australia, and New Zealand)	310,283	2,073 incident CHD and 3,332 stroke	A linear relationship between baseline BMI and risk of CHD and stroke. Each 2 kg/m^2 increment in BMI was associated with a 11% (95% CI: 9% to 13%) higher risk of CHD; 12% (95% CI: 9% to 15%) higher risk of ischemic stroke; and 8% (95% CI: 4% to 12%) higher risk of hemorrhagic stroke. The association was stronger for younger participants. No significant difference was found between Asian and Australian cohorts.	The mean baseline BMIs were low (23.6 for the overall population, 22.9 for Asian cohorts, and 26.4 for Australian and New Zealand cohorts). Mean duration of follow-up was relatively short (average 6.9 y). Analyses were adjusted for age, sex, and smoking status. Events within 3 y of follow-up were excluded from the analyses to minimize potential bias caused by prevalent disease.
The Diverse Populations Collaboration[2]	26 (most cohorts from the United States)	388,622	17,708 CHD deaths and 27,099 CVD deaths	For CHD mortality, the summary RRs for overweight groups compared with the normal-weight group were 1.10 (95% CI: 1.00 to 1.20) for women and 1.16 (95% CI: 1.09 to 1.24) for men. The summary RRs for the obese groups relative to those of normal weight were 1.62 (1.46 to 1.81) for females and 1.51 (1.36 to 1.67) for males. These RRs were slightly weaker for CVD mortality.	The years of follow-up ranged from 3 to 36 (average 17 y). The end points were CHD and CVD mortality rather than incidence. Smoking status was adjusted in the analyses. No stratified analyses by age or smoking were presented.
Rogers et al.[3]	31 (from Europe to United States)	389,239	20,652 incident CHD	Incident CHD was significantly elevated with increasing BMI levels. Overweight was associated with a RR of 1.33 (95% CI: 1.24 to 1.43) and obesity with a RR of 1.69 (95% CI: 1.44 to 1.99) compared with normal weight after adjustment for age, sex, and smoking habit. Underweight was not significantly associated with CHD risk. These RRs were somewhat attenuated after adjustment for blood pressure and cholesterol levels, but they still remained significant.	The vast majority of the participants were Caucasian. The meta-analyses found that the association between BMI and CHD was stronger for studies with longer follow-up time (>15 y) than those with a shorter follow-up. No significant difference in the summary RRs was found between studies using self-reported BMI and those with measured BMI values. The association was stronger for never smokers than current and former smokers.

1.10 (95% CI: 1.00 to 1.20); for overweight men, it was 1.16 (1.09 to 1.24). For obese females and males, the RRs were 1.62 (1.46 to 1.81) and 1.51 (1.36 to 1.67), respectively. Associations were somewhat weaker for CVD mortality—1.03 (0.95 to 1.12) for overweight women and 1.10 (1.03 to 1.16) for overweight men. The RRs for the female and male obese groups were 1.53 (1.38 to 1.69) and 1.45 (1.33 to 1.59), respectively. There were no stratified analyses by age or smoking, and persons with chronic diseases at baseline were not excluded.

The third meta-analysis, conducted by Bogers et al.,[3] included 389,239 persons and 20,652 CHD events from 31 prospective cohorts. After adjustment for age, sex, and smoking, the pooled RR for underweight participants (BMI < 18.5) compared with those of normal weight was 1.11 (95% CI: 0.91 to 1.36); for overweight and obese individuals, the figures were 1.33 (1.24 to 1.43) and 1.69 (1.44 to 1.99), respectively. The pooled RR per increment of five BMI units was higher for longer follow-up times (at least 15 years) (RR = 1.35; 95% CI: 1.29 to 1.42) than shorter ones (RR = 1.21; 95% CI: 1.14 to 1.29). RRs were higher in never-smokers (RR = 1.40; 95% CI: 1.29 to 1.52) than in ever-smokers (RR = 1.20; 95% CI: 1.09 to 1.32). There was also a significantly stronger association for younger participants compared with older ones. These meta-analyses indicate that overweight and obesity (but not underweight) are associated with increased risk of CHD. The association was appreciably stronger in studies with longer follow-up and analyses restricted to never-smokers.

These three meta-analyses of more than 1.1 million people provide strong evidence of significant associations between overweight and obesity and increased risk of CHD. There appears to be a linear relationship between BMI and CHD, with no clear threshold for elevated risk. This relationship was particularly evident in Asian populations. South Koreans made up the largest cohort in the Asian Pacific Cohort Studies Collaboration (Korea Medical Insurance Corporation Study [KMIC]). Jee et al.[4] published an updated analysis of BMI and CHD incidence among 133,740 KMIC participants during 9 years of follow-up. After adjustment for age, sex, and smoking status, each unit increase in BMI was associated with a 14% (95% CI: 12% to 16%) increased risk of incident CHD. Compared with a BMI of 18-18.9, even a normal BMI of 24 to 24.9 was associated with a 2-fold increased risk of CHD. There was no evidence of threshold effects for men, women, smokers, or nonsmokers. In a recent much larger study of more than 1 million Koreans in the Korean Cancer Prevention Study (KCPS), there was a linear relationship between increasing BMI and death from atherosclerotic cardiovascular causes.[5]

Chen et al.[6] examined the relationship between BMI and CHD deaths among 222,000 Chinese men aged 40 to 79. During 10 years of follow-up, 1,942 CHD deaths were documented. Overall, there was a J-shaped relationship between BMI and CHD mortality. Using a BMI of 20 as the reference, both BMI over and lower than 20 were associated with significantly elevated CHD mortality. This study did not examine CHD incidence.

An updated 20-year follow-up analysis of the Nurses' Health Study (NHS) cohort showed a graded relationship between increasing BMI and incidence of CHD[7] (Fig. 9.2). Compared with women of normal weight, the RR of CHD in overweight women was 1.43 (95% CI: 1.26 to 1.63). For obese women it was 2.44 (2.17 to 2.74). The association between increasing BMI and CHD was substantially stronger among never-smokers than past and current smokers. In the Women's Health Initiatives, overweight and obesity were significantly associated with CHD incidence in both white and black women.[8]

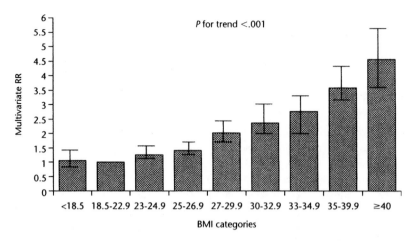

Figure 9.2 RRs of CHD according to BMI categories at baseline. Adjusted for age, parental history of myocardial infarction (MI), postmenopausal status, and hormone use (never-use, past, current), physical activity, aspirin use, smoking, and alcohol consumption. Adapted from Li TY, Rana JS, Manson JE, et al. Obesity as compared with physical activity in predicting risk of coronary heart disease in women. *Circulation*. 2006;113:499-506.[7]

Relative Importance of BMI and Body Fat Distribution

There has long been a debate on the relative importance of BMI and body fat distribution in predicting CHD. As a measure of adiposity, BMI does not distinguish fat mass from lean body mass, and its validity varies by age, sex, and ethnicity. Waist circumference, a surrogate measure of upper body or abdominal obesity, is considered central to metabolic syndrome and a root cause of the clustering of multiple cardiovascular risk factors (e.g., hypertension, dyslipidemia, and type 2 diabetes; see Chapter 8). Conceptually, waist circumference or waist-to-hip ratio (WHR) should be superior to BMI in predicting CVD risk. However, there are caveats when interpreting such data. First, the high correlation (from 0.80 to 0.90) between BMI and waist circumference seen in most studies makes it difficult to separate the effects of overall adiposity from abdominal obesity. Second, when BMI and waist circumference are included in the same model, the latter accounts for abdominal fatness, while BMI reflects lean body mass more than overall fatness (see Chapter 5). Thus, with simultaneous adjustment for waist circumference or WHR, the association between BMI and CHD becomes attenuated or even inverse. Finally, because WHR can reflect both increased visceral fat mass and/or reduced gluteofemoral muscle mass, its interpretation is complex.

Recent work from the INTERHEART study, a case-control study of 12,461 cases of first MI and 14,637 age- and sex-matched controls from 52 countries, found a much stronger association between WHR and MI than between BMI and MI, especially with simultaneous inclusion of both variables in the model.[9] Waist circumference was also a better predictor of MI than BMI, although its association with MI was weaker than that of WHR. These findings were remarkably consistent across different countries and ethnic groups. However, these outcomes should be interpreted cautiously. Despite a large number of cases, the INTERHEART was retrospective, which may have affected the relationship between BMI and MI. It is quite possible that many patients had already lost weight before the diagnosis of MI. Thus, BMI measured after diagnosis of MI may not have adequately reflected exposure to relevant levels of adiposity over the years, long before the diagnosis of CHD. Another problem, discussed earlier, is the change in the biological meaning of BMI when it is included in the same model with waist circumference or WHR. Such a change in meaning also occurs when hip circumference is adjusted for BMI or waist circumference. In the INTERHEART and other studies,[10] there was an inverse association between BMI-adjusted hip circumference and CVD morbidity and mortality. A large hip measurement may have reflected a greater amount of subcutaneous fat, more gluteal muscle mass, or larger bone structure. After adjustment for BMI or waist circumference, hip circumference is more likely to reflect the effects of lean body mass. Thus, the increased risk of MI with smaller hip circumference seen in the INTERHEART study may, in part, have reflected loss of muscle mass.

At least two dozen prospective studies have investigated the relationship between waist circumference or WHR and risk of CHD. In most of these studies, the association with BMI was also examined in parallel. Overall, findings showed that central or abdominal obesity plays an important role in predicting risk of CHD. However, the literature was inconsistent regarding the relative impact of BMI and body fat distribution. Some studies reported that waist circumference was more predictive of CHD risk than BMI or WHR.[11,12] Others found WHR a stronger predictor than waist circumference or BMI,[13-17] while still others suggested that BMI was as at least as predictive (if not more so) of CHD risk than waist circumference or WHR.[18-20] Reasons for the discrepancies are not clearly identified. However, they are probably related to different population characteristics (e.g., age, sex, and ethnicity) or ways of modeling the relative contributions of BMI and fat distribution (i.e., whether to include them in the same model) in different studies. Several studies have found significant associations between subscapular skinfold alone or the ratio of subscapular-to-triceps skinfold and risk of CVD, demonstrating the importance of regional fat distribution.[21-24]

To adjust for frame size, the waist circumference-to-height ratio (WHtR) has been proposed as an alternative to the WHR. Several cross-sectional studies have suggested that WHtR is a better predictor of metabolic disturbances and cardiovascular risk factors than WHR or waist circumference.[25-27] However, a prospective analysis from the NHS did not find statistically significant differences in predicting CHD risk between WHtR and WHR or waist circumference.[28]

Aging is associated with a loss of lean body mass and an increase in abdominal adiposity. Because of this relationship, it has been suggested that waist circumference or WHR are better than BMI as measures of obesity in the elderly (see Chapter 5). Using data from the Health Professionals' Follow-up Study (HPFS), Rimm et al.[29] examined differential effects of BMI and fat distribution on risk of CHD by age group. In men under 65, BMI appeared to be a stronger predictor of CHD than WHR, while in those over 65, WHR was a much stronger predictor than BMI. These results suggest that in older individuals, fat distribution may be a more important risk factor for CHD than overall adiposity or that BMI is a less valid measure of overall adiposity in older persons.

Nicklas et al.[30] examined the association between visceral adipose tissue measured by CT scans and incident MI in well-functioning men ($n = 1,116$) and women ($n = 1,387$) aged 70 to 79 years enrolled in the Health, Aging and Body Composition Study. During an average follow-up of 4.6 years, there were 116 new MI events (71 in men, 45 in women). The association between visceral adipose tissue and increased risk of MI was significant in women (adjusted RR = 1.67; 95% CI: 1.28 to 2.17 per standard deviation increase; $P <$ .001), but not in men. The association in women remained significant even after adjusting

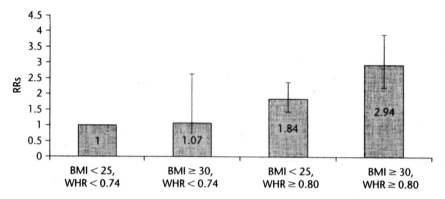

Figure 9.3 Joint associations of WHR and BMI with CHD. Adjusted for age, parental history of MI, postmenopausal status, and hormone use (never, past, current), physical activity, aspirin use, smoking, and alcohol consumption. Adapted with from Li TY, Rana JS, Manson JE, et al. Obesity as compared with physical activity in predicting risk of coronary heart disease in women. *Circulation.* 2006;113:499-506.[7]

for blood lipids, diabetes, and hypertension. This study demonstrated the importance of visceral fat in predicting MI in elderly women. The small number of events and a relatively short duration of follow-up, however, hampered the interpretation of results.

The strong correlation between BMI and waist circumference (typically greater than 0.8) means that relatively few individuals have a low BMI and a large waist, or a high BMI and a relatively small waist. However, analysis of those individuals can help distinguish the effects of overall adiposity from those of central obesity. Most likely, people with a low BMI but a large waist have more visceral adiposity, while those with a high BMI but a relatively small waist have more lean body mass. Recently, we examined the RRs of CHD according to joint classifications of BMI and WHR in the NHS cohort.[7] Obese women in the highest category of WHR ($\geq$0.8) had nearly 3-fold increased risk of CHD (adjusted RR = 2.94, 95% CI: 2.21 to 3.90) compared to normal-weight women who had a lower WHR (<0.74; Fig. 9.3). Of note, normal-weight women with central obesity (WHR $\geq$ 0.8) had a significantly higher RR of CHD (RR = 1.84; 95% CI: 1.42 to 2.38) than overweight or obese women in the lowest category of WHR (<0.74). Individuals with a higher BMI but a low WHR were more likely to be *muscular.* However, there were very few women (<1%) in that group. These results suggest that measures of fat distribution are of value in predicting risk of CHD beyond BMI. In normal-weight individuals, increased waist circumference or WHR is clearly associated with increased risk of CHD.

The Role of Intermediate Cardiovascular Risk Factors

Metabolic variables, such as hypertension, high cholesterol, and diabetes, are considered intermediate factors on the pathway between excess body weight and CHD, and thus, should not be adjusted when assessing the overall relationship between measures of obesity and CHD risk. However, adjustment for these variables in further analyses is useful in two ways: for testing the degree to which these factors mediate the effects of obesity; and for testing whether BMI or body fat distribution add to the prediction of CHD independent of their effects on intermediate metabolic factors.

Although obesity is a recognized risk factor for CHD, it is not included in global risk assessment tools, such as the Framingham risk score,[31] because many believe that the effects of obesity are indirect. In the development of the Framingham risk algorithm, BMI did not appear to be an independent predictor of CHD after incorporation of intermediate variables into the regression model. However, other studies have reported that overweight and obesity significantly predicted incident CHD even after adjustment for hypertension, high cholesterol, and diabetes. In the Johns Hopkins Sibling Study, Mora et al.[32] examined the relationship between BMI and incident CHD in 827 apparently healthy siblings of probands <60 years of age with premature CHD. Multivariate analyses indicated that BMI significantly predicted risk of CHD independent of the Framingham score ($P = .02$). The association was also independent of race, familial correlations, and triglyceride levels. Obese subjects with a higher Framingham score were at dramatically increased risk of CHD, suggesting that in addition to established risk factors (e.g., high cholesterol, hypertension, and diabetes), obesity should be included in standard CHD risk assessment. In the Chicago Heart Association Detection Project in Industry study, Yan et al.[33] examined whether midlife BMI predicted risk of CHD among those with low or moderate coronary risk profile based on blood pressure, serum cholesterol, and smoking. Results showed that even in individuals without any or only one cardiovascular risk factor at baseline, obesity was associated with a significantly higher risk of hospitalization and mortality from CHD, CVD, and diabetes in older age compared with normal-weight individuals. This study underscores the importance of including obesity in global risk assessment of CVD in apparently healthy middle-aged persons.

The impact of adjustment for intermediate metabolic risk factors on estimates of the association between BMI and risk of CHD has been examined in two meta-analyses. In the Asian Pacific Cohort Studies Collaboration,[1] adjustment for systolic blood pressure attenuated the risk estimate by approximately 33%; the increase in CHD risk for each two-unit BMI increment changed from 11% (95% CI: 9% to 13%) to 8% (95% CI: 6% to 10%). However, adjustment for serum cholesterol did not alter the risk estimate. In a meta-analysis of 21 cohort studies including over 300,000 persons, Bogers et al.[34] found that adjusting for blood pressure and cholesterol decreased the RR of CHD from 1.23 (95% CI: 1.18 to 1.29) to 1.11 (95% CI: 1.07 to 1.16) per five BMI units. These analyses suggest that hypertension and high cholesterol are important mechanisms through which obesity increases risk of CHD, but neither completely explains the excess risk.

Sufficient evidence demonstrates that the detrimental effects of excess weight are not entirely mediated through established cardiovascular risk factors. This is not surprising considering that obesity can affect other pathways, such as inflammation, endothelial dysfunction, and insulin resistance. From both clinical and public health points of view, there is an urgent need to incorporate obesity into CHD risk assessment tools.

Weight Gain and CHD Risk

Weight gain since young adulthood is common in the United States and other Western populations. For most people, accumulation of fat results from decreased physical activity and/or increased energy intake relative to energy expenditure. Thus, assessing changes in weight since young adulthood (approximately 21 years of age for men, when growth ends, and 18 years of age for women) is a useful way to examine the impact of increased adiposity on subsequent health outcomes. There is convincing evidence that even modest weight gain during adulthood is associated with increased risk of hypertension and type 2 diabetes (see Chapter 8). In a prospective study, weight gain from age 25 predicted increased carotid artery wall thickness.[35]

Several large prospective studies have evaluated the association between weight gain and long-term risk of CHD. The Framingham Heart Study reported a dose-response relationship between increase in Metropolitan Relative Weight between age 25 and baseline and incident CVD over 26 years of follow-up.[36] The relationship was independent of initial body weight and other cardiovascular risk factors. In the Western Electric Study,[37] the positive association between weight gain and CHD mortality was substantially stronger among never smokers than current smokers, suggesting that cigarette smoking may have masked the adverse effects of weight gain on risk of CHD. Among smokers, weight loss appeared to signal a greater amount of smoking. In addition, smoking appeared to be associated with increased abdominal fatness even without an increase in BMI.[37]

Willett et al.[38] examined the association between modest weight gain within the normal range of BMI (e.g., an increase of BMI from 20 to 24 kg/m^2) in 30- to 55-year-old women and subsequent incident CHD during 14 years of follow-up. Compared with stable-weight (±5 kg) women, RRs were 1.25 (95% CI: 1.01 to 1.55) for a 5- to 7.9-kg gain; 1.64 (1.33 to 2.04) for an 8 to 10.9 kg gain; 1.92 (1.61 to 2.29) for an 11 to 19 kg gain; and 2.65 (2.17 to 3.22) for a gain of 20 kg or more. The graded association between weight gain and CHD was consistent across different levels of BMI at age 18; of the women who gained weight, even those who remained within the normal range of BMI in midlife were at higher risk of CHD. These data provide strong evidence that weight gain after 18 years of age increases risk of CHD independent of current BMI. It is worth noting that weight gain since young adulthood provides a sensitive clinical measure to detect adverse effects of increasing adiposity early.

Two studies have suggested that the relationship between weight gain and CHD risk is stronger in younger men than it is in older men. In the HPFS, Rimm et al.[29] found that weight gain from age 21 significantly predicted CHD risk in men under 65 years of age, but not among older men. In the Honolulu Heart Program, Galanis et al.[39] observed a substantially stronger positive association between weight gain from age 25 and CHD in men aged 45 to 54 years compared with those 55 years or older at baseline.

The differential effects of weight gain on CHD risk in younger and older adults deserve careful consideration. Weight gain earlier in life consists primarily of an accumulation in body fat. In later life, body fat can increase without substantial weight gain, making its effects more difficult to study, because in older men, muscle mass is gradually replaced by fat, particularly within the abdomen (a phenomenon reflected by an increase in waist circumference or WHR with no change, or even a decrease in BMI). Unless lean body mass is preserved through weight training exercise or other means, stable weight in older men does not necessarily mean a lower risk of CHD compared with men who gain weight.

Intentional versus Unintentional Weight Loss

Substantial weight gain during young and middle adulthood is generally considered to be detrimental to health, but the effects of weight loss on CHD incidence and mortality remain controversial. Short-term clinical trials have unequivocally shown that modest weight loss (5% to 10%) leads to significant improvements in cardiovascular risk factors, such as blood pressure, lipids, inflammatory markers, insulin sensitivity, and glucose intolerance.[40] Weight loss induced by bariatric surgery in morbidly obese patients has also produced significant improvement or resolution of type 2 diabetes, hyperlipidemia, hypertension, and obstructive sleep apnea.[41] In the general population, however, confounding by unintentional weight loss from existing diseases and aging makes it more difficult to evaluate the effects of weight loss on CHD. So far, most epidemiologic studies do not distinguish between intentional and unintentional weight loss.

In the Iowa Women's Health Study,[42] unintentional weight loss was associated with increased CVD mortality, but only among women with existing chronic diseases. This finding reflects a well-known phenomenon called "reverse causation" (weight loss caused by existing diseases rather than the reverse; discussed in Chapter 4). Eilat-Adar et al.[43] reported that intentional weight loss after 6 months of dietary counseling was associated with lower incidence of CHD over 4 years of follow-up, but there may have been confounding from other health-related behaviors associated with attempted weight loss. Other studies that did not distinguish intentional from unintentional weight loss found that weight loss since young adulthood was, in general, not significantly associated with risk of CHD.[29,38] However, more recent weight loss in older individuals has been associated with increased CHD risk.[39] More often than not, weight loss in older individuals reflects loss in lean body mass due to aging and existing chronic diseases, a condition termed *fragility*. In Chapter 11, we will discuss the relationship between intentional and unintentional weight loss and total mortality.

Fatness versus Fitness in Predicting CHD

As discussed in Chapter 8, the *fat and fit* hypothesis suggests that higher levels of physical fitness reduce the adverse impact of overweight and obesity on health, making obesity a less important determinant of morbidity and mortality than fitness. In that most people find it difficult to sustain weight loss, the hypothesis has appeal; even without weight loss, physical fitness can be improved by increasing physical activity levels. So far, evidence to support this hypothesis has been limited largely to data from the Aerobics Center Longitudinal Study (ACLS).[44] The ACLS measured physical fitness using a maximal treadmill exercise test and found that low fitness conferred greater total and CVD mortality risk compared with fatness, and that fitness eliminated excess risk associated with fatness in men. Data also showed that lean men with lower cardiorespiratory fitness had a higher risk of all-cause and CVD mortality than did more physically fit men with higher overall or abdominal fat mass. This study, however, included only 428 deaths, and was unable to investigate the effects of adiposity among never-smokers. In an examination of the joint effects of fitness and fatness on mortality in 2506 women and 2860 men followed for more than 22 years in the Lipid Research Clinics Study, Stevens et al.[45] found that both fitness and fatness predicted total and CVD mortality, and that physical fitness did not eliminate the association between obesity and excess mortality.

Three additional studies examined the relative importance of physical activity and obesity on CHD risk without testing physical fitness (Table 9.2). Physical activity is the main nongenetic determinant of physical fitness as well as the primary focus of public health recommendations. It is useful, therefore, to evaluate the *fat and fit* hypothesis by studying the role of physical activity in modifying the relationship between obesity and mortality. Wessel et al.[46] found a significant association between self-reported physical function score (rather than BMI) and lower incidence of coronary artery disease among 906 women undergoing coronary angiography for suspected ischemia. However,

Table 9.2 A Summary of Prospective Studies on the Relative Importance of Obesity and Physical Fitness or Activity

First Author	Cohort	Participants	Follow-up Years	End Points	Physical Activity/ Fitness Measures	Adiposity Measures	Main Findings
Lee et al.[44]	Aerobics Center Longitudinal Study in Dallas, Texas	21,925 men	8 y	CVD and all-cause mortality	Cardiorespiratory fitness	Percentage of body fat and waist circumference	Low fitness was associated with a greater mortality risk compared with fatness; fitness removed the excess CVD and total mortality associated with fatness.
Stevens et al.[45]	Lipid Research Clinics Study	2,860 men and 2,506 women	26 y	All-cause mortality, cardiovascular disease mortality	Cardiorespiratory fitness	BMI	Both high levels of fatness and low levels of fitness independently predicted total and CVD mortality; being fit did not entirely alleviate the adverse effects of fatness.
Hu et al.[47]	Three independent population surveys established in Finland in 1987, 1992, and 1997.	8,928 men and 9,964 women	9.8 y	Cardiovascular disease	Self-reported physical activity, including occupational activity and leisure-time activity	BMI, waist circumference, and WHR	Regular physical activity and normal weight reduced the risk of CVD. Physical inactivity seems to have an independent effect on CVD risk, whereas obesity increased the risk partly through the modification of other risk factors.

Study	Population	Duration	Outcome	Physical activity measure	Adiposity measure	Findings
Wessel et al.[46]	Women's ischemic syndrome evaluation (WISE) study	936 women enrolled at 4 U.S. academic medical centers at the time of clinically indicated coronary angiography.	3.9 y	Incidence of adverse CVD events (all-cause death or hospitalization for nonfatal myocardial infarction, stroke, congestive heart failure, unstable angina, or other vascular events)	Self-reported Duke Activity Status Index (DASI) and Postmenopausal Estrogen-Progestin Intervention questionnaire (PEPI-Q) scores	BMI, waist circumference, WHR	Among women undergoing coronary angiography for suspected ischemia, higher self-reported physical activity and functional capacity were more important predictors of major adverse CVD events than overall or abdominal adiposity.
Li et al.[7]	Nurses' Health Study	88,393 healthy women	20 y	Coronary heart disease, including nonfatal myocardial infarction, and fatal CHD	Self-reported physical activity, including vigorous and moderate activities	BMI, waist circumference, WHR	Obesity and physical inactivity independently contributed to CHD in women. Normal-weight and active women had the lowest incidence of CHD, whereas obese and sedentary women had the highest risk. Obese active women had higher risk than normal-weight women who were inactive.

BMI, body mass index; CHD, coronary heart disease; WHR, waist-to-hip ratio.

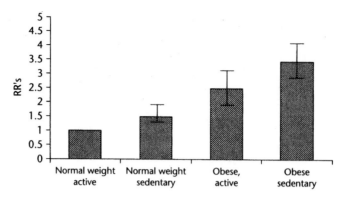

Figure 9.4 Joint associations of body mass index (BMI) and physical activity with coronary heart disease (CHD). Normal weight is defined as BMI of 18.5-24.9 kg/m^2, and obesity is defined as BMI $\geq$ 30 kg/m^2. Being active is defined as moderate to vigorous exercise at least 3.5 hours per week, and being sedentary is defined as less than 1 hour per week of exercise. Adjusted for age, parental history of myocardial infarction (MI), postmenopausal status, and hormone use (never-use, past, current), physical activity, aspirin use, smoking, and alcohol consumption. Adapted from Li TY, Rana JS, Manson JE, et al. Obesity as compared with physical activity in predicting risk of coronary heart disease in women. *Circulation.* 2006;113:499-506.[7]

this study had a relatively small sample size and short follow-up (4 years). Many women had already had coronary disease at baseline, which may have inhibited exercise. In a Finnish study of 18,892 men and women 25 to 74 years of age without a history of CVD at baseline,[47] obesity and physical activity independently predicted incidence of CHD during 10 years of follow-up, and physical activity only partly mitigated excess risk from obesity. Similarly, in the NHS cohort, physical activity and adiposity (measured by BMI or WHR) independently predicted risk of CHD.[7] Being physically active moderately attenuated but did not eliminate the adverse effects of obesity on coronary health, and being lean did not counteract the increased risk associated with physical inactivity. Lean and physically active women had the lowest risk of CHD (Fig. 9.4) as well as total mortality (see Chapter 11). These results indicate that leanness, accompanied or achieved by an active lifestyle, is the optimal way to reduce risk of CHD, and that excess adiposity remains a concern even in active individuals.

Obesity and Stroke

Stroke, a leading cause of death and disabilities, shares many risk factors with CHD, for example, age, smoking, hypertension, diabetes, physical inactivity, and dyslipidemia.[48] The risk of stroke is substantially increased after an MI.[49] Insulin resistance has also been associated with risk of stroke.[50] Though obesity has long been considered a risk factor for stroke, literature on obesity and stroke remains limited (despite substantial growth in the past several years) compared with that for CHD. In general, results have shown a positive association between higher BMI and increased risk of total and ischemic stroke, but the association with hemorrhagic stroke has been less consistent. In the Asian Pacific Cohort Studies Collaboration,[1] there were linear positive associations between baseline BMI and the risks of both ischemic and hemorrhagic stroke: each 2 kg/m^2 increase in BMI was associated with a 12% (95% CI: 9% to 15%) higher risk of ischemic stroke and an 8% (95% CI: 4% to 12%) higher risk of hemorrhagic stroke. However, in categorical analyses of BMI, the increased risk of hemorrhagic stroke with BMI was confined to the obese group.

In the largest study conducted so far, Song et al.[51] followed 234,863 Korean men aged 40 to 64 years for approximately 10 years and documented 7,444 total strokes, 3,981 ischemic strokes, and 1,806 hemorrhagic strokes (including 412 subarachnoid hemorrhages). Compared to men with BMI 22.0 to 23.9, the age-adjusted RRs of total stroke were 1.2 (95% CI: 1.1 to 1.2) for BMI 24.0 to 25.9; 1.4 (1.3 to 1.5) for BMI 26.0 to 27.9; 1.6 (1.3 to 2.1) for BMI 28.0 to 29.9; and 1.6 (1.3 to 2.1) for BMI $\geq$ 30 kg/m². Adjustment for intermediate variables, including blood pressure, glucose, and cholesterol, substantially attenuated these RRs, but the test for linear trend remained statistically significant. Of note, the elevated RR in the obese group was stronger for hemorrhagic stroke (age-adjusted RR = 2.5, 1.7 to 3.7) than for ischemic stroke (age-adjusted RR = 1.4, 1.0 to 1.9). In lower BMI categories (<20 kg/m²), there was a significantly lower risk of ischemic stroke but a significantly elevated risk of hemorrhagic stroke. Higher BMI has also been consistently associated with total and ischemic stroke in Western populations.[52-56] The Physicians' Health Study[54] found a significantly elevated risk of hemorrhagic stroke with increasing BMI, but this association has not been consistently observed in other studies. Because the relative proportion of hemorrhagic stroke versus ischemic stroke was much smaller in Western populations than in Asian populations, most studies of Western populations have limited power to examine the association between obesity and hemorrhagic stroke.

Rexrode et al.[53] examined the relationship between weight change since young adulthood and stroke incidence in the NHS cohort. In multivariate analyses that also adjusted for BMI at age 18, weight gain for women who maintained stable weight from age 18 until 1976 was associated with a RR for ischemic stroke of 1.69 (1.26 to 2.29) for a gain of 11 to 19.9 kg and 2.52 (1.80 to 3.52) for a gain of 20 kg or more (P for trend <.001) compared with women who maintained stable weight (loss or gain <5 kg). There was no relationship between weight change and risk of hemorrhagic stroke.

Several studies examined waist circumference or WHR in relation to stroke risk. In a prospective study of 789 Swedish men, WHR rather than BMI significantly predicted risk of stroke over 18.5 years of follow-up.[57] Similarly, Walker et al.[58] found that WHR was a stronger predictor of stroke than either waist circumference or BMI in men in the HPFS. In the Iowa Women's Health Study, a strong association between WHR and risk of stroke was largely mediated through hypertension and diabetes.[59] However, a 15-year follow-up of an elderly population in Sweden showed that BMI and waist circumference were equally predictive of stroke risk in men, and that the association remained significant even after adjustment for baseline diabetes, serum cholesterol, systolic blood pressure, and coronary disease.[20]

In summary, substantial evidence indicates that excess adiposity is an important risk factor for stroke in both Asian and Western populations. The association between BMI and ischemic stroke appears to be linear; it mimics the association with CHD but seems to have less strength. Similar to CHD, weight gain since young adulthood is associated with increased risk of ischemic stroke. The positive association between obesity and both CHD and ischemic stroke reflects shared pathophysiology between the two conditions. The relationship between obesity and hemorrhagic stroke is not as well established. However, results from the Asian Pacific Cohort Studies Collaboration and other Asian studies indicate that higher BMI is associated with a substantial increase in hemorrhagic stroke. There is some suggestion that very low BMI is associated with increased risk of hemorrhagic stroke in both Asian and Western populations, but the mechanism underlying this association is unknown. Cumulative evidence indicates that abdominal adiposity reflected by WHR is as good, if not better, than BMI in predicting stroke. Clearly, all three variables (BMI, weight gain since young adulthood, and body fat distribution) should be considered for risk assessment and prevention of CHD and stroke.

Obesity and CHF

Considerable evidence indicates that obesity is an independent risk factor for CHF.[60-65] In the NHANES I epidemiologic follow-up study,[60] after adjustment for hypertension, diabetes, CHD, and other cardiovascular risk factors at baseline, overweight was associated with a 23% (95% CI: 9% to 38%) higher risk of CHF. In that hypertension, diabetes, and CHD are all strongly related to obesity, a model adjusted for these variables would certainly underestimate the effects of BMI.

In the Framingham Heart Study, Kenchaiah et al.[62] reported a 39% (12% to 72%) increased risk of CHF in the overweight group and a nearly 2-fold (1.54 to 2.56) increased risk among the obese compared to the normal-weight group. After adjustment for other cardiovascular risk factors at baseline (e.g., hypertension, diabetes, left ventricular hypertrophy, and MI), each unit increment in BMI was associated with a 5% increase in CHF risk for men and a 7% increase for women. Clearly, this is overadjustment as the adjusted factors are intermediate variables in the pathway between obesity and CHF. The estimated population-attributable risk of CHF due to overweight and obesity was 28% in women and 30% in men.

Nicklas et al.[63] examined overall and abdominal obesity in relation to risk of CHF in older men and women in the Health, Aging and Body Composition study. In the analyses adjusting for demographic variables and smoking, all adiposity measurements—including BMI, percentage of body fat, total fat mass, waist circumference, and visceral and subcutaneous abdominal adipose tissue measured by CT scans—significantly predicted CHF risk. However, waist circumference appeared to be the most robust predictor of CHF when included with other adiposity variables in multivariate models. Further adjustment for inflammation, hypertension, insulin resistance, and diabetes mellitus did not materially alter the association for waist circumference. This study underscores the importance of abdominal obesity in the development of CHF.

The observed link between obesity and CHF is not surprising given that major risk factors for CHF (e.g., CHD, hypertension, and diabetes) are all strongly associated with obesity. The association between obesity and CHF remained significant, however, even after adjustment for these risk factors, suggesting additional mechanisms. Obesity has been associated with left ventricular hypertrophy and dilatation, both important precursors to CHF.[66,67] In a Swedish study, Ingelsson et al.[64] reported that insulin resistance measured by euglycemic insulin clamp significantly predicted incidence of CHF independent of BMI and waist circumference, whereas positive associations between BMI or waist circumference and CHF became nonsignificant after adjustment for insulin resistance. This study suggests that at least part of the association between excess adiposity and CHF is mediated through insulin resistance.

"Obesity Paradox" in CHF

Obesity is clearly an important risk factor for the development of CHF, but it has also been associated with improved survival in patients with established CHF—a phenomenon referred to as "reverse epidemiology"[68] or "obesity paradox."[69] In CHF, the direction of association between other cardiovascular risk factors (e.g., blood pressure and serum cholesterol) and mortality is also reversed. In other words, hypercholesterolemia and high blood pressure are associated with improved rather than decreased survival among patients with CHF.[68] The inverse association between higher BMI and lower mortality has been consistent in many small studies. A recent large study of 7767 CHF patients, with a mean follow-up of 37 months,[69] found that overweight patients had 12% (95% CI: 4% to 20%) lower mortality and obese patients 19% (95% CI: 8% to 28%) lower mortality compared with normal-weight patients. Underweight patients had 21% increased mortality.

Improved survival associated with high BMI levels has also been observed in other chronic conditions, such as end-stage renal disease, advanced malignancies, and AIDS.[70] In a recent meta-analysis of 250,152 patients with existing CHD, overweight and moderate obesity were associated with improved survival, whereas low BMI was associated with significantly increased mortality.[71] Besides its relatively short follow-up (average follow-up of 3.8 years), this study, like other epidemiologic studies of CHF, did not consider weight loss caused by the disease.

The mechanisms for the inverse association between BMI and mortality in CHF and other advanced diseases are not well understood. It has been suggested that metabolic and nutritional reserve among obese patients may be beneficial for survival.[68] This hypothesis, however, has yet to be tested.

Several methodological problems have been suggested to explain the "obesity paradox" in CHF. In patients with CHF or other chronic diseases, BMI becomes a poor measure of body fat because of involuntary weight loss and reduction in muscle mass. In addition, it is difficult to evaluate the relationship between BMI and mortality among these patients because of intractable confounding by severity of diseases and treatment modalities. "Reverse causation" is the most serious problem in such analyses. Here, low BMI and other cardiovascular risk factors (e.g., serum cholesterol and blood pressure) in lean individuals often result from more severe forms of the disease that lead to greater weight loss and decreased survival. Cachexia and wasting, common problems among patients with CHF and end-stage renal disease, are associated with increased mortality.[72] This may explain increased mortality among the underweight. Given that the BMI range for normal weight is quite large, some patients at the lower range of "normal weight" may also suffer from malnutrition and wasting.

Survival bias is another methodological problem in analyzing BMI and mortality in patients with CHF. Because of its high case fatality rate, CHF patients who are obese may die earlier, leading to "depletion of the susceptible." Thus, obese patients with stable CHF who enroll in most studies are a select group with a survival advantage. Survival bias is more evident in short-term rather than long-term studies. So far, there have been no studies on the effects of obesity on short- versus long-term survival in patients with CHF. Nigam et al.[73] reported significantly lower 6-month mortality among overweight and obese patients following MI compared with normal-weight patients. After 1 year, however, the survival advantage of obesity disappeared, and overweight and obese patients were more likely to develop recurrent MI and die from cardiac causes than normal-weight patients.

Thus, the "reverse epidemiology" observed in CHF is most likely due to methodological problems (e.g., reverse causation, confounding, and survival bias), although potential benefits of nutritional reserve in overweight patients are also possible. From a public health point of view, it is not desirable to recommend that most CHF patients, who are already overweight or obese, gain weight. Conversely, obese patients may benefit from weight management through proper nutrition and exercise. For very lean patients, adequate nutritional support is important for improving immune function and perhaps survival, but there is no evidence that weight gain per se is beneficial.

Obesity and Other Cardiovascular Conditions

Obesity has been associated with new onset of atrial fibrillation (AF), the most common form of cardiac arrhythmia. The Framingham Heart Study[74] found a linear relationship between increasing BMI and new onset of AF (a 4% increase in AF risk per 1-unit increase in BMI after adjusting for cardiovascular risk factors and interim MI or CHF). Compared with normal-weight participants, obesity was associated with a 52% (95% CI: 9% to 113%) increase in AF risk in men and a 46% (95% CI: 3% to 107%) increase in women. The increased risk associated with obesity became nonsignificant after further adjustment for echocardiographic left atrial diameter, suggesting that the association is mainly mediated through left atrial dilation, a known precursor to AF. Retrospective cohort analyses have demonstrated a significant association between increasing BMI and greater risk for new-onset AF after cardiac surgery.[75]

Hippocrates noted the link between obesity and sudden death more than 2500 years ago: "Sudden death is more common in those who are naturally fat than in the lean."[76] This observation from ancient times has now been confirmed by large epidemiologic studies. Using data from the NHS cohort, Albert et al.[77] reported a positive association between obesity and SCD in women. In this study, 88% of SCDs were classified as arrhythmic. The age-adjusted RR of SCD was 2.65 (95% CI: 1.82 to 3.85) for obese women compared with normal-weight women. This RR was attenuated to 1.63 (95% CI: 1.10 to 2.43) after adjustment for hypertension, diabetes, and other cardiovascular risk factors. In the same analyses, hypertension, diabetes, and smoking were strong predictors of SCD. These data indicate that obesity and its related effects play important roles in the pathophysiology of SCD.

Summary

More than 100 prospective studies have examined the relationship between BMI and risk of CHD. Persuasive evidence indicates that overweight and obesity confer significantly elevated risk of CHD, and that greater BMI adds to the prediction of CHD beyond measurements of traditional risk factors. Unfortunately, assessment of obesity is not among the standard tools (e.g., the Framingham risk score) used in overall coronary risk assessments. Considering the strength of the evidence and the public health burden of obesity, there is an urgent need to reevaluate the role of obesity in global risk assessment of CHD.

Convincing evidence demonstrates that increasing BMI is associated with greater risk of total and ischemic stroke in both Asian and Western populations, but the relationship between obesity and hemorrhagic stroke is not as well established. As with CHD, the association between obesity and stroke is partly mediated through hypertension and diabetes. At a molecular level, inflammation, endothelial dysfunction, and insulin resistance may underlie the common pathway linking obesity and CHD and stroke.

Substantial evidence indicates that obesity is also an independent risk factor for CHF. Among patients with CHF and other advanced diseases, however, obesity appears to confer a survival advantage. While there are no convincing explanations for this "obesity paradox," methodological problems (e.g., reverse causation, confounding, and survival bias) probably play an important role. Such problems, which are difficult to address in epidemiologic studies, are also common in the analyses of BMI and mortality in older populations (see Chapter 11). Although it is useful to understand the "reverse epidemiology" phenomenon in CHF and other chronic conditions, one should not be distracted from the overwhelming evidence that obesity causes CHD, CHF, and other cardiovascular conditions.

The relative importance of body fat distribution and overall adiposity may vary with age, gender, and ethnicity. Still, body fat distribution measured by WHR or waist circumference has been associated with both CHD and stroke independent of BMI and other cardiovascular risk factors. Moderate weight gain since young adulthood (age 18 for women and 21 for men) has been associated with increased risk of CHD and stroke, independent of BMI at a young age. Thus, all three variables in the *adiposity triad* (BMI, waist circumference, and weight gain since young adulthood) are important in assessing the relationship between adiposity and CHD risk, because each adds information to the risk prediction and indicates the potential for prevention.

References

1. Ni Mhurchu C, Rodgers A, Pan WH, Gu DF, Woodward M, Asia Pacific Cohort Studies Collaboration. Body mass index and cardiovascular disease in the Asia-Pacific Region: an overview of 33 cohorts involving 310 000 participants. *Int J Epidemiol.* 2004;33:751-758.
2. McGee DL, Diverse Populations Collaboration. Body mass index and mortality: a meta-analysis based on person-level data from twenty-six observational studies. *Ann Epidemiol.* 2005;15:87-97.
3. Bogers RP, Bemelmans WJE, Hoogenveen RT, et al. Overweight and risk of coronary heart disease in a pooled analysis of 31 cohorts involving almost 400 000 persons: assessing increased risk and exploring impact of study characteristics. Submitted 2007.
4. Jee SH, Pastor-Barriuso R, Appel LJ, Suh I, Miller ER III, Guallar E. Body mass index and incident ischemic heart disease in South Korean men and women. *Am J Epidemiol.* 2005;162:42-48.
5. Jee SH, Sull JW, Park J, et al. Body-mass index and mortality in Korean men and women. *N Engl J Med.* 2006;355:779-787.
6. Chen Z, Yang G, Zhou M, et al. Body mass index and mortality from ischaemic heart disease in a lean population: 10 year prospective study of 220 000 adult men. *Int J Epidemiol.* 2006;35:141-150.
7. Li TY, Rana JS, Manson JE, et al. Obesity as compared with physical activity in predicting risk of coronary heart disease in women. *Circulation.* 2006;113:499-506.
8. McTigue K, Larson JC, Valoski A, et al. Mortality and cardiac and vascular outcomes in extremely obese women. *JAMA.* 2006;296:79-86.
9. Yusuf S, Hawken S, Ounpuu S, et al. Obesity and the risk of myocardial infarction in 27 000 participants from 52 countries: a case-control study. *Lancet.* 2005;366: 1640-1649.
10. Heitmann BL, Frederiksen P, Lissner L. Hip circumference and cardiovascular morbidity and mortality in men and women. *Obes Res.* 2004;12:482-487.
11. Higgins M, Kannel W, Garrison R, Pinsky J, Stokes J III. Hazards of obesity—the Framingham experience. *Acta Med Scand Suppl.* 1988;723:23-36.
12. Wang Z, Hoy WE. Waist circumference, body mass index, hip circumference and waist-to-hip ratio as predictors of cardiovascular disease in aboriginal people. *Eur J Clin Nutr.* 2004;58:888-893.
13. Lapidus L, Bengtsson C, Larsson B, Pennert K, Rybo E, Sjostrom L. Distribution of adipose tissue and risk of cardiovascular disease and death: a 12 year follow up of participants in the population study of women in Gothenburg, Sweden. *BMJ (Clin Res Ed).* 1984;289:1257-1261.
14. Larsson B, Svardsudd K, Welin L, Wilhelmsen L, Bjorntorp P, Tibblin G. Abdominal adipose tissue distribution, obesity, and risk of cardiovascular disease and death: 13 year follow up of participants in the study of men born in 1913. *BMJ. (Clin Res Ed).* 1984;288:1401-1404.

15. Prineas RJ, Folsom AR, Kaye SA. Central adiposity and increased risk of coronary artery disease mortality in older women. *Ann Epidemiol.* 1993;3:35-41.

16. Folsom AR, Stevens J, Schreiner PJ, McGovern PG. Body mass index, waist/hip ratio, and coronary heart disease incidence in African Americans and whites. Atherosclerosis Risk in Communities Study Investigators. *Am J Epidemiol.* 1998;148:1187-1194.

17. Welborn TA, Dhaliwal SS, Bennett SA. Waist-hip ratio is the dominant risk factor predicting cardiovascular death in Australia. *Med J Aust.* 2003;179:580-585.

18. Rexrode KM, Buring JE, Manson JE. Abdominal and total adiposity and risk of coronary heart disease in men. *Int J Obes Relat Metab Disord.* 2001;25:1047-1056.

19. Rexrode KM, Carey VJ, Hennekens CH, et al. Abdominal adiposity and coronary heart disease in women. *JAMA.* 1998;280:1843-1848.

20. Dey DK, Lissner L. Obesity in 70-year-old subjects as a risk factor for 15-year coronary heart disease incidence. *Obes Res.* 2003;11:817-827.

21. Donahue RP, Abbott RD, Bloom E, Reed DM, Yano K. Central obesity and coronary heart disease in men. *Lancet.* 1987;1:821-824.

22. Kannel WB, Cupples LA, Ramaswami R, Stokes J III, Kreger BE, Higgins M. Regional obesity and risk of cardiovascular disease; the Framingham Study. *J Clin Epidemiol.* 1991;44:183-190.

23. Freedman DS, Williamson DF, Croft JB, Ballew C, Byers T. Relation of body fat distribution to ischemic heart disease. The National Health and Nutrition Examination Survey I (NHANES I) Epidemiologic Follow-up Study. *Am J Epidemiol.* 1995;142:53-63.

24. Yarnell JW, Patterson CC, Thomas HF, Sweetnam PM. Central obesity: predictive value of skinfold measurements for subsequent ischaemic heart disease at 14 years follow-up in the Caerphilly Study. *Int J Obes Relat Metab Disord.* 2001;25:1546-1549.

25. Hsieh SD, Yoshinaga H. Abdominal fat distribution and coronary heart disease risk factors in men-waist/height ratio as a simple and useful predictor. *Int J Obes Relat Metab Disord.* 1995;19:585-589.

26. Savva SC, Tornaritis M, Savva ME, et al. Waist circumference and waist-to-height ratio are better predictors of cardiovascular disease risk factors in children than body mass index. *Int J Obes Relat Metab Disord.* 2000;24:1453-1458.

27. Tseng CH. Waist-to-height ratio is independently and better associated with urinary albumin excretion rate than waist circumference or waist-to-hip ratio in chinese adult type 2 diabetic women but not men. *Diabetes Care.* 2005;28:2249-2251.

28. Page JH, Rexrode KM, Hu FB, Albert CM, Chae CU, Manson JE. Waist-to-height ratio as a predictor of Coronary Artery Disease among women. Submitted 2007

29. Rimm EB, Stampfer MJ, Giovannucci E, et al. Body size and fat distribution as predictors of coronary heart disease among middle-aged and older US men. *Am J Epidemiol.* 1995;141:1117-1127.

30. Nicklas BJ, Penninx BW, Cesari M, et al. Association of visceral adipose tissue with incident myocardial infarction in older men and women: the health, aging and body composition study. *Am J Epidemiol.* 2004;160:741-749.

31. Wilson PW, D'Agostino RB, Levy D, Belanger AM, Silbershatz H, Kannel WB. Prediction of coronary heart disease using risk factor categories. *Circulation.* 1998;97:1837-1847.

32. Mora S, Yanek LR, Moy TF, Fallin MD, Becker LC, Becker DM. Interaction of body mass index and framingham risk score in predicting incident coronary disease in families. *Circulation.* 2005;111:1871-1876.

33. Yan LL, Daviglus ML, Liu K, et al. Midlife body mass index and hospitalization and mortality in older age. *JAMA.* 2006;295:190-198.

34. Bogers RP, Bemelmans WJ, Hoogenveen RT, Boshuizen HC, Woodward M, Knekt P, van Dam RM, Hu FB, Visscher TL, Menotti A, Thorpe RJ Jr, Jamrozik K, Calling S, Strand BH, Shipley MJ; for the BMI-CHD Collaboration Investigators. Association of overweight with increased risk of coronary heart disease partly

independent of blood pressure and cholesterol levels: a meta-analysis of 21 cohort studies including more than 300 000 persons. *Arch Intern Med.* 2007;167(16): 1720-1728.

35. Stevens J, Tyroler HA, Cai J, et al. Body weight change and carotid artery wall thickness. The Atherosclerosis Risk in Communities (ARIC) Study. *Am J Epidemiol.* 1998;147:563-573.

36. Hubert HB, Feinleib M, McNamara PM, Castelli WP. Obesity as an independent risk factor for cardiovascular disease: a 26-year follow-up of participants in the Framingham Heart Study. *Circulation.* 1983;67:968-977.

37. Fulton JE, Shekelle RB. Cigarette smoking, weight gain, and coronary mortality: results from the Chicago Western Electric Study. *Circulation.* 1997;96:1438-1444.

38. Willett WC, Manson JE, Stampfer MJ, et al. Weight, weight change, and coronary heart disease in women. Risk within the 'normal' weight range. *JAMA.* 1995;273:461-465.

39. Galanis DJ, Harris T, Sharp DS, Petrovitch H. Relative weight, weight change, and risk of coronary heart disease in the Honolulu Heart Program. *Am J Epidemiol.* 1998;147:379-386.

40. Clinical Guidelines on the Identification, Evaluation, and Treatment of Overweight and Obesity in Adults. The Evidence Report. *Obes Res.* 1998;6(Suppl):51S-209S.

41. Buchwald H, Avidor Y, Braunwald E, et al. Bariatric surgery: a systematic review and meta-analysis. *JAMA.* 2004;292:1724-1737.

42. French SA, Folsom AR, Jeffery RW, Williamson DF. Prospective study of intentionality of weight loss and mortality in older women: the Iowa Women's Health Study. *Am J Epidemiol.* 1999;149:504-514.

43. Eilat-Adar S, Eldar M, Goldbourt U. Association of intentional changes in body weight with coronary heart disease event rates in overweight subjects who have an additional coronary risk factor. *Am J Epidemiol.* 2005;161:352-358.

44. Lee CD, Blair SN, Jackson AS. Cardiorespiratory fitness, body composition, and all-cause and cardiovascular disease mortality in men. *Am J Clin Nutr.* 1999;69:373-380.

45. Stevens J, Cai J, Evenson KR, Thomas R. Fitness and fatness as predictors of mortality from all causes and from cardiovascular disease in men and women in the lipid research clinics study. *Am J Epidemiol.* 2002;156:832-841.

46. Wessel TR, Arant CB, Olson MB, et al. Relationship of physical fitness vs body mass index with coronary artery disease and cardiovascular events in women. *JAMA.* 2004;292:1179-1187.

47. Hu G, Tuomilehto J, Silventoinen K, Barengo N, Jousilahti P. Joint effects of physical activity, body mass index, waist circumference and waist-to-hip ratio with the risk of cardiovascular disease among middle-aged Finnish men and women. *Eur Heart J.* 2004;25:2212-2219.

48. Goldstein LB, Adams R, Becker K, et al. Primary prevention of ischemic stroke: a statement for healthcare professionals from the Stroke Council of the American Heart Association. *Circulation.* 2001;103:163-182.

49. Witt BJ, Brown RD Jr, Jacobsen SJ, Weston SA, Yawn BP, Roger VL. A community-based study of stroke incidence after myocardial infarction. *Ann Intern Med.* 2005;143:785-792.

50. Kernan WN, Inzucchi SE, Viscoli CM, Brass LM, Bravata DM, Horwitz RI. Insulin resistance and risk for stroke. *Neurology.* 2002;59:809-815.

51. Song YM, Sung J, Davey Smith G, Ebrahim S. Body mass index and ischemic and hemorrhagic stroke: a prospective study in Korean men. *Stroke.* 2004;35:831-836.

52. Shinton R, Shipley M, Rose G. Overweight and stroke in the Whitehall study. *J Epidemiol Community Health.* 1991;45:138-142.

53. Rexrode KM, Hennekens CH, Willett WC, et al. A prospective study of body mass index, weight change, and risk of stroke in women. *JAMA.* 1997;277:1539-1545.

54. Kurth T, Gaziano JM, Berger K, et al. Body mass index and the risk of stroke in men. *Arch Intern Med.* 2002;162:2557-2562.

55. Kurth T, Gaziano JM, Rexrode KM, et al. Prospective study of body mass index and risk of stroke in apparently healthy women. *Circulation.* 2005;111:1992-1998.

56. Jood K, Jern C, Wilhelmsen L, Rosengren A. Body mass index in mid-life is associated with a first stroke in men: a prospective population study over 28 years. *Stroke.* 2004;35:2764-2769.

57. Welin L, Svardsudd K, Wilhelmsen L, Larsson B, Tibblin G. Analysis of risk factors for stroke in a cohort of men born in 1913. *N Engl J Med.* 1987;317:521-526.

58. Walker SP, Rimm EB, Ascherio A, Kawachi I, Stampfer MJ, Willett WC. Body size and fat distribution as predictors of stroke among US men. *Am J Epidemiol.* 1996;144:1143-1150.

59. Folsom AR, Prineas RJ, Kaye SA, Munger RG. Incidence of hypertension and stroke in relation to body fat distribution and other risk factors in older women. *Stroke.* 1990;21:701-706.

60. He J, Ogden LG, Bazzano LA, Vupputuri S, Loria C, Whelton PK. Risk factors for congestive heart failure in US men and women: NHANES I epidemiologic follow-up study. *Arch Intern Med.* 2001;161:996-1002.

61. Wilhelmsen L, Rosengren A, Eriksson H, Lappas G. Heart failure in the general population of men—morbidity, risk factors and prognosis. *J Intern Med.* 2001; 249:253-261.

62. Kenchaiah S, Evans JC, Levy D, et al. Obesity and the risk of heart failure. *N Engl J Med.* 2002;347:305-313.

63. Nicklas BJ, Cesari M, Penninx BW, et al. Abdominal obesity is an independent risk factor for chronic heart failure in older people. *J Am Geriatr Soc.* 2006;54:413-420.

64. Ingelsson E, Sundstrom J, Arnlov J, Zethelius B, Lind L. Insulin resistance and risk of congestive heart failure. *JAMA.* 2005;294:334-341.

65. Murphy NF, MacIntyre K, Stewart S, Hart CL, Hole D, McMurray JJ. Long-term cardiovascular consequences of obesity: 20-year follow-up of more than 15 000 middle-aged men and women (the Renfrew-Paisley study). *Eur Heart J.* 2006;27:96-106.

66. Hammond IW, Devereux RB, Alderman MH, Laragh JH. Relation of blood pressure and body build to left ventricular mass in normotensive and hypertensive employed adults. *J Am Coll Cardiol.* 1988;12:996-1004.

67. Lauer MS, Anderson KM, Kannel WB, Levy D. The impact of obesity on left ventricular mass and geometry. The Framingham Heart Study. *JAMA.* 1991;266: 231-236.

68. Kalantar-Zadeh K, Block G, Horwich T, Fonarow GC. Reverse epidemiology of conventional cardiovascular risk factors in patients with chronic heart failure. *J Am Coll Cardiol.* 2004;43:1439-1444.

69. Curtis JP, Selter JG, Wang Y, et al. The obesity paradox: body mass index and outcomes in patients with heart failure. *Arch Intern Med.* 2005;165:55-61.

70. Kalantar-Zadeh K, Abbott KC, Salahudeen AK, Kilpatrick RD, Horwich TB. Survival advantages of obesity in dialysis patients. *Am J Clin Nutr.* 2005;81:543-554.

71. Romero-Corral A, Montori VM, Somers VK, et al. Association of bodyweight with total mortality and with cardiovascular events in coronary artery disease: a systematic review of cohort studies. *Lancet.* 2006;368:666-678.

72. Morley JE, Thomas DR, Wilson MM. Cachexia: pathophysiology and clinical relevance. *Am J Clin Nutr.* 2006;83:735-743.

73. Nigam A, Wright RS, Allison TG, et al. Excess weight at time of presentation of myocardial infarction is associated with lower initial mortality risks but higher long-term risks including recurrent re-infarction and cardiac death. *Int J Cardiol.* 2006;110:153-159.

74. Wang TJ, Parise H, Levy D, et al. Obesity and the risk of new-onset atrial fibrillation. *JAMA.* 2004;292:2471-2477.

75. Zacharias A, Schwann TA, Riordan CJ, Durham SJ, Shah AS, Habib RH. Obesity and risk of new-onset atrial fibrillation after cardiac surgery. *Circulation*. 2005;112:3247-3255.
76. Chadwick J, Mann WN. *Medical Works of Hippocrates*. Boston, MA: Blackwell Scientific Publications; 1950:154.
77. Albert CM, Chae CU, Grodstein F, et al. Prospective study of sudden cardiac death among women in the United States. *Circulation*. 2003;107:2096-2101.

10

Obesity and Cancer

Eugenia E. Calle

Introduction

Obesity has long been recognized to be an important cause of type 2 diabetes mellitus, hypertension, and dyslipidemia (see Chapter 8). The adverse metabolic effects of excess body fat are known to accelerate atherogenesis and increase the risk of coronary heart disease, stroke, and early death (see Chapters 9 and 11). The relationship of obesity to cancer has received less attention than its cardiovascular effects. Results from epidemiologic studies that largely began in the 1970s indicate that adiposity contributes to the increased incidence and/or death from cancers of the colon, female breast (in postmenopausal women), endometrium, kidney (renal cell), esophagus (adenocarcinoma), gastric cardia, pancreas, gallbladder, liver, and possibly others. It has been estimated that 15% to 20% of all cancer deaths in the United States can be attributed to overweight and obesity.[1] At present, the strongest empirical support for mechanisms to link obesity and cancer risk involves the metabolic and endocrine effects of obesity, and the alterations they induce in production of peptide and steroid hormones[2] (Table 10.1). As the worldwide obesity epidemic has shown no signs of abating, insight into the mechanisms by which obesity contributes to tumor formation and progression is urgently needed, as are new approaches to intervene in this process.

Epidemiology of Adiposity and Cancer Risk

Historical Perspective of Epidemiologic Studies of Weight

The association of overweight and obesity with noncancer outcomes is generally stronger than the association with all cancer or specific cancer sites. In populations experiencing temporal increases in the prevalence of obesity, increases in hypertension, hyperlipidemia, and diabetes emerge earlier than increases in cancer outcomes. Because the incidence and mortality of specific types of cancer are less common than these noncancer outcomes, the relation of obesity to particular cancer sites has been more difficult to study. Moreover, a biological mechanism that clearly links obesity to forms of cancer without an endocrine component has not been established.

For these reasons, understanding the associations between overweight, obesity, and a wide variety of cancers, as well as the biological mechanisms contributing to these

Table 10.1 Associations of Obesity with Selected Hormones and Proteins

Hormone or Binding Globulin	Obesity vs. Normal Weight
Insulin	Increased levels with obesity
IGF-1	Nonlinear relation, with peak levels in people with BMIs of 24-27 kg/m^2
Free IGF-1	Increased levels with obesity
IGFBP1	Decreased levels with obesity
IGFBP3	Increased levels with obesity or no observed effect
SHBG	Decreased levels with obesity
Total testosterone	Decreased levels with obesity (men); no observed effect (women); increased levels with obesity (premenopausal women with polycystic ovary syndrome)
Free testosterone	No observed effect or decreased levels with obesity (men); increased levels with obesity (women)
Total estradiol	Increased levels with obesity (men and postmenopausal women); no observed effect (premenopausal women)
Free estradiol	Increased levels with obesity (men and postmenopausal women); no observed effect (premenopausal women)
Progesterone	No observed effect or decreased levels with obesity in women with a susceptibility to develop ovarian hyperandrogenism (premenopausal women only)

BMI, body mass index; IGF-1, insulin-like growth factor; IGFBP, IGF-binding protein; SHBP, sex-hormone-binding globulin. Adapted with permission from Calle EE, Kaaks R. Overweight, obesity and cancer: epidemiological evidence and proposed mechanisms. *Nat Rev Cancer.* 2004;4:579-591.[2]

associations, remains an evolving and currently very active area of research. Accumulating research on obesity and cancer suggests that this relationship is not confined to just a few forms of cancers.

Evaluation by the International Agency for Research on Cancer

The International Agency for Research on Cancer (IARC) Working Group on the Evaluation of Cancer-Preventive Strategies published a comprehensive evaluation of the available literature on weight and cancer that considered epidemiologic, clinical, and experimental data.[3] Their 2002 report concluded that there is "sufficient evidence" in humans for a cancer-preventive effect of avoidance of weight gain for cancers of the endometrium, female breast (postmenopausal), colon, kidney (renal cell), and esophagus (adenocarcinoma).[3] Regarding premenopausal breast cancer, the report concluded that available evidence on the avoidance of weight gain "suggests lack of a cancer-preventive effect." For all other sites, IARC characterized the evidence for a cancer-preventive effect of avoidance of weight gain as inadequate in humans.

The conclusions regarding the evidence in humans were based on epidemiologic studies of overweight and/or obese individuals compared to leaner individuals, not on studies of individuals who had lost weight. Unfortunately, few individuals lose and maintain significant amounts of weight, making it difficult to examine cancer outcomes in large populations of weight losers, although such studies are starting to appear. Consequently, the IARC report concluded that there is "inadequate evidence" in humans for a cancer-preventive effect of intentional weight loss for any cancer site. However, recent studies of the impact of weight loss on breast cancer,[4,5] endometrial cancer,[6,7] and prostate cancer[8] suggest that weight loss over the course of adult life may substantially reduce the risk for several cancers.[9]

Obesity-Related Cancers

Endometrial cancer (cancer of the uterine lining) was the first cancer to be recognized as being obesity related. There is convincing and consistent evidence from both case-control and cohort studies that overweight and obesity are associated strongly with endometrial cancer.[2,3] A linear increase in the risk of endometrial cancer with increasing weight or body mass index (BMI) has been observed in most studies.[1,3,6,10-13] The increase in risk generally ranges from 2- to 3.5-fold in overweight and/or obese women (Table 10.2), and might be somewhat higher in studies of mortality than incidence.

The probable mechanism for the increase in risk of endometrial cancer associated with obesity in postmenopausal women is the obesity-related increase in circulating estrogens.[2,3] Many studies have shown large increases in endometrial cancer risk among postmenopausal women who take unopposed estrogen replacement therapy (i.e., estrogen in the absence of progesterone), as well as increases in risk among women with higher circulating levels of total and bioavailable estrogens. In premenopausal women, endometrial cancer risk is also increased among women with polycystic ovary syndrome, which is characterized by chronic hyperinsulinemia as well as progesterone deficiency. Thus, in both pre- and postmenopausal women, endometrial cancer is increased by the mitogenic effects of estrogens on the endometrium when these effects are not counterbalanced by sufficient levels of progesterone.

Mechanisms involving the insulin pathway may also play a role in endometrial cancer. Blood levels of adiponectin, an insulin-sensitizing protein, secreted exclusively by adipocytes are lower in obese individuals and those with insulin-resistant conditions,[14] and are inversely associated with endometrial cancer independent of BMI.[15,16] This is entirely consistent with studies showing a positive association between type 2 diabetes and endometrial cancer,[2] and another showing upper body fat to be significantly associated with

Table 10.2 Relative Risks Associated with Overweight and Obesity and the Percentage of Cases Attributable to Overweight and Obesity in the United States

Type of Cancer	Relative Risk* BMI		PAF% for US Adults 2000†
	≥25-<30	30+	
Colorectal (men)	1.5	2.0	35.4
Colorectal (women)	1.2	1.5	20.8
Female breast (post)	1.3	1.5	22.6
Endometrium	2.0	3.5	56.8
Kidney (renal cell)	1.5	2.5	42.5
Esophagus (adeno)	2.0	3.0	52.4
Pancreas	?	1.7	—‡
Liver	?	1.5-4.0	—‡
Gallbladder	1.5	2.0	35.5
Gastric cardia (adeno)	1.5	2.0	35.5

* Relative risk estimates are summarized from the literature cited.
† Data on prevalence of overweight and obesity are from the National Health and Nutrition Examination Survey (NHANES) (1999-2000)[156] for U.S. men and women 50 to 69 years of age.
‡ PAFs were not estimated because the magnitude of the relative risks across studies is not sufficiently consistent.
BMI, body mass index in kg/m²; RR, relative risk; PAF, population attributable fraction.
Adapted with permission from Calle EE, Kaaks R. Overweight, obesity and cancer: epidemiological evidence and proposed mechanisms. *Nat Rev Cancer.* 2004;4:579-591.[2]

endometrial cancer, with a more pronounced effect among premenopausal than post-menopausal women.[17]

Many epidemiologic studies since the 1970s have assessed the association between anthropometric measures and *female breast cancer* occurrence and/or prognosis.[2,3] Early studies established that the association between body size and risk of breast cancer varied based on menopausal status—that heavier women were at increased risk of postmeno-pausal, but not premenopausal, breast cancer. In fact, among premenopausal women, there is consistent evidence of a modest reduction in risk among women with high (≥28) BMI. Mechanisms underlying the inverse association between premenopausal breast cancer and obesity have not yet been clearly identified, but researchers have long hypothesized that the reduction in risk could be due to the increased tendency for young obese women to have anovulatory menstrual cycles and lower levels of circulating steroid hormones, notably progesterone and estradiol. However, results from a recent large longitudinal study examining BMI and premenopausal breast cancer while controlling for menstrual cycle irregularities and ovulatory infertility did not support this hypothesis.[18] A recent systematic review suggests that central adiposity, rather than general adiposity, may be a predictor for premenopausal breast cancer.[19]

Obesity has been shown consistently to increase rates of breast cancer in postmeno-pausal women by 30% to 50% (Table 10.2).[2,20-22] A recent systematic review suggests that central adiposity is not an independent predictor of postmenopausal breast cancer risk beyond the risk attributed to overweight alone.[19] In addition, adult weight gain has generally been associated with a considerably larger increase in risk of postmenopausal breast cancer than has BMI, in studies that examined both.[23-26] Women experiencing weight gain in adulthood of 50 or more pounds have a 2-fold higher risk of breast cancer compared to women with stable weight.[23,26]

Recent prospective studies suggest that intentional weight loss in healthy women is associated with decreased risk of postmenopausal breast cancer.[4,9,27,28] The magnitude of the inverse association varies between studies and according to age at which the weight loss took place. Estimates of decreased risk often do not reach statistical significance due to the small numbers of women who lose weight. Many more studies are needed before the presumed benefits of weight loss can be quantified.

High levels of circulating estrogens and low levels of sex hormone binding globulin (SHBG) have been shown to be associated with increased risk of breast cancer in post-menopausal women.[29] Another mechanism by which obesity may affect the risk of breast cancer involves insulin and/or insulin growth factors (IGFs). IGF-I is a potent mitogen for normal and transformed breast epithelial cells and is associated with mammary gland hyperplasia and mammary cancer in animals.[2] In addition, IGF-I receptors are present in most human breast tumors and in normal breast tissue. A systematic review and meta-analysis of epidemiologic studies found that both serum or plasma IGF-I and IGF-binding protein 3 (IGFBP-3) are positively associated with risk of breast cancer in premenopausal, but not postmenopausal, women.[30] That the association with IGF-I is stronger in studies of premenopausal than postmenopausal breast cancer has been interpreted as suggesting that IGF-I may increase risk only in the presence of high levels of endogenous estrogens.[3]

Studies of circulating insulin or C-peptide (a marker of insulin secretion) levels and breast cancer have had inconsistent results.[2] A recent prospective cohort study found that postmeno-pausal, but not premenopausal, women with type 2 diabetes were at greater risk of breast cancer than those without diabetes; the association was particularly evident among women with estrogen receptor-positive breast cancer.[31] Prediagnostic levels of plasma leptin were not found to be associated with postmenopausal breast cancer in one study,[32] whereas an inverse association has been seen with serum adiponectin and postmenopausal breast cancer.[33]

Obesity has also been consistently associated with higher risk of *colorectal cancer* in men (relative risks of approximately 1.5 to 2.0) and women (relative risks of approximately 1.2 to 1.5) in both case-control and cohort studies (Table 10.2).[3,10,11,34-39] In studies that were able to examine separately the colon and rectum, relative risks have been generally higher for the colon.[3,12,36-40] Similar relationships are seen for colon adenomas, with stronger associations observed between obesity and advanced adenomas.

A gender difference, in which obese men are more likely to develop colorectal cancer than obese women, has been observed consistently across studies and populations. The reasons for this gender difference are speculative. One hypothesis is that central adiposity, which occurs more frequently in men, is a stronger predictor of colon cancer risk than peripheral adiposity or general overweight. Support for the role of central obesity on colorectal cancer comes from studies reporting that waist circumference and waist-to-hip ratio (WHR) are related strongly to risk of colorectal cancer and large adenomas in men. Three recent prospective cohort studies examining the predictive value of anthropometric measurements for risk of colon cancer specifically, found waist circumference[41] or WHR[36,42] to be associated with colon cancer risk, independent of, and with greater magnitude than, BMI, and this result was seen in women as well as in men. These results suggest that abdominal obesity is a more important predictor of colon cancer than general overweight and that measures of central adiposity are better indicators of risk in women than BMI.

Another explanation is that there might be an offsetting beneficial effect of obesity on colorectal cancer risk in women based on the evidence that exogenous estrogens (in the form of postmenopausal hormone therapy) reduce the risk of colorectal cancer in women.[43] In one large prospective study, when the data were stratified by postmenopausal hormone use, the positive association between WHR and colon cancer in women was completely attenuated among the hormone users.[36] However, this hypothesis also is speculative, as circulating levels of endogenous estrogens are higher in obese men as well as obese women, compared to lean subjects and oral intake of exogenous estrogens could have different effects than endogenous estrogens on the risk of colon cancer.

Giovannucci[44] was the first to propose the mechanistic hypothesis that high body mass, and central obesity in particular, increased colon cancer risk through their effect on insulin production. Insulin and IGFs have been shown to promote the growth of colonic mucosal cells and colonic carcinoma cells in in vitro studies. This hypothesis has received recent support from many epidemiologic studies. Higher risk of colorectal cancer has been associated with elevated fasting plasma glucose and insulin levels following a standard dose of oral glucose challenge, with elevated serum insulin or C-peptide levels, and with factors associated with insulin resistance syndrome.[2,37,45,46] Several prospective cohort and case-control studies have found increased risk of colorectal cancer and large adenomas with increasing absolute levels of IGF-I, and decreasing levels of IGFBP-3. A recent meta-analysis of six case-control and nine cohort studies found diabetes mellitus, which is preceded by many years of hyperinsulinemia, to be associated with a 30% increase in risk of colorectal cancer.[47] This association was also evident among a population of Chinese men and women, despite their relative leanness.[48] Elevated levels of serum leptin recently have been found to be associated with increased risk of colon cancer,[49] independent of circulating insulin levels.[50,51] Low levels of plasma adiponectin have also been found to be associated with increased risk of colorectal cancer[52] and colorectal adenoma.[53]

The risk of *kidney cancer* (specifically, renal cell cancer) is 1.5- to 3-fold higher in overweight and obese persons than in normal weight men and women in study populations worldwide (Table 10.2); most studies have found a dose-response relationship with increasing weight or BMI.[2,3,11,39,40,54,55] In several studies, the increase in risk with increasing BMI was greater in women than in men,[2,56] though at present this finding remains unexplained and was not confirmed in a review of published studies, nor in a recent prospective cohort study.[11] Importantly, the obesity-associated risk of renal cell cancer appears to be independent of blood pressure, indicating that hypertension and obesity might influence renal cell cancer through different mechanisms. The hypothesis that chronic hyperinsulinemia contributes to the association of BMI and renal cell cancer is supported indirectly by the increased risk of kidney cancer seen in diabetics.

The incidence of *adenocarcinoma of the esophagus* has been rapidly increasing in westernized countries in recent decades, while rates for the other main histologic subtype, squamous cell carcinoma, have remained stable or decreased. Thus, an increasing proportion of all esophageal cancers in Western countries are adenocarcinomas. Obesity is consistently associated with a 2- to 3-fold increase in risk for adenocarcinoma of the esophagus (Table 10.2),[2,3,39,57-59] with stronger associations seen in nonsmokers.[1,60] Obesity is not associated with an increased risk of squamous cell carcinoma of the esophagus.

Independent of obesity, gastroesophageal reflux disease (GERD) has been associated with esophageal adenocarcinoma and with its metaplastic precursor, Barrett's esophagus. Obesity has been hypothesized to increase the risk of adenocarcinoma of the esophagus indirectly, by increasing the risk of GERD and Barrett's esophagus. The association between obesity and esophageal adenocarcinoma has been shown in some studies to be independent of reflux.[57] Thus, obesity might increase the risk of esophageal adenocarcinoma through mechanisms other than, or in addition to, reflux.

Cancers Likely to Be Obesity Related

Risk for *adenocarcinoma of the gastric cardia* has been found to be obesity related,[2,57-59] but the magnitude of the association is not as great as for adenocarcinoma of the esophagus. Relative risks are in the range of 1.5 to 2.0. It is unclear at present why risks associated with obesity are greater for esophageal adenocarcinoma than for gastric cardia adenocarcinoma. It is possible that reflux mechanisms are more closely related to adenocarcinoma of the esophagus than of the gastric cardia. Data are limited for noncardia cancers of the stomach, but there is no suggestion of increased risk with obesity.

There have been a limited number of studies of *gallbladder cancer* and obesity, and most have been relatively small, as gallbladder cancer is quite rare, especially in men. However, these few studies have consistently found elevated risks of about 2-fold (Table 10.2).[2,38,40] One study found a greater than 4-fold increase in risk for the highest category of BMI ($\geq$30), but only among women in this Japanese cohort.[12] Obesity is thought to operate indirectly to increase the risk of gallbladder cancer by increasing the risk of gallstones, which in turn causes chronic inflammation and increased risk of biliary tract cancer.

Eight studies that have examined obesity and *liver cancer* or hepatocellular carcinoma (HCC) found excess relative risk in both men and women in the range of 1.5 to 4.0;[2,10,35,39,40] however, two studies did not find any suggestion of an increased risk.[12,61] Taken together, these studies suggest that obesity increases the risk of liver cancer, but the magnitude of the observed relative risk from existing studies is not consistent.

Obesity, and especially visceral adiposity, is strongly associated with nonalcoholic fatty liver disease, a chronic liver disease that occurs in nondrinkers but which is histologically similar to alcohol-induced liver disease.[62] NAFLD is an emerging clinical problem among obese patients and is now recognized as the most common cause of abnormal liver tests. Disorders of glucose regulation are significantly associated with NAFLD, indicating that insulin resistance is the link between NAFLD and metabolic diseases.[63]

NAFLD is characterized by a spectrum of liver tissue changes ranging from accumulation of fat in the liver to nonalcoholic steatohepatitis (NASH), cirrhosis, and HCC at the most extreme end of the spectrum. Progression to NASH appears to represent the turning point from a seemingly nonprogressive condition to fibrosis, necrosis, and inflammation, and multiple cellular adaptations to the resulting oxidative stress.[62] Visceral adiposity likely contributes to the risk of HCC by promoting NAFLD and NASH.

Several recent studies suggest that high body mass is associated with increased risk for *pancreatic cancer* in men and women, with relative risk estimates for obesity generally in the range of 1.5 to 2.0 (Table 10.2).[2,10,39,64-66] However, other studies found smaller positive associations[12,67,68] or in some cases, no association.[40] Further research is needed to refine the magnitude of the risk in both men and women and to explain the inconsistency in current estimates of risk. Many of these studies are based on small numbers of cases, and retrospective studies of adiposity are hampered by weight loss that accompanies pancreatic cancer and that often begins before diagnosis. There is some evidence that the relationship between adiposity and pancreatic cancer is not linear and that increased risk is not observed until levels of BMI $\geq$ 30.[66] In addition, smoking is an important potential confounder of the relationship between adiposity and pancreatic cancer, and the smoking habits of the various study populations and differential adequacy of control for smoking may partly explain differences across studies. It is thought that chronic hyper-insulinemia and glucose intolerance may contribute to an increased risk of pancreatic cancer, as suggested by the well-established positive association between diabetes and pancreatic cancer in prospective studies. A recent study suggests that individuals with the highest versus lowest quartiles of fasting serum levels of glucose and insulin, and insulin resistance, have more than a 2-fold increased risk of pancreatic cancer.[69] Another study found that a tendency toward central (vs. peripheral) weight gain was associated with a 45% increase in risk of pancreatic cancer, after adjustment for the independent effects of general adiposity.[66]

Several studies have examined the relationship between *hematopoietic cancers* and BMI, but results from most of these studies are based on relatively small numbers of events. Still, most of the available studies have observed modest obesity-associated increases in the risk of non-Hodgkin's lymphoma,[2,10,11,35,40,70-72] multiple myeloma,[2,70,73,74] and leukemia.[2,40,70,75-77] Relative risks from these studies have been generally in the range of 1.2 to 2.0.

There are many studies that do not support an association between body mass and incident *prostate cancer*.[3,10-12,35,78] However, four recent large studies found small but statistically significant increased risk of prostate cancer among obese men[61,79,80] or a significant trend toward increasing risk with increasing BMI.[40] The authors of a recent meta-analysis of 31 cohort and 25 case-control studies concluded that obesity is weakly associated with an increased risk of prostate cancer (RR of 1.05 per 5 BMI units).[81] A single prospective study has examined adult weight loss and risk of prostate cancer; this study suggests that weight loss may decrease the risk of being diagnosed with prostate cancer.[8]

Other Cancers

Studies on BMI and *cervical cancer* are limited and inconclusive.[2,3] Two prospective studies of mortality from cervical cancer found it was associated with high BMI (2- to 3-fold increased risk) whereas much lower relative risks were observed in two cohorts of hospitalized patients diagnosed with obesity, compared to general populations, and no association was observed in three cohort studies.[10,12] A recent case-control study that controlled for human papilloma virus infection found about a 2-fold increased risk of cervical adenocarcinoma among overweight and obese women; smaller increases in risk were seen for cervical squamous cell carcinoma. However, differential screening behavior (obese women are less likely to be screened on a regular basis than women of normal weight) could also bias and explain some of these observations.

Although endogenous hormones are believed to be involved in the etiology of *ovarian cancer*, and obesity is a well-established risk factor for other hormone-related cancers in women (e.g., breast and endometrial cancers), ovarian cancer has not been linked consistently to obesity.[2,3,10-12,82-87] Some studies have reported an association between obesity and ovarian cancer, and relative risks in these studies have been in the range of 1.5-2.0 for the highest categories of BMI studied. However, several large studies have not found an association between ovarian cancer and obesity, so no solid conclusions should be drawn at this time. It is not clear what factors might explain the divergent results among studies. Weight loss several years previous to the time of cancer diagnosis would bias the relative risk downward in case-control studies, but such a bias would not be operative in several prospective cohort studies that found no association. It is possible that obesity increases the risk of specific histologic subtypes of ovarian cancer (e.g., endometroid) but not others. Most studies have not examined risk by histologic subtype of ovarian cancer, and this may contribute to the inconsistent findings.

Effects of Adiposity on Cancer Outcomes

Results from a large prospective mortality study of over 1 million individuals suggest that overweight and obesity are associated with increased death rates from cancers at multiple specific sites in men and women.[1] Studies examining the specific impact of adiposity on prognostic factors, recurrence, and/or survival are most prevalent for cancer of the female breast, and more recently, cancer of the prostate. Studies specifically related to adiposity and prognosis are limited for other cancer sites.

There are at least 40 published studies of adiposity and *breast cancer* prognosis, and results from the majority of these studies show that overweight and obese women have poorer prognosis and shorter survival than do normal weight or lean women after adjustment for stage and treatment.[88-100] Very obese postmenopausal women (BMI $\geq$ 40.0) have breast cancer death rates that are three times higher than very lean (BMI < 20.5) women.[101] Unlike the positive association between adiposity and incident breast cancer, which is only observed in postmenopausal women, the adverse effect of adiposity on prognosis is seen irrespective of menopausal status. The observation that adiposity is associated with poorer prognosis in the premenopause, coupled with the observation that WHR and BMI may have independent effects on survival from breast cancer,[100] suggest that more than one biological pathway may play a role in the relationship between obesity and breast cancer progression.

The greater risk of death among heavier women likely reflects both a true biological effect of adiposity on survival and delayed diagnosis in heavier women. There are substantial data to suggest that adiposity is associated with a more aggressive tumor; obese women are more likely than lean to have increased tumor size, lymph node involvement, and later-stage disease at diagnosis.[91-93,95,97,102,103] Among a large prospective cohort of postmenopausal women, adult weight gain was associated more strongly with risk for breast cancer diagnosis at advanced stage than risk for localized disease.[102]

In addition to the direct effects of adiposity, there is evidence that heavier women are less likely to receive mammography screening.[104] Recent studies suggest that mammography screening is not a confounder of the relationship between adiposity and poor prognosis,[92,94,103,105] nor is mammography any less sensitive among heavier women.[106] Thus, the impact of obesity on prognosis is unlikely to be solely, or even largely, an artifact of delayed diagnosis.

Another important area of research is the impact of treatment-related weight gain on prognosis for women with breast cancer. Weight gain after diagnosis is common in breast cancer patients who receive adjuvant chemotherapy as part of their treatment. Results from available studies suggest that weight gain after diagnosis exerts an adverse impact on prognosis, and research in this area is active.[107-109]

There is accumulating evidence that obesity is associated with an increase in risk of advanced *prostate cancer* or death from prostate cancer.[2,8,81,110-114] Recent studies consistently indicate that obese men with prostate cancer are more likely to have aggressive disease that recurs after radical prostatectomy than nonobese men.[115-118] While still speculative, the mechanisms by which obesity predicts for advanced prostate cancer likely involve the insulin pathway. Several studies suggest that insulin acts to promote prostate cancer development and growth.[119-122] High concentrations of IGF-I[30] and overexpression of type 1 IGF-I receptor[123,124] are associated with prostate cancer. Studies of circulating leptin levels and prostate cancer risk are not consistent; while three studies have linked increased leptin levels to more advanced, higher-grade tumors,[125-127] three other studies have not found an association.[78,128,129] Decreased adiponectin levels, which indicate decreased insulin sensitivity, have also been linked to high-grade, advanced prostate cancer.[130]

As with breast cancer, nonbiological issues of screening, detection, and treatment are important to the evaluation of the impact of adiposity on prostate cancer prognosis. It can be harder to perform a digital rectal examination in obese men because of their general adiposity in combination with larger prostate size.[131,132] In addition, despite larger prostate sizes, obese men may have lower serum levels of prostate-specific antigen (PSA),[133-136] potentially biasing them toward later stage at diagnosis even with regular PSA screening. Surgery is more difficult to perform in obese men with a greater risk of positive surgical margins. Still, mortality from prostate cancer was found to be increased in obese men in a prospective cohort study conducted from 1950 to 1972,[137] long before PSA screening, and at a time when surgery was rarely done. These results suggest that the adverse impact of adiposity on prognosis is rooted in biological characteristics of the tumor.

Studies on BMI and prognosis among women with *endometrial cancer* suggest that heavier women have a better prognostic profile, as indicated by more favorable pathological features, and longer survival.[138-142] This finding lends additional support to the mechanistic hypothesis of unopposed estrogens, as it mirrors the better prognostic profile seen in women whose endometrial cancer was induced by estrogen replacement therapy.

There are several studies examining the impact of adiposity on prognosis among *colorectal* cancer patients. Available studies suggest that adiposity may have an adverse effect on prognosis,[143-147] although results are somewhat inconsistent by gender and for colon versus rectal cancer. While obesity is not consistently associated with increased risk of *ovarian cancer*, studies among ovarian cancer patients suggest that obesity may adversely impact survival.[148-150]

For breast, prostate, and other cancer patients, obesity may bring added complications of multiple comorbidities, resulting in poorer overall survival. In addition, obesity may compromise efficacy of cancer treatment, both surgery and chemotherapy. Additional work is needed to understand the impact of adiposity on prognosis across a wider range of cancer sites.

Methodologic Issues

Confounding by Smoking

For smoking-related cancers, it can be very difficult to assess the association between adiposity and the cancer. Smoking generally begins early in life, and is associated with a lower BMI over a period of decades of the adult lifespan. It also strongly predicts for some cancers, such as lung, esophagus, and pancreas cancers. For smoking-related cancers, the prospective effects of adiposity on the risk of cancer among smokers cannot be separated from the prospective effects of smoking—namely, decreased BMI and increased cancer risk. Residual confounding between smoking behavior and BMI can bias downward the estimate of the association between adiposity and cancer risk. Earlier analyses demonstrated that the apparent inverse association of BMI and mortality due to lung cancer was incrementally attenuated with increasingly complex statistical control for smoking in multivariate models, and it disappeared entirely when the analysis was restricted to those who had never smoked.[151] For smoking-related cancers, estimates of relative risk based on the total population are likely to be underestimates, and those based on nonsmokers are more likely to result in valid estimates of the risk between adiposity and cancer.

BMI has been reported to be inversely associated with lung cancer in several study populations that did not exclude smokers from the analysis,[3] while no association is seen between BMI and lung cancer in nonsmoking populations.[1,39,61] Relative risks for BMI and esophageal cancer are lower when based on total rather than nonsmoking populations,[1,60] as are relative risks for pancreatic cancer.[1,39]

Reverse Causation by Undiagnosed Disease

While not true of all cancers, some cancers (e.g., pancreas, liver, lung, esophagus, renal cell, lymphoma, colon), especially when diagnosed at late stage, can cause weight loss before the time of diagnosis. In studies of these cancers, weight measured shortly before or at the time of diagnosis may not reflect typical weight. This reverse causation will bias the risk of obesity downward and inflate the risk of leanness. This is more of a problem in case-control study designs than in cohort studies. Analyses conducted in cohort studies often exclude the first year or two of follow-up to assess and eliminate this potential misclassification of weight.

Measure of Exposure

There are many ways to estimate adiposity as a risk factor in epidemiologic studies. The measure that has been most often used is BMI, usually measured at some time in adulthood. Some studies have examined measures of central adiposity such as WHR or waist circumference. More recently, and especially in prospective cohorts, investigators are examining the impact of weight gain and weight loss as predictors of cancer. The potential differences between these measures in predicting cancer risk depend on the individual cancer site under investigation and on the hypothesized mechanism for the relationship between adiposity and the specific cancer site.

Measures of central adiposity rather than overall adiposity are better predictors of risk for those cancers where obesity increases risk through its impact on insulin production and the resulting insulin resistance syndrome. For example, colorectal cancer is better predicted by measures of central adiposity than by BMI. This is most clear in studies in women, where BMI is a weak predictor of colorectal cancer (because women are more likely than men to carry adiposity peripherally rather than centrally). However, recent studies show that waist circumference and WHR are strong predictors of colorectal cancer in women, as they are in men.[36-38] In contrast, for postmenopausal breast cancer, where risk is largely driven by the increased levels of circulating estrogens, central adiposity is not a better predictor of risk than overall adiposity as estimated by BMI.[21] It is quite likely that the variability across studies in estimates of risk associated with BMI for pancreas and liver cancer is partly due to the use of BMI as the measure of exposure rather than a measure of central adiposity.

Adult weight gain is a stronger predictor of postmenopausal breast cancer than BMI.[22-25] BMI reflects both lean body mass and adipose, whereas weight gain throughout adult life reflects primarily the accumulation of excess adipose tissue. Thus, weight gain is likely a more precise measure of the relevant exposure (e.g., adipose) than BMI. In addition, because obesity before the menopause is associated with a lower risk of breast cancer, women who are obese throughout their life have their lifetime risk pulled in two opposite directions. The women at greatest lifetime risk of breast cancer are those who are lean in the premenopausal period and become heavier in the postmenopausal period. Adult weight gain measures this, whereas a single BMI does not.

Effect Modification

While the impact of adiposity on cancer risk generally operates across all subgroups of individuals, there are documented exceptions. The most obvious is the well-documented modification by menopausal status of the effect of adiposity on breast cancer risk. Another is the apparent difference by gender for colorectal cancer risk as noted already. However, when the correct measure of central adiposity is used rather than general adiposity, the risks in both men and women are stronger and more similar to one another.[36]

Another subgroup difference relates to adiposity, exogenous hormone use, and risk of postmenopausal breast cancer. Both BMI and weight gain are related to risk of breast cancer only among postmenopausal women who have never used (or in some cases not currently using) hormone replacement therapy (HRT).[20,23,27,152-156] This finding has been replicated consistently and lends support to the hypothesis that adiposity increases postmenopausal breast cancer risk through its estrogenic effects. Lean women who are not using HRT have the lowest levels of circulating estrogens and the lowest risk of breast cancer. In HRT users, both lean and heavy women have high levels of circulating estrogens by virtue of their HRT use and have similar risk of breast cancer; against this background, the estrogenic effect of obesity is imperceptible and does not increase risk further.

The impact of adiposity may also vary according to characteristics of the cancer, including stage, tumor characteristics, subsite, or histology. Adiposity predicts for advanced but not local prostate cancer. Adiposity is associated with more aggressive breast cancers but with less aggressive endometrial cancers. Several studies suggest that the association between adiposity and breast cancer varies by estrogen and progesterone receptor status.[26,156] Adiposity predicts more strongly for colon cancer than for rectal cancer, and is a strong risk factor for adenocarcinoma of the esophagus but not for squamous cell carcinoma of the esophagus. To the extent possible, studies should examine the impact of adiposity by subgroups of individuals and by subtypes of cancer outcome.

Control for Screening and Tumor Characteristics in Analyses of Prognosis and Survival

Control for nonbiological factors of screening and detection is essential in analyses of cancer prognosis or survival in order to disentangle potential ascertainment differences related to adiposity from a biological impact of adiposity on tumor growth or characteristics. An important question remains: how appropriate is control for tumor-related prognostic factors (e.g., stage at diagnosis) in analyses of obesity and cancer? Clearly, if poorer prognostic features of tumors are due to delayed screening and diagnosis (ascertainment bias), then these features should be included in multivariate models. However, if poorer prognostic features of tumors are due to biological effects of adiposity, then they are in the causal pathway and should not be included in multivariate models. The ideal method of control is not for tumor characteristics but for history of screening before diagnosis and for clinical characteristics that are obesity related, and that influence the likelihood of finding an existent cancer.[132]

Population Attributable Fraction

The proportion or percentage of disease in a population that can be attributed to a risk factor is termed the "population attributable fraction" (PAF) and is used as a measure of the public health impact of the risk factor (see Chapter 4). The PAF is sometimes referred to as the population attributable risk, population attributable risk percent, and excess fraction. The magnitude of the PAF depends on both the magnitude of the association between the risk factor and the disease (i.e., the size of the relative risk) and the prevalence of the risk factor in the population of interest. The PAF will increase as either one of its component increases. Because the PAF is very sensitive to the population prevalence of the risk factor, in this case overweight and obesity, it is not generalizable to populations with different distributions of the risk factor. The PAFs presented in Table 10.2 are estimates of the percentage of cancer cases at each indicated site that could be attributed to excess adiposity, defined as a BMI > 25.0. These estimates were calculated for each cancer site that is obesity related or likely to be obesity related. The calculations were based on summary relative risks estimated from the existing published literature and on the distribution of BMI in adults in the United States in 2000.

Research Questions

Further research defining the causal role of obesity and cancers of specific sites is needed, including mechanistic research, and studies that are able to separate the effects of obesity and several highly correlated factors such as physical activity and dietary composition. At present, the biological mechanisms clearly linking overweight and obesity to many forms of cancer, other than those with an endocrine component, are poorly understood. In addition to causing changes in hormone metabolism (insulin, IGF-I, sex steroids), proteins secreted by adipose tissue also contribute to the regulation of immune response (leptin), inflammatory response (TNF-α, IL-6, serum amyloid A) vasculature and stromal interactions and angiogenesis (vascular endothelial growth factor-1), and extracellular matrix components (type 4 collagen).[5] Obesity-associated dysregulation of multiple adipokines is likely to be of great significance for the occurrence, promotion, and metastatic potential of human cancers.

References

1. Calle E, Rodriguez C, Walker-Thurmond K, Thun MJ. Overweight, obesity, and mortality from cancer in a prospectively studied cohort of U.S. adults. *N Engl J Med.* 2003;348:1625-1638.
2. Calle EE, Kaaks R. Overweight, obesity and cancer: epidemiological evidence and proposed mechanisms. *Nat Rev Cancer.* 2004;4:579-591.
3. IARC. *IARC Handbooks of Cancer Prevention. Weight Control and Physical Activity.* Lyon: International Agency for Research on Cancer, 2002.
4. Harvie M, Howell A, Vierkant RA, et al. Association of gain and loss of weight before and after menopause with risk of postmenopausal breast cancer in the Iowa women's health study. *Cancer Epidemiol Biomarkers Prev.* 2005;14:656-661.
5. Rajala MW, Scherer PE. Minireview: the adipocyte—at the crossroads of energy homeostasis, inflammation, and atherosclerosis. *Endocrinology.* 2003;144:3765-3773.
6. Xu WH, Xiang YB, Zheng W, et al. Weight history and risk of endometrial cancer among Chinese women. *Int J Epidemiol.* 2006;35:159-166.
7. National Center for Health Statistics CfDCaP. National Health and Nutrition Examination Survey 1999-2000, online. 2002.
8. Rodriguez C, Freedland SJ, Deka A, et al. Body Mass Index, Weight Change, and Risk of Prostate Cancer in the Cancer Prevention Study II Nutrition Cohort. *Cancer Epidemiol Biomarkers Prev.* 2006.
9. Parker ED, Folsom AR. Intentional weight loss and incidence of obesity-related cancers: the Iowa Women's Health Study. *Int J Obes.* 2003;27:1447-1452.
10. Rapp K, Schroeder J, Klenk J, et al. Obesity and incidence of cancer: a large cohort study of over 145,000 adults in Austria. *Br J Cancer.* 2005;93:1062-1067.
11. Lukanova A, Bjor O, Kaaks R, et al. Body mass index and cancer: results from the Northern Sweden Health and Disease Cohort. *Int J Cancer.* 2006;118:458-466.
12. Kuriyama S, Tsubono Y, Hozawa A, et al. Obesity and risk of cancer in Japan. *Int J Cancer.* 2005;113:148-157.
13. Trentham-Dietz A, Nichols HB, Hampton JM, Newcomb PA. Weight change and risk of endometrial cancer. *Int J Epidemiol.* 2006;35:151-158.
14. Snijder MB, Heine RJ, Seidell JC, et al. Associations of adiponectin levels with incident impaired glucose metabolism and type 2 diabetes in older men and women: the hoorn study. *Diabetes Care.* 2006;29:2498-2503.
15. Soliman PT, Wu D, Tortolero-Luna G, et al. Association between adiponectin, insulin resistance, and endometrial cancer. *Cancer.* 2006;106:2376-2381.
16. Dal Maso L, Augustin LS, Karalis A, et al. Circulating adiponectin and endometrial cancer risk. *J Clin Endocrinol Metab.* 2004;89:1160-1163.
17. Xu WH, Matthews CE, Xiang YB, et al. Effect of adiposity and fat distribution on endometrial cancer risk in Shanghai women. *Am J Epidemiol.* 2005;161:939-947.
18. Michels KB, Terry KL, Willett WC. Longitudinal study on the role of body size in premenopausal breast cancer. *Arch Intern Med.* 2006;166:2395-2402.
19. Harvie M, Hooper L, Howell A. Central obesity and breast cancer risk: a systematic review. *Obes Rev.* 2003;4:157-173.
20. Lahmann PH, Hoffmann K, Allen N, et al. Body size and breast cancer risk: findings from the European Prospective Investigation into Cancer and Nutrition (EPIC). *Int J Cancer.* 2004;111:762-771.
21. Tehard B, Clavel-Chapelon F. Several anthropometric measurements and breast cancer risk: results of the E3N cohort study. *Int J Obes (Lond).* 2006;30:156-163.
22. Chang SC, Ziegler RG, Dunn B, et al. Association of energy intake and energy balance with postmenopausal breast cancer in the prostate, lung, colorectal, and ovarian cancer screening trial. *Cancer Epidemiol Biomarkers Prev.* 2006;15:334-341.
23. Feigelson H, Jonas C, Teras L, Thun M, Calle EE. Weight gain, body mass index, hormone replacement therapy, and postmenopausal breast cancer in a large prospective study. *Cancer Epidemiol Biomark Prev.* 2004;13:220-224.

24. Sweeney C, Blair CK, Anderson KE, Lazovich D, Folsom AR. Risk factors for breast cancer in elderly women. *Am J Epidemiol.* 2004;160:868-875.

25. Han D, Nie J, Bonner MR, et al. Lifetime adult weight gain, central adiposity, and the risk of pre- and postmenopausal breast cancer in the Western New York exposures and breast cancer study. *Int J Cancer.* 2006;119:2931-2937.

26. Rosenberg LU, Einarsdottir K, Friman EI, et al. Risk factors for hormone receptor-defined breast cancer in postmenopausal women. *Cancer Epidemiol Biomarkers Prev.* 2006;15:2482-2488.

27. Eliassen AH, Colditz GA, Rosner B, Willett WC, Hankinson SE. Adult weight change and risk of postmenopausal breast cancer. *JAMA.* 2006;296:193-201.

28. Lahmann PH, Schulz M, Hoffmann K, et al. Long-term weight change and breast cancer risk: the European prospective investigation into cancer and nutrition (EPIC). *Br J Cancer.* 2005;93:582-589.

29. The Endogenous Hormones and Breast Cancer Collaborative Group. Endogenous sex hormones and breast cancer in postmenopausal women: reanalysis of nine prospective studies. *J Natl Cancer Inst.* 2002;94:606-616.

30. Renehan AG, Zwahlen M, Minder C, O'Dwyer ST, Shalet SM, Egger M. Insulin-like growth factor (IGF)-I, IGF binding protein-3, and cancer risk: systematic review and meta-regression analysis. *Lancet.* 2004;363:1346-1353.

31. Michels KB, Solomon CG, Hu FB, et al. Type 2 diabetes and subsequent incidence of breast cancer in the Nurses' Health Study. *Diabetes Care.* 2003;26:1752-1758.

32. Stattin P, Soderberg S, Biessy C, et al. Plasma leptin and breast cancer risk: a prospective study in northern Sweden. *Br Cancer Res Treat.* 2004;86:191-196.

33. Mantzoros C, Petridou E, Dessypris N, et al. Adiponectin and breast cancer risk. *J Clin Endocrinol Metab.* 2004;89:1102-1107.

34. Lin J, Zhang SM, Cook NR, Rexrode KM, Lee IM, Buring JE. Body mass index and risk of colorectal cancer in women (United States). *Cancer Causes Control.* 2004;15:581-589.

35. Batty GD, Shipley MJ, Jarrett RJ, Breeze E, Marmot MG, Smith GD. Obesity and overweight in relation to organ-specific cancer mortality in London (UK): findings from the original Whitehall study. *Int J Obes (Lond).* 2005;29:1267-1274.

36. Pischon T, Lahmann PH, Boeing H, et al. Body size and risk of colon and rectal cancer in the European Prospective Investigation Into Cancer and Nutrition (EPIC). *J Natl Cancer Inst.* 2006;98:920-931.

37. Bowers K, Albanes D, Limburg P, et al. A prospective study of anthropometric and clinical measurements associated with insulin resistance syndrome and colorectal cancer in male smokers. *Am J Epidemiol.* 2006;164:652-664.

38. Engeland A, Tretli S, Austad G, Bjorge T. Height and body mass index in relation to colorectal and gallbladder cancer in two million Norwegian men and women. *Cancer Causes Control.* 2005;16:987-996.

39. Samanic C, Chow WH, Gridley G, Jarvholm B, Fraumeni JF Jr. Relation of body mass index to cancer risk in 362,552 Swedish men. *Cancer Causes Control.* 2006;17:901-909.

40. Oh SW, Yoon YS, Shin SA. Effects of excess weight on cancer incidences depending on cancer sites and histologic findings among men: Korea National Health Insurance Corporation Study. *J Clin Oncol.* 2005;23:4742-4754.

41. Moore LL, Bradlee ML, Singer MR, et al. BMI and waist circumference as predictors of lifetime colon cancer risk in Framingham Study adults. *Int J Obes Relat Metab Disord.* 2004;28:559-567.

42. MacInnis RJ, English DR, Hopper JL, Gertig DM, Haydon AM, Giles GG. Body size and composition and colon cancer risk in women. *Int J Cancer.* 2005;118:1496-1500.

43. Writing Group for the Women's Health Initiative Investigators. Risks and benefits of estrogen plus progestin in healthy postmenopausal women: principal results from the Women's Health Initiative randomized controlled trial. *JAMA.* 2002;288: 321-333.

44. Giovannucci E, Ascherio A, Rimm E, Colditz GA, Stampfer MJ, Willett W. Physical activity, obesity, and risk for colon cancer and adenoma in men. *Ann Intern Med.* 1995;122:327-334.

45. Wei EK, Ma J, Pollak MN, et al. A prospective study of C-peptide, insulin-like growth factor-I, insulin-like growth factor binding protein-1, and the risk of colorectal cancer in women. *Cancer Epidemiol Biomarkers Prev.* 2005;14:850-855.

46. Wei EK, Ma J, Pollak MN, et al. C-peptide, insulin-like growth factor binding protein-1, glycosylated hemoglobin, and the risk of distal colorectal adenoma in women. *Cancer Epidemiol Biomarkers Prev.* 2006;15:750-755.

47. Larsson SC, Orsini N, Wolk A. Diabetes mellitus and risk of colorectal cancer: a meta-analysis. *J Natl Cancer Inst.* 2005;97:1679-1687.

48. Seow A, Yuan JM, Koh WP, Lee HP, Yu MC. Diabetes mellitus and risk of colorectal cancer in the Singapore Chinese Health Study. *J Natl Cancer Inst.* 2006;98:135-138.

49. Tamakoshi K, Toyoshima H, Wakai K, et al. Leptin is associated with an increased female colorectal cancer risk: a nested case-control study in Japan. *Oncology.* 2005;68:454-461.

50. Stattin P, Lukanova A, Biessy C, et al. Obesity and colon cancer: does leptin provide a link? *Int J Cancer.* 2004;109:149-152.

51. Stattin P, Palmqvist R, Soderberg S, et al. Plasma leptin and colorectal cancer risk: a prospective study in northern Sweden. *Oncol Rep.* 2003;6:2015-2021.

52. Wei E, Giovannucci E, Fuchs CS, Willett WC, Mantzoros C. Low plasma adiponectin levels and risk of colorectal cancer in men: a prospective study. *J Natl Cancer Inst.* 2005;97:1688-1694.

53. Otake S, Takeda H, Suzuki Y, et al. Association of visceral fat accumulation and plasma adiponectin with colorectal adenoma: evidence for participation of insulin resistance. *Clin Cancer Res.* 2005;11:3642-3646.

54. van Dijk BA, Schouten LJ, Kiemeney LA, Goldbohm RA, van den Brandt PA. Relation of height, body mass, energy intake, and physical activity to risk of renal cell carcinoma: results from the Netherlands Cohort Study. *Am J Epidemiol.* 2004;160:1159-1167.

55. Pan SY, DesMeules M, Morrison H, Wen SW. Obesity, high energy intake, lack of physical activity, and the risk of kidney cancer. *Cancer Epidemiol Biomarkers Prev.* 2006;15:2453-2460.

56. Pischon T, Lahmann PH, Boeing H, et al. Body size and risk of renal cell carcinoma in the European Prospective Investigation into Cancer and Nutrition (EPIC). *Int J Cancer.* 2006;118:728-738.

57. Lindblad M, Rodriguez LA, Lagergren J. Body mass, tobacco and alcohol and risk of esophageal, gastric cardia, and gastric non-cardia adenocarcinoma among men and women in a nested case-control study. *Cancer Causes Control.* 2005;16:285-294.

58. Kubo A, Corley DA. Body mass index and adenocarcinomas of the esophagus or gastric cardia: a systematic review and meta-analysis. *Cancer Epidemiol Biomarkers Prev.* 2006;15:872-878.

59. Ryan AM, Rowley SP, Fitzgerald AP, Ravi N, Reynolds JV. Adenocarcinoma of the oesophagus and gastric cardia: male preponderance in association with obesity. *Eur J Cancer.* 2006;42:1151-1158.

60. Chow W-H, Blot W, Vaughan T, et al. Body mass index and risk of adenocarcinomas of the esophagus and gastric cardia. *J Natl Cancer Inst.* 1998;90:150-155.

61. Pan S, Johnson K, Ugnat A-M, Wen S, Mao Y, Group CCRER. Association of obesity and cancer risk in Canada. *Am J Epidemiol.* 2004;159:259-268.

62. Harrison S, Diehl A. Fat and the liver—a molecular overview. *Seminars in Gastrointestinal Disease.* 2002;13:3-16.

63. Festi D, Colecchia A, Sacco T, Bondi M, Roda E, Marchesini G. Hepatic steatosis in obese patients: clinical aspects and prognostic significance. *Obes Rev.* 2004;5:27-42.

64. Larsson SC, Permert J, Hakansson N, Naslund I, Bergkvist L, Wolk A. Overall obesity, abdominal adiposity, diabetes and cigarette smoking in relation to the risk of pancreatic cancer in two Swedish population-based cohorts. *Br J Cancer.* 2005;93:1310-1315.
65. Fryzek JP, Schenk M, Kinnard M, Greenson JK, Garabrant DH. The association of body mass index and pancreatic cancer in residents of southeastern Michigan, 1996-1999. *Am J Epidemiol.* 2005;162:222-228.
66. Patel AV, Rodriguez C, Bernstein L, Chao A, Thun MJ, Calle EE. Obesity, recreational physical activity, and risk of pancreatic cancer in a large U.S. Cohort. *Cancer Epidemiol Biomarkers Prev.* 2005;14:459-466.
67. Berrington de Gonzalez A, Spencer EA, Bueno-de-Mesquita HB, et al. Anthropometry, physical activity, and the risk of pancreatic cancer in the European prospective investigation into cancer and nutrition. *Cancer Epidemiol Biomarkers Prev.* 2006; 15:879-885.
68. Sinner PJ, Schmitz KH, Anderson KE, Folsom AR. Lack of association of physical activity and obesity with incident pancreatic cancer in elderly women. *Cancer Epidemiol Biomarkers Prev.* 2005;14:1571-1573.
69. Stolzenberg-Solomon R, Graubard B, Chari S, et al. Insulin, glucose, insulin resistance, and pancreatic cancer in male smokers. *JAMA.* 2005;294:2872-2878.
70. Chiu BC, Gapstur SM, Greenland P, Wang R, Dyer A. Body mass index, abnormal glucose metabolism, and mortality from hematopoietic cancer. *Cancer Epidemiol Biomarkers Prev.* 2006;15:2348-2354.
71. Willett EV, Skibola CF, Adamson P, et al. Non-Hodgkin's lymphoma, obesity and energy homeostasis polymorphisms. *Br J Cancer.* 2005;93:811-816.
72. Cerhan JR, Bernstein L, Severson RK, et al. Anthropometrics, physical activity, related medical conditions, and the risk of non-Hodgkin lymphoma. *Cancer Causes Control.* 2005;16:1203-1214.
73. Bosetti C, Negri E, Gallus S, Dal Maso L, Franceschi S, La Vecchia C. Anthropometry and multiple myeloma. *Epidemiology.* 2006;17:340-341.
74. Blair CK, Cerhan JR, Folsom AR, Ross JA. Anthropometric characteristics and risk of multiple myeloma. *Epidemiology.* 2005;16:691-694.
75. Kasim K, Levallois P, Abdous B, Auger P, Johnson KC. Lifestyle factors and the risk of adult leukemia in Canada. *Cancer Causes Control.* 2005;16:489-500.
76. MacInnis RJ, English DR, Hopper JL, Giles GG. Body size and composition and the risk of lymphohematopoietic malignancies. *J Natl Cancer Inst.* 2005;97:1154-1157.
77. Ross JA, Parker E, Blair CK, Cerhan JR, Folsom AR. Body mass index and risk of leukemia in older women. *Cancer Epidemiol Biomarkers Prev.* 2004;13:1810-1813.
78. Baillargeon J, Platz EA, Rose DP, et al. Obesity, adipokines, and prostate cancer in a prospective population-based study. *Cancer Epidemiol Biomarkers Prev.* 2006; 15:1331-1335.
79. Samanic C, Gridley G, Chow W-H, Lubin J, Hoover R, Fraumeni J. Obesity and cancer risk among white and black United States veterans. *Cancer Causes Control.* 2004;15:35-43.
80. Engeland A, Tretli S, Bjorge T. Height, body mass index, and prostate cancer: a follow-up of 950000 Norwegian men. *Br J Cancer.* 2003;89:1237-1242.
81. MacInnis RJ, English DR. Body size and composition and prostate cancer risk: systematic review and meta-regression analysis. *Cancer Causes Control.* 2006;17: 989-1003.
82. Peterson NB, Trentham-Dietz A, Newcomb PA, et al. Relation of anthropometric measurements to ovarian cancer risk in a population-based case-control study (United States). *Cancer Causes Control.* 2006;17:459-467.
83. Rossing MA, Tang MT, Flagg EW, Weiss LK, Wicklund KG, Weiss NS. Body size and risk of epithelial ovarian cancer (United States). *Cancer Causes Control.* 2006;17:713-720.

84. Greer JB, Modugno F, Ness RB, Allen GO. Anthropometry and the risk of epithelial ovarian cancer. *Cancer*. 2006;106:2247-2257.

85. Anderson JP, Ross JA, Folsom AR. Anthropometric variables, physical activity, and incidence of ovarian cancer: The Iowa Women's Health Study. *Cancer*. 2004; 100:1515-1521.

86. Hoyo C, Berchuck A, Halabi S, et al. Anthropometric measurements and epithelial ovarian cancer risk in African-American and White women. *Cancer Causes Control*. 2005;16:955-963.

87. Zhang M, Xie X, Holman CD. Body weight and body mass index and ovarian cancer risk: a case-control study in China. *Gynecol Oncol*. 2005;98:228-234.

88. Rock C, Demark-Wahnefried W. Nutrition and survival after the diagnosis of breast cancer: a review of the evidence. *J Clin Oncol*. 2002;20:3302-3316.

89. Chlebowski R, Aiello E, McTiernan A. Weight loss in breast cancer patient management. *J Clin Oncol*. 2002;20:1128-1143.

90. Stephenson G, Rose D. Breast cancer and obesity: an update. *Nutr Cancer*. 2003;45:1-16.

91. Dignam JJ, Wieand K, Johnson KA, Fisher B, Xu L, Mamounas EP. Obesity, tamoxifen use, and outcomes in women with estrogen receptor-positive early-stage breast cancer. *J Natl Cancer Inst*. 2003;95:1467-1476.

92. Berclaz G, Li S, Price KN, et al. Body mass index as a prognostic feature in operable breast cancer: the International Breast Cancer Study Group experience. *Ann Oncol*. 2004;15:875-884.

93. Maehle BO, Tretli S, Thorsen T. The associations of obesity, lymph node status and prognosis in breast cancer patients: dependence on estrogen and progesterone receptor status. *Apmis*. 2004;112:349-357.

94. Baumgartner KB, Hunt WC, Baumgartner RN, et al. Association of body composition and weight history with breast cancer prognostic markers: divergent pattern for Hispanic and non-Hispanic White women. *Am J Epidemiol*. 2004;160:1087-1097.

95. Carmichael AR, Bendall S, Lockerbie L, Prescott RJ, Bates T. Does obesity compromise survival in women with breast cancer? *Breast*. 2004;13:93-96.

96. Whiteman MK, Hillis SD, Curtis KM, McDonald JA, Wingo PA, Marchbanks PA. Body mass and mortality after breast cancer diagnosis. *Cancer Epidemiol Biomarkers Prev*. 2005;14:2009-2014.

97. Loi S, Milne RL, Friedlander ML, et al. Obesity and outcomes in premenopausal and postmenopausal breast cancer. *Cancer Epidemiol Biomarkers Prev*. 2005;14:1686-1691.

98. Tao MH, Shu XO, Ruan ZX, Gao YT, Zheng W. Association of overweight with breast cancer survival. *Am J Epidemiol*. 2006;163:101-107.

99. Dignam JJ, Wieand K, Johnson KA, et al. Effects of obesity and race on prognosis in lymph node-negative, estrogen receptor-negative breast cancer. *Breast Cancer Res Treat*. 2006;97:245-254.

100. Abrahamson PE, Gammon MD, Lund MJ, et al. General and Abdominal Obesity and Survival among Young Women with Breast Cancer. *Cancer Epidemiol Biomarkers Prev*. 2006;15:1871-1877.

101. Petrelli JM, Calle EE, Rodriguez C, Thun MJ. Body mass index, height, and post-menopausal breast cancer mortality in a prospective cohort of US women. *Cancer Causes Control*. 2002;13:325-332.

102. Feigelson HS, Patel AV, Teras LR, Gansler T, Thun MJ, Calle EE. Adult weight gain and histopathologic characteristics of breast cancer among postmenopausal women. *Cancer*. 2006;107:12-21.

103. Porter GA, Inglis KM, Wood LA, Veugelers PJ. Effect of obesity on presentation of breast cancer. *Ann Surg Oncol*. 2006;13:327-332.

104. Ostbye T, Taylor DH Jr, Yancy WS Jr, Krause KM. Associations between obesity and receipt of screening mammography, Papanicolaou tests, and influenza

vaccination: results from the Health and Retirement Study (HRS) and the Asset and Health Dynamics among the Oldest Old (AHEAD) Study. *Am J Public Health.* 2005;95:1623-1630.

105. Daling JR, Malone KE, Doody DR, Johnson LG, Gralow JR, Porter PL. Relation of body mass index to tumor markers and survival among young women with invasive ductal breast carcinoma. *Cancer.* 2001;92:720-729.

106. Elmore JG, Carney PA, Abraham LA, et al. The association between obesity and screening mammography accuracy. *Arch Intern Med.* 2004;164:1140-1147.

107. Kroenke CH, Chen WY, Rosner B, Holmes MD. Weight, weight gain, and survival after breast cancer diagnosis. *J Clin Oncol.* 2005;23:1370-1378.

108. Camoriano JK, Loprinzi CL, Ingle JN, Therneau TM, Krook JE, Veeder MH. Weight change in women treated with adjuvant therapy or observed following mastectomy for node-positive breast cancer. *J Clin Oncol.* 1990;8:1327-1334.

109. Chlebowski RT. Obesity and early-stage breast cancer. *J Clin Oncol.* 2005;23: 1345-1347.

110. Rohrmann S, Roberts WW, Walsh PC, Platz EA. Family history of prostate cancer and obesity in relation to high-grade disease and extraprostatic extension in young men with prostate cancer. *Prostate.* 2003;55:140-146.

111. Neugut AI, Chen AC, Petrylak DP. The "skinny" on obesity and prostate cancer prognosis. *J Clin Oncol.* 2004;22:395-398.

112. Freedland SJ. Obesity and prostate cancer: a growing problem. *Clin Cancer Res.* 2005;11:6763-6766.

113. Gong Z, Neuhouser ML, Goodman PJ, et al. Obesity, diabetes, and risk of prostate cancer: results from the prostate cancer prevention trial. *Cancer Epidemiol Biomarkers Prev.* 2006;15:1977-1983.

114. Wright ME, Chang S-C, Schatzkin A, et al. Prospective study of adiposity and weight change in relation to prostate cancer incidence and mortality. *Cancer.* 2007;109:675-684.

115. Amling C, Riffenburgh R, Sun L, et al. Pathologic variables and recurrence rates as related to obesity and race in men with prostate cancer undergoing radical prostatectomy. *J Clin Oncol.* 2004;22:439-445.

116. Freedland S, Aronson W, Kane C, et al. Impact of obesity on biochemical control after radical prostatectomy for clinically localized prostate cancer: a report by the Shared Equal Access Regional Cancer Hospital Database Study Group. *J Clin Oncol.* 2004;22:446-453.

117. Strom SS, Wang X, Pettaway CA, et al. Obesity, weight gain, and risk of biochemical failure among prostate cancer patients following prostatectomy. *Clin Cancer Res.* 2005;11:6889-6894.

118. Strom SS, Kamat AM, Gruschkus SK, et al. Influence of obesity on biochemical and clinical failure after external-beam radiotherapy for localized prostate cancer. *Cancer.* 2006;107:631-639.

119. Hammarsten J, Hogstedt B. Hyperinsulinaemia: a prospective risk factor for lethal clinical prostate cancer. *Eur J Cancer.* 2005;41:2887-2895.

120. Hsing AW, Gao YT, Chua S Jr, Deng J, Stanczyk FZ. Insulin resistance and prostate cancer risk. *J Natl Cancer Inst.* 2003;95:67-71.

121. Hsing AW, Chua S Jr, Gao YT, et al. Prostate cancer risk and serum levels of insulin and leptin: a population-based study. *J Natl Cancer Inst.* 2001;93:783-789.

122. Tulinius H, Sigfusson N, Sigvaldason H, Bjarnadottir K, Tryggvadottir L. Risk factors for malignant diseases: a cohort study on a population of 22,946 Icelanders. *Cancer Epidemiol Biomarkers Prev.* 1997;6:863-873.

123. Hellawell GO, Turner GD, Davies DR, Poulsom R, Brewster SF, Macaulay VM. Expression of the type 1 insulin-like growth factor receptor is up-regulated in primary prostate cancer and commonly persists in metastatic disease. *Cancer Res.* 2002;62:2942-2950.

124. Kawada M, Inoue H, Masuda T, Ikeda D. Insulin-like growth factor I secreted from prostate stromal cells mediates tumor-stromal cell interactions of prostate cancer. *Cancer Res.* 2006;66:4419-4425.

125. Ho E, Boileau TW, Bray TM. Dietary influences on endocrine-inflammatory interactions in prostate cancer development. *Arch Biochem Biophys.* 2004;428:109-117.

126. Chang S, Hursting SD, Contois JH, et al. Leptin and prostate cancer. *Prostate.* 2001;46:62-67.

127. Stattin P, Soderberg S, Hallmans G, et al. Leptin is associated with increased prostate cancer risk: a nested case-referent study. *J Clin Endocrinol Metab.* 2001; 86:1341-1345.

128. Freedland SJ, Sokoll LJ, Mangold LA, et al. Serum leptin and pathological findings at the time of radical prostatectomy. *J Urol.* 2005;173:773-776.

129. Stattin P, Kaaks R, Johansson R, et al. Plasma leptin is not associated with prostate cancer risk. *Cancer Epidemiol Biomarkers Prev.* 2003;12:474-475.

130. Goktas S, Yilmaz MI, Caglar K, Sonmez A, Kilic S, Bedir S. Prostate cancer and adiponectin. *Urology.* 2005;65:1168-1172.

131. Presti JC Jr, Lee U, Brooks JD, Terris MK. Lower body mass index is associated with a higher prostate cancer detection rate and less favorable pathological features in a biopsy population. *J Urol.* 2004;171:2199-2202.

132. Freedland SJ, Terris MK, Platz EA, Presti JC Jr. Body mass index as a predictor of prostate cancer: development versus detection on biopsy. *Urology.* 2005;66:108-113.

133. Fowke JH, Signorello LB, Chang SS, et al. Effects of obesity and height on prostate-specific antigen (PSA) and percentage of free PSA levels among African-American and Caucasian men. *Cancer.* 2006;107:2361-2367.

134. Baillargeon J, Pollock BH, Kristal AR, et al. The association of body mass index and prostate-specific antigen in a population-based study. *Cancer.* 2005;103:1092-1095.

135. Barqawi AB, Golden BK, O'Donnell C, Brawer MK, Crawford ED. Observed effect of age and body mass index on total and complexed PSA: analysis from a national screening program. *Urology.* 2005;65:708-712.

136. Kristal AR, Chi C, Tangen CM, Goodman PJ, Etzioni R, Thompson IM. Associations of demographic and lifestyle characteristics with prostate-specific antigen (PSA) concentration and rate of PSA increase. *Cancer.* 2006;106:320-328.

137. Rodriguez C, Patel A, Calle E, Jacobs E, Chao A, Thun M. Body mass index, height, and prostate cancer mortality in two large cohorts of adult men in the United States. *Cancer Epidemiol Biomark Prev.* 2001;10:345-353.

138. Everett E, Tamimi H, Greer B, et al. The effect of body mass index on clinical/ pathologic features, surgical morbidity, and outcome in patients with endometrial cancer. *Gynecol Oncol.* 2003;90:150-157.

139. Pavelka JC, Ben-Shachar I, Fowler JM, et al. Morbid obesity and endometrial cancer: surgical, clinical, and pathologic outcomes in surgically managed patients. *Gynecol Oncol.* 2004;95:588-592.

140. Duska LR, Garrett A, Rueda BR, Haas J, Chang Y, Fuller AF. Endometrial cancer in women 40 years old or younger. *Gynecol Oncol.* 2001;83:388-393.

141. Anderson B, Connor JP, Andrews JI, et al. Obesity and prognosis in endometrial cancer. *Am J Obstet Gynecol.* 1996;174:1171-1178; discussion 1178-1179.

142. Temkin SM, Pezzullo JC, Hellmann M, Lee Y-C, Abulafia O. Is body mass index an independent risk factor of survival among patients with endometrial cancer? *Am J Clin Oncol.* 2007;30:8-14.

143. Meyerhardt JA, Catalano PJ, Haller DG, et al. Influence of body mass index on outcomes and treatment-related toxicity in patients with colon carcinoma. *Cancer.* 2003;98:484-495.

144. Meyerhardt JA, Tepper JE, Niedzwiecki D, et al. Impact of body mass index on outcomes and treatment-related toxicity in patients with stage II and III rectal cancer: findings from Intergroup Trial 0114. *J Clin Oncol.* 2004;22:648-657.

145. Haydon AM, MacInnis RJ, English DR, Giles GG. Effect of physical activity and body size on survival after diagnosis with colorectal cancer. *Gut.* 2006;55:62-67.

146. Doria-Rose VP, Newcomb PA, Morimoto LM, Hampton JM, Trentham-Dietz A. Body mass index and the risk of death following the diagnosis of colorectal cancer in postmenopausal women (United States). *Cancer Causes Control.* 2006;17:63-70.

147. Dignam JJ, Polite BN, Yothers G, et al. Body mass index and outcomes in patients who receive adjuvant chemotherapy for colon cancer. *J Natl Cancer Inst.* 2006;98:1647-1654.

148. Pavelka JC, Brown RS, Karlan BY, et al. Effect of obesity on survival in epithelial ovarian cancer. *Cancer.* 2006;107:1520-1524.

149. Kjarrbye-Thygesen A, Frederiksen K, Hogdall EV, et al. Smoking and overweight: negative prognostic factors in stage III epithelial ovarian cancer. *Cancer Epidemiol Biomarkers Prev.* 2006;15:798-803.

150. Zhang M, Xie X, Lee AH, Binns CW, Holman CD. Body mass index in relation to ovarian cancer survival. *Cancer Epidemiol Biomarkers Prev.* 2005;14:1307-1310.

151. Henley SJ, Flanders WD, Manatunga A, Thun MJ. Leanness and lung cancer risk: fact or artifact? *Epidemiology.* 2002;13:268-276.

152. Collaborative Group on Hormonal Factors in Breast Cancer. Breast cancer and hormone replacement therapy: collaborative reanalysis of data from 51 epidemiological studies of 52 705 women with breast cancer and 108 411 women without breast cancer. *Lancet.* 1997;350:1047-1059.

153. Huang Z, Hankinson SE, Colditz GA, et al. Dual effects of weight and weight gain on breast cancer risk. *JAMA.* 1997;278:1407-1411.

154. Schairer C, Lubin J, Troisi R, Sturgeon S, Brinton L, Hoover R. Menopausal estrogen and estrogen-progestin replacement therapy and breast cancer risk. *JAMA.* 2000;283:485-491.

155. Morimoto LM, White E, Chen Z, et al. Obesity, body size, and risk of postmenopausal breast cancer: the Women's Health Initiative (United States). *Cancer Causes Control.* 2002;13:741-751.

156. Suzuki R, Rylander-Rudqvist T, Ye W, Saji S, Wolk A. Body weight and postmenopausal breast cancer risk defined by estrogen and progesterone receptor status among Swedish women: a prospective cohort study. *Int J Cancer.* 2006;119:1683-1689.

11

Obesity and Mortality

Frank B. Hu

The relationship between body weight and mortality has long been a subject of debate. In particular, considerable controversy has surrounded the shape of the curve for the association between body mass index (BMI) and mortality and the effects of moderate overweight on mortality. Epidemiologic studies have variously found J-shaped, U-shaped, and linear relationships.[1] In some studies, overweight was associated with increased mortality, but in others, overweight individuals had no excess mortality or even slightly decreased mortality as compared with those who were normal weight. In addition, wide variations in the estimated numbers of deaths attributable to overweight and obesity have further fueled debate.[2,3] These divergent findings have not only caused a great deal of confusion among the general public, but also been used by commercial interest groups to downplay the importance of obesity as a public health issue.[4] Discrepancies in study findings underscore many methodological challenges in analyses of the relationship between BMI and mortality. These include reverse causation, confounding by smoking, overcontrol of intermediate variables, effect modification by age, and imperfect measures of adiposity.

In this chapter, we first discuss these methodological issues in analyses of obesity and mortality (Table 11.1). Then, we review recent literature on obesity and mortality, paying special attention to body fat distribution, intentionality of weight loss, and the relative impact of fatness and fitness. Finally, we discuss the impact of obesity on years of life lost and life expectancy.

Methodological Issues in Analyzing the Relationship between Obesity and Mortality

Reverse Causation

Reverse causation—when a low BMI is the result of underlying illness rather than the cause—is a major concern in the analysis of the relationship between obesity and mortality[5] (Fig. 11.1A). Most people, even those who are obese, die after age 65. By the time they reach older ages, many of those who were previously obese have already lost weight because of underlying diseases. Weight loss can result from the direct effects of disease on weight, or sometimes from conscious weight loss motivated by a diagnosis of serious illness. Many conditions that cause weight loss, such as chronic obstructive pulmonary disease (COPD) and depression, may remain undiagnosed for years. Because populations of lean individuals include smokers, healthy active people, and

Table 11.1 Epidemiologic Studies of Body Weight and Mortality: Methodological Factors that Can Bias Results

- Weight loss due to antecedent disease (*reverse causation*), especially in studies of older populations and studies with short follow-up periods
- Confounding by cigarette smoking
- *Overcontrol* for intermediate variables in the causal pathway (e.g., blood pressure, lipids, glucose)

Methodological factors of particular concern in studies of the elderly:
- High prevalence of comorbidity, preexisting disease, and illness-related weight loss
- BMI* less reliable marker of adiposity due to differential loss of muscle and lean body mass
- Depletion of *susceptibles*
- High baseline risk of death and dilution of individual risk factors

* BMI = body mass index.
Reproduced with permission from Manson JE, Bassuk SS, Hu FB, Stampfer MJ, Colditz GA, Willett WC. Estimating the number of deaths due to obesity: can the divergent findings be reconciled? *J Women's Health.* 2007;16:168-176.[1]

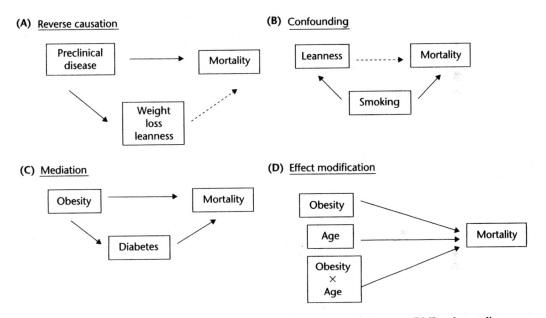

Figure 11.1 Methodological issues in the analyses of the relationship between BMI and mortality.

those with chronic illness, disentangling various influences on cause and effect can be challenging.

Reverse causation increases with older age because of the accumulation of chronic illness, making the relationship between BMI and mortality less clear among the elderly than among middle-aged adults. Although there is no perfect way to deal with this problem, one way to minimize the impact of reverse causation is to exclude subjects with existing cardiovascular disease and cancer at baseline.[5] Still, residual confounding by preclinical or undiagnosed conditions (which are more common among older persons) may attenuate the effects of obesity. Excluding deaths during the first few years of follow-up can also be a useful way to reduce bias due to reverse causation. However, chronic conditions (e.g., cirrhosis, COPD, and some neurodegenerative diseases) may cause weight loss and precede death by many years, thwarting even careful attempts to reduce bias due to reverse causation, especially in older populations. However, the analyses of midlife BMI and subsequent mortality can help to reduce reverse causation bias because of low prevalence of undiagnosed chronic diseases in middle-aged adults.

Reverse causation is most evident in studies of subjects with wasting conditions (e.g., congestive heart failure, end-stage renal disease, advanced malignancies, COPD, and AIDS), in whom obesity is associated with improved survival or decreased mortality (see Chapter 9). In these individuals, traditional risk factors, such as high blood pressure and serum cholesterol, are also associated with better survival.[6] The biological basis for this "obesity paradox" is unclear. Although high BMI levels among the chronically ill may confer survival benefits by providing a "metabolic or nutritional reserve," methodological bias from reverse causation may also be a plausible explanation, because those with low BMI and decreased blood pressure and cholesterol usually have more severe forms of disease that result in undernutrition and weight loss. Thus, the mortality risk in many lean subjects, especially those who are underweight, is substantially elevated, leading to the apparent survival advantage observed with higher BMI levels.

Confounding by Smoking

Confounding by smoking is of concern, because smokers tend to weigh less than non-smokers but have much higher mortality rates,[5] which can combine to produce an arti-fact of an elevated mortality risk among leaner individuals (Fig. 11.1B). In the Nurses' Health Study (NHS) cohort, smoking-related deaths (e.g., from lung cancer and emphy-sema) were clearly elevated among leaner women.[7] Although adjustment for smoking can reduce the impact of confounding, variations in duration of smoking and degrees of inhalation typically make statistical adjustment inadequate. Among past smokers, duration of quitting may also influence future risk of morbidity and mortality. Thus, the best way to deal with smoking is to restrict the analyses of obesity and mortality to never-smokers. In studies that found a J-shaped relationship between BMI and overall mortality in the overall cohorts, a stronger and monotonic relationship between BMI and mortality emerged when the analyses were restricted to never-smokers.[8-11] Because the problems of reverse causation and confounding by smoking typically coexist, it is impor-tant to simultaneously exclude both persons with known chronic disease and smokers from analytic samples.

Overcontrol of Intermediate Variables

In the study of obesity and mortality, diabetes, hypertension, and dyslipidemia are considered biological intermediates in the pathway[5] (Fig. 11.1C). Controlling for these variables usually reduces estimated relative risks (RRs) relating obesity to mortality, leading to overcontrol in the statistical models and underestimation of obesity's effects on morbidity and mortality. Some studies have controlled for intermediate variables to assess the degree to which these variables mediate the effects of obesity on mortality. However, these estimates should not be used to reflect overall effects of obesity.

Effect Modification by Age

In studying obesity and mortality, age appears to be one of the most important effect modifiers (Fig. 11.1D). Typically, the positive association of mortality with increasing BMI tends to decline with age. In the Cancer Prevention Study II, stratified analyses by three age groups (30 to 64 years, 65 to 74 years, and ≥75 years) showed stronger RR of mortality associated with increasing BMI in younger than older participants.[8] However, because overall mortality is much higher in the elderly, the absolute increase in death rates associated with higher BMIs was much greater in older people than in middle-aged individuals[12] (Fig. 11.2). Thus, the reduced relative impact of obesity on mortality does not mean that obesity is not detrimental in the elderly.

The declining relative impact of BMI on mortality with increasing age may also reflect several methodological issues: (a) greater bias due to higher prevalence of existing and occult chronic diseases in the elderly; (b) lower validity of BMI in measuring excess body fat in older people; or (c) survival bias or depletion of the susceptible, which relates to the deaths of those most vulnerable to obesity-related complications. These difficult methodological problems can affect the ability to obtain valid estimates of the relationship between BMI and mortality.

Future research may address these problems in part by reporting both relative and absolute risks associated with obesity. In addition, it is imperative to include measures of body fat distribution (discussed later). Moreover, it is important to evaluate the effects of obesity on functional disability in older individuals. Data have shown that even though BMI has a diminished impact on mortality in individuals 65 years or older, overweight and obesity were associated with significantly increased functional disabilities.[13] Given the methodological issues related to BMI and mortality, public health guidelines for

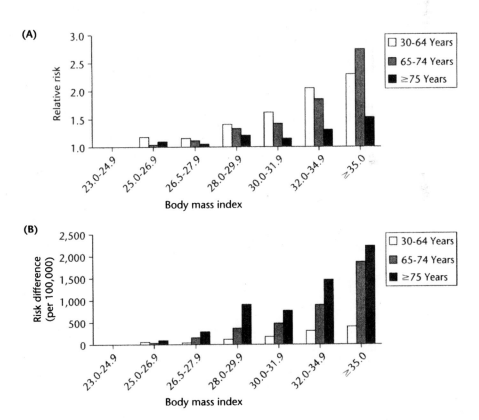

Figure 11.2 Risk of death associated with BMI among male nonsmokers without chronic health conditions, according to age. The annual risk of death is expressed as both the RR (A) and the absolute amount of additional risk (risk difference) (B) per 100,000 population, as reported in the American Cancer Society Cancer Prevention Study 2. Reproduced with permission from Byers T. Overweight and mortality among baby boomers—now we're getting personal. *N Engl J Med.* 2006;355:758-760.[12]

healthy weights should be based largely on studies conducted among people younger than 75 years of age.

Adiposity Measurements

Many large epidemiologic studies depend on self-reported height and weight to calculate BMI values. It is well-known that participants tend to overreport height and underreport weight, which leads to underestimates of obesity's prevalence, especially among those who are obese.[14] However, numerous epidemiologic studies have demonstrated a very high correlation between self-reported and technician-measured BMI values ($r > .90$), with the mean difference being relatively small.[15] In an analysis of 10,639 NHANES III participants,[16] self-reported or technician-measured BMI values produced virtually identical correlation coefficients with biomarkers of obesity and cardiovascular disease (see Chapter 5).

To address underreporting of BMI, van Dam et al.[17] conducted a sensitivity analysis using lower BMI cutoff points: 24.5 kg/m^2 to reflect a measured BMI of 25.0 kg/m^2, and 29.0 kg/m^2 to reflect a measured BMI of 30.0 kg/m^2. The RRs of mortality from this analysis were very similar to those from the original analysis, which used the standard BMI categories. Thus, self-reported height and weight values can lead to underestimates of obesity prevalence in population surveys, but there is no evidence that they cause substantial biases in the relationship between adiposity and mortality, especially when the validity of self-reported values has been demonstrated in the study population.

Another related measurement issue is the regression-dilution bias caused by intraindividual (within-person) variation in a single observation of a variable (e.g., BMI at baseline).[18] Such bias typically leads to attenuation of the estimated association between an exposure and outcomes. Greenberg et al.[18] demonstrated that correcting regression-dilution bias by using the average BMI of three visits instead of baseline BMI to predict mortality risk substantially strengthened the association between obesity and mortality in the Atherosclerosis Risk in Communities Study. Correcting for reverse causation bias by excluding ever-smokers and participants with serious illness further strengthened this association. The improvement in risk estimates by using average BMI rather than a single BMI measurement is likely due to two reasons: first, the average BMI accounts for intraindividual variation in BMI data and second, it reflects the usual amount of adiposity, which is less likely to be affected by underlying diseases. Because random within-person errors in BMI measurements are typically small, the second reason may account for a greater amount of regression deattenuation when average BMI is used in the analyses.

BMI and Mortality

A Summary of Meta-analyses and Systematic Reviews

The relationship between BMI and mortality has been examined in numerous epidemiologic studies. Although differences in study populations (e.g., age, sex, race, health status, and follow-up periods) and analytic approaches (e.g., different BMI categories and reference groups) make it difficult to synthesize the literature, several authors have conducted qualitative and quantitative reviews of the published data. Here, we briefly summarize these systematic reviews before discussing more recent studies.

Manson et al.[5] conducted one of the first systematic qualitative reviews of published studies on obesity and mortality. This review, conducted in 1987, examined 25 prospective cohort studies and found that the relationship of weight to all-cause mortality varied among linear, J-shaped, and even U-shaped curves. The authors identified three major methodological biases in most of the studies: inadequate control (or failure to control) for cigarette smoking; overcontrol of biologic intermediate variables (e.g., hypertension and hyperglycemia); and failure to control for weight loss due to preexisting or subclinical disease. The authors concluded that in most studies, these biases led to systematic underestimation of the association between obesity and mortality.

In 1996, Troiano et al.[19] analyzed 17 prospective cohort studies that included 356,747 men and 247,501 women. For the meta-analysis, categorical BMI was converted to a continuous variable, with the midpoint of BMI assigned to each category. The authors found a U-shaped relationship between BMI and mortality for both men and women. The positive association between increasing BMI and mortality in men was stronger with 30 years of follow-up than with 10 years of follow-up. Studies with 30 years of follow-up showed the lowest mortality at BMI of 24 kg/m². Smokers could not be separated from nonsmokers because the data were extracted from published reports, many of which did not distinguish between the two groups.

Allison et al.[20] conducted a meta-analysis in 1999 to examine the impact of excluding early deaths on the relationship between BMI and mortality. The meta-analysis, which included 29 studies and 1,954,345 subjects, was based on either published data or raw data obtained from the original investigators. The authors found that mortality risk started to increase at BMI of 25 kg/m² in both men and women. Overall, elimination of early deaths reduced BMI associated with minimum mortality by an estimated 0.4 units for men and 0.6 units for women at age 50. Thus, the authors concluded that excluding early deaths had a significant but relatively small impact on the shape of the curve. It should be noted, however, that the definition of *early death* varied across studies included in the meta-analysis.

Allison et al.,[2] also in 1999, conducted a pooled analysis of estimated number of deaths attributable to obesity based on six large cohort studies (the Alameda Community Health Study, the Framingham Heart Study, the Tecumseh Community Health Study, the American Cancer Society Cancer Prevention Study I, the National Health and Nutrition Examination Survey I Epidemiologic Follow-up Study, and the NHS). Using BMI of 23 to 24.9 kg/m² as the reference group, the authors found increased mortality for overweight and obese groups in most of the studies, especially among nonsmokers. They estimated 280,000 deaths per year in the United States were attributable to overweight and obesity. Using the RR estimates from nonsmokers, the approximate number of deaths due to obesity increased to 325,000.

In 2003, Katzmarzyk et al.[21] conducted a systematic review of the literature on physical activity, obesity, and premature mortality. The meta-analysis compared mortality rates in the highest category of BMI with the reference category in the published studies (both the highest and reference categories of BMI varied across studies). In 13 studies that included physical activity as a covariate, the summary RR of all-cause mortality for an elevated BMI was 1.23 (95% CI: 1.18 to 1.29). In 36 studies that did not include physical activity as a covariate, the summary RR of all-cause mortality for an elevated BMI was 1.24 (95% CI: 1.21 to 1.28). The authors concluded that the positive association between increasing BMI and mortality risk was independent of physical activity levels.

In 2005, McGee[22] reported a pooled analysis of BMI and mortality based on individual-level data from 26 observational studies (including 388,622 individuals, with 60,374 deaths during follow-up) from the Diverse Populations Collaboration. Compared with normal-weight men and women, obese individuals had significantly elevated total and CVD mortality. Overweight was associated with significantly elevated coronary heart disease mortality, but a slightly lower risk of total mortality. This study, however, did not report stratified analysis by smoking status, age, or race.

For practical reasons, it is not possible for the meta-analyses or systematic reviews to include all published studies, or a random sample of the studies. Because most data are provided in aggregate form, it is likewise impossible for meta-analyses to simultaneously minimize reverse causation and account for cigarette smoking. Thus, the findings from these systematic reviews or meta-analyses should be interpreted in the context of large cohort studies that have carefully addressed methodological issues.

A Summary of Individual Cohort Studies

A recent analysis of three NHANES surveys heightened the long-standing controversy regarding the relationship between BMI and mortality. The study, by Flegal et al.,[3] found that excess mortality due to obesity was much lower than earlier reports, and that overweight was associated with lower mortality compared with normal weight. They estimated 112,000 obesity-related deaths per year, substantially fewer than in earlier reports.[2] In a secondary analysis, the authors excluded persons according to smoking status and baseline diseases, but the exclusions were not simultaneous. They speculated that improved treatment of obesity-related conditions might have accounted for the dramatic decline in the estimated number of deaths over time. In subsequent analysis of the same datasets, the investigators reported cause-specific excess deaths associated with different weight categories.[23] Overweight was associated with significantly decreased mortality from noncancer, non-CVD causes (including chronic respiratory disease, infections, injuries, and neurodegenerative diseases), but it was not associated with cancer or CVD mortality. Obesity was associated with increased CVD mortality, but not total cancer mortality. As with the earlier study, the primary analyses of this study included all participants, including smokers and those with preexisting chronic diseases.

These results are best interpreted in the context of other studies, especially large cohort studies that have carefully addressed methodological biases in the relationship between obesity and mortality. In one of the largest studies conducted to date, Calle et al.[8] examined the relationship between BMI and mortality in an American Cancer Society cohort of more than 1 million adults (Cancer Prevention Study II or CPS II) followed from 1982 to 1996. The study showed a clear pattern of increasing mortality with increasing weight after excluding baseline smokers and those with prevalent diseases. Among healthy people with stable weight who had never smoked, the lowest mortality occurred at BMI of 23.5 to 24.9 kg/m^2 for men and 22.0 to 23.4 kg/m^2 for women (Fig. 11.3). Similarly, a 16-year follow-up study of 115,000 female nurses aged 30 to 55 without CVD or cancer at baseline also demonstrated that the gradient between increasing BMI and total mortality became substantially steeper with simultaneous accounting for reverse causation and smoking status (Fig. 11.3). In addition, overweight was associated with significantly elevated risk of both CVD and cancer mortality among never-smokers.

An updated analysis of the CPS II, with 20 years of follow-up, showed a persistent linear association between BMI and mortality, with no evidence that the impact of overweight and obesity on total mortality declined over time.[24] Data indicated that the RRs of mortality associated with a high BMI did not change substantially between time periods spanning a total of 20 years (1982-1991, 1992-1997, and 1998-2002). Thus, these analyses did not support the hypothesis that the relative impact of obesity on mortality has decreased over time.

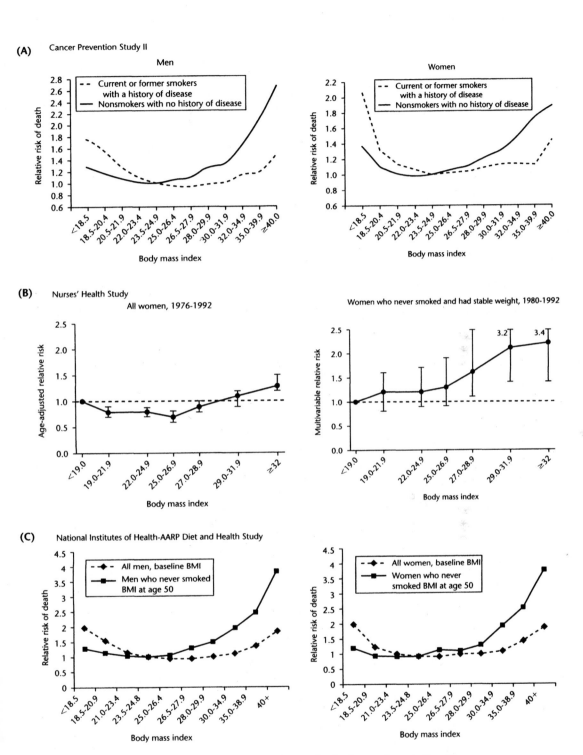

Figure 11.3 The relationships between BMI and mortality in three cohort studies: Cancer Prevention Study II, Nurses' Health Study, and National Institute of Health-AARP Diet and Health Study. Reproduced with permission from Manson JE, Bassuk SS, Hu FB, Stampfer MJ, Colditz GA, Willett WC. Estimating the number of deaths due to obesity: can the divergent findings be reconciled? *Women's Health*. 2007;16(2):168-176.[1]

In the updated analysis of the NHS,[7] the association between BMI and mortality became even stronger over 24 years of follow-up in middle-aged women than was in the earlier study. When the analyses were restricted to women who had never smoked, there was a direct monotonic relationship between BMI and total CVD and cancer mortality. The lowest overall mortality was observed among never-smoking women with a BMI of <23 kg/m^2. Several other large cohort studies have shown an approximately monotonic relationship between increasing BMI and mortality after elimination of current smokers and subjects with baseline diseases. These studies include the Harvard Alumni Study,[9] the Health Professionals' Follow-up Study (HPFS),[25] the Physicians' Health Study,[10] the Adventist Health Study,[26] the Canada Fitness Survey,[27] a 22-year prospective cohort study of 2 million Swedish men between the ages of 20 and 74,[28] and a prospective nationwide cohort study of 83,740 U.S. radiologic technologists followed for an average of 14.7 years.[29]

During 12 years of follow-up, van Dam et al.[17] examined the relationship between BMI at age 18 and mortality in a cohort of 102,400 women from the NHS II who were 24 to 44 years of age and free of cancer in 1989. Because prevalent and occult diseases are rare in this age group, potential bias due to reverse causation was likely to be minimal, especially with baseline diseases excluded. In this cohort, overweight at both age 18 and at the beginning of follow-up were associated with significantly elevated risk of total mortality and mortality from CVD and cancer. Overweight at age 18 was also associated with increased suicide risk in these women.

Recently, Adams et al.[30] examined BMI in relation to the risk of all-cause mortality in the National Institutes of Health-AARP cohort of 527,265 U.S. men and women who were 50 to 71 years old at enrollment in 1995-1996. During the 10 years of follow-up, 61,317 deaths (42,173 men and 19,144 women) occurred. Overall analyses showed a U-shaped relationship between BMI and mortality. However, when the analysis was restricted to healthy people who never smoked, the association between higher BMI and increasing mortality became much stronger (Fig. 11.3). BMI at midlife (age 50 years) had an approximately linear relationship with mortality. In this age group, overweight was associated with a 20% to 40% increase in mortality, while obesity was associated with 2- to 3-fold increase in mortality compared to those with BMI of 23.0 to 24.9 kg/m^2. The stronger relationship observed with midlife BMI probably reflects less confounding by existing or occult chronic diseases, which are relatively uncommon in this age group.

Taken together, cumulative evidence demonstrates that overweight and obesity in middle life are associated with significantly increased total, CVD, and cancer mortality. There is no evidence that the relative impact of obesity on mortality has decreased over time. In evaluating the evidence on obesity and mortality, it is important to distinguish studies focusing on statistical predictions (e.g., the analyses using the NHANES datasets[3]) from those that aim at identifying optimal BMI for disease prevention and health promotion. It is critical for the latter analyses to address confounding and reverse causation biases so that the "true" relationship between BMI and mortality can be estimated.

Ethnic and Racial Differences

Most research on the relationship between BMI and mortality has been conducted among Caucasian samples in the United States or Europe. Although there is increasing evidence that minority populations in the United States are more susceptible to the development of obesity-related metabolic disorders and type 2 diabetes than whites (see Chapter 8), the relationship between obesity and mortality is less well defined in minority populations. Several studies have suggested that the relative impact of BMI on mortality is weaker in African Americans compared with whites.[8,31-33] In particular, moderate overweight did not appear to predict mortality in African Americans, while severe obesity predicted increased mortality in African Americans to a lesser extent than in whites. Using data from the NHANES I Epidemiologic Follow-up Study, Durazo-Arvizu et al.[34] estimated that BMI values associated with minimum mortality in African-American men and women were at least two units higher than those in white men and women. However, the Women's Health Initiative Observational Study, with 7 years of follow-up, showed no significant difference in the relationship between obesity and mortality among black and white women.[35] In the AARP cohort,[30] the overall BMI-mortality relationship did not appear to differ appreciably across different ethnic groups (whites, blacks, Hispanics, and Asian or Pacific Islanders).

Because the number of minority participants in most studies is relatively small, the statistical power to study ethnic-specific effects is generally low. In addition, lower estimates in African Americans may reflect, in part, ethnic differences in the reliability of BMI as a measure of excess body fat. As discussed in Chapter 5, for a given BMI, blacks tend to have lower adiposity and percent body fat but higher muscle mass and bone mineral density than do whites. However, this difference in body composition does not completely explain the flatter relationship between BMI and mortality in blacks, because BMI is equally (or more strongly) related to several metabolic conditions and cardiovascular diseases in African Americans compared to whites (see Chapter 8).

The relationship between BMI and mortality has been studied in several Asian populations. Yuan et al.[36] followed a cohort of 18,244 Chinese men 45 to 64 years of age in Shanghai for up to 10 years and found a U-shaped relationship between BMI and total mortality among lifelong nonsmokers. Compared to men with BMI 21.0 to 23.5 kg/m^2, the RR for all-cause mortality was 1.73 (95% CI: 1.23 to 2.42) for men with BMI < 18.5 kg/m^2 and 1.48 (95% CI: 1.07 to 2.03) for men at or above a BMI of 26 kg/m^2 after adjustment for age, level of education, and alcohol intake. Whereas cardiovascular and cerebrovascular diseases accounted for most of the elevated risk in overweight and obese men, the increased overall mortality risk in underweight men was primarily due to infectious diseases.

Gu et al.[37] examined the relationship between BMI and mortality in a cohort study of a nationally representative sample of 169,871 Chinese men and women 40 years of age or older. After adjustment for age, sex, cigarette smoking, and other covariates, the authors observed a U-shaped association between BMI and all-cause mortality, with both underweight and obesity associated with increased mortality. Being moderately overweight did not appear to increase mortality risk, and eliminating smokers or those with chronic diseases did not appreciably alter the results. One unique feature of this study—the high prevalence of underweight (11.6% compared with 2% to 3% in most Western populations)—reflected the fact that when the cohort started in 1991, undernutrition was fairly common in rural areas of China.

Jee et al.[38] examined the association between BMI and the risk of death in a 12-year prospective cohort study of 1,213,829 Koreans between the ages of 30 and 95 years, including 82,372 deaths from any cause. Overall, there was a J-shaped association between BMI and mortality, with increased mortality observed in underweight, overweight, and obese groups. Consistent with earlier studies conducted in Western populations, the association between higher BMI and increasing mortality was stronger among never-smokers than smokers, and among younger than older participants. The lowest mortality was observed among participants with a BMI of 23.0 to 24.9 kg/m^2. There was a strong linear relationship between increasing BMI and deaths from atherosclerotic cardiovascular disease or cancer, even at the low end of BMI. Underweight was associated with a higher mortality from respiratory causes (including tuberculosis, pneumonia, COPD, and asthma), while higher BMI was associated with lower mortality from these causes. The biological mechanisms for these findings are unclear. However, increased respiratory mortality in very lean subjects may reflect residual confounding by smoking or reverse causation due to weight loss caused by these chronic conditions.

The studies conducted in Asian populations provide strong evidence that overweight and obesity are associated with increased mortality. Asians develop type 2 diabetes and cardiovascular disease at much lower BMI values than Caucasians (Chapters 8 and 9) because of differences in body composition, but current evidence does not suggest that the BMI values associated with minimum mortality are substantially lower in Asians than in whites. In developing countries that undergo economic and epidemiologic transitions, such as China, underweight and the low end of normal weight are more likely to reflect malnutrition, while the high end of normal weight and modest overweight reflect higher socioeconomic status. Thus, in these populations, it may be difficult to separate the effects of body weight from socioeconomic developments, even with control for levels of education and urbanization. Also, because cigarette smoking is highly prevalent in Asian males, analyses are more susceptible to residual confounding effects by smoking, even if cigarette smoking is carefully controlled for or only nonsmokers are included in the analyses.

Fat Distribution and Mortality

Abdominal or central obesity, reflected by a higher waist circumference (WC) and waist-to-hip ratio (WHR), is an important determinant of the metabolic syndrome, diabetes, cardiovascular disease, and several forms of cancer (see Chapters 8 to 10). Although most of the large cohort studies discussed earlier did not include a measure of body fat distribution, several cohort studies have demonstrated an important role for abdominal obesity in predicting all-cause mortality, especially in older populations. In the Iowa Women's Health Study, Folsom et al.[39] found that WC and WHR were better predictors of mortality than BMI among women 55 to 69 years of age. After adjusting for age, BMI, smoking, and other covariates, a 0.15-unit increase in WHR was associated with a 60% greater risk of death. The HPFS reported a significant association between BMI and total mortality among men younger than 65 years of age but not among older men.[25] On the other hand, WC predicted total and cardiovascular mortality in both younger and older men.

In a large Danish cohort, there was a strong association between WC and all-cause mortality after adjustment for body fat assessed by bioimpedance; each 10% increment in WC was associated with a 36% (95% CI: 22% to 52%) increase in mortality in men and a 30% (95% CI: 17% to 44%) increase in mortality in women.[40] In addition, WC accounted for a positive association between body fat mass and mortality. In the Rotterdam study, a large WC was more predictive of increased mortality than BMI in never-smoking men.[41] In Japanese Americans 71 to 93 years of age, there was a positive association between WHR and increased mortality, while higher BMI and skinfold thickness predicted lower mortality.[42]

In one of the largest studies conducted so far, both BMI and body fat distribution were significant predictors of mortality.[43] In particular, higher WHR and WC were significantly associated with increased mortality, even after adjustment for BMI, physical activity, and other covariates: RRs of total mortality across the lowest to the highest WC quintiles were 1.00, 1.11, 1.16, 1.29, and 1.69 (95% CI: 1.45 to 1.95) (P value for trend <.001). Similar associations were found for WHR and waist-to-height ratio. Even among women with a normal weight according to BMI (18.5 kg/m^2 ≤ BMI < 25 kg/m^2), abdominal obesity (WC ≥ 88 cm or WHR ≥ 0.88) was associated with significantly higher risk for CVD mortality (RR associated with higher WC was 3.02 (1.31, 6.99); for WHR it was 3.74 (2.02, 6.92)). Interestingly, increasing hip circumference was significantly associated with lower total and CVD mortality after adjusting for WC.

Recently, Zhang et al.[44] reported a significant positive association between WHR and mortality in the Shanghai Women's Health Study among 72,773 Chinese women 40 to 70 years of age. This population is quite lean according to Western standards, with relatively low prevalence of obesity (5%). In stratified analyses, the positive association was even stronger in women with a lower BMI. In a comparison of the extreme WHR quintiles, the RRs of total mortality were 2.36 (95% CI: 1.71 to 3.27), 1.60 (1.10 to 2.34), and 1.46 (0.97 to 2.20), respectively, for women with BMI < 22.3 kg/m², between 22.3 and 25.1 kg/m², and ≥25.2 kg/m². The strong association between WHR and mortality in lean women underscores that a relatively high degree of abdominal adiposity in a lean population is deleterious.

These results clearly demonstrate the importance of abdominal obesity in predicting mortality. However, the studies do not diminish the importance of overall adiposity, particularly in younger and middle-aged people. There is often a strong correlation between BMI and WC (r > .80), and in many situations, it is difficult to separate the effects of central obesity from overall adiposity, especially in underpowered studies. Also, some studies included BMI and WC simultaneously in the same model to compare the effects of BMI and WC. As discussed in Chapter 5, such analysis leads to attenuation of the effects of BMI and also alters the interpretation of BMI (WC-adjusted BMI largely reflects the effects of lean body mass rather than overall adiposity).

There is some evidence that WC may be superior to WHR as a surrogate measure of central obesity (see Chapter 5). WC is easier to measure than WHR and it is associated with fewer measurement errors. WHR is also more difficult to interpret because it is the ratio of two complex variables, such that increased WHR may reflect both greater intraabdominal fat mass (reflected by higher WC) and/or reduced gluteofemoral muscle mass (reflected by lower hip circumference). This may explain why waist and hip circumferences, when mutually adjusted, appeared to have opposite effects on metabolic and cardiovascular risk factors as well as mortality in several studies.[43,45]

Weight Change and Mortality

Many cohort studies have shown that weight loss is associated with increased mortality, especially among the elderly. However, weight loss in nonexperimental settings, especially in older individuals, is often caused by existing or preclinical chronic conditions (see Chapter 5). Such weight loss is largely due to loss in muscle mass (a phenomenon known as *sarcopenia*). Many studies exclude participants with diagnosed chronic diseases, but some conditions can be present for several years before clinical diagnosis. Thus, in many studies, the elevated mortality risk associated with unexplained weight loss is most likely due to methodological bias from reverse causation. Excluding deaths in the first few years can reduce such bias, but it may not be possible to completely eliminate it because chronic conditions may go undiagnosed for long periods of time. In the Honolulu Heart Study, weight loss was associated with increased mortality in the overall cohort but was unrelated to death in healthy men who had never smoked.[46] The observed positive associations between weight loss or weight fluctuation and mortality were explained, in part, by confounding by smoking and the presence of preexisting disease. As with the analyses on BMI and mortality, the least biased way to study the effects of weight change on mortality is to do so among middle-aged people who have never smoked and have no known preexisting diseases.

We examined the association between a change in weight during adulthood and overall and cause-specific mortality in the NHS. Results showed a strong positive and graded association between weight gain and mortality among never-smokers.[7] The increased mortality associated with weight gain was not modified by higher levels of physical activity. Weight loss was not associated with mortality. Thus, this study provides strong evidence that weight gain since young adulthood increases risk of premature death in middle-aged and older adults. These results are consistent with those of studies on the adverse effects of weight gain on metabolic diseases, cardiovascular disease, and cancer (see Chapters 8 to 10).

Lack of information on the magnitude of fat versus muscle loss poses a major problem in studying weight loss in older individuals. Some evidence indicates that among moderately obese individuals, weight loss is associated with increased mortality, while fat loss measured by changes in skinfold thickness is associated with a decreased mortality rate.[47] In most large epidemiologic studies, however, it is not feasible to differentiate fat loss from muscle loss. As discussed in Chapter 5, weight loss in the elderly is often accompanied by a substantial loss in muscle mass. Thus, it is not surprising that many studies have found that weight loss has detrimental effects on mortality in older individuals.

Several studies have suggested that intentional and unintentional weight loss have different effects on mortality. In the Iowa Women's Health Study, unintentional weight loss was associated with higher mortality, but the finding was limited to women with prevalent chronic disease.[48] Conversely, intentional weight loss was not associated with total or cardiovascular mortality. Similarly, Wannamethee et al.[49] found that unintentional (but not intentional) weight loss was associated with significantly increased risk of all-cause mortality in men. While men who lost weight intentionally as a result of personal choice showed significant benefit in all-cause mortality, those who lost weight owing to ill health had significantly elevated mortality.

Gregg et al.[50] examined the relationship between self-reported intentional weight loss and mortality among 6391 overweight and obese persons who were at least 35 years of age. The analyses were adjusted for age, sex, ethnicity, education, smoking, health status, health care utilization, and initial BMI. Compared with individuals who were not trying to lose weight and reported no weight change, those with intentional weight loss had a 24% lower mortality rate, while those with unintentional weight loss had a 31% higher mortality rate. Regardless of actual weight change, mortality rates were significantly lower among those who reported trying to lose weight compared with those who reported no effort to lose weight. Other studies have also found potential benefits of intentional weight loss on premature mortality, but the effects appeared to depend on the presence of chronic conditions at baseline.[51,52] Among overweight women with obesity-related conditions (but not among healthy women), intentional weight loss seemed to be associated with lower mortality.

A major challenge in studying intentionality of weight loss and mortality is confounding by healthy dietary and lifestyle behaviors associated with weight loss attempts. Although some studies controlled for health-related behavioral variables, such as smoking and physical activity, unmeasured and residual confounding remain highly probable, because a wide range of health-seeking behaviors (e.g., increased screening and preventive care) may be associated with attempted weight loss, especially among those with existing conditions. Ideally, this issue should be addressed in large randomized clinical trials with hard endpoints. However, it is still difficult to attribute the observed benefits or harmful effects from clinical trials to weight loss per se or to interventions used to induce weight loss. Nonetheless, well-designed prospective cohort studies that carefully differentiate intentional from unintentional weight loss, combined with results from randomized clinical trials, should provide the best possible evidence on the health effects of weight loss.

Fatness versus Fitness and Mortality

Earlier chapters discussed the relative impact of obesity and physical fitness or activity on risk of type 2 diabetes and CHD (see Chapters 8 and 9). Similar analyses have also been conducted to examine whether physical fitness or activity can mitigate the effects of obesity on mortality. The Aerobics Center Longitudinal Study (ACLS),[53] which measured physical fitness using a maximal treadmill exercise test, found that low fitness conferred higher risk of mortality compared with fatness, and that fitness eliminated the excess risk associated with fatness in men. These results, however, were not consistent with a Lipid Research Clinics Study analysis that found that both fitness and fatness were independent risk factors for mortality, and that being fit did not abolish the relationship between obesity and mortality.[54]

Because physical activity is the primary modifiable determinant of fitness, we examined the combined effects of physical activity and obesity on mortality in the NHS. Results showed that excess adiposity (reflected by BMI or WHR) and lower physical activity were independent predictors of overall and cause-specific mortality.[7] The adverse effects of body fatness on mortality were consistent in both lower and higher physical activity categories, and being physically active did not mitigate the mortality risk associated with body fatness. This study demonstrated that regardless of a woman's physical activity levels, even modest weight gain during adulthood significantly increased mortality risk. It also showed that the benefits of physical activity were not limited to lean women. Among those who were overweight or obese, physically active women tended to have lower mortality compared with sedentary women. Women who were both lean and physically active had the lowest risk. Thus, maintaining a healthy weight and being physically active are both important for longevity. Even among those who are physically active, it is important to minimize weight gain during adulthood.

Classifying lean people based on physical activity levels offers a useful way to differentiate between active and inactive members of the lean group. Compared with the normal weight group in the HPFS cohort, there was increased mortality among lean inactive men but not among lean active men.[24] The lean inactive group probably included many participants with preexisting or subclinical chronic diseases that had led to decreased physical activity levels. Excluding of subjects with existing diagnoses of chronic diseases, and eliminating deaths that occur early in the follow-up period can help reduce, but not completely eliminate, biases due to reverse causation. Cross-classification of physical activity and BMI can also be a useful way to separate healthy, lean groups from the unhealthy ones.

Obesity, Years of Life Lost, and Life Expectancy

Several recent studies have estimated years of life lost (YLL) associated with obesity or the impact of obesity on life expectancy in the general population. As a way to measure the health effects of obesity, YLL offers the advantages of simplicity and intuitive appeal. However, statistical methods used to estimate YLL, or life expectancy reduction associated with obesity, have varied across studies, as have the estimates. Using a cohort life table derived from the Framingham Heart Study, Peeters et al.[55] estimated that overweight 40-year-old female nonsmokers lost 3.3 years and that overweight 40-year-old male nonsmokers lost 3.1 years of life expectancy. In comparison, obese 40-year-old female nonsmokers lost 7.1 years and obese 40-year-old male nonsmokers lost 5.8 years. The YLL associated with obesity was similar to that observed with smoking.

Fontaine et al.[56] estimated the expected number of YLL due to overweight and obesity using data from the 1999 U.S. life tables and NHANES I and II epidemiologic follow-up studies. Overall, a BMI of 33 kg/m^2 at age 40 was associated with a loss of life expectancy of 2 to 3 years. The estimated YLL associated with severe obesity (BMI > 45) was 13 years for white men aged 20 to 30 years, representing a 22% reduction in expected remaining life span. The corresponding YLL for severely obese white women was 8 years. The YLL estimates were substantially lower in blacks than in whites.

Olshansky et al.[57] estimated the impact of obesity on overall life expectancy in the U.S. population using U.S. life tables and NHANES data sets. Data from this study indicated that obesity would reduce overall life expectancy at birth in the United States by 0.33 to 0.93 year for white males; 0.30 to 0.81 year for white females; 0.30 to 1.08 years for black males; and 0.21 to 0.73 year for black females. The authors suggested that this reduction in life expectancy was comparable to that caused by all accidental deaths combined.

The different estimates obtained from the studies are probably due to variations in statistical methods and population characteristics. It should be noted that the studies by Peeters et al.[55] and Fontaine et al.[56] estimated YLL among overweight and obese people, whereas Olshansky et al.[57] estimated the reduction in life expectancy in the entire population and thus, the latter estimates were substantially lower than the former ones. Nonetheless, these estimates underscore the substantial life-shortening effects of obesity, which may manifest to a greater degree in future generations if childhood obesity continues to rise.

Summary

Numerous epidemiologic studies have examined the relationship between BMI and mortality. Although obesity is clearly associated with increased mortality, the health consequences of being moderately overweight remain controversial. There has been much debate regarding the shape of the weight-mortality curve and optimal BMI for longevity. Although BMI is an imperfect measure of body fat, compelling evidence from recent large prospective cohort studies indicates that both overweight and obesity in midlife are associated with increased total, CVD, and cancer mortality in later life.

Although total mortality is a simple and appealing endpoint, epidemiologic studies of body weight and mortality are particularly prone to biases resulting from methodological problems, such as reverse causation (e.g., low BMI being the result of underlying illness rather than the cause) and confounding by smoking. These artifacts can lead to J-shaped or U-shaped relationships between BMI and mortality, and to systematic underestimation of the impact of obesity on premature mortality. Reverse causation bias is particularly problematic and difficult to address in studies of the elderly because of high prevalence of undiagnosed diseases and reduced accuracy of BMI as a reflection of adiposity. Thus, the best estimates of the impact of obesity on mortality should derive from cohort studies with large sample sizes and long follow-up periods from midlife or earlier. In fact, many large studies that were conducted among middle-aged subjects have shown a monotonic relationship between increasing BMI and elevated mortality risk, especially when analyses were restricted to healthy participants who had never smoked. In these studies, BMI values associated with the lowest mortality were clearly below 25.

There is increasing evidence that abdominal or central obesity reflected by higher WC or WHR predicts increased premature mortality independent of BMI, especially in older populations. Existing evidence suggests that various measurements of fat distribution including WC, WHR, and waist-to-height ratios provide similar predictions of mortality. Because measurement of WC is more practical and simple to interpret than other measures of fat distribution, it should be monitored routinely for most people, including those who are of normal weight.

Weight gain since young adulthood has been associated with increased mortality in later life. On the other hand, intentional weight loss is associated with decreased mortality, although lifestyle factors associated with weight loss attempts may confound the relationship. Thus, future studies on obesity and mortality should also assess midlife weight gain and intentionality of weight loss.

Although mortality is an important end point, studies of BMI and mortality may not provide the best estimates of the impact of obesity on health because of methodological issues examined in this chapter. Thus, it is equally important to study incidence of chronic diseases as endpoints. As discussed in earlier chapters, overweight and obesity are clearly associated with major chronic diseases, such as hypertension, diabetes, cardiovascular diseases, and major forms of cancer. These conditions not only lead to increased risk of premature death, but also lead to impaired quality of life and increased healthcare costs. Thus, assessment of the overall public health burden of obesity should consider multiple endpoints including mortality, morbidities, functional disabilities, quality of life, and obesity-related economic costs. Indeed, functional impairment and limitations in activities of daily living have increased over time in the older, obese U.S. population.[58] In addition, obesity is associated with a reduction in both total life expectancy and disability-free life expectancy.[13] As with prediction and prevention of chronic diseases, a comprehensive evaluation of the public health impact of obesity on mortality should include the assessment of all three variables in the *adiposity triad* (BMI, WC, and weight gain since young adulthood).

References

1. Manson JE, Bassuk SS, Hu FB, Stampfer MJ, Colditz GA, Willett WC. Estimating the number of deaths due to obesity: can the divergent findings be reconciled? *J. Women's Health*. 2007;16:168-176.
2. Allison DB, Fontaine KR, Manson JE, Stevens J, VanItallie TB. Annual deaths attributable to obesity in the United States. *JAMA*. 1999;282:1530-1538.
3. Flegal KM, Graubard BI, Williamson DF, Gail MH. Excess deaths associated with underweight, overweight, and obesity. *JAMA*. 2005;293:1861-1867.
4. Couzin J. Public health. A heavyweight battle over CDC's obesity forecasts. *Science*. 2005;308:770-771.
5. Manson JE, Stampfer MJ, Hennekens CH, Willett WC. Body weight and longevity. A reassessment. *JAMA*. 1987;257:353-358.
6. Curtis JP, Selter JG, Wang Y, et al. The obesity paradox: body mass index and outcomes in patients with heart failure. *Arch Intern Med*. 2005;165:55-61.
7. Hu FB, Willett WC, Li T, Stampfer MJ, Colditz GA, Manson JE. Adiposity as compared with physical activity in predicting mortality among women. *N Engl J Med*. 2004;351:2694-2703.
8. Calle EE, Thun MJ, Petrelli JM, Rodriguez C, Heath CW Jr. Body-mass index and mortality in a prospective cohort of U.S. adults. *N Engl J Med*. 1999;341:1097-1105.
9. Lee IM, Manson JE, Hennekens CH, Paffenbarger RS Jr. Body weight and mortality. A 27-year follow-up of middle-aged men. *JAMA*. 1993;270:2823-2828.
10. Ajani UA, Lotufo PA, Gaziano JM, et al. Body mass index and mortality among US male physicians. *Ann Epidemiol*. 2004;14:731-739.
11. Engeland A, Bjorge T, Selmer RM, Tverdal A. Height and body mass index in relation to total mortality. *Epidemiology*. 2003;14:293-299.
12. Byers T. Overweight and mortality among baby boomers—now we're getting personal. *N Engl J Med*. 2006;355:758-760.
13. Al Snih S, Ottenbacher KJ, Markides KS, Kuo YF, Eschbach K, Goodwin JS. The effect of obesity on disability vs mortality in older Americans. *Arch Intern Med*. 2007;167:774-780.
14. Gillum RF, Sempos CT. Ethnic variation in validity of classification of overweight and obesity using self-reported weight and height in American women and men: the Third National Health and Nutrition Examination Survey. *Nutr J*. 2005;4:27.
15. Willett WC. *Nutritional Epidemiology*. 2nd ed. New York: Oxford University Press; 1998.
16. McAdams MA, Van Dam RM, Hu FB. Comparison of self-reported and measured BMI as correlates of disease markers in US adults. *Obesity (Silver Spring)*. 2007; 15:188-196.

17. van Dam RM, Willett WC, Manson JE, Hu FB. The relationship between overweight in adolescence and premature death in women. *Ann Intern Med.* 2006;145:91-97.

18. Greenberg JA, Fontaine K, Allison DB. Putative biases in estimating mortality attributable to obesity in the US population. *Int J Obes (Lond).* 2007;31:1449-1455.

19. Troiano RP, Frongillo EA Jr, Sobal J, Levitsky DA. The relationship between body weight and mortality: a quantitative analysis of combined information from existing studies. *Int J Obes Relat Metab Disord.* 1996;20:63-75.

20. Allison DB, Faith MS, Heo M, Townsend-Butterworth D, Williamson DF. Meta-analysis of the effect of excluding early deaths on the estimated relationship between body mass index and mortality. *Obes Res.* 1999;7:342-354.

21. Katzmarzyk PT, Janssen I, Ardern CI. Physical inactivity, excess adiposity and premature mortality. *Obes Rev.* 2003;4:257-290.

22. McGee DL. Diverse Populations Collaboration. Body mass index and mortality: a meta-analysis based on person-level data from twenty-six observational studies. *Ann Epidemiol.* 2005;15:87-97.

23. Flegal KM, Graubard BI, Williamson DF, Gail, MH. Cause-specific excess deaths associated with underweight, overweight, and obesity. *JAMA.* 2007;298(17):2028-2037.

24. Calle EE, Teras LR, Thun MJ. Obesity and mortality. *N Engl J Med.* 2005; 353: 2197-2199.

25. Baik I, Ascherio A, Rimm EB, et al. Adiposity and mortality in men. *Am J Epidemiol.* 2000;152:264-271.

26. Singh PN, Lindsted KD, Fraser GE. Body weight and mortality among adults who never smoked. *Am J Epidemiol.* 1999;150:1152-1164.

27. Katzmarzyk PT, Craig CL, Bouchard C. Original article underweight, overweight and obesity: relationships with mortality in the 13-year follow-up of the Canada Fitness Survey. *J Clin Epidemiol.* 2001;54:916-920.

28. Heitmann BL, Erikson H, Ellsinger BM, Mikkelsen KL, Larsson B. Mortality associated with body fat, fat-free mass and body mass index among 60-year-old Swedish men—a 22-year follow-up. The study of men born in 1913. *Int J Obes Relat Metab Disord.* 2000;24:33-37.

29. Freedman DM, Ron E, Ballard-Barbash R, Doody MM, Linet MS. Body mass index and all-cause mortality in a nationwide US cohort. *Int J Obes.* 2006;30:822-829.

30. Adams KF, Schatzkin A, Harris TB, et al. Overweight, obesity, and mortality in a large prospective cohort of persons 50 to 71 years old. *N Engl J Med.* 2006;355:763-778.

31. Stevens J, Keil JE, Rust PF, Tyroler HA, Davis CE, Gazes PC. Body mass index and body girths as predictors of mortality in black and white women. *Arch Intern Med.* 1992;152:1257-1262.

32. Durazo-Arvizu R, Cooper RS, Luke A, Prewitt TE, Liao Y, McGee DL. Relative weight and mortality in U.S. blacks and whites: findings from representative national population samples. *Ann Epidemiol.* 1997;7:383-395.

33. Stevens J, Plankey MW, Williamson DF, et al. The body mass index-mortality relationship in white and African American women. *Obes Res.* 1998;6:268-277.

34. Durazo-Arvizu RA, McGee DL, Cooper RS, Liao Y, Luke A. Mortality and optimal body mass index in a sample of the US population. *Am J Epidemiol.* 1998;147:739-749.

35. McTigue K, Larson JC, Valoski A, et al. Mortality and cardiac and vascular outcomes in extremely obese women. *JAMA.* 2006;296:79-86.

36. Yuan JM, Ross RK, Gao YT, Yu MC. Body weight and mortality: a prospective evaluation in a cohort of middle-aged men in Shanghai, China. *Int J Epidemiol.* 1998;27:824-832.

37. Gu D, He J, Duan X, et al. Body weight and mortality among men and women in China. *JAMA.* 2006;295:776-783.

38. Jee SH, Sull JW, Park J, et al. Body-mass index and mortality in Korean men and women. *N Engl J Med.* 2006;355:779-787.

39. Folsom AR, Kaye SA, Sellers TA, et al. Body fat distribution and 5-year risk of death in older women. *JAMA*. 1993;269:483-487.
40. Bigaard J, Frederiksen K, Tjonneland A, et al. Waist circumference and body composition in relation to all-cause mortality in middle-aged men and women. *Int J Obes (Lond)*. 2005;29:778-784.
41. Visscher TL, Seidell JC, Molarius A, van der Kuip D, Hofman A, Witteman JC. A comparison of body mass index, waist-hip ratio and waist circumference as predictors of all-cause mortality among the elderly: the Rotterdam study. *Int J Obes Relat Metab Disord*. 2001;25:1730-1735.
42. Kalmijn S, Curb JD, Rodriguez BL, Yano K, Abbott RD. The association of body weight and anthropometry with mortality in elderly men: the Honolulu Heart Program. *Int J Obes Relat Metab Disord*. 1999;23:395-402.
43. Zhang C, Rexrode K, Li TY, Van Dam RM, Hu FB. Abdominal adiposity and mortality in women: 16-year follow-up of the Nurses' Health Study. *Circulation*. In press.
44. Zhang X, Shu XO, Yang G, et al. Abdominal adiposity and mortality in Chinese women. *Arch Int Med*. 2007;167(9):886-892.
45. Bigaard J, Frederiksen K, Tjonneland A, et al. Waist and hip circumferences and all-cause mortality: usefulness of the waist-to-hip ratio? *Int J Obes Relat Metab Disord*. 2004;28:741-747.
46. Iribarren C, Sharp DS, Burchfiel CM, Petrovitch H. Association of weight loss and weight fluctuation with mortality among Japanese American men. *N Engl J Med*. 1995;333:686-692.
47. Allison DB, Zannolli R, Faith MS, et al. Weight loss increases and fat loss decreases all-cause mortality rate: results from two independent cohort studies. *Int J Obes Relat Metab Disord*. 1999;23:603-611.
48. French SA, Folsom AR, Jeffery RW, Williamson DF. Prospective study of intentionality of weight loss and mortality in older women: the Iowa Women's Health Study. *Am J Epidemiol*. 1999;149:504-514.
49. Wannamethee SG, Shaper AG, Lennon L. Reasons for intentional weight loss, unintentional weight loss, and mortality in older men. *Arch Intern Med*. 2005;165: 1035-1040.
50. Gregg EW, Gerzoff RB, Thompson TJ, Williamson DF. Intentional weight loss and death in overweight and obese U.S. adults 35 years of age and older. *Ann Intern Med*. 2003;138:383-389.
51. Williamson DF, Pamuk E, Thun M, Flanders D, Byers T, Heath C. Prospective study of intentional weight loss and mortality in never-smoking overweight US white women aged 40-64 years. *Am J Epidemiol*. 1995;141:1128-1141.
52. Williamson DF, Pamuk E, Thun M, Flanders D, Byers T, Heath C. Prospective study of intentional weight loss and mortality in overweight white men aged 40-64 years. *Am J Epidemiol*. 1999;149:491-503.
53. Lee CD, Blair SN, Jackson AS. Cardiorespiratory fitness, body composition, and all-cause and cardiovascular disease mortality in men. *Am J Clin Nutr*. 1999;69:373-380.
54. Stevens J, Cai J, Evenson KR, Thomas R. Fitness and fatness as predictors of mortality from all causes and from cardiovascular disease in men and women in the lipid research clinics study. *Am J Epidemiol*. 2002;156:832-841.
55. Peeters A, Barendregt JJ, Willekens F, et al. Obesity in adulthood and its consequences for life expectancy: a life-table analysis. *Ann Intern Med*. 2003;138: 24-32.
56. Fontaine KR, Redden DT, Wang C, Westfall AO, Allison DB. Years of life lost due to obesity. *JAMA*. 2003;289:187-193.
57. Olshansky SJ, Passaro DJ, Hershow RC, et al. A potential decline in life expectancy in the United States in the 21st century. *N Engl J Med*. 2005;352:1138-1145.
58. Alley DE, Chang VW. The changing relationship of obesity and disability, 1988-2004. *JAMA*. 2007;298(17):2020-2027.

12

Obesity and Health-Related Quality of Life

Daniel Kim and Ichiro Kawachi

Introduction

Obesity rates have reached epidemic proportions in the United States, affecting nearly a third of adults,[1] and more than doubling among children and adolescents since the 1970s.[2] Obesity has also rapidly become an epidemic in many developed and developing nations.[3] Defined as a body mass index (BMI) $\geq$ 30 kg/m², obesity has been established as a predictor of mortality from a number of chronic diseases. In adults, obesity has been associated with a 1.5 to 2 times greater risk of premature mortality from all causes, compared to those in the healthy BMI range (20 to 25 kg/m²).[4]

In the wake of the obesity epidemic, increasing concern has focused on the effects of obesity on morbidity and health-related quality of life (HRQOL). HRQOL is a multidimensional construct that reflects how a person subjectively evaluates his/her own well-being in the domains of physical, psychological and social functioning, as influenced by a person's experiences, expectations, and perceptions.[5]

Why Focus on HRQOL?

The relevance of the concept of quality of life can be traced back to the World Health Organization's definition of health as "a state of complete physical, mental and social well-being and not merely the absence of disease or infirmity."[6] More recently, the significance of quality of life is reflected in the U.S. Department of Health and Human Services' Healthy People 2010, for which an overarching goal is "to help individuals of all ages increase life expectancy *and* to improve their quality of life."[7]

HRQOL summarizes the impact of a risk factor such as obesity on a person's overall level of well-being. Analogous to studies that utilize all-cause mortality as the outcome, studies of HRQOL provide an integrated approach to evaluating the impact of obesity on health status. For example, the "jolly fat" hypothesis[8-10] has posited that obese individuals may be at *reduced* risk of depression and anxiety compared to normal weight individuals (with one suggested explanation being a mood-enhancing effect of carbohydrate consumption, while also contributing to weight gain[9]). This hypothesis has been supported by empirical studies, particularly among men, although such studies have not distinguished between different classes/levels of obesity.[8-10] A recent investigation has similarly found higher BMI to be significantly associated with *lower* suicide risk among young and middle-aged men[11] (while in a study among young women, a significant association between overweight/obesity and higher suicide risk was observed[12]). On the other hand, many studies have also documented the social stigma associated with the condition of being obese (e.g., references 13 and 14), which would place affected individuals at increased risk of low self-esteem and negative affect. Examining the impact of obesity on generically-assessed HRQOL provides additional insight into these apparently contradictory findings. Furthermore, most studies of "hard" health outcomes associated with obesity (such as cardiovascular disease, diabetes, hypertension, and gallstones) provide only a narrow window through which to examine the impact of this risk factor on people's lives. Although examining specific health outcomes are of etiologic interest, they are the "tip of the iceberg" when it comes to assessing the true extent of the population burden of morbidity associated with overweight and obesity. People care about the consequences of health risks (such as obesity) on their ability to perform their daily activities and social roles, and studies of HRQOL thus provide valuable information for consumers, clinicians, and policy makers.

Mechanisms Linking Obesity to HRQOL

Obesity can adversely affect HRQOL because of the symptoms and treatments associated with the specific diseases that it causes (e.g., pain from arthritis, functional limitations due to cardiovascular disease). However, obesity may deleteriously affect HRQOL above and beyond the effects that are mediated by established diagnoses. First, obesity may limit a person's ability to function *even in the absence* of established disease. An overweight individual may not have been diagnosed with hypertension or diabetes, and yet report significant limitations in daily activities such as walking up a flight of stairs, bending or stooping, or carrying groceries. Second, the stigma associated with being obese may compromise an individual's ability to function in social settings. There is interest in documenting both the direct and indirect (i.e., mediated by established diagnoses) consequences of obesity for HRQOL.

In observational studies linking obesity to HRQOL, causal inference is complicated by the fact that health behaviors, such as sedentarism, may act simultaneously as both confounders and mediators of the association. In other words, lack of physical activity may mediate the association between obesity and low HRQOL. Alternatively, a sedentary lifestyle may be a common prior cause of both weight gain as well as lower HRQOL. A similar concern applies to markers of socioeconomic status (SES). Low socioeconomic position (e.g., low educational attainment and low income) is a well-established risk factor for obesity as well as low HRQOL, that is, it is a potential confounder of the relationship between obesity and HRQOL. On the other hand, studies have also documented that obesity earlier in life is a predictor of subsequent social mobility,[15,16] such that lower socioeconomic position may mediate the relationship between obesity and low HRQOL. In the systematic review of the literature in this chapter, we have noted the occasions when observational studies attempted to measure and control for potential confounding variables when describing the relationship between obesity and HRQOL.

In the following sections, we provide an overview of commonly used instruments to measure HRQOL in adult and child and adolescent populations, and summarize how well these measures have performed in psychometric evaluations. In addition to presenting findings from a systematic review of the existing epidemiologic literature on obesity and HRQOL in the section "Obesity, Weight Change, and HRQOL," we comment on methodological issues and knowledge gaps in these studies that should be addressed in future investigations.

Measurement of HRQOL

Measures in Adult Populations

A variety of instruments have been used to assess the relationship between obesity and HRQOL. In this section, we describe some of the most commonly applied instruments, as well as their psychometric properties.

The Short-Form 36 (SF-36) is a widely used 36-item questionnaire originally applied in the RAND Medical Outcomes Study.[17] The SF-36 taps into eight core domains: physical functioning (PF), role limitations due to physical health problems (RP), bodily pain (BP), general health (GH), vitality (VT), social functioning (SF), role limitations due to emotional health (RE), and mental health (MH). Each scale is scored from 0 to 100, with higher scores indicating higher HRQOL. The PF, RP, BP, and GH scales can be used in turn to construct a Physical Component Summary (PCS) score, while the VT, SF, RE, and MH scales are used to calculate a Mental Component Summary (MCS) score. The original English version of the SF-36 has been translated into other languages, including Spanish, Swedish, and Chinese. Good internal consistency reliability, test-retest reliability, and construct validity have been documented for the SF-36 in both clinical and general population samples across multiple countries.[18-22]

The Short-Form 12 (SF-12) and Health Status Questionnaire (HSQ-12) are both 12-item shortened versions of the SF-36, which measure the same eight domains as the SF-36, and which likewise enable PCS and MCS scores to be calculated. Like the SF-36, psychometric studies have demonstrated the reliability and validity of these measures in general population samples, including in older age groups.[23-25]

The Obesity Specific Quality of Life (OSQOL) scale is an 11-item scale that encompasses four dimensions of self-rated health: physical state, vitality, relations with other people, and psychological state. In a random sample of 500 obese and 500 nonobese individuals in the general population, the scale exhibited acceptable internal consistency reliability (Cronbach's alpha = 0.77) as well as content and construct validity.[26]

Four items comprise the Centers for Disease Control and Prevention HRQOL-4 instrument,[27] corresponding to general health status, recent physical health status based on the number of physically unhealthy days during the past month, recent mental health status, and recent number of days of activity limitation during the past month. In both healthy and disabled populations, each of these items has been shown to possess good construct and criterion validity,[28-30] as well as moderate-to-high 2-week test-retest reliability.[31]

The Quality of Well-Being (QWB) scale quantifies HRQOL by combining preference-weighted values for symptoms and functioning, and yields a numerical expression of well-being, ranging from 0 for death to 1 for optimal functioning.[32] Internal consistency reliability, test-retest reliability, along with content, construct, and criterion validity have all been demonstrated in general population and clinical samples.[33-35]

The World Health Organization Quality of Life Questionnaire abbreviated version (WHOQOL-BREF) is a 26-item instrument comprised of four domains (physical, psychological, social relations, and the environment) that can also be used to assess HRQOL. Each of the domains has a possible score ranging from 0 (poor HRQOL) to 20 (excellent HRQOL). Cross-cultural surveys of adult respondents in 23 countries have shown the WHOQOL-BREF to possess good to excellent psychometric properties of reliability as well as validity in both general population and clinical samples.[36]

The EuroQol EQ-5D categorizes a respondent's health according to the following dimensions: mobility, self-care, usual activities, pain/discomfort, and anxiety/depression.[37] This measure can be used to provide a self-rating of health status based on a visual analogue scale (EQ VAS), with anchoring at 0 (worst imaginable health) and 100 (best imaginable health).[37,38] Test-retest reliability has been satisfactory in clinical samples, and reasonable construct and criterion validity have been demonstrated in population-based samples. However, some evidence suggests that the EQ-5D is less sensitive than the SF-36 in detecting differences associated with less severe morbidity.[39]

HRQOL Measures in Child and Adolescent Populations

Several survey instruments specific to the measurement of HRQOL in child and adolescent populations have also been developed and undergone psychometric testing.

The CHQ-PF50 is a parent-report version of the Child Health Questionnaire, a multidimensional measure of child HRQOL. It consists of 50 items, encompassing domains of physical, emotional, social, and family functioning (activities and cohesion), and comprising subscales of physical functioning, role/social limitations due to physical problems, role/social limitations due to emotional/behavioral problems, bodily pain, general behavior, mental health, self-esteem, general health, emotional impact on parent, impact on parental time for child's needs, family activities, and family cohesion. Each scale is scored from 0 to 100, with 100 representing the best possible health and 0 the worst possible health.[40] Internal consistency, 2-week test-retest reliability, and concurrent and construct validity of the scales were generally supported in an Australian representative sample of parents of children and adolescents aged 5 to 18 years.[41] Notably, however, factor analysis revealed a different two-factor solution for physical and psychosocial summary measures in this sample versus that in a U.S. sample.[41]

The PedsQL 4.0 is a 23-item questionnaire developed for children and adolescents (aged 2 to 18 years), spanning physical, emotional, social, and school functioning domains, and from which total, physical, and psychosocial health summary scores (ranging from 0 to 100) can be derived. Nearly identical parent-proxy and child self-report versions are available. High levels of internal consistency as well as acceptable construct validity (based on comparisons of children with chronic health conditions and healthy children) have been previously shown for both versions.[42]

The KINDL survey instrument is a 24-item instrument that contains six subscales (from which scores of 0 to 100 are calculated) to assess HRQOL in children and adolescents: physical functioning, emotional well-being, self-esteem, family functioning, social functioning, and school functioning. Internal consistency reliability and construct validity of the self-report version of the questionnaire have been generally found to be satisfactory among children with and without chronic illnesses in English (in the country of Singapore), and in other languages, including German and Norwegian.[43-45] Nevertheless, the parent-proxy version in Western English-speaking populations has yet to be psychometrically evaluated.

Obesity, Weight Change, and HRQOL

Systematic Literature Review

We conducted a systematic literature review of all studies in English that have examined obesity or weight change in relation to HRQOL measures. Citations were searched using the PubMed database (which includes citations from MEDLINE and other life science journals for biomedical articles) for the period between 1966 and April 1, 2007, with the keyword combinations of "obesity" and "quality of life"; "weight change" and "quality of life"; "weight gain" and "quality of life"; and "weight loss" and "quality of life." Articles were then obtained and reviewed. We included studies that applied measures corresponding to at least two domains of HRQOL, and also included studies that solely examined physical functioning or disability. Studies were further restricted to those based on representative, population-based samples, as opposed to clinical or nonrepresentative samples. The reference sections of retrieved articles were searched to identify additional potential articles for inclusion. Based on the ages of study participants, studies were divided into those conducted in adults (i.e., aged 18 years and older) and in children and adolescents (i.e., aged less than 18 years).

Obesity, Weight Change, and HRQOL in Adults

A total of 31 studies in adults met our inclusion criteria. Tables 12.1 and 12.2 (for BMI/ waist circumference/body fat percentage and weight change as predictors of HRQOL, respectively) show the salient characteristics from these studies, listed chronologically by year of publication. We summarize the study authors and year of publication, dataset analyzed, age range of study participants, study design (cross-sectional vs prospective/ longitudinal), measure of obesity (for Table 12.1 only), HRQOL instrument and its domains, control for potential confounders, and key significant findings (from the fully adjusted models). When reported, measures of overweight and their corresponding findings were also abstracted.

Among adults, the first study of obesity/weight change and HRQOL appeared in 1994, using the outcome of mobility disability. More than a third of the studies (13 of 31 studies) have been published since 2004. The largest sample analyzed to date was in the study by Hassan et al.,[73] with 182,372 adults from 50 U.S. states, using data from the Behavioral Risk Factor Surveillance System (BRFSS) survey. Other large datasets analyzed include the Nurses' Health Study and the Health Professionals Follow-up Study, with analyses of 40,098 female nurses and 46,755 male health professionals in the United States, respectively, and the National Population Health Survey, with a total sample of 38,151 adults from all 10 Canadian provinces.

Across studies, study participants varied widely in age, from 18 to 96 years, with six studies exclusively focusing on elderly populations (i.e., aged 60 years and older). The vast majority of studies sampled U.S. populations (at the national, state, or regional/local level), while other studies sampled populations in Canada, England, Spain, France, the Netherlands, Turkey, and Taiwan.

Twenty-seven of the 31 studies used BMI to measure obesity. Only three studies used waist circumference, one study analyzed body fat percentage, and three studies examined weight change as a predictor of HRQOL.

The most commonly applied measure of HRQOL has been the SF-36, including versions in different languages to survey non-English speaking study populations. Other instruments have also been utilized, including all of the adult measures described in the section "Measurement of HRQOL."

All but three of the studies that applied BMI/waist circumference as the measure of obesity were cross-sectional in design, whereas all studies on weight change were prospective (with follow-up times ranging from two years in the study by Leon-Munoz et al.[72] to up to 16 years in the study by Launer et al.[70]). Most studies controlled for multiple key potential confounders, including socio-demographic characteristics (e.g., age and race/ethnicity), SES (e.g., income or education), and lifestyle behaviors and comorbid conditions, through adjustment in statistical models, stratification, or matching. Nonetheless, several studies did not adjust or stratify for race/ethnicity (e.g., reference 51) or SES

Table 12.1 Studies of Obesity and Health-Related Quality of Life (HRQOL) in Adults

Authors (Year)	Dataset, Source, Years	Sample Size, Population, Setting	Age Range	Study Design	Measure of Obesity Status	HRQOL Measure and Domains*	Control for Potential Confounders	Key Findings
Coakley et al. (1998)[17]	Nurses' Health Study (1992)	69,902 female nurses in United States	46 to 72 y	Cross-sectional	BMI	Physical function in SF-36 (PF, RP, BP, and VT)	Age, minority status, smoking, physical activity, alcohol, menopausal status, hormone replacement use	Higher BMI associated with worse PF (all 4 domains)
Han et al. (1998)[46] and Lean et al. (1998)[47]	Monitoring Risk Factors and Health in The Netherlands (MORGEN) project (1995)	1,885 men and 2,156 women randomly selected from civil registries in Maastricht, Amsterdam, and Doetinchem, all in Netherlands	20 to 59 y	Cross-sectional	BMI, waist circumference	SF-36 questionnaire (Dutch version): PF, SF, RP, RE, MH, VT, BP, GH, health change in past year	Age, marital status, employment status, household composition, education, smoking, alcohol, physical activity, parity; analyses stratified by gender	(1) Highest tertiles of BMI and waist circumference associated with worse PF (both sexes) (2) Highest tertile of BMI associated with BP (both sexes) and poor GH (women)

(continued)

Table 12.1 continued

Authors (Year)	Dataset, Source, Years	Sample Size, Population, Setting	Age Range	Study Design	Measure of Obesity Status	HRQOL Measure and Domains*	Control for Potential Confounders	Key Findings
Stafford et al. (1998)[48]	Whitehall II study (1985-1993)	4,918 men and 2,194 women working as civil servants in London in United Kingdom	39 to 63 y	Cross-sectional	BMI	SF-36: PF	Age, employment grade, physical activity, smoking, alcohol, menopausal status, steady weight change, comorbid conditions; analyses stratified by gender	BMI $\geq$ 29 kg/m² associated with poor PF (significant for women); significant linear trend across BMI categories (both sexes)
Le Pen et al. (1998)[26]	—	391 overweight/ obese and 462 matched nonobese adults randomly selected from cohort of 20,000 households in France	>18 y	Cross-sectional	BMI	(1) OSQOL scale (physical state, vitality, relations with other people, psychological state) (2) SF-36 (9 domains including reported health transition)	Matching of overweight/obese and nonobese individuals on age, gender, employment status	(1) OSQOL: overweight and obesity associated with worse physical state and vitality; obesity also associated with worse psychological state (2) SF-36: overweight and obesity associated with worse PF; obesity also associated with worse RP, BP, GH, and VT

Study	Data source	Sample	Age	Design	Measure	Outcome	Covariates	Results
Brown et al. (1998)[49]	Australian Longitudinal Study on Women's Health	13,431 middle-aged women randomly selected in Australia	45 to 49 y	Cross-sectional	BMI	SF-36: 8 domains + PCS and MCS	Education, smoking, physical activity, menopausal status, area of residence	Overweight and obesity associated with worse PF, BP, and PCS; obesity also associated with worse RP, GH, and VT
Lean et al. (1999)[50]	Monitoring Risk Factors and Health in The Netherlands (MORGEN) project (1995)	1,885 men and 2,156 randomly selected from civil registries in Maastricht, Amsterdam and Doetinchem, all in Netherlands	20 to 59 y	Cross-sectional	BMI	SF-36: PF	Age, employment status, household composition, education, smoking, alcohol, physical activity, parity; analyses stratified by gender	Obesity associated with poor PF (both sexes)
Doll et al. (2000)[51]	1997	13,800 adults in four counties in England	18 to 64 y	Cross-sectional	BMI	SF-36: 8 domains + PCS and MCS	Age, gender, frequency of health service utilization	Obesity associated with worse outcomes for each domain and PCS and MCS
Brown et al. (2000)[52]	Australian Longitudinal Study on Women's Health	14,779 young women selected randomly in Australia	18 to 23 y	Cross-sectional	BMI	SF-36: 8 domains	Age, education, smoking, physical activity, area of residence	Overweight and obesity associated with worse PF, GH, and VT

(continued)

Table 12.1 continued

Authors (Year)	Dataset, Source, Years	Sample Size, Population, Setting	Age Range	Study Design	Measure of Obesity Status	HRQOL Measure and Domains*	Control for Potential Confounders	Key Findings
Sturm and Wells (2001)[53]	Healthcare for Communities survey (1997/1998)	9,585 adults randomly sampled in 60 randomly selected communities in United States	18+ y	Cross-sectional	BMI	SF-12: physical health scale; Mental Health Inventory (from Medical Outcomes Study)	Age, marital status, race/ethnicity, smoking, alcohol; analyses stratified by gender	Obesity associated with worse physical health but not mental health (both sexes)
Trakas et al. (2001)[54]	National Population Health Survey (1996-1997)	38,151 adults in all 10 provinces of Canada	20 to 64 y	Cross-sectional	BMI	Health Utility Index-Mark III (HUI3): vision, hearing, speech, mobility, dexterity, emotion, cognition, pain	Analyses stratified by age and gender	Class II/III obesity† associated with worse mean HUI3 in all age groups in women and all age groups except 30 to 39, 40 to 49 y in men; obesity associated with worse outcomes for each domain
Ford et al. (2001)[55]	Behavioral Risk Factor Surveillance System (BRFSS) survey (1996)	109,076 adults randomly sampled in 50 states of United States	18+ y	Cross-sectional	BMI	HRQOL-4	Age, gender, race/ethnicity, education, employment status, smoking, physical activity	Overweight and obesity associated with poor self-rated health; obesity (but not overweight) associated with 14+ recent poor physical health days, mental health days, and days of activity limitation

Study	Data source	Sample	Age	Design	Measure	Outcome	Covariates	Results
Damush et al. (2002)[56]	Health and Retirement Surveys (1992, 1994, 1996)	7895 adults randomly sampled from U.S. areas	51 to 61 y in 1992	Prospective cohort	BMI	Self-rated general health, mobility	Age, gender, race/ethnicity, income, net worth, smoking, alcohol consumption, physical activity, comorbid condition disease severity	Obesity at baseline significantly associated with worsening of self-rated health and mobility
Larsson et al. (2002)[57]	1997	1,685 men and 1,790 women in 25 municipalities in western Sweden	16 to 64 y	Cross-sectional	BMI	SF-36 (Swedish version): 8 domains + PCS and MCS	Age, gender, physical activity, sick leave/disability pension	Ages 16 to 34 y: overweight and obesity associated with worse PF, GH, PCS (both sexes); obesity also associated with worse BP in women, and worse RP, BP, VT, SF, and MCS in men Ages 35 to 64 y: obesity associated with worse PF and GH in men, and worse outcomes on all domains and PCS, MCS in women

(continued)

Table 12.1 continued

Authors (Year)	Dataset, Source, Years	Sample Size, Population, Setting	Age Range	Study Design	Measure of Obesity Status	HRQOL Measure and Domains*	Control for Potential Confounders	Key Findings
Lopez-Garcia et al. (2003)[58]	—	3,605 adults randomly sampled in 420 randomly selected census sections in Spain	60+ y	Cross-sectional	BMI, waist circumference	SF-36 (Spanish version): 8 domains	Age, education, living alone, size of town of residence, smoking, alcohol, leisure-time physical activity, comorbid conditions; analyses stratified by gender	*Men:* overweight and obesity *inversely* associated with poor VT, MH; waist circumference associated with poor PF *Women:* obesity associated with poor PF, BP; waist circumference associated with poor PF, RP
Heo et al. (2003)[59] and Hassan et al. (2003)[60]	Behavioral Risk Factor Surveillance System (BRFSS) survey (1999)	154,074 /182,372 adults randomly sampled in 50 states of United States	18+ y	Cross-sectional	BMI	HRQOL-4	Age, gender, race/ethnicity, marital status, income, education, employment status, smoking, comorbid conditions	All obesity classes associated with poor general health; Class II, III obesity† associated with recent unhealthy physical days; overweight and Class I, III obesity† associated with recent unhealthy mental days
Goins et al. (2003)[61]	Behavioral Risk Factor Surveillance System (2000)	1,542 adults in Appalachian region of United States	65+ y	Cross-sectional	BMI	HRQOL-4	Age, gender, race/ethnicity, marital status, education	Obesity associated with worse self-rated health, greater mean number of days with poor physical health

Study	Study name	Sample	Age	Design	Exposure	Outcome measure	Covariates	Findings
Daviglus et al. (2003)[62]	Chicago Heart Association Detection Project in Industry Study (1996)	3,830 men and 2,936 women employed in 84 Chicago-area companies and organizations in United States	65+ y	Cross-sectional	BMI	12-item Health Status Questionnaire (HSQ-12): same eight domains as SF-36; overall summary score	Age, race/ethnicity, education, smoking, electrocardiogram abnormalities; analyses stratified by gender	Significant trend of higher weight categories associated with worse outcomes for each domain and summary scores (both sexes)
He and Baker (2004)[63] and Damush et al. (2002)[56]	Health and Retirement Study (1992-1996)	7867/7895 adults in random sample of areas in the United States	51 to 61 y at baseline	Prospective cohort	BMI	Decline in general health status, new mobility difficulty	Age, gender, race/ethnicity, marital status, income, education, smoking, alcohol, physical activity, general health, mobility, health insurance status	Overweight and obesity associated with decline in general health and new mobility difficulty
Yan et al. (2004)[64]	Chicago Heart Association Detection Project in Industry Study (1996)	3981 men and 3099 women employed in 84 Chicago-area companies and organizations in the United States	65+ y	Cross-sectional	BMI	12-item Health Status Questionnaire (HSQ-12): same eight domains as SF-36; overall summary score	Age, race/ethnicity, education, smoking, alcohol, comorbid conditions; analyses stratified by gender	Overweight associated with worse PF but better MH in women, and better GH, RP, RE, SF and summary scores in men. Obesity associated with worse outcomes on most domains in women, and fewer domains in men
Groessl et al. (2004)[32]	Rancho Bernardino study (1992-1995)	1326 adults in community of Rancho Bernardino, United States	55+ y	Cross-sectional	BMI	QWB Scale: symptoms/complex, mobility, physical activity, and social activity	Age, gender, smoking, physical activity	Obesity associated with worse QWB scores

(continued)

Table 12.1 continued

Authors (Year)	Dataset, Source, Years	Sample Size, Population, Setting	Age Range	Study Design	Measure of Obesity Status	HRQOL Measure and Domains*	Control for Potential Confounders	Key Findings
Jia and Lubetkin (2005)[37]	Medical Expenditure Panel Survey (2000)	13,646 adults randomly sampled in United States	18+ y	Cross-sectional	BMI	SF-12 (8 domains + PCS and MCS, PCS-12, MCS-12); EuroQol EQ-5D and EQ VAS (based on mobility, self-care, usual activities, pain/discomfort, anxiety/depression)	Age, gender, race/ethnicity, income, smoking, physical activity, comorbid conditions	Overweight and obesity associated with worse PCS-12 and EQ-5D; Class I and II obesity associated with worse EQ VAS; Class II obesity† associated with worse MCS-12
Huang et al. (2006)[65]	Taiwan National Health Interview Survey (2001)	14,221 adults in seven regions of Taiwan	18 to 96 y	Cross-sectional	BMI	SF-36 (Taiwan version): 8 domains + PCS and MCS	Age, gender, education, income, smoking, comorbid conditions	Overweight associated with *better* SF, GH, VT, MH and MCS; obesity associated with worse PF and PCS, and *better* MH and MCS

Study	Data source	Sample/population	Age	Study design	Exposure measure	Outcome measure	Covariates	Findings
Dinc et al. (2006)[66]	Manisa Demographic and Health Survey (2000)	1,602 reproductive-age women in city of Manisa, Turkey	15 to 49 y	Cross-sectional	BMI	WHOQOL-BREF (physical health, psychological health, social relations, environment)	Age, education, comorbid conditions	Obesity associated with worse outcomes for each domain except environment
Kruger et al. (2006)[67]	National Physical Activity and Weight Loss Study (2002-2003)	9,173 adults randomly sampled in United States	18+ y	Cross-sectional	BMI	HRQOL-4	Age-standardization of prevalence estimates	Obesity associated with less favorable age-adjusted prevalence estimates for all four HRQOL outcomes
Kostka and Bogus (2007)[68]	—	300 adults in one district of city of Lodz, Poland	66 to 79 y	Cross-sectional	BMI, body fat percentage	EuroQol EQ-5D (based on mobility, self-care, usual activities, pain/discomfort, anxiety/depression)	Age, comorbid conditions, number of medications, activities of daily living	Higher BMI associated with mobility problems Higher body fat percentage associated with pain/discomfort and anxiety/depression
Mukamal et al. (2007)[69]	Health Professionals Follow-Up Study	46,755 male health professionals in United States	40 to 75 y	Prospective cohort	BMI	SF-36: PCS and MCS	Age, marital status, smoking, alcohol, geographic region, physical activity	Obesity associated with *better* MCS Significant trend for relations of higher BMI with *better* MCS

* PF = physical functioning; RP = role limitations due to physical health problems; RE = role limitations due to emotional health problems; BP = bodily pain; GH = general health; VT = vitality; SF = social functioning; MH = mental health; PCS = Physical Component Summary score; MCS = Mental Component Summary score.

† Class I obesity: BMI = 30-34.9 kg/m²; Class II obesity: BMI = 35-39.9 kg/m²; Class III obesity: BMI ≥ 40 kg/m².

Table 12.2 Studies of Weight Change and Health-Related Quality of Life (HRQOL) in Adults

Authors (Year)	Dataset, Source, Years	Sample Size, Population, Setting	Age Range	Study Design	HRQOL Measure and Domains	Control for Potential Confounders	Key Findings*
Launer et al. (1994)[70]	Epidemiologic Follow-Up Study of National Health and Nutrition Examination Survey (1971-1987)	1,124 women randomly sampled in United States	45+ y	Prospective cohort	Mobility disability	Age, education, smoking, time to follow-up, comorbid conditions; analyses stratified into two age groups (45 to 59, 60 to 74 y)	Weight *loss* associated with incident disability in ages 60 to 74 y; high past BMI associated with incident disability in both age groups; high current BMI associated with incident disability in ages 45 to 59 y
Fine et al. (1999)[71]	Nurses' Health Study (1992-1996)	40,098 female nurses in the United States	46 to 71 y	Prospective cohort	SF-36: 8 domains + PCS and MCS	Smoking, physical activity, alcohol, comorbid conditions; analyses stratified by age group (<65, 65+ y) and BMI category†	*Weight gain* In both women ages <65, 65+ y: 20+ pound weight gain over 4 y associated with worse PF, VT, BP, MH (not significant in those 65+ y) in each BMI category *Weight loss* In women ages <65 y: 20+ pound weight loss associated with better PF among those with Class II/III obesity; better VT among those overweight and with Class I,

					II/III obesity; and better BP among those with class I obesity In women ages 65+ y: 20+ pound weight loss associated with better PF among those with Class I, II/III obesity; better BP among those with Class I obesity; *worse* MH among those with Class I obesity; and *worse* MH and VT among overweight women
Leon-Munoz et al. (2005)[72]	2001-2003	3,605 adults randomly sampled in 420 randomly selected census sections in Spain	60+ y	Prospective cohort	SF-36 (Spanish version): eight domains	Age, education, comorbid conditions, voluntariness of weight change, baseline scores; analyses stratified by obesity at baseline and gender	In those not obese at baseline: weight gain associated with worse PF, RP in men; and worse GH in women In those obese at baseline: weight gain associated with worse VT in men; and worse RP, RE, SF, BP in women

---

* PF = physical functioning; RP = role limitations due to physical health problems; RE = role limitations due to emotional health problems; BP = bodily pain; GH = general health; VT = vitality; SF = social functioning; MH = mental health; PCS = Physical Component Summary score; MCS = Mental Component Summary score.

† Normal weight = <25 kg/m²; Overweight = 25-29.9 kg/m²; Class I obesity: BMI = 30-34.9 kg/m²; Class II obesity: BMI = 35-39.9 kg/m²; Class III obesity: BMI ≥ 40 kg/m².

indicators (e.g., reference 54) in samples that were heterogeneous on these characteristics, thereby potentially contributing to residual confounding bias in the estimates.

In spite of their application to diverse populations and settings, the majority of studies found obesity (vs. normal weight) status to be significantly associated (at a 5% significance level) with a range of adverse HRQOL outcomes. There was some evidence to suggest that overweight status ($25 \leq$ BMI < 30 kg/m²) was similarly associated with worse HRQOL outcomes, although these associations were generally weaker in magnitude and less significant than for obesity associations. Furthermore, in several studies (e.g., references 53 and 61), associations with poor physical health outcomes were stronger and more frequently significant than for mental health outcomes. Nevertheless, other studies have found obesity to be significantly associated with worse mental health (e.g., references 51 and 55). Meanwhile, Lopez-Garcia et al.[58] found obesity (as well as overweight) in elderly men and women in Spain to be associated with *better* MH, respectively, compared to normal weight status, findings which are consistent with the "jolly fat" hypothesis. Similarly, a study in Taiwan[65] observed overweight and obesity to be significantly associated with better MH and MCS scores in both sexes combined, and a study among male health professionals in the United States found a significant inverse trend between higher BMI and better MCS scores.[69] In the latter study, a significant inverse trend between higher BMI and risk of suicide mortality was also seen, and was not affected by additional adjustment for glycemic load.

In investigations that stratified their analyses by gender, comparable findings associated with obesity were obtained between men and women in selected studies.[47,50,53,62] In other studies,[48,64,72] findings were consistent with obesity or weight gain having a significant adverse effect on additional HRQOL domains (such as GH, SF, and/or role limitations due to physical and emotional functioning domains) in women rather than in men. Women may pay a higher penalty than men from being obese, possibly due to the greater stigma and discrimination associated with obesity that women face. However, empirical evidence to support the latter is mixed to date.[14] In the study by Larsson et al.,[57] obesity was more significantly associated with worse physical, mental, and social scores in women than men among middle-aged and older adults (ages 35 to 64), whereas the reverse (i.e., with men faring worse than women) was true among younger adults (ages 16 to 34).

Four other studies in adults stratified their analyses by age.[54,65,70,71] Trakas et al.[54] found significant associations for severely or morbidly obese (vs normal weight) individuals (BMI ≥ 35 kg/m²) in both young and older age groups in women, and significant associations in all age groups except for 30- to 39- and 40- to 49-year olds in men. Huang et al.[65] determined significant PCS scores associated with obesity across all age groups (18 to 44.9, 45 to 64.9, 65+ years), with slightly larger effect sizes being seen in older age groups. This pattern might plausibly be ascribed to the lower physiologic reserve among older (compared to younger) individuals to compensate for the added demands of excess weight.[65] In the large, prospective Nurses' Health Study, Fine et al.[71] observed weight gain of 20 or more pounds over a 4-year period to be significantly associated with decreased PF, VT, and BP in overweight and obese women aged 45 to 64 and 65 or greater years at baseline, and to be significantly associated with worse MH scores among overweight and obese women aged 45 to 64 (but not those aged 65+) years. Similarly, weight loss of 20 pounds or more was significantly associated with increased VT scores among obese women in the younger age group (45 to 64 years) only. Such age-specific findings for certain domains of HRQOL might possibly be attributed to a higher social stigma of obesity in younger versus older adults, as suggested in some surveys,[73] and warrant further study.

Contrary to expected, the study by Fine et al.[71] also determined that the small subsample of women of normal weight at baseline who lost 20 or more pounds over 4 years and were aged 45 to 64 years had significantly *worse* MH scores by the end of follow-up. Women who lost 20 or more pounds over 4 years and were aged 65 or greater years had significantly *worse* MH, PF, VT, and BP scores by the end of follow-up (Table 12.2). However, these subsamples of women were found to possess greater comorbidity and worse self-rated health, and were more likely to practice unhealthy behaviors (including sedentarism) at baseline than women in the other weight groups. These differences would suggest that the weight loss may have been involuntary, such as due to an underlying physical or mental illness.[71]

Among studies that accounted for the presence of comorbid conditions in their analyses (e.g., references 48, 58, 59, 64, and 65), there was evidence of attenuation in the magnitude of effect estimates with this adjustment, in some instances to nonsignificance (e.g., references 59 and 64). This would be compatible with a partial mediation of the effects of obesity on HRQOL by these conditions, such that estimates that were adjusted for comorbid conditions would underestimate the combined (i.e., mediated and nonmediated) effects of obesity on HRQOL. At the same time, Huang et al.[65] demonstrated that associations for particular HRQOL domains (VT, MH) became larger in magnitude and statistically significant after controlling for comorbidity, consistent with comorbidity acting as a potential confounder of the association between obesity and HRQOL.

Obesity, Weight Change, and HRQOL in Children and Adolescents

Only five studies of obesity and HRQOL in children and adolescents were identified. Table 12.3 summarizes the relevant characteristics observed for each study.

The first study in children or adolescents was published in 2002. By contrast to several large studies conducted in adults, the largest sample consisted of 5530 children and adolescents in randomly sampled households in the western part of the state of Texas in the United States (and for a nationally representative sample, 4826 adolescents in the United States, based on data from the National Longitudinal Study of Adolescent Health). Across studies, study participants ranged in age from 3 to 20 years. Three studies corresponded to US populations, while the other two studies sampled representative populations in Australia.

All studies used BMI as the measure of obesity (frequently termed *overweight* in children and adolescents), while no studies applied other anthropometric measures or weight change.

HRQOL measures consisted of the parent-report version of the Child Health Questionnaire (CHQ-PF50); the PedsQL 4.0 (both parent-proxy and self-report); a self-report measure that approximated the PedsQL measure; and the KINDL survey (parent-proxy).

Studies were solely cross-sectional in design, and adjusted for multiple potential confounders. However, the two earliest studies[40,74] did not control for SES, and Wake et al.[74] did not adjust for several socio-demographic characteristics of the child, including gender and race/ethnicity.

Most studies found obesity (vs. normal weight) status to be significantly associated with worse HRQOL outcomes. Across studies, the significance of the associations spanned physical, mental, and social functioning domains. In individual studies, however, significant associations were not present across all domains. There was some evidence that overweight (vs. normal weight) status was associated with worse HRQOL outcomes, with these associations being weaker in magnitude and less significant than for being obese. By contrast to adults, impaired emotional/social functioning and self-esteem due

Table 12.3 Studies of Obesity and HRQOL in Children and Adolescents

Authors (Year)	Dataset, Source, Years	Sample Size, Population, Setting	Age Range	Study Design	Obesity Measure	HRQOL Measure	Control for Potential Confounders	Key Findings
Wake et al. (2002)[74]	Health of Young Victorians Study (2000)	2,863 children in 24 randomly selected schools in state of Victoria, Australia	5 to 14 y	Cross-sectional	Overweight and obesity (cut-points based on age- and gender-specific curves passing through adult BMI cut-points for overweight and obesity)	Parent-report version of Child Health Questionnaire (CHQ-PF50)	Child age, parent respondent gender	Overweight associated with poor mental health in boys, and role/social limitations due to emotional/ behavioral problems and poor self-esteem in girls. Obesity associated with bodily pain, poor physical functioning, mental health, self-esteem, and general health in boys; and poor self-esteem and general health in girls
Friedlander et al. (2003)[40]	Cleveland Children's Sleep and Health Study	371 children randomly selected from birth records of 3 Cleveland-area hospitals for period	8 to 11 y	Cross-sectional	"At-risk for overweight" (BMI = 85th percentile-94th percentile); "overweight" (BMI ≥ 95th percentile)	Parent-report version of Child Health Questionnaire (CHQ-PF50)	Age, gender, race/ethnicity, comorbid conditions	"At-risk for overweight" associated with poor physical functioning "Overweight" associated with poor

Study	Sample	Age	Design	Weight classification	QoL measure	Covariates	Findings
	1988-1993 in United States						physical functioning, self-esteem, emotional impact on parent, and overall poor psychosocial health
Williams et al. (2005)[75]	1,456 children in 24 randomly selected schools in state of Victoria, Australia	9 to 12 y	Cross-sectional	Overweight and obesity (cut-points based on age- and gender-specific curves passing through adult BMI cut-point for obesity)	PedsQL 4.0: parent-proxy, self-report	Age, gender, maternal education, socioeconomic disadvantage	Overweight associated with worse parent-proxy total PedsQL scores and self-reported social functioning Obesity associated with worse parent-proxy summary physical scores, social functioning, total PedsQL scores, and self-reported physical summary scores and social functioning
Swallen et al. (2005)[76]	4,827 adolescents randomly sampled in the United States	12 to 20 y	Cross-sectional	Overweight (95th percentile-97th percentile plus 2 BMI units); obesity (≥97th percentile of BMI plus 2 BMI units for age and gender)	Approximated PedsQL measure (self-reported general health, functional limitations, illness symptoms	Age, gender, race/ethnicity, family structure, income, father's education, mother's education	Overweight and obesity associated with poor general health, functional limitations

(continued)

Table 12.3 continued

Authors (Year)	Dataset, Source, Years	Sample Size, Population, Setting	Age Range	Study Design	Obesity Measure	HRQOL Measure	Control for Potential Confounders	Key Findings
						depression, self-esteem, school and social functioning)		
Arif et al. (2006)[77]	Childhood Health and Diabetes Survey (2002)	Parents/ guardians of 5,530 children and adolescents in randomly sampled households in west Texas, United States	3 to 18 y	Cross-sectional	"At-risk for over-weight" (85th percentile–95th percentile for age and gender); "overweight" (>95th percentile of BMI for age and gender)	Parent-proxy KINDL instrument (physical-functioning, emotional well-being, self-esteem, family function-ing, friends, and school functioning)	Age, gender, race/ethnicity, income, language acculturation, hyperglycemia symptoms, fam-ily history of diabetes	"At-risk for overweight" associated with worse scores on friends scale "Overweight" associated with worse scores on self-esteem and friends scales

to obesity appeared to figure more prominently in children and adolescents, consistent with greater stigma attached to perceptions of obesity in children and adolescents than in adults that have been found in other studies.[78,79]

Key Methodological Issues and Knowledge Gaps

Waist circumference is an infrequently applied measure of obesity in HRQOL studies. It has been proposed that BMI may be a less desirable measure of obesity at older ages, because height begins to decline as of middle age, and body weight, muscle mass (due to age-related degeneration [i.e., sarcopenia]), and BMI tend to decrease after approximately 60 years of age (see Chapter 5). By contrast, intra-abdominal fat increases progressively with age.[58] Some evidence suggests that among male never-smokers, waist circumference (but not BMI or waist-to-hip ratio) predicts an increased risk of all-cause mortality,[80] whereas other evidence indicates that waist circumference does not confer an advantage over BMI for predicting disease risk at older ages.[81] Nonetheless, comparing alternative measures of obesity in future studies would be useful in establishing the relative sensitivities of these measures with HRQOL within and across diverse study populations.

A critique of studies to date that concerns the valid interpretation of findings is the predominance of cross-sectional studies. A key criterion for making valid causal inferences is *temporality*, with measured exposures preceding the measured outcomes. Cross-sectional studies are subject to the threat to internal validity of *reverse causation*, whereby, in reference to the focus of our review, spurious associations could result from poor health causing low body weight, as opposed to body weight having an effect on health/HRQOL. Particularly in the elderly, lean individuals may have lost weight due to pre-existing or pre-clinical diseases (with associated poor HRQOL), such that obesity might appear to have a beneficial effect on health/HRQOL. The cross-sectional study by Lopez-Garcia et al.[58] that determined associations between obesity (as well as overweight) status with better MH in elderly men and women in Spain could well be susceptible to such bias. Similarly, the seemingly harmful effects of weight loss on HRQOL in the study by Fine et al.[71] could be attributed to this bias, if the small subsample of women of normal weight at baseline who subsequently lost weight had suffered from pre-existing physical or mental illnesses that caused the weight loss. Prospective studies have the advantage of being able to satisfy the temporality criterion, and to allow for weight *change* to be examined as a predictor of HRQOL *change*. In observational studies (which include all studies on this topic thus far), examining such changes helps to reduce (although may not necessarily eliminate) bias due to reverse causation and confounding.

Given the burgeoning obesity epidemic in children and adolescents, the limited number of studies conducted in younger age groups suggests an urgent need for additional empirical investigations. These studies should also ideally be based on prospective study designs to strengthen causal inference, and because of their potential usefulness in tracking HRQOL over formative years of development, and into adulthood.

Future research should continue to explore variations in HRQOL according to age and gender, and should examine variations according to other population characteristics, including racial/ethnicity and SES. Plausibly, obesity may follow different trajectories for HRQOL according to one's income and race/ethnicity. For instance, obesity status, independent of its effects on chronic diseases, may have a less adverse impact on HRQOL in blacks compared to whites, because of a potentially greater social acceptance of obesity among Blacks.[82] Despite the fact that HRQOL measures used to date in studies of the associations between obesity or weight change have been shown to be generally reliable and valid in population samples, future studies that focus on population subgroups will require psychometric validation of the measures within the subgroups analyzed.

Conclusions

In summary, assessing the consequences of obesity on HRQOL plays an important role in evaluating the impact of obesity on individual and population health. To date, a variety of studies, conducted primarily in adults and using cross-sectional designs, has attempted to evaluate the associations between obesity and HRQOL. The general validity of the HRQOL instruments used in these studies has been demonstrated, while the majority of studies conducted in general population samples suggest deleterious effects of obesity across multiple dimensions of HRQOL.

Additional studies in children and adolescents, and the application of prospective study designs, including assessments of weight change as a predictor of HRQOL change, would be particularly valuable. Future epidemiologic studies should also further explore possible effect modification of the associations of obesity with HRQOL by age and gender, as well as test for heterogeneous effects according to race/ethnicity and SES. Given the stigma and prejudice faced by obese individuals in society, it is important to document which groups of individuals (e.g., women, racial minorities, as well as individuals from lower SES groups) are at particular risk of paying the psychosocial penalty of being overweight. Interventions to reduce "fat bias," and to assist vulnerable individuals to lose weight, should be targets of priority.

References

1. Flegal KM, Carroll MD, Ogden CL, Johnson CL. Prevalence and trends in obesity among US adults, 1999-2000. *JAMA*. 2002;288:1723-1727.
2. Institute of Medicine. *Preventing Childhood Obesity: Health in the Balance*. Washington, DC: The National Academies Press; 2004.
3. James PT, Leach R, Kalamara E, Shayeghi M. The worldwide obesity epidemic. *Obes Res*. 2001;9(Suppl 4);228S-233S.
4. National Institutes of Health. *Clinical Guidelines on the Identification, Evaluation, and Treatment of Overweight and Obesity in Adults*. Bethesda, MD: US Department of Health and Human Services; 1998.
5. Testa MA, Simonson DC. Assessment of quality-of-life outcomes. *N Engl J Med*. 1996;334:835-840.
6. World Health Organization. *Constitution and Charter*. Geneva: World Health Organization; 1948.
7. US Department of Health and Human Services. *Healthy People 2010: Understanding and Improving Health*. 2nd ed. Washington, DC: US Government Printing Office; 2000.
8. Roberts RE, Strawbridge WJ, Deleger S, Kaplan GA. Are the fat more jolly? *Ann Behav Med*. 2002;24:169-180.
9. Palinkas LA, Wingard DL, Barrett-Connor E. Depressive symptoms in overweight and obese older adults: a test of the "jolly fat" hypothesis. *J Psychosom Res*. 1996;40:59-66.
10. Crisp AH, McGuiness B. Jolly fat: relations between obesity and psychoneurosis in general population. *BMJ*. 1976;1:7-9.
11. Magnusson PK, Rasmussen F, Lawlor DA, Tynelius P, Gunnell D. Association of body mass index with suicide mortality: a prospective cohort study of more than one million men. *Am J Epidemiol*. 2006;163:1-8.

12. van Dam RM, Willett WC, Manson JE, Hu FB. The relationship between overweight in adolescence and premature death in women. *Ann Intern Med.* 2006;145:91-97.

13. Carr D, Friedman MA. Is obesity stigmatizing? Body weight, perceived discrimination, and psychological well-being in the United States. *J Health Soc Behav.* 2005;46:244-259.

14. Puhl RM, Brownell KD. Confronting and coping with weight stigma: an investigation of overweight and obese adults. *Obesity.* 2006;14:1802-1815.

15. Gortmaker SL, Must A, Perrin JM, Sobol AM, Dietz WH. Social and economic consequences of overweight in adolescence and young adulthood. *N Engl J Med.* 1993;329:1008-1012.

16. Conley D, Glauber R. *Gender, Body Mass and Economic Status.* Cambridge, MA: National Bureau of Economic Research Working Paper 11343. Available at: http://www.nber.org/papers/w11343. Accessed November 15, 2006.

17. Coakley EH, Kawachi I, Manson JE, Speizer FE, Willett WC, Colditz GA. Lower levels of physical functioning are associated with higher body weight among middle-aged and older women. *Int J Obes.* 1998;22:958-965.

18. McHorney CA, Ware JE, Raczek AE. The MOS 36-item short-form health survey (SF-36): II. Psychometric and clinical tests of validity in measuring physical and mental health constructs. *Med Care.* 1993;31:247-263.

19. McHorney CA, Ware JE, Lu JFR, Sherbourne CD. The MOS 36-item short-form health survey (SF-36): III. Test of data quality, scaling assumptions, and reliability across diverse patient groups. *Med Care.* 1994;32:40-66.

20. Lu JF, Tseng HM, Tsai YJ. Assessment of health-related quality of life in Taiwan (I): development and psychometric testing of SF-36 Taiwan version. *Taiwan J Public Health.* 2003;22:501-511.

21. Sullivan M, Karlsson J, Ware JE Jr. The Swedish SF-36 Health Survey—I. Evaluation of data quality, scaling assumptions, reliability and construct validity across general populations in Sweden. *Soc Sci Med.* 1995;41:1349-1358.

22. Gandek B, Ware JE Jr, Aaronson NK, et al. Tests of data quality, scaling assumptions, and reliability of the SF-36 in eleven countries: results from the IQOLA Project. International Quality of Life Assessment. *J Clin Epidemiol.* 1998;51:1149-1158.

23. Ware JE, Kosinski M, Keller SD. A 12-item short-form health survey: construction of scales and preliminary tests of reliability and validity. *Med Care.* 1996;34:220-233.

24. Bowling A, Windsor J. Discriminative power of the health status questionnaire 12 in relation to age, sex, and longstanding illness: findings from a survey of households in Great Britain. *J Epidemiol Community Health.* 1997;51:564-573.

25. Pettit T, Livingston G, Manela M, Kitchen G, Katona C, Bowling A. Validation and normative data of health status measures in older people: the Islington study. *Intl J Geriatr Psych.* 2001;16:1061-1070.

26. Le Pen C, Levy E, Loos F, Banzet MN, Basdevant A. "Specific" scale compared with "generic" scale: a double measurement of the quality of life in a French community sample of obese subjects. *J Epidemiol Community Health.* 1998;52;445-450.

27. Moriarty DG, Zack MM, Kobau R. The Centers for Disease Control and Prevention's Healthy Days Measures—Population tracking of perceived physical and mental health over time. *Health Qual Life Outcomes.* 2003;1:37.

28. Verbrugge LM, Merrill SS, Liu X. Measuring disability with parsimony. *Disabil Rehab.* 1999;21:295-306.

29. Currey SS, Rao JK, Winfield JB, Callahan LF. Performance of a generic health-related quality of life measure in a clinic population with a rheumatic disease. *Arth Care Res.* 2003;49:658-664.

30. Ounpuu S, Chambers LW, Patterson C, Chan D, Yusuf S. Validity of the US Behavioral Risk Factor Surveillance System's Health Related Quality of Life survey tool in a group of older Canadians. *Chronic Dis Can.* 2001;22:93-101.

31. Andresen EM, Catlin TK, Wyrwich KW, Jackson-Thompson J. Retest reliability of surveillance questions on health-related quality of life. *J Epidemiol Community Health*. 2003;57:339-343.

32. Groessl EJ, Kaplan RM, Barrett-Connor E, Ganiats TG. Body mass index and quality of well-being in a community of older adults. *Am J Prev Med*. 2004;26:126-129.

33. Anderson JP, Kaplan RM, Berry CC, Bush JW, Rumbaut RG. Interday reliability of function assessment for a health status measure. The quality of well-being scale. *Med Care*. 1989:27;1076-1083.

34. Anderson JP, Bush JW, Berry CC. Internal consistency analysis: a method for studying the accuracy of function assessment for health outcome and quality of life evaluation. *J Clin Epidemiol*. 1988:41;127-137.

35. Kaplan RM, Bush JW, Berry CC. Health status: types of validity and the index of well-being. *Health Serv Res*. 1976:11;478-507.

36. Skevington SM, Lotfy M, O'Connell KA. The World Health Organization's WHO-QOL-BREF quality of life assessment: psychometric properties and results of the international field trial. A report from the WHOQOL group. *Qual Life Res*. 2004;13:299-310.

37. Jia H, Lubetkin EI. The impact of obesity on health-related quality-of-life in the general adult US population. *J Public Health*. 2005;27:156-164.

38. Rabin R, de Charro F. EQ-5D: a measure of health status from the EuroQol Group. *Ann Med*. 2001;33:337-343.

39. Coons SJ, Rao S, Keininger DL, Hays RD. A comparative review of generic quality-of-life instruments. *Pharmacoeconomics*. 2000;17:13-35.

40. Friedlander SL, Larkin EK, Rosen CL, Palermo TM, Redline S. Decreased quality of life associated with obesity in school-aged children. *Arch Pediatr Adolesc Med*. 2003;157:1206-1211.

41. Waters E, Salmon L, Wake M. The parent-form Child Health Questionnaire in Australia: comparison of reliability, validity, structure, and norms. *J Pediatr Psychol*. 2000;25:381-391.

42. Varni JW, Burwinkle TM, Seid M, Skarr D. The PedsQL 4.0 as a pediatric population health measure: feasibility, reliability, and validity. *Ambulatory Pediatr*. 2003;3:329-341.

43. Wee HL, Lee WW, Ravens-Sieberer U, Erhart M, Li SC. Validation of the English version of the KINDL generic children's health-related quality of life instrument for an Asian population—results from a pilot test. *Qual Life Res*. 2005;14:1193-1200.

44. Ravens-Sieberer U, Bullinger M. Assessing health-related quality of life in chronically ill children with the German KINDL: first psychometric and content analytical results. *Qual Life Res*. 1998;7:399-407.

45. Helseth S, Lund T, Christophersen KA. Health-related quality of life in a Norwegian sample of healthy adolescents: some psychometric properties of CHQ-CF87-N in relation to KINDL-N. *J Adolesc Health*. 2006;38:416-425.

46. Han TS, Tijhuis MAR, Lean MEJ, Seidell JC. Quality of life in relation to overweight and body fat distribution. *Am J Public Health*. 1998;88:1814-1820.

47. Lean MEJ, Han TS, Seidell JC. Impairment of health and quality of life in people with large waist circumference. *Lancet*. 1998;351:853-856.

48. Stafford S, Hemingway H, Marmot M. Current obesity, steady weight change and weight fluctuation as predictors of physical functioning in middle aged office workers: the Whitehall II study. *Int J Obes*. 1998;22:23-31.

49. Brown WJ, Dobson AJ, Mishra G. What is a healthy weight for middle aged women? *Int J Obes*. 1998;22:520-528.

50. Lean ME, Han TS, Seidell JC. Impairment of health and quality of life using new US federal guidelines for the identification of obesity. *Arch Intern Med*. 1999;159:837-843.

51. Doll HA, Petersen SEK, Stewart-Brown SL. Obesity and physical and emotional well-being: associations between body mass index, chronic illness, and the physical and mental components of the SF-36 questionnaire. *Obes Res*. 2000;8:160-170.

52. Brown WJ, Mishra G, Kenardy J, Dobson A. Relationships between body mass index and well-being in young Australian women. *Int J Obes*. 2000;24:1360-1368.

53. Sturm R, Wells KB. Does obesity contribute as much to morbidity as poverty or smoking? *Public Health*. 2001;115:229-235.

54. Trakas K, Oh PI, Singh S, Risebrough N, Shear NH. The health status of obese individuals in Canada. *Int J Obes Relat Metab Disord*. 2001;25:662-668.

55. Ford ES, Moriarty DG, Zack MM, Mokdad AH, Chapman DP. Self-reported body mass index and health-related quality of life: findings from the Behavioral Risk Factor Surveillance System. *Obes Res*. 2001;9:21-31.

56. Damush TM, Stump TE, Clark DO. Body mass index and 4-year change in health-related quality of life. *J Aging Health*. 2002;14:195-210.

57. Larsson U, Karlsson J, Sullivan M. Impact of overweight and obesity on health-related quality of life—a Swedish population study. *Int J Obes Relat Metab Disord*. 2002;26:417-424.

58. Lopez-Garcia E, Banegas Banegas JR, Gutierrez-Fisac JL, Perez-Regadera AG, Ganan LD, Rodriguez-Artalejo F. Relation between body weight and health-related quality of life among the elderly in Spain. *Int J Obes Relat Metab Disord*. 2003;27:701-709.

59. Heo M, Allison DB, Faith MS, Zhu S, Fontaine KR. Obesity and quality of life: mediating effects of pain and comorbidities. *Obes Res*. 2003;11:209-216.

60. Hassan MK, Joshi AV, Madhavan SS, Amonkar MM. Obesity and health-related quality of life: a cross-sectional analysis of the US population. *Int J Obes*. 2003;27:1227-1232.

61. Goins RT, Spencer SM, Krummel DA. Effect of obesity on health-related quality of life among Appalachian elderly. *South Med J*. 2003;96:552-7.

62. Daviglus ML, Liu K, Yan LL, et al. Body mass index in middle age and health-related quality of life in older age: the Chicago heart association detection project in industry study. *Arch Intern Med*. 2003;163:2448-2455.

63. He XZ, Baker DW. Body mass index, physical activity, and the risk of decline in overall health and physical functioning in late middle age. *Am J Public Health*. 2004;94:1567-1573.

64. Yan LL, Daviglus ML, Liu K, et al. BMI and health-related quality of life in adults 65 years and older. *Obes Res*. 2004;12:69-76.

65. Huang IC, Frangakis C, Wu AW. The relationship of excess body weight and health-related quality of life: evidence from a population study in Taiwan. *Int J Obes*. 2006;30:1250-1259.

66. Dinc G, Eser E, Saatli GL, et al. The relationship between obesity and health-related quality of life of women in a Turkish city with a high prevalence of obesity. *Asia Pac J Clin Nutr*. 2006;15:508-515.

67. Kruger J, Bowles HR, Jones DA, Ainsworth BE, Kohl HW. Health-related quality of life, BMI and physical activity among US adults (≥18 years): National Physical Activity and Weight Loss Survey. *Int J Obes (Lond)*. 2007;31:321-327.

68. Kostka T, Bogus K. Independent contribution of overweight/obesity and physical inactivity to lower health-related quality of life in community-dwelling older subjects. *Z Gerontol Geriat*. 2007;40:43-51.

69. Mukamal KJ, Kawachi I, Miller M, Rimm EB. Body mass index and risk of suicide among men. *Arch Intern Med*. 2007;167:468-475.

70. Launer LJ, Harris T, Rumpel C, Madans J. Body mass index, weight change, and risk of mobility disability in middle-aged and older women. The epidemiologic follow-up study of NHANES I. *JAMA*. 1994;271:1093-1098.

71. Fine JT, Colditz GA, Coakley EH, et al. A prospective study of weight change and health-related quality of life in women. *JAMA*. 1999;282:2136-2142.

72. Leon-Munoz LM, Guallar-Castillon P, Banegas JR, et al. Changes in body weight and health-related quality-of-life in the older adult population. *Int J Obes (Lond)*. 2005;29:1385-1391.

73. Rand CS, Wright BA. Continuity and change in the evaluation of ideal and acceptable body sizes across a wide age span. *Int J Eat Disord.* 2000;28:90-100.

74. Wake M, Salmon L, Waters E, Wright M, Hesketh K. Parent-reported health status of overweight and obese Australian primary school children: a cross-sectional population survey. *Int J Obes (Lond).* 2002;26:717-724.

75. Williams J, Wake M, Hesketh K, Maher E, Waters E. Health-related quality of life of overweight and obese children. *JAMA.* 2005;293:70-76.

76. Swallen KC, Reither EN, Haas SA, Meier AM. Overweight, obesity, and health-related quality of life among adolescents: the National Longitudinal Study of Adolescent Health. *Pediatrics.* 2005;115:340-347.

77. Arif AA, Rohrer JE. The relationship between obesity, hyperglycemia symptoms, and health-related quality of life among Hispanic and non-Hispanic white children and adolescents. *BMC Fam Pract.* 2006;7:3.

78. Latner JD, Stunkard AJ. Getting worse: the stigmatization of obese children. *Obes Res.* 2003;11:452-456.

79. Latner JD, Stunkard AJ, Wilson GT. Stigmatized students: age, sex, and ethnicity effects in the stigmatization of obesity. *Obes Res.* 2005;13:1226-1231.

80. Visscher TL, Seidell JC, Molarius A, van der Kuip D, Hofman A, Witteman JC. A comparison of body mass index, waist-hip ratio and waist circumference as predictors of all-cause mortality among the elderly: the Rotterdam study. *Int J Obes Relat Metab Disord.* 2001;25:1730-1735.

81. Iwao S, Iwao N, Muller DC, Elahi D, Shimokata H, Andres R. Does waist circumference add to the predictive power of the body mass index for coronary risk? *Obes Res.* 2001;9:685-695.

82. Wilfley DE, Schreiber GB, Pike KM, Streigel-Moore RH, Wright DJ, Rodin J. Eating disturbances and body image: a comparison of a community sample of adult black and white women. *Int J Eat Disord.* 1996;20:377-387.

13

Economic Costs of Obesity

Graham A. Colditz and Y. Claire Wang

Introduction

As the prevalence of overweight and obesity continues to climb, the challenges of quantifying the impact of this epidemic to inform public policies and health services become more pressing. The consequences of obesity on population health are far-reaching—as extensively discussed in Chapters 8 to 12: the society bears its burden from premature mortality, morbidity associated with numerous chronic conditions, and negative impacts on health-related quality of life. One useful metric to summarize the overall burden from such broad impact on the health care system and the society at large is the economic costs of obesity. Such metric can encompass the financial consequences of medical resources devoted to treating all obesity-related fatal and nonfatal conditions, productivity loss, and the psychosocial burden from suffering and poorer quality of life, forgone job opportunities, and other disruptions in life plans. Laying out the economic consequences of obesity in monetary terms tells us how much the population is paying for obesity-related costs (expenditure or opportunity costs). Subsequently it identifies the components of such burden and the share of these costs borne by each sector in the society. It is argued that such information can highlight research and funding priorities and help build political will to address the obesity epidemic.

In the 2001 U.S. Surgeon General's call to action to prevent and decrease overweight and obesity, the costs of obesity to the United States were cited to be $117 billion in 2000[1]—a figure likely much greater today. This estimate includes $61 billion in direct costs (costs incurred in the health care process) and $56 billion in indirect costs (forgone wages and productivity).[1,2] Details on these two components of economic costs of obesity as well as some less tangible aspects of obesity's burden will be provided in the section "Components of Economic Burden of Obesity." Methods adopted in the studies aimed to estimate costs of obesity can generally be classified to two types: the prevalence- and incidence-based approaches. The prevalence-based approach is the most common; it estimates the total costs incurred in a given year attributable to obesity. The incidence-based approach, on the other hand, often involves calculating the lifetime costs. The section "Methods of Quantifying Economic Cost" surveys the literature to describe these two approaches and discusses the strengths and weaknesses of each method. The section "Who Bears the Economic Costs of Obesity?" reviews studies for insights on who shoulders the overall cost burden of obesity. Finally, the section "Knowledge Gap and Future Research" addresses criticisms and limitations of the cost-of-illness estimates and discusses key knowledge gaps and future research directions.

Components of Economic Burden of Obesity

Direct Costs

The direct costs of a disease or a risk factor, in our case, obesity, consist of the resources used within the health care system, which can include the costs incurred by excess utilization of ambulatory care, hospitalization, pharmacotherapy, radiological or laboratory tests, and long-term care (including nursing home) for diseases that are attributable to excess body weight. Unsurprisingly, the disease burden is largely driven by the devastating consequences from elevated risks of cardiovascular diseases and cancer (evidently suggested by numerous epidemiological studies mentioned in Chapters 9 and 10) as well as some nonfatal, yet costly, conditions such as osteoarthritis. Nonetheless, rapidly increasing evidence now indicates that many additional conditions are also linked to obesity and, as a result, may be also contributing to its costs, such as benign prostate hypertrophy,[3] infertility,[4] asthma,[5,6] and sleep apnea.[7] Thorpe et al.[8] examined the relation between obesity trend and increase in U.S. health expenditure. They found that the combination of rising obesity prevalence and increased spending among the obese accounts for 27% of the growth in U.S. health care expenditure between 1987 and 2001. The latter effect signifies the changes in standard care for diabetes, hypertension, hyperlipidemia, and heart disease. It is worth noting, however, that the increase in medical costs and health services utilization differ substantially by moderate versus severe obesity[9,10] and by demographic factors such as age and race.[11]

Depending on methodology, data source, and calendar period, the annual medical costs of obesity in the United States are estimated to amount to $75 billion (in 2003 dollars)[12] and responsible for between 4.3% and 7% of total health care expenditure.[10,13-15] Levy et al.[16] estimated that the costs of obesity in France were approximately 2% of health care costs in 1992. In the Netherlands, Seidell estimated that the cost was 4%,[17] and Segal et al. estimated that obesity was responsible for 2% of health care costs in Australia.[18] The application of similar methodology to all member states of the European Union has provided estimates for the combined direct and indirect costs of obesity in 2002 of approximately €33 billion a year.[19,20]

Indirect Costs

In addition to direct costs, there are significant indirect costs due to decreased years of disability-free life and increased mortality before retirement, early retirement, work absenteeism or reduced productivity, and disability pensions as a result of chronic conditions attributable to obesity. Though research in this area is more limited, some suggest that the magnitude of indirect costs can be even larger than direct medical costs.[21] Many studies on productivity loss were conducted in Scandinavian countries.[22,23] For example, in Sweden,[23] obese subjects are found 1.5 to 1.9 times more likely to take sick leave, and 12% of obese women had disability pensions attributable to obesity, costing some U.S. $300 for every adult female in the population.

In the United States, Thompson et al. estimated that absenteeism due to obesity cost employers $2.4 billion in 1998.[24] The estimated workday loss among the very obese (BMI $\geq$ 40 or BMI $\geq$ 35 and with comorbidities) derived from the 2002 National Health Interview Survey amounts to approximately 4 days/year for men and 5.5 days/year for women.[25] Using data from the Duke Health and Safety Surveillance System, Østbye et al.[26] found a dose-response relationship between BMI and the number of workers' compensation claims, associated costs, and lost workdays. In terms of disability and restricted activity days, Wolf and Colditz[2] estimated that obesity resulted in 239 million restricted activity days and 89.5 million bed days every year. Overall, the indirect costs attributable to obesity in the United States amounted to at least $48 billion in 1995 dollars.[13] The major contributor to these costs is coronary heart disease (CHD; 48%), which accounts for a large portion of premature mortality. As the treatment improves for CHD and its precursor risk factors and as mortality decreases, the impact of CHD on the indirect costs of obesity will likely decline and that on the direct costs will perhaps increase. Other significant contributors to indirect costs were type 2 diabetes (17.5%) and osteoarthritis (17.1%), the latter largely due to excess bed days, workdays lost, and restricted activity days.

Psychosocial Toll and Disparity

Unlike direct and indirect costs that are relatively easier to quantify in monetary terms, obesity also has serious psychosocial consequences and negative impacts on the general well-being that are less straightforward to tally in an economic framework. Obesity has been linked to reduced vitality[27] and (in particular health-related) quality of life;[28] it also increases the risk of social discrimination and downward social mobility.[1,29] From individuals' point of view, several studies have evaluated salary according to BMI levels and have shown that more obese subjects have lower wages. Reduced household income is also associated with overweight and obesity.[30] The mechanism that drives such wage differential remains debated. Gortmaker et al.[30] evaluated this problem through a prospective analysis of the national longitudinal study of adolescents and observed that, over a 7-year period, women who were overweight in adolescence had delay in marriage and lower household income than women with weight within the normal range. They also reported that men who are overweight as adolescents have 9% ($2876) lower annual household incomes 7 years later than do men of normal weight. This work also suggested that overweight during adolescence could impact one's trajectory to occupation and future earnings from early in life. Further, it has been suggested that obese women tend to work in lower-paying occupations.[31] Evidence for men is somewhat less compelling.[32]

Although the prevalence of overweight and obesity has increased in all segments of the US population, certain groups have experienced a greater increase than others. For example, the prevalence of obesity is approximately 15% higher among non-Hispanic black women and Mexican American women than among non-Hispanic white women. Among men, the prevalence of obesity is comparable across ethnic groups but overweight was more common among Mexican American men than among non-Hispanic white and non-Hispanic black men.[33] Whether such trend is sufficient to address obesity as a top priority of minority population's health and what would be the ultimate mean to address the issue without stigmatization are difficult questions.[34] Moreover, obesity and its consequences, such as diabetes, continue to disproportionally affect low-income populations in the United States.[35] This trend implies that obesity's overall burden might be greatest for people who are the least able to afford it, making these conditions possible sources of widening disparities. Notably, income and race-ethnic disparity emerges before adulthood and might be even more striking among children and adolescents, for whom health consequences might lay further into the future (except for asthma), yet there exist immediate psychosocial issues such as low self-esteem, discrimination, and psychiatric well-being.

Methods of Quantifying Economic Costs

One can look cross-sectionally at the economic burden in terms of current health care costs through a prevalence-based approach, or use a prospective incidence-based approach. Each approach has its own methodological challenges that are summarized in the following sections.

Prevalence-Based Approach

The economic costs of obesity have been estimated for several countries using a prevalence-based approach. There are two major types of cost-of-illness studies using such an approach: the first method specifies a list of obesity-related conditions and estimates the proportion of total treatment costs to be attributable to obesity; the second method directly investigates the differences in annual medical expenditure between obese and nonobese individuals. Both methods generally use data inputs that are cross-sectional in nature to provide prevalence estimates on obesity and medical conditions.

The majority of total direct cost studies follow the first method, developed by Colditz in 1992.[10] For direct costs, this method requires a comprehensive listing of all diseases caused by obesity, average medical costs per case of each disease, and estimated proportion of that disease attributable to obesity (population attributable risk [PAR], see Chapter 4). To estimate PAR for each disease, relative risks are typically determined from literature of prospective studies, and the prevalence of overweight and obesity is taken from cross-sectional estimates. Treatment costs are taken from medical expenditure data,[36] often updated to more recent currency value by adjusting for inflation using the medical component of the consumer price index. The PAR estimate for each disease, which represents the proportion of disease burden that is due to obesity, is then multiplied by the average medical expenditure to care among all prevalent cases in a given year. Summing across all listed diseases, this is then a cross-sectional summary of the economic costs of obesity incurred in the medical care setting.

Using this method, Wolf and Colditz[2] calculated the obesity-attributable direct costs from type 2 diabetes, cardiovascular disease, hypertension, gallbladder disease, postmenopausal breast cancer, endometrial cancer, colon cancer, and osteoarthritis. Using prevalence estimates based on National Health and Nutrition Examination Survey III (NHANES III; 22.4% overall obesity in the United States and 24.9% among women for breast and endometrial cancers), they estimated that the economic costs of obesity amount to $99 billion in 1995, of which $52 billion are direct medical costs, which is equivalent to 5.7% of national health expenditure at the time. Colditz[13] updated the costs attributable to obesity and inactivity. Overall, the direct health care costs of obesity and the lack of leisure-time physical activity were approximately $7,094 billion or 9.4% of total health care costs in 1995.

Note that these cross-sectional estimates of economic burden are extremely conservative given the range of health conditions examined. Rapidly expanding evidence now indicates that many additional conditions beyond those included in the analyses of the early 1990s should also be added to the list. For example, increased abdominal adiposity causes benign prostatic hypertrophy,[3] and infertility is clearly related to higher BMI categories among young women in prospective studies.[4] Asthma risk is directly related to adiposity among children[5] and possibly also among adults.[6] Sleep apnea is directly related to adiposity and has also been omitted from cost estimates to date.[7]

The selection of cancers to be included in the cost estimates has also evolved over time. The most recent review by the International Agency for Research on Cancer (IARC)[37] concluded that excess adiposity causes cancers of the colon, postmenopausal breast, esophagus (adenocarcinoma), kidney, and endometrium. Subsequent data from the American Cancer Society (ACS) Cancer Prevention Study II suggest that an even broader range of cancers is directly related to obesity and may account for 14% to 20% of cancer mortality.[38] Recent prospective cohort data, for incidence, support the ACS mortality findings, indicating that non-Hodgkin's lymphoma, multiple myeloma,[39] and pancreatic cancer[40,41] should also be added to the list, further increasing the proportion of cancer due to overweight and obesity to approximately 10%. The *best estimate* of the economic costs of obesity will obviously be a moving target.

Critics of the prevalence-based method point out that the correlation among the conditions is often not considered, which therefore poses the potential of double counting of expenditures. For example, an obese individual can have both high blood pressure and diabetes, and the medical visits may treat more than one condition. An alternative approach that avoids this potential source of bias is to use existing health services data systems to obtain direct estimates of utilization for insured users, stratified according to BMI. An increasing number of recent studies examine the financial impact of overweight and obesity by directly contrasting medical expenditure or health services utilization among individuals at different BMI levels. These studies avoid having to enlist medical conditions that are attributable to excess body weight and oftentimes employ regression methods to adjust for confounders (e.g., smoking).

For example, Finkelstein et al.[15] used the Medical Expenditure Panel Survey (MEPS) linked with National Health Interview Survey (NHIS) data to estimate the total medical care cost attributable to obesity. They found that obese individuals had substantially higher health care costs—35% to 40% higher than individuals of normal weight. As a result, the total medical costs of obesity at the population level amount to $78.5 billion in 1998 U.S. dollars.[15]

The estimation of indirect costs is often carried out in a similar manner using the concept of PAR. Wolf and Colditz's[2] estimates of $3.9 billion and 39.2 million days of lost work attributable to obesity in 1998 are based on such an approach using a cross-sectional survey.

Incidence-Based Approach

An incidence-based approach to costs of illness often uses a database following a population over time and recording health service utilization. Regression modeling is often adopted to adjust for demographic variables such as age, race, and smoking. Following this strategy, investigators linked the Chicago Heart Association Detection Project in Industry to Medicare data from 1984 to 2002 and calculated total Medicare charges from age 65 to death. They evaluated the relation between BMI at an average of age 46 years and subsequent health care expenditure after age 65.[42] Total cumulative charges for inpatient and outpatient care from age 65 to death or age 83 were between $30,000 and $100,000 higher among overweight or obese women and between $9,000 and $76,000 higher among overweight or obese men compared to their normal-weight counterparts.

Using an HMO data systems approach, Thompson et al. used longitudinal data from a nonsmoking and disease-free population and examined the relation of BMI and subsequent health care costs in the Kaiser Permanente Northwest Division.[43] Costs were higher for outpatient, inpatient, and prescription drugs for overweight and obese members compared with normal-weight members. In a larger study in the same population, Elmer et al.[44] related a large weight gain (>20 lb) in middle-aged overweight and obese adults to subsequent total medical care costs and compared these costs to those of weight maintainers. In this adult population, weight gain was associated with a significant increase in health care costs.[44]

Although straightforward, this method is also very data intensive. Cohort studies can rarely follow up the subjects long enough to answer questions such as lifetime costs of obesity. An alternative approach is therefore to use a modeling approach that projects both future risk of diseases and their associated costs. Such models typically use epidemiologic data to simulate the disease process using estimated incidence as a function of different levels of BMI in hypothetical cohorts. The associated costs of care again come from either a national estimate of a modeling study or actual costs of services used in a database study. In the modeling approach, future costs are discounted using standard economic approaches to bring future expenses to current dollar values before summing costs over the life course.[45]

Gorsky et al.[46] simulated three hypothetical cohorts to estimate the costs of health care according to level of obesity over a 25-year period, discounting future costs at 3% per year to a single present value. They estimated that 16 billion additional dollars would be spent over the next 25 years treating obesity-related illness among middle-aged women. Thompson et al.[47] estimated the excess lifetime costs of health services according to level of obesity at baseline from a small list of conditions—hypertension, high cholesterol, diabetes, CHD, and stroke. The per-person costs for obesity were comparable to those for smoking. Discounted per capita medical care costs for treatment of the five conditions were $10,000-15,000 higher in current dollars for the obese compared to normal weight men and women.

The incidence-based approach can circumvent the potential bias introduced by weight loss due to disease that plagues the prevalence-based approaches. However, most of the studies to date have not modeled future weight gain but, instead, have held weight constant from baseline. Given the substantial increase in weight over time throughout one's lifetime, these estimates are extremely conservative.

Methodological Considerations

The prevalence-based approach identifies the costs incurred during a given year, which is particularly informative in estimating the magnitude of disease burden on an annual basis. However, this approach does not quantify the long-term consequences of current BMI. For such purposes, the incidence-based approach would become more appropriate.

An important methodologic issue involves the lack of consistency in the literature with regard to the cutpoint for obesity and the BMI definition of the reference category. This issue is particularly prevalent in earlier publications. For example, reflecting the epidemiologic practices of the time, the earliest estimates defined obesity as greater than 27 kg/m²; subsequent analyses have used the current World Health Organization (WHO) recommended definition of obesity as BMI of 30 kg/m² or greater. This transition in definition partially explains why numerous estimates have omitted the direct and indirect costs among those who are overweight (BMI 25 to 29.9 kg/m²).[48] The definition for the reference category also impacts the relative risk estimate, which is in turn applied to the PAR estimate. Because the risk for many conditions such as diabetes and hypertension increases even before the WHO cutpoint of 25 kg/m²,[48] the true impact of adiposity is underestimated by including the population up to BMI 25 in the reference group. Moreover, studies evaluating only the costs for BMI at 30 or greater provide a mere lower bound of economic burden from excess adiposity because there are adverse health effects associated with a BMI of 30.[49,50] In other words, there are substantial additional costs incurred among those who are overweight but not obese.

Pertinent to prevalence-based approach and modeling methods that rely on the PAR framework, Allison et al.[14] argue that biases arise to inflate the costs of obesity as higher mortality rates among obese individuals compared to normal weight individuals are not accounted for. They argue that eliminating obesity would extend life and thereby increase lifetime aggregate health care costs. Contrasting such possibilities, some have suggested that the average costs of treating conditions such as heart disease may be greater for obese subjects who tend to have more complications.[51]

Alternative approaches to prevalence-based methods have been proposed that evaluate the attributable risk among cases of a given disease who are currently in the population, using BMI of those with the condition. While this method of estimating attributable risk can be legitimate for some settings, using BMI at the time of diagnosis or among those who survive from a condition will obviously lead to biased relative risk estimates for the many diseases that weight loss is a manifestation of the pre-diagnosis period or is a consequence of the disease management or progress. For obesity, this approach is immediately confounded by disease and does not reflect the burden of obesity that led to the development and diagnosis of the condition of interest.

Who Bears the Economic Costs of Obesity?

Most of the early cost estimates took a societal perspective; nonetheless, partitioning the total burden of obesity to different sectors that share the costs provides the incentives to address the distribution issue and to adopt preventive strategies.

More recently, costs for employers have been reported by Finkelstein et al.[32] and by Thompson et al.[24] Finkelstein et al. used data from two national samples of full-time employed adults. They estimated that overweight- and obesity-attributable costs ranged from $175 to $2,485 dollars per year depending on the degree of overweight and gender; approximately 30% of these costs result from increased absenteeism. Although those with Class-III obesity represent only 3% of the employed population, they account for 21% of the costs. Another important work by Finkelstein et al.[15] quantifies the costs to tax payers. They found that, in 1998, total medical bill due to overweight and obesity might have been as high as $78.5 billion in the United States. Medicare and Medicaid finance approximately half of these costs, private insurance pays 30% to 40%, and roughly 15% is paid out of pocket.[15] The increase in the medical conditions (such as hypertension and hyperlipidemia) treated among obese individuals has been suggested to be a key determinant of increased spending from private health insurance.[8]

Compared to developed countries, individuals in poorer countries are more likely to shoulder a considerable share of the economic consequences of the global obesity epidemic.[52] It is of particular significance because the high costs of diabetes, stroke, or CHD can often impoverish people in developing countries, and their financial difficulties can in turn force one to forgo medical treatments.[53,54]

Knowledge Gap and Future Research

Cost-of-illness estimates aim to enhance the understanding of the scope of the burden as well as to advocate for building the political will to address obesity as a clinical and public health priority.[55-58] Dr. Hubbard of the U.S. National Institutes of Health commissioned the first economic estimate for a presentation at an NIH Consensus Conference, in part to provide a summary measure of the impact of severe obesity.[10] Space precludes a detailed timeline of this shift, but commissioning of major reviews by leading medical journals in the late 1990s[48] and changing dietary guidelines all point to the growing recognition of the impact of obesity on health and society. The economic metric allows direct comparison of the burden, medical or otherwise, with other conditions (eg, smoking)—forcing the discussion of changing disease coding and insurance coverage decisions. International organizations such as the World Bank and the World Health Organization also utilize these cost burden estimates to make comparative assessments of health risks.

Nonetheless, the value of cost-of-obesity studies is not without debate.[59,60] The wide variation of cost-of-illness estimates raises serious questions of the comparability, accuracy, validity, and usefulness of these studies.[61] Roux and Donaldson[62] criticized the value of economic estimates of obesity's burden and argued for a greater focus on formal economic evaluations of alternative strategies to prevent and treat obesity. They suggested that a cost-effectiveness framework, which evaluates the relative value of investing in different interventions, better informs the allocation of resources for pubic health and clinical responses.[45] They also argued that the assumptions underlying cost-of-illness studies are flawed with the assumption that there will be cost savings through weight loss. They focused on the fact that not all diseases can be eliminated. This is a classic argument around PAR calculations, which assume a causal relationship between obesity and disease outcomes and form the baseline for future savings by eliminating obesity. Moreover, there remains no consensus on whether monetary terms provide superior information than other metrics, such as disability-adjusted life-years, as the prime outcome measure for resource prioritization decisions.

In the face of the childhood obesity epidemic, an increasing number of recent studies started to document its economic burden. Wang and Dietz[63] showed that obesity-associated conditions, notably asthma, sleep apnea, diabetes, and gall bladder diseases, have driven a threefold increase between 1979-1981 and 1997-1999 (from $35 million to $127 million) in hospital costs. While evidence on the health consequences has continued to grow over the past few years, many of which are outlined in Chapters 8 to 12 and 20, the full picture of the economic costs of this epidemic awaits future research efforts.

The evidence is overwhelming that excess weight is associated with increased morbidity and mortality. Current estimates of economic expenses related to excess weight clearly underestimate the true costs to society. To date, the majority of these estimates have evaluated only a narrow range of overweight- and obesity-related illness; they have not included factors such as the impact of reduced physical functioning,[27, 28, 64] and many have not accounted for the effects on those who are overweight but not obese. With the rising prevalence of overweight and obesity, we will continue to see growing effects and mounting costs on the individual, our communities, and our society as a whole.

References

1. US Department of Health and Human Services. *The Surgeon General's Call to Action to Prevent and Decrease Overweight and Obesity.* Rockville, MD: US Department of Health and Human Services, Public Health Service, Office of the Surgeon General 2001.
2. Wolf A, Colditz GA. Current estimates of the economic cost of obesity in the United States. *Obes Res.* 1998;6:97-106.
3. Giovannucci E, Rimm EB, Chute CG, et al. Obesity and benign prostatic hyperplasia. *Am J Epidemiol.* 1994;140:989-1002.
4. Rich-Edwards JW, Garland MT, Hunter DJ, et al. Physical activity, body mass index, and ovulatory disorder infertility (abstract). *Am J Epidemiol.* 1998;147:S57.
5. Camargo CA Jr, Wentowski CC, Field A, Gillman M, Frazier AA, Colditz GA. Prospective cohort study of body mass index and risk of asthma in children. *Ann Epidemiol.* 2003;13:565.

6. Camargo CA Jr, Weiss ST, Zhang S, Willett WC, Speizer FE. Prospective study of body mass index, weight change, and risk of adult-onset asthma in women. *Arch Intern Med.* 1999;159:2582-2588.

7. Rossner S, Lagerstrand L, Persson HE, Sachs C. The sleep apnoea syndrome in obesity: risk of sudden death. *J Intern Med.* 1991;230:135-141.

8. Thorpe KL, Florence CS, Howard DH, Joski PJ. The impact of obesity on rising medical spending. *Health Aff (Millwood).* 2004:Suppl Web Exclusives:W4-480-W4-486.

9. Andreyeva TA, Sturm RA, Ringel JS. Moderate and severe obesity have large differences in health care costs. *Obes Res.* 2004;12:1936-1943.

10. Colditz GA. Economic costs of obesity. *Am J Clin Nutr.* 1992;55:503S-507S.

11. Wee CC, Phillips RS, Legedza AT, et al. Health care expenditures associated with overweight and obesity among US adults: importance of age and race. *Am J Public Health.* 2005;95:159-165.

12. Finkelstein EA, Fiebelkorn IC, Wang G. State-level estimates of annual medical expenditures attributable to obesity. *Obes Res.* 2004;12:18-24.

13. Colditz GA. Economic costs of obesity and inactivity. *Med Sci Sports Exerc.* 1999;31:S663-S667.

14. Allison DB, Zannolli R, Narayan KM. The direct health care costs of obesity in the United States. *Am J Public Health.* 1999;89:1194-1199.

15. Finkelstein EA, Fiebelkorn IC, Wang G. National medical spending attributable to overweight and obesity: how much, and who's paying? *Health Aff (Millwood).* 2003:Suppl Web Exclusives:W3-219-W3-226.

16. Levy E, Levy P, Le Pen C, Basdevant A. The economic cost of obesity: the French situation. *Int J Obes Relat Metab Disord.* 1995;19:788-792.

17. Seidell JC. The impact of obesity on health status—some implications for health care costs. *Int J Obes.* 1995;19 (Suppl 6):S13-S16.

18. Segal L, Carter R, Zimmet P. The cost of obesity. The Australian perspective. *PharmacoEconomics.* 1994;5(Suppl):45-52.

19. Comptroller and Auditor General. *Tackling Obesity in England. Appendix 6: Estimating the Cost of Obesity in England.* London: Stationery Office, 2001.

20. Fry J, Finley W. The prevalence and costs of obesity in the EU. *Proc Nutr Soc.* 2005;64:359-362.

21. Popkin BM, Kim S, Rusev ER, Du S, Zizza C. Measuring the full economic costs of diet, physical activity and obesity-related chronic diseases. *Obes Rev.* 2006;7:271-293.

22. Biering-Sorensen F, Lund J, Hoydalsmo OJ, et al. Risk indicators of disability pension. A 15 year follow-up study. *Dan Med Bull.* 1999;46:258-262.

23. Narbro K, Jonsson E, Larsson B, Waaler H, Wedel H, Sjostrom L. Economic consequences of sick-leave and early retirement in obese Swedish women. *Int J Obes Relat Metab Disord.* 1996;20:895-903.

24. Thompson D, Edelsberg J, Kinsey KL, Oster G. Estimated economic costs of obesity to U.S. business. *Am J Health Promot.* 1998;13:120-127.

25. Finkelstein EA, Ruhm CJ, Kosa KM. Economic causes and consequences of obesity. *Ann Rev Public Health.* 2005;26:239-257.

26. Østbye T, Dement JM, Krause KM. Obesity and workers' compensation: results from the Duke Health and Safety Surveillance System. *Arch Intern Med.* 2007;167:766-773.

27. Coakley EH, Kawachi I, Manson JE, Speizer FE, Willett WC, Colditz GA. Lower levels of physical functioning are associated with higher body weight among middle-aged and older women. *Int J Obes.* 1998;22:958-996.

28. Fine JT, Colditz GA, Coakley EH, et al. A prospective study of weight change and health-related quality of life in women. *JAMA.* 1999;282:2136-2142.

29. Sarlio-Lahteenkorva S, Stunkard A, Rissanen A. Psychosocial factors and quality of life in obesity. *Int J Obes Real Metab Disord.* 1995;19:S1-S5.

30. Gortmaker SL, Must A, Perrin JM, Sobol AM, Dietz WH. Social and economic consequences of overweight in adolescence and young adulthood. *N Engl J Med.* 1993;329:1008-1012.

31. Pagan JA, Davila A. Obesity, occupational attainment, and earnings. *Soc Sci Q.* 1997; 78:756-770.
32. Finkelstein E, Fiebelkorn C, Wang G. The costs of obesity among full-time employees. *Am J Health Promot.* 2005;20:45-51.
33. Flegal KM, Carroll MD, Kuczmarski RJ, Johnson CL. Overweight and obesity in the United States: prevalence and trends, 1960-1994. *Int J Obes Real Metab Disord.* 1998;22:39-47.
34. Kumanyika SK. Obesity, health disparities, and prevention paradigms: hard questions and hard choices. *Prev Chronic Dis.* 2005;2:A02.
35. Zhang Q, Wang Y. Trends in the association between obesity and socioeconomic status in U.S. adults: 1971 to 2000. *Obes Res.* 2004;12:1622-1632.
36. Hodgson TA. Costs of illness in cost-effectiveness analysis. A review of methodology. *Pharmacoeconomics.* 1994;6:536-552.
37. International Agency for Research on Cancer. *Weight Control and Physical Activity,* 2002.
38. Calle EE, Rodriguez C, Walker-Thurmond KA, Thun MJ. Overweight, obesity, and mortality from cancer in a prospectively studied cohort of U.S. adults. *N Engl J Med.* 2003;348:1625-1638.
39. Blair CK, Cerhan JR, Folsom AR, Ross JA. Anthropometric characteristics and risk of multiple myeloma. *Epidemiology.* 2005;16:691-694.
40. Michaud DS, Giovannucci E, Willett WC, Colditz GA, Stampfer MJ, Fuchs CS. Physical activity, obesity, height, and the risk of pancreatic cancer. *JAMA.* 2001;286:921-929.
41. Patel AV, Rodriguez C, Bernstein L, Chao A, Thun MJ, Calle EE. Obesity, recreational physical activity, and risk of pancreatic cancer in a large U.S. Cohort. *Cancer Epidemiol Biomarkers Prev.* 2005;14:459-466.
42. Daviglus ML, Liu K, Yan LL, et al. Relation of body mass index in young adulthood and middle age to Medicare expenditures in older age. *JAMA.* 2004;292:2743-2749.
43. Thompson D, Brown JB, Nichols GA, Elmer PJ, Oster G. Body mass index and future healthcare costs: a retrospective cohort study. *Obes Res.* 2001;9:210-218.
44. Elmer PJ, Brown JB, Nichols GA, Oster G. Effects of weight gain on medical care costs. *Int J Obes Relat Metab Disord.* 2004;28:1365-1373.
45. Gold MR, Siegel JE, Russell LB, Weinstein MC. *Cost-Effectiveness in Health and Medicine.* New York: Oxford University Press, 1996.
46. Gorsky RD, Pamuk E, Williamson DF, Shaffer PA, Koplan JP. The 25-year health care costs of women who remain overweight after 40 years of age. *Am J Prev Med.* 1996;12:388-394.
47. Thompson D, Edelsberg J, Colditz GA, Bird AP, Oster G. Lifetime health and economic consequences of obesity. *Arch Intern Med.* 1999;159:2177-2183.
48. Willett WC, Dietz WH, Colditz GA. Guidelines for healthy weight. *N Engl J Med.* 1999;341:427-434.
49. NHLBI Obesity Education Initiative Expert Panel on the Identification, Evaluation and Treatment of Overweight and Obesity in Adults. *Clinical Guidelines on the Identification, Evaluation and Treatment of Overweight and Obesity in Adults.* Bethesda, MD: National Heart, Lung, and Blood Institute, National Institutes of Health, 1998:228.
50. U.S. Department of Agriculture, U.S. Department of Health and Human Services. *Nutrition and Your Health: Dietary Guidelines for Americans.* 4th ed. Washington, DC: U.S. Government Printing Office, 1995.
51. Lahey SJ, Borlase BC, Lavin PT, Levitsky S. Preoperative risk factors that predict hospital length of stay in coronary artery bypass patients > 60 years old. *Circulation.* 1992;86:181-185.
52. Yach D, Stuckler D, Brownell KD. Epidemiologic and economic consequences of the global epidemics of obesity and diabetes. *Nat Med.* 2006;12:62-66.
53. Wang L, Kong L, Wu F, Bai Y, Burton R. Preventing chronic diseases in China. *Lancet.* 2005;366:1821-1824.

54. Barcelo A, Aedo C, Rajpathak S, Robles S. The cost of diabetes in Latin America and the Caribbean. *Bull World Health Organ.* 2003;81:19-27.

55. Richmond JB, Kotelchuck M. Coordination and development of strategies and policy for public health promotion in the United States. In: Holland W, Detel R, Know G, eds. *Oxford Textbook of Public Health.* Oxford: Oxford University Press, 1991.

56. Atwood K, Colditz GA, Kawachi I. Implementing prevention policies: relevance of the Richmond model to health policy judgments. *Am J Public Health.* 1997;87:1603-1606.

57. Sturm R. The effects of obesity, smoking, and drinking on medical problems and costs. *Health Aff (Millwood).* 2002;21:245-253.

58. Institute of Medicine. *Weighing the Options: Criteria for Evaluating Weight-Management Programs.* Washington, DC: National Academy Press, 1995.

59. Rice DP. Cost-of-illness studies: fact or fiction? *Lancet.* 1994;344:1519-1520.

60. Shiell A, Gerard K, Donaldson C. Cost of illness studies—an aid to decision-making. *Health Policy.* 1987;8:317-323.

61. Bloom BS, Bruno DJ, Maman DY, Jayadevappa R. Usefulness of US cost-of-illness studies in healthcare decision making. *Pharmacoeconomics.* 2001;19:207-213.

62. Roux L, Donaldson C. Economics and obesity: costing the problem or evaluating solutions. *Obes Res.* 2004;12:173-179.

63. Wang G, Dietz WH. Economic burden of obesity in youths aged 6 to 17 years: 1979-1999. *Pediatrics.* 2002;109:E81-1.

64. Fontaine KR, Cheskin LJ, Barofsky I. Health-related quality of life in obese persons seeking treatment. *J Fam Pract.* 1996;43:265-270.

Part III

Epidemiologic Studies
of Determinants of Obesity

14

Diet, Nutrition, and Obesity

Frank B. Hu

Weight gain and obesity in free-living populations result from cumulative effects of small changes in daily energy balance. Many dietary factors can directly and indirectly tip the balance in energy intake and expenditure and thus effect changes in body weight. Numerous epidemiologic studies and clinical trials have investigated the role of dietary factors in weight control and obesity prevention. However, the relative influence of major metabolic fuels (fat, carbohydrate, and protein) on body fatness is unclear, and popular diets designed to promote weight loss remain controversial.[1] Many methodological issues can complicate the interpretation of results in both epidemiologic studies and clinical trials. Epidemiologic studies, even those with a prospective cohort design, are subject to measurement errors in dietary assessment as well as to residual and unmeasured confounding. Most clinical trials also suffer from serious limitations, such as short duration, small sample size, and inadequate adherence to dietary interventions (see Chapter 4).

Large epidemiologic studies have only recently been launched to investigate consumption of foods and food groups as well as overall eating patterns in relation to long-term weight gain. These efforts appear to have yielded more fruitful results than traditional epidemiologic studies focusing on individual nutrients (e.g., fat or carbohydrate) and obesity. Recent prospective cohort studies, for example, suggest that sugar-sweetened soft drinks have adverse effects on body weight. They also indicate that higher consumption of whole grains is associated with reduced weight gain. Increasing evidence suggests that overall dietary patterns influence long-term weight gain.

In this chapter, we will briefly review evidence from epidemiologic studies and clinical trials regarding the effects of macronutrients on body weight. We will then describe epidemiologic studies with respect to individual foods or beverages (including whole grains, fruits and vegetables, nuts, dairy products, coffee and caffeine, and alcoholic beverages). Finally, we will discuss studies on overall eating patterns (including fast-food habits and skipping breakfast) and dietary energy density in relation to body weight.

Macronutrients

Dietary Fats

Because of the high energy density of fat and the enhanced palatability of high-fat foods, it is widely believed that intake of dietary fat leads to weight gain and obesity, while reduced consumption of dietary fat promotes weight loss. Thus, prevailing weight-loss guidelines recommend a fat- and calorie-restricted diet high in carbohydrates. However, epidemiologic and clinical-trial evidence on the relationship between fat intake and obesity is mixed. Several authors have conducted detailed reviews of the literature on dietary fat and body fatness.[1-8] We briefly summarize the epidemiologic and clinical-trial evidence in the following sections.

Epidemiologic Evidence

Ecological studies have shown a strong positive association between percentage of energy intake from fat and prevalence of obesity across countries.[3] However, intractable confounding by differences in economic development, availability of foods, and levels of physical activity can make these comparisons misleading. Comparisons among populations with similar levels of economic development have found little association between percentage of fat intake and obesity rates in either European countries (percentages of energy from fat ranged from 25% to 47%) or 65 counties in China (percentages of energy from fat ranged from 8% to 25%).[5] In developing countries undergoing economic and nutritional transitions, there appears to be a positive correlation between increased fat intake and body fatness.[9] However, such analyses (e.g., cross-cultural correlations) are complicated by confounding from changes in food availability and other aspects of diet and physical activity levels. Secular trends in the United States in the last 2 decades suggest a correspondence between a substantial decrease in the percentage of dietary energy from fat and a considerable increase in obesity,[5] suggesting that fat reduction per se is unlikely to stem the obesity trend. However, it should be noted that physical activity levels in the U.S. population have also decreased substantially during the same time period (see Chapter 15).

Many cross-sectional studies have found a positive association between dietary fat and body fatness.[2] However, this correlation could reflect changes made by health-conscious individuals to reduce fat intake and modify other aspects of diet and lifestyle. Such factors are difficult to measure and control for statistically. Unlike other health conditions (e.g., high blood pressure and high cholesterol), body weight is a readily apparent end point that participants can affect by altering diet and lifestyle in response to changes in weight status.[10]

Relatively few prospective cohort studies have examined long-term relationships between dietary fat and body fatness or weight gain, and among those that have, the results have been highly inconsistent.[2,4] These studies have varied considerably in size, duration of follow-up, age groups, covariates adjusted in the statistical analyses, and dietary assessment methods.

Prospective analyses of dietary fat and body weight are also subject to confounding by health-conscious behaviors. The problem can be mitigated somewhat by using repeated measures of diet and weight over time to examine the impact of specific dietary changes on body weight. Most studies, however, measure diet at baseline only and therefore lack information on changes in important confounders (e.g., smoking, alcohol use, and physical activity) during the course of follow-up.

In a 6-year study of 361 Swedish women, Heitmann et al.[11] found a significant association between high-dietary fat intake and body mass index (BMI) in obese women with a family history of obesity ($P = .003$) but not obese women with lean parents or lean women with or without obese parents. These outcomes suggest that "high-dietary fat intake may have an obesity-promoting effect in women with a genetic predisposition." However, a much larger study of 41,518 women by Field et al.[12] found no evidence that parental weight status modified the relationship between dietary fat and weight gain.

In terms of types of fat, there was a weak positive association between saturated and trans fat consumption and weight gain, but no association with increases in percentages of energy from mono- or polyunsaturated fats. The different associations with specific types of fat may reflect different biological actions of these fats on insulin resistance and fat accumulation.[13] Given that the amount of energy provided by different types of fat is the same, the varied effects may also reflect confounding by other dietary and lifestyle factors associated with intakes of different types of fat.

Only one prospective study has examined the association between dietary fat intake and changes in waist circumference. Multivariate analyses by Koh-Banerjee et al.[14] found that total fat intake was not associated with gain in waist circumference. However, a significant association was found between increasing consumption of trans fat and gain in waist circumference during 9 years of follow-up, even after further adjustment for concurrent changes in BMI. Although confounding by other dietary factors related to a higher intake of trans fat (e.g., fast-food habits) cannot be ruled out, these data suggest potentially detrimental effects of trans fat on abdominal fat accumulation.

Clinical-Trial Evidence on Fat Reduction and Weight Loss

Numerous clinical trials have been conducted to examine the effects of fat reduction diets on weight loss in overweight and obese individuals. A meta-analysis of 28 mainly short-term trials demonstrated that a 10% decrease in total energy from fat can reduce body weight by 16 g/day (which extrapolates to a weight reduction of 8.8 kg by 18 months).[3] Longer-term trials, however, have not substantiated these findings.

Willett[5] conducted a systematic review of several longer-term intervention trials on the effect of low-fat diets on weight, including nine trials ranging from 12 to 24 months. The data showed that diets lower in fat can result in modest short-term reductions in body weight. However, studies lasting 1 year or more showed that variation from 18% to 40% of energy intake from fat has a negligible effect on body weight.

The Women's Health Initiative Dietary Modification Trial (WHI), the largest randomized dietary intervention trial, compared an ad libitum low-fat dietary pattern with usual diet in 48,835 postmenopausal women in the United States. The mean follow-up was 7.5 years.[15] Those in the intervention group were instructed to reduce total fat intake to 20% of total energy and increase consumption of fruits, vegetables, and grain products; they also received intensive behavioral modification sessions led by nutritionists. The control group received a copy of the Dietary Guidelines for Americans and followed their usual diet. The intervention group lost more weight in the first year than the control group (2.2 kg; $P < .01$), but the difference between the two groups was negligible and not significant at the end of follow-up (0.4 kg at 7.5 years). This study provides the strongest evidence to date against the use of low-fat diets to achieve appreciable long-term weight loss.

Carbohydrates

The obesity epidemic in the United States has continued unabated despite a decreasing percentage of energy intake from fat. This has drawn attention to the alternative hypothesis that compensatory increases in carbohydrate consumption may be fueling the obesity epidemic.[16] However, few epidemiologic studies have directly examined the relationship between carbohydrates and body fatness. Because of a reciprocal relationship between energy from fat and carbohydrates in most diets, based on the epidemiologic and clinical-trial evidence reviewed earlier, one can conclude that substitution of carbohydrates for fat is unlikely to have an appreciable effect on body fat.

Cross-sectional analyses have shown an inverse association between sugar intake and BMI,[8] but this relationship most likely reflects reverse causation; that is, the fact that overweight subjects are more likely to attempt weight control by reducing sugar consumption. Overweight individuals also tend to underreport their sugar consumption. The inverse association between total carbohydrate intake and BMI observed in cross-sectional studies may also reflect confounding by health-conscious behaviors used to control weight.[1]

Carbohydrate restriction has recently been promoted as an alternative strategy for weight loss. Several clinical trials have evaluated the effects of low-carbohydrate diets on weight loss. A meta-analysis of five randomized controlled trials with 6-12 months of follow-up compared the effects on weight loss of ad libitum low-carbohydrate diets with those of low-fat, energy-restricted diets on weight loss.[17] The authors found that, after 6 months, participants randomized to low-carbohydrate diets had lost more weight than those randomized to low-fat diets (weighted mean difference, –3.3 kg; 95% CI, –5.3 to –1.4 kg). However, there was no difference in weight loss after 12 months. This meta-analysis also compared the effects of the two dietary patterns on cardiovascular disease risk factors. After 6 months, changes in triglyceride and high-density lipoprotein (HDL) cholesterol were more favorable in the low-carbohydrate diet group but that changes in total cholesterol and low-density lipoprotein (LDL) cholesterol were more favorable in the low-fat group. It is worth noting that although these trials indicate greater short-term (within 6 months) weight loss with low-carbohydrate diets versus low-fat diets, the studies were very small and suffered from low compliance to the intervention diets and high dropout rates during follow-up.

Recently, Gardner et al.[18] compared the effects of four popular diets (Atkins, Zone, Ornish, and LEARN diets) on weight loss in a randomized trial of 311 free-living, overweight/obese premenopausal women. Mean 12-month weight loss was 4.7 kg for the Atkins group, 1.6 kg for the Zone group, 2.6 kg for the LEARN group, and 2.2 kg for the Ornish group. At 12 months, the Atkins group had greater reductions in triglycerides with only a small and nonsignificant increase in LDL cholesterol. Unlike other low-carbohydrate dietary intervention trials, this study had a relatively low dropout rate at one year (approximately 20%), although the degree of dietary adherence in all the groups was generally low. The data from this study provide the strongest evidence so far that more severe carbohydrate restriction may be moderately effective for weight loss. Whether such a strategy is beneficial for preventing weight gain is unclear.

Quality of Carbohydrates

Traditionally, carbohydrates are classified as simple or complex on the basis of chemical structures. Since simple sugars are thought to be digested and absorbed more quickly than complex carbohydrates, and thus to induce a more rapid postprandial glucose response, prevailing dietary recommendations have promoted intake of complex carbohydrates or starches and avoidance of simple carbohydrates or sugars.[1] However, it is now recognized that many starchy foods (e.g., baked potatoes and white bread) produce even higher glycemic responses than do simple sugars.[19] To quantify glycemic responses induced by different carbohydrate foods, Jenkins et al.[20] developed the concept of glycemic index (GI). The index is based on the increase in blood glucose levels (the area under the curve for blood glucose levels) after the ingestion of 50 g of carbohydrate from a test food compared with a standard amount (50 g) of reference carbohydrate (glucose or white bread). To represent both the quality and quantity of carbohydrates consumed, Salmeron et al.[21] developed the concept of glycemic load (GL, the product of the GI value of a food and its carbohydrate content).

Several prospective studies have demonstrated that dietary GI and GL predict incidence of type 2 diabetes and cardiovascular disease,[22] but few epidemiologic studies have evaluated their relationship to body weight. A cross-sectional analysis of the Insulin Resistance Atherosclerosis Study found no significant association between dietary GI and BMI or waist circumference.[23] However, a 4-year longitudinal study by Ma et al.[24] indicated a positive association between dietary GI (but not total carbohydrates or GL) and BMI. In a systematic review,[25] most of the short-term feeding studies in humans (lasting for a single meal or a single day) demonstrated a direct association between consumption of high-GI foods/liquids and increased subsequent hunger and/or decreased satiety. Voluntary energy intake also increased after consumption of high-GI meals compared with low-GI meals. These observations suggest that long-term consumption of high-GI diets may promote excess energy intake and thus contribute to weight gain or maintenance of excess body weight, especially among susceptible individuals (e.g., sedentary or overweight subjects).

Several recent longer-term clinical trials on the role of GI/GL in weight loss have yielded mixed results. In a 10-week parallel, randomized intervention trial, a low-GI diet induced greater weight and fat loss as compared with a high-GI diet, but the difference did not achieve statistical significance.[26] A 12-week randomized trial with a larger sample size found that a low-GI diet, especially when combined with a higher amount of protein, resulted in significantly greater fat loss (but not greater weight loss) compared with a high-GI diet.[27] However, a randomized trial of 203 healthy Brazilian women with BMI of 23 to 30 found no difference in weight loss between isocaloric high- and low-GI diets during 18 month of follow-up.[28] These studies suggest that altering types of carbohydrates alone without substantial reduction in total GL may not have appreciable effects on weight loss. In a recent randomized trial of obese young adults (aged 18 to 35 years; $n = 73$), Ebbeling et al.[29] found that as compared with a low-fat diet, reducing dietary GL was more effective in achieving weight loss among individuals with higher insulin secretion measured by serum insulin concentration at 30 minutes after a 75 g dose of oral glucose at baseline. These intriguing results need to be confirmed in future weight loss intervention studies.

Protein

The popularity of low-carbohydrate diets, most of which are high in protein, has focused increased attention on the role of protein in weight control. A review of 15 short-term studies found that diets higher in protein exert a larger thermic effect than those with less protein.[30] In addition, higher-protein diets may reduce subsequent energy intake. Skov et al.[31] found that free-living subjects randomized to a high-protein diet consumed an average of 8,956 kJ/day compared with a mean of 10,907 kJ/day for those on a low-protein diet during a 6-month period. These data, which are consistent with those from other ad libitum studies,[30] support the hypothesis that high-protein diets produce greater satiety and lower subsequent energy intake as compared with lower protein diets.

Cross-sectional analyses show an inverse association between protein intake and abdominal obesity,[32] but prospective data on the relationship between protein intake and body fatness are lacking. In randomized clinical trials of low-carbohydrate diets discussed earlier, simultaneous increases in consumption of protein and dietary fat as percentages of energy make it difficult to attribute the effects of weight loss to any particular macronutrients. In the 6-month trial mentioned earlier,[31] protein was used to replace carbohydrates while fat intake remained constant at 30% of energy. At the end of the study, subjects randomized to high-protein intake (25% energy from protein) lost significantly more weight (8.8 vs. 5.1 kg) and fat (7.6 vs. 4.3 kg) than those on the low-protein diet (12% energy from protein).

Overall, there is some evidence that high-protein diets enhance short-term weight loss as compared with lower-protein diets. Possible mechanisms include increased satiety and decreased subsequent energy intake, increased thermogenesis, and reduced GL.[33] However, larger and longer-term studies are clearly needed to draw firm conclusions about the role of protein in weight control.

Foods and Food Groups

Recent studies have examined the relationship between consumption of specific foods or overall dietary patterns and body fatness. Such analyses are of value for identifying dietary determinants of obesity that can be useful in making practical dietary recommendations.

Whole Grains and Fiber

Whole-grain products (e.g., whole wheat breads, brown rice, oats, and barley) usually have lower GI values and are richer in fiber, antioxidant vitamins, magnesium, and phytochemicals than are refined-grain products, which lose substantial amounts of dietary fiber and other beneficial nutrients during processing. Several studies have found an inverse association between consumption of whole-grain foods and risk of type 2 diabetes and cardiovascular disease.[22] However, there are few epidemiologic studies on whole-grain foods and risk of obesity. At 7-year follow-up, the Coronary Artery Risk Development in Young Adults (CARDIA) study showed an inverse relationship between whole-grain intake and BMI, but no association between whole-grain intake and waist-to-hip ratio.[34]

During 12 years of follow-up in the Nurses' Health Study (NHS), Liu et al.[35] examined the relationship between changes in intakes of dietary fiber and whole- or refined-grain products and weight gain. Increased consumption of whole grains was associated with a lower mean 4-year weight gain (1.58 kg in the lowest quintile and 1.07 kg in the highest quintile; P for trend <.0001). In contrast, increased intake of refined grains was related to greater weight gain (from 0.99 to 1.65 kg; P for trend <.0001). These findings are consistent with those in a related study on associations between whole-grain, bran, and cereal-fiber consumption and weight gain in a cohort of men.[36]

Whole grains are rich in many nutrients and compounds, but the fiber component is thought to be responsible for most of the beneficial effects on body weight.[37,38] Because of their bulk and relatively low energy density, high-fiber foods may promote satiety, leading to decreased energy intake.[38] A systematic review of 27 experimental studies showed beneficial effects of dietary fiber on satiety and subsequent energy intake.[39]

Approximately 20% to 50% of fiber in whole-grain products is in a soluble or viscous form.[38] Viscous fiber with gel-like properties can delay gastric emptying and/or intestinal absorption. Thus, short-term clinical trials have suggested that substitution of whole grains for refined grains improves insulin sensitivity, probably by blunting postprandial glycemic and insulinemic responses.[40] Decreased glycemic and insulinemic responses may also reduce hunger and subsequent energy intake.

Several prospective studies have reported an inverse association between fiber consumption and adiposity. In the NHS, women with the greatest increase in intake of dietary fiber gained a mean of 1.52 kg less weight than subjects with the smallest increase in fiber intake (P for trend <.0001),[35] after adjusting for body weight at baseline, age, and changes in covariate status. In a cohort of men, increasing fiber consumption was associated with decreased central obesity; each 12 g increase in total fiber per day produced a 0.63 cm decrease in waist circumference ($P < .001$).[14] The CARDIA study identified a significant association between dietary fiber intake at baseline and lower body weight, waist-to-hip ratio, and fasting insulin levels in both whites and blacks during 10 years of follow-up.[41]

Soluble-fiber supplements (e.g., guar gum and psyllium), however, were not efficacious for weight loss in short-term randomized trials.[42] This finding suggests that the long-term benefits of fiber on body weight seen in epidemiologic studies may be due to the combined effects of multiple components in whole-grain products rather than to fiber alone. It is also possible that fiber from foods has different biological effects than fiber from supplements.

Fruits and Vegetables

Although fruits and vegetables have been consistently associated with lower risk of cardiovascular disease, data on the long-term relationship between fruit and vegetable intake and body weight are limited. He et al.[43] examined changes in fruit and vegetable intake in relation to risk of obesity and weight gain in 74,063 middle-aged women in the NHS during 12 years of follow-up. Women with the largest increase in fruit and vegetable intake had a 24% lower risk of obesity (BMI $\geq$ 30 kg/m^2) than women with the largest decrease in intake, after adjustment for age, physical activity, smoking, total energy intake, and other lifestyle variables (relative risk, 0.76; 95% CI, 0.69 to 0.86; P for trend $< .0001$). Women with the largest increase in fruit and vegetable intake also had a 28% lower risk of major weight gain ($\geq$25 kg) compared with those with the lowest increase (relative risk, 0.72; 95% CI, 0.55 to 0.93; $P = .01$). Separate analyses of changes in fruit and vegetable consumption yielded similar results. These promising results need to be confirmed in future prospective cohort studies and randomized clinical trials.

Nuts

Substantial evidence from epidemiologic studies and clinical trials indicates that high nut consumption has beneficial effects on blood lipids and cardiovascular disease risk.[22] A major concern is that because of their high-fat content and high energy density, increased consumption of nuts may cause weight gain and obesity. However, several cross-sectional analyses of large cohort studies, including the Adventist Health Study[44] and the NHS,[45] have shown that individuals who consume nuts regularly tend to weigh less than those who rarely consume them.

A 28-month prospective study conducted in Spain found an association between higher nut consumption and lower risk of weight gain.[46] Compared with those who never or almost never ate nuts, participants who ate nuts two or more times per week had a 31% (relative risk, 0.69; 95% CI, 0.53 to 0.90) lower risk of gaining at least 5 kg during the follow-up. In the NHS, nut consumption was inversely associated with risk of type 2 diabetes,[47] and 16-year average weight gain was also slightly lower among those who consumed nuts at least five times per week compared with those who rarely ate them (6.2 vs. 6.5 kg, respectively).

Several clinical trials of nut consumption without constraints on body weight showed no significant weight changes in groups assigned to higher consumption of nuts.[48] During 3 months of follow-up in the PREDIMED study, a Mediterranean diet supplemented with tree nuts improved cardiovascular risk factors but did not lead to weight gain as compared with a low-fat diet.[49] Wien et al.[50] demonstrated that substitution of almonds (84 g/day) for carbohydrates in a formula-based low-calorie diet resulted in greater weight loss during a 24-week intervention among 65 overweight and obese adults.

These epidemiologic and clinical-trial data indicate that in free-living subjects, higher nut consumption does not cause greater weight gain; rather, incorporating nuts into hypocaloric diets may be beneficial for weight control. The mechanisms for these observations are unclear but could be related to higher amounts of protein and fiber in nuts, which may enhance satiety and suppress hunger.[51] In dietary practice, the majority of energy contained in nuts appears to be balanced by reductions in other sources of energy, especially carbohydrates. This may explain lower body weight in regular nut consumers observed in epidemiologic studies and the lack of predicted weight gain in nut-supplemented diets.[52] Another potential contributing factor for the lack of expected weight gain among those who eat a higher amount of nuts is the incresed fecal loss of fat due to incomplete mastication of nuts, leading to loss of available energy in nuts.[48]

Dairy Products and Calcium

The potential benefits of calcium, especially dairy calcium, on weight regulation have recently attracted a great deal of attention. Calcium is an essential nutrient that plays a role in regulating lipogenesis.[53] Low calcium intake stimulates formation of 1,25 dihydroxyvitamin D [1,25(OH)2D] and secretion of parathyroid hormone or calciotropic hormones that cause increased intestinal calcium uptake. The rise in intracellular calcium promotes lipogenesis and reduces lipolysis, leading to adipocyte hypertrophy and increased fat mass.[53] Thus, higher calcium intake could potentially have an antiobesity effect. However, the role of calcium in weight control remains controversial.

Zemel et al.[54] first suggested the potential effect of calcium intake on body weight in a clinical trial that investigated the antihypertensive effect of calcium in obese African Americans. In that study, the investigators reported that increasing calcium intake from 400 mg/day to 1,000 (two cups of yogurt) mg/day for 1 year resulted in a 4.9 kg reduction in body fat. A subsequent review of several clinical trials on the role of calcium or dairy products on body weight concluded that there was not enough evidence to support the claim of weight-loss benefits from calcium or dairy products.[55] However, most of the studies in the review were not designed or powered to study weight change as the outcome variable.

Several recent weight-loss trials evaluated the role of calcium or dairy supplementation with weight as the primary outcome. In a 24-week randomized clinical trial of 32 obese adults (27 women and 5 men) who were maintained on a 500 kcal/day deficit diet,[56] weight loss was enhanced among those who were assigned to high calcium and high-dairy diets. This finding, however, has not been confirmed by subsequent larger trials. In a 25-week double-blind, randomized clinical trial of weight loss in 100 overweight and obese women, Shapses et al.[57] reported that calcium supplementation of 1 g/day had no effect on body weight. Lorenzen et al.[58] also found that calcium supplementation (500 mg/day) for 1 year did not reduce body weight or fat mass in 110 young girls. Similarly, Gunther et al.[59] reported no significant differences in mean 1-year changes in body weight and fat mass in an isocaloric dairy supplement intervention among 155 normal-weight women (aged 18 to 30 years) randomized to one of three groups: usual diet; medium-dairy diet with calcium intake of 1,000 to 1,100 mg/day; or high-dairy diet with calcium intake of 1,300 to 1,400 mg/day.

Epidemiologic studies on the relationship between calcium intake and body weight have also yielded mixed results. So far, most epidemiologic studies on this association have been cross-sectional in design and thus vulnerable to reverse causation bias, that is, reduced consumption of dairy products by overweight individuals. Most prospective studies have not found beneficial effects of calcium or dairy products on weight gain.

A 10-year study by Gonzalez et al.[60] found an association between calcium supplementation and significantly lower weight gain in middle-aged women but not men. Dietary calcium, however, was not associated with weight change in either men or women. In a longitudinal study of healthy perimenopausal women, dietary calcium was not associated with 5- to 7-year weight change.[61] Rajpathak et al.[62] conducted a detailed study of the association between calcium and dairy intakes and 12-year weight change in men and found no significant association between body weight and baseline or change in total calcium intake. In addition, there was no relationship between weight change and dietary, dairy, or supplemental calcium intake when evaluated separately. In a longitudinal study of 12,829 U.S. children aged 9 to 14 years at baseline, Berkey et al.[63] actually found a positive association between milk consumption and weight gain. Excessive caloric intake resulting from higher milk consumption was suggested to be the reason.

These prospective data, together with those from randomized clinical trials, do not support the hypothesis that increased intake of calcium or dairy products reduces weight gain. Although several studies have suggested a potential beneficial effect of dairy consumption on insulin resistance[64] and type 2 diabetes,[65] these inverse associations appear to be independent of BMI.

Sugar-Sweetened Beverages

The time-trend data over the past three decades have shown a close parallel between a dramatic increase in consumption of caloric sweetener in soft drinks and the obesity epidemic in the United States.[66] However, simultaneous changes in other dietary and lifestyle factors make such data subject to a variety of interpretations. To examine the relationship between consumption of sugar-sweetened beverages, particularly carbonated soft drinks and weight gain, Malik et al.[67] conducted a systematic review of 30 studies on this topic (15 cross-sectional, 10 prospective, and 5 experimental). Because of the well-known limitations of cross-sectional studies, the authors gave greater weight to data from large prospective studies and randomized clinical trials.

Several studies,[68-71] but not all,[72,73] reported a significant positive association between the intake of sugar-sweetened beverages and increases in overweight or obesity in children. During a 3-year follow-up of 11,654 children, Berkey et al.[68] demonstrated a significant association between soda consumption and weight gain in both boys and girls. In a smaller investigation, with 19 months of follow-up, Ludwig et al.[69] found that baseline consumption of sugar-sweetened beverages and change in intake independently predicted change in BMI. In the fully adjusted model, BMI increased by 0.18 from baseline for each serving consumed per day (95% CI: 0.09 to 0.27; $P = .02$). For each additional serving of sugar-sweetened drink per day, BMI increased by 0.24 (95% CI: 0.10 to 0.39, $P = .03$) and the odds ratio of obesity increased by 60% (95% CI: 14% to 124%; $P = .02$).

Several prospective studies have examined the relationship between the intake of sugar-sweetened beverages and weight gain in adults. In the largest study, Schulze et al.[74] evaluated the association between intake of sugar-sweetened beverages and weight gain in a large cohort of young and middle-aged women. After adjustment for lifestyle and dietary confounders, women who increased their consumption of sugar-sweetened soft drinks from 1 or fewer drinks per week to 1 or more drinks per day gained the most weight (multivariate adjusted means, 4.69 kg for 1991-1995 and 4.20 kg for 1995-1999), while those who decreased their intake gained the least amount of weight (1.34 and 0.15 kg for the two periods, respectively) (Fig. 14.1). A recent cohort study of 7,194 Spanish men and women found a positive association between higher consumption of sugar-sweetened beverages and risk of weight gain, especially among those with a history

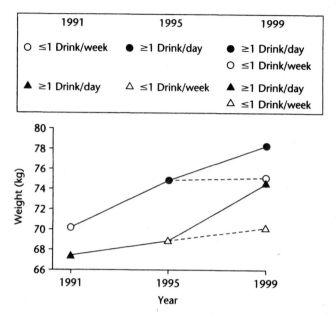

Figure 14.1 Mean weight in 1991, 1995, and 1999 according to "Trends in sugar-sweetened soft-drink consumption in 1969 women who changed consumption from 1991 to 1995 and either changed or maintained level of consumption until 1999." Low and high intakes were defined as 1 drink or less per week and 1 drink or more per day, respectively. Means were adjusted for age, alcohol intake, physical activity, smoking, postmenopausal hormone use, oral contraceptive use, cereal-fiber intake, and total fat intake at each point in time. Reproduced with permission from Schulze MB, Manson JE, Ludwig DS, et al. Sugar-sweetened beverages, weight gain, and incidence of type 2 diabetes in young and middle-aged women. *JAMA*. 2004;292:927-934.[74]

of weight gain.[75] Two smaller studies identified a positive but nonsignificant association between soft-drink consumption and increases in body weight.[76,77]

Findings from short-term feeding trials in adults suggest that intake of sugar-sweetened beverages induces positive energy balance and promotes weight gain.[78-80] Raben et al.[79] randomized overweight men and women to daily supplements of either sucrose or artificial sweeteners for 10 weeks. Body weight and fat mass increased in the sucrose group (by 1.6 and 1.3 kg, respectively) and decreased in the sweetener group (by 1.0 and 0.3 kg, respectively). Tordoff and Alleva[80] observed similar findings in a 3 × 3 crossover trial in which normal-weight subjects received 1150 g of soda per day sweetened with aspartame or high-fructose corn syrup or no soda for 3 weeks. DiMeglio and Mattes[78] conducted a crossover trial in which subjects received 1883 kJ/day of carbohydrate loads in either liquid (soda) or solid (jelly beans) form. During the solid phase, subjects compensated for energy provided by reducing free-feeding intake, but there was no compensation observed in the liquid phase.

Two intervention studies evaluated the effects of reducing soft-drink consumption on body weight among children. James et al.[81] conducted a cluster-randomized controlled trial on schoolchildren to evaluate the efficacy of a school-based educational program aimed at reducing consumption of carbonated drinks. At 12 months, the proportion of overweight and obese children in the control group increased by 7.5%, while those in the intervention group decreased by 0.2%. Recently, Ebbeling et al.[82] conducted a 25-week pilot randomized controlled trial to evaluate the effect of sugar-sweetened drinks on body weight among 103 adolescents 13 to 18 years of age who regularly consumed sugar-sweetened beverages (≥ 1 serving per day). They were randomly assigned to either the intervention group, which received weekly home deliveries of noncaloric beverages, or the control group, which continued usual beverage consumption throughout the follow-up period. Decreasing sugar-sweetened drink consumption had a significant beneficial effect on body weight only among those in the upper tertile of baseline BMI.

Although the overall results were not entirely consistent, the weight of epidemiologic and experimental evidence indicates that greater consumption of sugar-sweetened beverages is associated with weight gain and obesity in children and adults. However, the existing studies suffer from many methodological limitations, including cross-sectional design, small sample size, short follow-up, inadequate dietary assessment, and lack of repeated measures of diet and lifestyle.[67] Future epidemiologic studies should include a prospective design with repeated measures of diet and weight and should also investigate obesity-related end points such as diabetes and cardiovascular disease.

Coffee and Caffeine

Clinical trials in humans have demonstrated that the combination of caffeine and ephedrine produce a modest short-term weight loss.[83-85] Ephedrine, an alkaloid extracted from the plant ma huang (*Ephedrine silica*), exhibits thermogenic and appetite-suppressant properties.[86] Caffeine is often combined with ephedrine to boost the thermogenic effect of ephedrine.[87] However, dietary supplements containing ephedra alkaloids have been associated with increased cardiovascular events.[88] For this reason, National Institutes of Health (NIH) guidelines do not recommend the use of ephedra-containing products for weight loss.[89]

Caffeine is a nonselective antagonist of adenosine receptor, which is present in many tissues.[90] Caffeine ingestion has been shown to stimulate fat utilization in muscle tissue during prolonged exercise.[91] In addition, several studies have demonstrated that caffeine ingestion stimulates thermogenesis and increases basal energy expenditure in healthy subjects.[92,93] These data suggest a short-term beneficial effect of caffeine on energy metabolism. However, the long-term effects of chronic caffeine consumption on energy balance and body weight are unclear.

The association between caffeine consumption and weight change has been examined in only one prospective study. Lopez-Garcia et al.[94] followed 18,417 men and 39,740 women from 1986 to 1998 and observed less weight gain in those who increased caffeine consumption than in those who decreased it. However, differences between extreme quintiles were small: -0.43 kg (95% CI: -0.17 to -0.69) in men and -0.41 kg (95% CI: -0.20 to -0.62) in women. In addition, a modest inverse association between decaffeinated coffee and reduced weight gain was also observed, suggesting that the effects of coffee could be due to compounds other than caffeine. For example, chlorogenic acid in coffee has been shown to attenuate glucose absorption in the digestive tract, which might help control weight.[95] Numerous epidemiologic studies have found an inverse association between coffee consumption and risk of type 2 diabetes,[96] even after adjusting for BMI. These results suggest that the beneficial effects of coffee on type 2 diabetes are unlikely to be due to improved weight control.

Alcohol

Alcohol is the second most energy-dense nutrient after dietary fat (7 cal/g of alcohol). Short-term metabolic studies have shown that alcohol stimulates appetite and food intake, leading to elevated 24-hour energy intake.[97] Adding ethanol to the diet decreases lipid oxidation and thus may also induce lipid storage (ethanol is not stored in the body but is preferably oxidized over other fuels).[98] On the other hand, relatively high ethanol-induced thermogenesis (which accounts for approximately 20% of ethanol energy)[99] makes utilization of ethanol energy inefficient as compared with other macronutrients. In a randomized controlled trial, Davies et al.[100] found that moderate alcohol ingestion reduced fasting insulin and improved insulin sensitivity, outcomes that could affect body weight (see Chapter 18).

Numerous epidemiologic studies have examined the relationship between alcohol intake and body weight, but most are cross-sectional. In 1990, Hellerstedt et al.[101] conducted a systematic review of 29 cross-sectional studies of alcohol and weight. Most of these showed an inverse association between alcohol consumption and BMI in women, but results were highly inconsistent in men. Subsequent cross-sectional studies have revealed a similar pattern in gender differences.[102] The inverse association observed in women may reflect earlier weight gain among past drinkers who quit smoking. It is also possible that heavier women who are concerned about weight gain may abstain from drinking.

Only a few prospective studies have examined the relationship between alcohol and weight gain. Liu et al.[103] found that female drinkers with moderate alcohol consumption (up to two drinks per day) were significantly less likely than nondrinkers to have major weight gain ($\geq$10 kg); the association in men was not significant. A 5-year follow-up study of 7,608 British men 40 to 59 years of age found a significant association between high levels of alcohol intake ($\geq$30 g/day) and greater weight gain; lighter drinking was not associated with increased risk.[104] In other prospective studies, alcohol consumption did not appear to be an important predictor of weight gain.[75,105]

Wannamethee et al.[106] prospectively examined the relationship between alcohol and 8-year weight gain among 49,324 healthy women 27 to 44 years old. Multivariate analyses revealed a nonlinear relationship between alcohol and weight gain ($\geq$5 kg). The adjusted relative risks (95% CI) of weight gain as compared with the risk in nondrinkers were 0.94 (0.89 to 0.99) for those consuming 0.1 to 4.9 g/day; 0.92 (0.85 to 0.99) for 5 to 14.9 g/day; 0.86 (0.76 to 0.78) for 15 to 29.9 g/day; and 1.07 (0.89 to 1.28) for those consuming 30+ g/day ($P <$ .0001 for quadratic trend). Increased risk of weight gain among heavy drinkers was most evident in younger women (<35 years) (RR = 1.64; 95% CI: 1.03 to 2.61).

This association was observed for both beer and wine, suggesting that the type of alcoholic beverage consumed is less important than the quantity. It is unclear whether reduced weight gain seen in light and moderate female drinkers is an artifact due to residual confounding by a generally healthy diet and lifestyle among moderate drinkers or is the result of true physiological effects of alcohol (i.e., increased basal energy expenditure and inefficient energy utilization).[106] A gender difference in the relationship between alcohol and body weight has consistently been observed, but the biological mechanism is unclear. Despite these unknowns, evidence suggests that light-to-moderate alcohol consumption does not cause weight gain in free-living populations. Heavy consumption, however, may increase weight gain and other health risks and should thus be discouraged.

Dietary Patterns

Dietary pattern analysis has recently emerged as a complementary approach to traditional single-nutrient or food analysis (Chapter 6). Habitual intake patterns are typically characterized by statistical methods such as factor or cluster analysis or diet-quality indices based on prevailing dietary recommendations or healthful traditional diets (e.g., the Mediterranean diet).

Numerous cross-sectional studies have evaluated the relationship between dietary patterns and body weight. Togo et al.[107] conducted a systematic review of 30 cross-sectional studies using factor or cluster analysis or dietary indices to define dietary patterns. The authors concluded that no consistent associations could be identified between BMI and overall dietary patterns. As with other cross-sectional analyses of diet and body weight, concurrent examinations of dietary patterns and BMI are subject to the problem of reverse causation. In addition, variability in dietary patterns and dietary assessment methods may have contributed to heterogeneity of the results.

Relatively few prospective studies have examined associations between overall dietary patterns and weight change over time. Newby et al.[108] evaluated the relationship between dietary pattern and changes in BMI and waist circumference in the Baltimore Longitudinal Study of Ageing cohort among 219 women and 240 men. In women, there was an inverse association between a dietary pattern derived by factor analysis (i.e., low in white bread, refined grains, processed meats, potatoes, meat, and sugar-sweetened soft drinks and high in low-fat dairy products, cereal, fruit, fruit juice, nonwhite bread, nuts and seeds, and legumes) and annual changes in BMI and waist circumference. In men, there was an inverse association with change in waist circumference but not BMI. In the same cohort, a cluster of subjects with a diet high in potatoes and meat had the largest annual increase in BMI. A *healthy* dietary pattern—high in fruits, cereals, low-fat dairy products, and low in fast-food, sugar-sweetened soft drinks, and salty snacks—produced the smallest annual increase in BMI.[109]

In the EPIC-Potsdam Study, a dietary pattern characterized by high consumption of whole-grain bread, fruits, fruit juices, grain flakes/muesli, and raw vegetables and low consumption of processed meat, butter, high-fat cheese, margarine, and red meat was associated with lower weight gain in normal-weight individuals but not in obese individuals during 4 years of follow-up.[110] Schulze et al.[111] examined the association between adherence to dietary patterns and weight change in 51,603 women aged 26 to 46 years. This cohort was followed from 1991 to 1999, with dietary intake and body weight ascertained in 1991, 1995, and 1999. Two dietary patterns—a Western pattern characterized by high intakes of red and processed meats, refined grains, sweets and desserts, and potatoes; and a prudent pattern characterized by high intakes of fruits, vegetables, whole grains, fish, poultry, and salad dressing—were identified with factor analysis. Weight gain over an 8-year period was higher among women who consistently scored high on a Western pattern (5.62 kg) compared with those who scored low on a Western pattern (4.90 kg; $P < .001$). Women who decreased their prudent-pattern score while increasing their Western-pattern score had the largest weight gain between 1991 and 1995 (multivariate adjusted mean: 6.47 kg); the opposite change in patterns produced the smallest weight gain (1.32 kg; $P < .001$; Fig. 14.2). This study provides the strongest evidence to date regarding the role of overall dietary patterns in preventing midlife weight gain.

Breakfast Consumption

Regular breakfast consumption has been widely recommended for obesity prevention. Skipping breakfast may increase the production of appetite-stimulating hormones and thus lead to daytime overeating. During prolonged fasting, ghrelin levels rise[112] and insulin levels decline.[113] These hormonal changes can trigger hunger and stimulate eating.[114,115] In a randomized clinical trial, skipping breakfast led to increased energy intake during the day, increased total and LDL cholesterol, and impaired postprandial insulin and glucose responses.[116] Rapid rise and decline in blood glucose levels have been associated with increased hunger and meal requests, which may induce overeating.[117]

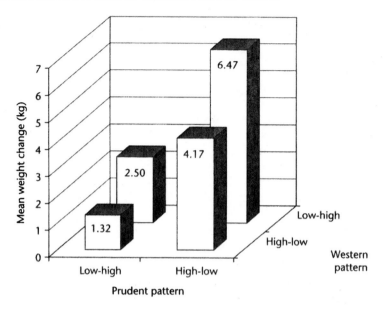

Figure 14.2 Mean weight change (kg) between 1991 and 1995 according to joint classifications in Prudent- and Western-pattern scores (low and high pattern scores were defined as the lower 2 and upper 2 quintiles, respectively). From Schulze MB, Fung TT, Manson JE, Willett WC, Hu FB. Dietary patterns and changes in body weight in women. *Obesity (Silver Spring)*. 2006;14:1444-1453.[111]

Several cross-sectional studies found a consistent association between skipping breakfast and a higher BMI or obesity.[118-122] For example, Ma et al.[119] found that skipping breakfast was associated with a 4.5 times (95% CI: 1.57 to 12.9) higher prevalence of obesity, even after adjusting for physical activity and total energy intake. This strong association, however, may reflect dieting behaviors among obese individuals. In a nationally representative sample, consumption of breakfast or ready-to-eat cereal was associated with significantly lower prevalence of overweight and lower BMI.[118]

Prospective studies on breakfast consumption and body weight are limited. Berkey et al.[123] found that normal-weight children who never ate breakfast gained more weight than peers who ate breakfast nearly every day. In the Physicians' Health Study, an inverse association was observed between consumption of breakfast cereal and the amount of weight regardless of the type of breakfast cereal used.[124] In contrast, increased frequency of breakfast consumption was associated with increases in waist circumference in Dutch men around the age of retirement.[125] This finding may have been confounded by other changes in lifestyle related to retirement.

van der Heijden et al.[126] examined the association between consumption of breakfast and 10-year weight gain in men who participated in the Health Professionals' Followup Study (HPFS). Breakfast consumption was inversely associated with the risk of 5-kg weight gain after adjustment for age (RR = 0.77; 95% CI: 0.72 to 0.82); the association was somewhat attenuated after adjusting for lifestyle and BMI at baseline (RR = 0.87; 95% CI: 0.82 to 0.93). The inverse association between breakfast consumption and weight gain was more pronounced in normal-weight men (RR = 0.78; 95% CI: 0.70 to 0.87) compared with those who were overweight at baseline (RR = 0.92; 95% CI: 0.85 to 1.00). Fiber and nutrient intakes did not explain the association between breakfast consumption and the risk of weight gain. Interestingly, the number of eating episodes added to three regular meals per day was associated with a slightly increased risk of weight gain, perhaps caused by increased caloric intake from snacking.

Fast-Food Consumption

Increased consumption of fast-foods is widely believed to be a major contributing factor to the obesity epidemic. Habitual intake of fast-foods—with their large portions, high palatability, and high sugar and trans fat content[127]—may lead to excess energy intake. Ebbeling et al.[128] found that children tend to overconsume fast-foods and that overweight children are less likely than lean ones to compensate for the added energy consumption. Taveras et al.[129] also found that children who consumed greater quantities of fried food away from home were heavier, had greater total energy intake, and had poorer diet quality.

In a prospective study among 3,031 young black and white adults in the CARDIA, Pereira et al.[130] investigated the association between reported fast-food habits and changes in body weight and insulin resistance over a 15-year period. Data showed strong positive associations between frequency of visits to fast-food restaurants and increases in body weight and insulin resistance. Those who visited fast-food restaurants frequently (≥ 2 times/week) gained an extra 4.5 kg of body weight and had a twofold greater increase in insulin resistance compared to infrequent consumers of fast food (<1 time/week). The associations were largely independent of other potentially confounding lifestyle factors (e.g., physical activity and television viewing). In addition, increasing consumption of fast-food over time conferred even greater weight gain for those who already consumed fast-food regularly at baseline (Fig. 14.3). French et al.[131] also found a positive association between more frequent use of fast-food restaurants and 3-year weight gain among 891 middle-aged women. In young adults, Duffey et al.[132] found that greater consumption of

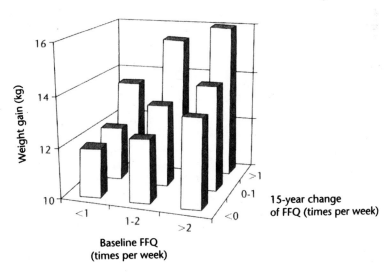

Figure 14.3 Joint association of year 0 frequency of fast-food consumption and 15-year changes in frequency of fast-food consumption with 15-year changes in body weight. From Pereira MA, Kartashov AI, Ebbeling CB, et al. Fast-food habits, weight gain, and insulin resistance (the CARDIA study): 15-year prospective analysis. *Lancet.* 2005;365:36-42.[130]

fast-food, but not restaurant food, was associated with higher BMI and greater 3-year weight gain.

The positive association between fast-food habits and obesity is likely to be due to large portion sizes, low prices, and palatability—a combination that results in overeating and positive energy balance. On the other hand, fast-food habits may be a marker of unhealthy diet and lifestyle or low individual and neighborhood socioeconomic status (SES). Some of these variables, especially neighborhood SES, have not been considered in most analyses. In addition, none of the analyses have controlled for overall eating patterns derived from factor or cluster analysis. Measuring fast-food habits also presents a challenge in epidemiologic studies because there is no standard definition of fast-food. In the CARDIA Study, fast-food habits were assessed by asking the participants, "How often do you eat breakfast, lunch, or dinner in a place such as McDonald's, Burger King, Wendy's, Arby's, Pizza Hut, or Kentucky Fried Chicken?" while restaurant food consumption was assessed with the question, "How many times in a week or month do you eat breakfast, lunch, or dinner at a restaurant or cafeteria?" The validity of these measurements has not been rigorously studied.

Portion Size

The past several decades have seen a marked increase in the size of food portions.[133] According to data from the Nationwide Food Consumption Survey (NFCS) and the Continuing Survey of Food Intakes by Individuals (CSFII), between 1977 and 1996, the caloric content and portion size of salty snacks increased by 93 kcal (from 1.0 to 1.6 oz); soft drinks increased by 49 kcal (from 13.1 to 19.9 fl oz); hamburgers by 97 kcal (from 5.7 to 7.0 oz); and french fries by 68 kcal (from 3.1 to 3.6 oz). The largest increases in portion sizes were found for foods consumed at fast-food establisments and at home.

Short-term experimental studies have demonstrated that subjects provided with large portions of food have significantly higher energy intake. Rolls et al.[134] found that adults served the largest of four portion sizes (500, 625, 750, or 1,000 g) of a macaroni and cheese entrée consumed 30% more energy than those served the smallest portion size. Diliberti et al.[135] also found an association between entrée size and energy intake in a natural setting. Standard- or large-size pasta entrees (248 and 377 g, respectively) were available for the same price in a cafeteria-style restaurant. Subjects who purchased the larger portion size increased their energy intake from the entrée by 43% (719 kJ; 172 kcal) and by 25% (664 kJ; 159 kcal) for the entire meal.

Despite short-term experimental evidence on the relationship between portion size and energy intake, epidemiologic studies on portion size and body weight are limited. One cross-sectional study found a positive relationship between larger portion sizes and increased energy intake and body weight among children.[136] Prospective studies are needed to examine whether large portion sizes predict future risk of weight gain independent of lifestyle and SES factors. However, it may be difficult to disentangle the effects of large portion sizes from high energy density and fast-food habits because these variables are likely to be highly correlated.

Energy Density

Increasing energy density of many foods may be another major contributor to the current obesity epidemic. Energy density is defined as "the amount of energy in a given weight of food (kcal/g or kJ/g)."[137] In that the amount of water added to a food increases food weight but not energy, it is a major determinant of energy density. Thus, soups, milk, and beverages typically have a low energy density, as do natural fruits and vegetables. Dry fruits and vegetables, however, tend to be energy dense. Many processed foods high in fat and sugar are both energy dense and palatable, which may lead to overeating. However, higher-fat diets are not necessarily energy dense. In the Nurses' Health Study II cohort,[138] dietary energy density was positively associated with intakes of saturated ($r = .16$) and trans fat ($r = .15$), dietary GI ($r = .16$), and snack foods, but inversely associated with vegetable protein ($r = -.30$) and intake of fruits and vegetables. Interestingly, dietary energy density was only minimally associated with total fat intake ($r = .08$). These results suggest that overall dietary energy density is primarily driven by consumption of foods high in saturated and trans fats and refined carbohydrates and reduced consumption of fruits and vegetables.

Several short-term feeding interventions showed an association between the energy density of test foods (ingested as preloads or incorporated into meals) and energy intake. In general, subjects tended to ingest more calories when consuming foods with a high energy density than those with a low energy density.[137] A 2-day study also showed that decreases in energy density and portion size had independent effects on reduction of ad libitum energy intake without increased hunger.[139] Despite a positive relationship between energy density and energy intake, it is unclear whether there is compensation over the long-term. So far, no long-term randomized trials have been conducted to evaluate the effects of lowered energy density on weight loss and maintenance. As discussed earlier in this chapter, low-fat diets (which presumably reduce energy density) are not particularly effective in sustaining long-term weight loss.

Ecological analyses suggest a close relationship between high energy density of foods and low cost (dollars per megajoule), which may explain higher obesity rates among socioeconomically disadvantaged groups.[140] Several cross-sectional studies found a positive relationship between energy density and body weight. In the Multiethnic Cohort, Howarth et al.[141] calculated energy density from responses to a food-frequency questionnaire (FFQ) and validated the measures against multiple 24-hour recalls. After adjusting for the amount of food consumed per day, age, current smoking status, physical activity, chronic disease, and education, a higher energy density was associated with increased current BMI in each ethnic group. Ledikwe et al.[142] conducted a cross-sectional survey of adults ($n = 7,356$) from the 1994-1996 CSFII. Using two 24-hour dietary recalls to calculate energy density (beverages were excluded from the calculations), the authors found that the energy density for obese subjects tended to be slightly higher than that for normal-weight people. A similar association was found among subjects from the NHANES III.[143] Another cross-sectional study found a positive correlation between energy density and energy intake but not BMI.[144]

Only two prospective studies have examined the relationship between energy density and weight gain over time. Iqbal et al.[145] examined the association between dietary energy density and 5-year weight gain among Danish men and women and found no overall association, although dietary energy density was positively associated with weight gain only among obese women. In a much larger study with 50,749 middle-aged women in the Nurses' Health Study II, Bes-Rastrollo et al.[138] found that women who moved from the lowest to the highest quintiles of dietary energy density during follow-up increased their body weight the most (1991-1999: 6.83 kg), whereas participants who moved from the highest to the lowest quintiles increased their body weight the least (1991-1999: 4.29 kg) during follow-up. These analyses suggest that reducing overall dietary energy density may have modest benefits on reducing weight gain in middle-aged women. Interestingly, the amount of weight change over time varied considerably according to energy density values of individual foods and beverages. Some foods/beverages with low energy density values, such as soda, fruit punches, and potatoes, were associated with greater weight gain. In contrast, some foods with higher energy-density values, such as olive oil and nuts, were associated with smaller weight gain. Thus, public health recommendations should focus on energy density of the total diet rather than energy density values of individual foods and beverages. Reduced consumption of saturated and trans fats and refined carbohydrates and increased consumption of fruits and vegetables can help to lower energy density and prevent weight gain.

Conclusions

Although diet is widely believed to play a major role in weight control, the impact of specific dietary factors remains elusive. Clearly, there is no "magic bullet" for weight control. Rather, many individual dietary factors exert a modest effect on body weight, and over time, cumulative effects of small changes in daily energy balance lead to weight gain and obesity. Although dietary fat has long been considered the main culprit behind obesity, large prospective cohort studies and longer-term randomized clinical trials do not support a major role of reducing dietary fat as percentage of energy in obesity prevention and weight control. In contrast, emerging evidence suggests potential weight control benefits by severely restricting carbohydrates and reducing GL, but long-term prospective data are limited.

The long-term relationship between intake of foods and beverages and body weight has received increased attention. Such analyses are particularly useful in making practical dietary recommendations. Several large prospective studies have demonstrated that increasing consumption of whole grains and fruits and vegetables predicts less weight gain over time in middle-aged and older adults. In addition, substantial evidence indicates that higher consumption of sugar-sweetened soft drinks induces greater weight gain in both children and adults. Although nuts are a high-fat food, epidemiologic studies and clinical trials show that increased consumption of nuts at the expense of other foods is beneficial for cardiovascular disease risk and does not cause weight gain.

The effects of dairy products and calcium on body weight remain controversial. More recent large epidemiologic studies and longer-term trials have failed to confirm the benefits of dairy or calcium on weight. Many epidemiologic studies have shown that light-to-moderate alcohol consumption is not associated with weight gain in men and may be beneficial in women. Heavy alcohol consumption, however, increases energy intake and results in greater weight gain. Reducing energy density of a diet by decreasing consumption of processed foods high in sugar and saturated and trans fats and increasing consumption of fruits and vegetables may help prevent weight gain.

The existing literature on diet and weight is fraught with methodological problems (Table 14.1). Experimental studies should provide some of the most rigorous evaluations of dietary intake and body weight. However, dietary intervention trials of long duration, while theoretically ideal, are seldom feasible because of high cost and lack of compliance by study participants. Most of existing trials are small in size and test only a limited number of nutrients or foods at single intake level. In addition, poor compliance and high dropout rates are common in dietary intervention trials. For these reasons, evaluation of the long-term relationship between various dietary factors and obesity have been largely based on epidemiologic studies. Interpretation of epidemiologic data, however, is complicated by multiple methodological issues, including measurement errors in assessing diet and physical activity, lack of repeated measures in dietary exposures and outcomes, reverse causation, and confounding by other diet and lifestyle factors.[67] In particular, small underpowered studies are likely to produce both false negative and false positive results. Various dietary instruments, including 24-hour recalls, dietary records, and FFQs, have

Table 14.1 Methodological Issues in Epidemiologic and Intervention Studies of Diet and Body Weight

Prospective Cohort Studies	• Small sample size • Short duration of follow-up • Lack of repeated measures of diet and lifestyle • Confounding by physical activity and other covariates • Reverse causation (e.g., overweight→change in diet) • Measurement errors in diet, physical activity, and adiposity • Multiple testing
Randomized Clinical Trials	• Small sample size • Short duration • Inadequate adherence to dietary interventions • Dropout • Different intensity of interventions between the treatment and control groups • Different flavor/taste between the intervention and control diets • Only a small number of nutrients/foods at a single intake level are studied

been used in epidemiologic studies. None of these instruments is perfect (see Chapter 6). However, carefully validated FFQs that are administered repeatedly during follow-up are considered best-suited for the assessment of long-term patterns in intake. Future studies, whether observational or interventional, should attend to these methodological problems.

In conclusion, the existing literature suggests that altering macronutrient composition is unlikely to have a substantial impact on long-term weight control. However, there is some evidence that more severe restriction of carbohydrate intake has modest benefits on weight loss. Nonetheless, any single dietary factor is unlikely to have a large effect on body weight. Rather, the combined effects of multiple dietary factors (including individual foods and beverages) can accumulate over time to have a substantial long-term impact on body weight. Therefore, prevention of weight gain and obesity should focus on both control of total caloric intake and adapting an overall healthy eating pattern.

References

1. Malik VS, Hu FB. Popular weight-loss diets: from evidence to practice. *Nat Clin Pract Cardiovasc Med.* 2007;4:34-41.
2. Lissner L, Heitmann BL. Dietary fat and obesity: evidence from epidemiology. *Eur J Clin Nutr.* 1995;49:79-90.
3. Bray GA, Popkin BM. Dietary fat intake does affect obesity! *Am J Clin Nutr.* 1998;68:1157-1173.
4. Seidell JC. Dietary fat and obesity: an epidemiologic perspective. *Am J Clin Nutr.* 1998;67(3 Suppl):546S-550S.
5. Willett WC. Dietary fat plays a major role in obesity: no. *Obes Rev.* 2002;3:59-68.
6. Willett WC, Leibel RL. Dietary fat is not a major determinant of body fat. *Am J Med.* 2002;113 (Suppl 9B):47S-59S.
7. Astrup A, Astrup A, Buemann B, Flint A, Raben A. Low-fat diets and energy balance: how does the evidence stand in 2002? *Proc Nutr Soc.* 2002;61:299-309.
8. Swinburn BA, Caterson I, Seidell JC, James WP. Diet, nutrition and the prevention of excess weight gain and obesity. *Public Health Nutr.* 2004;7:123-146.
9. Popkin BM. The nutrition transition: an overview of world patterns of change. *Nutr Rev.* 2004;62:S140-S143.

10. Willett WC. Is dietary fat a major determinant of body fat? *Am J Clin Nutr.* 1998;67(3 Suppl):556S-562S.

11. Heitmann BL, Lissner L, Sorensen TI, Bengtsson C. Dietary fat intake and weight gain in women genetically predisposed for obesity. *Am J Clin Nutr.* 1995;61:1213-1217.

12. Field AE, Willett WC, Lissner L, Colditz G. Dietary fat and weight gain among women in the Nurses' Health Study. *Obesity (Silver Spring).* 2007;15:967-976.

13. Hu FB, van Dam RM, Liu S. Diet and risk of type II diabetes: the role of types of fat and carbohydrate. *Diabetologia.* 2001;44:805-817.

14. Koh-Banerjee P, Chu NF, Spiegelman D, et al. Prospective study of the association of changes in dietary intake, physical activity, alcohol consumption, and smoking with 9-y gain in waist circumference among 16 587 US men. *Am J Clin Nutr.* 2003;78: 719-727.

15. Howard BV, Manson JE, Stefanick ML, et al. Low-fat dietary pattern and weight change over 7 years: the Women's Health Initiative Dietary Modification Trial. *JAMA.* 2006;295:39-49.

16. Ludwig DS. Clinical update: the low-glycaemic-index diet. *Lancet.* 2007;369:890-892.

17. Nordmann AJ, Nordmann A, Briel M, et al. Effects of low-carbohydrate vs low-fat diets on weight loss and cardiovascular risk factors: a meta-analysis of randomized controlled trials. *Arch Intern Med.* 2006;166:285-293.

18. Gardner CD, Kiazand A, Alhassan S, et al. Comparison of the Atkins, Zone, Ornish, and LEARN diets for change in weight and related risk factors among overweight premenopausal women: the A TO Z Weight Loss Study: a randomized trial. *JAMA.* 2007;297:969-977.

19. Ludwig DS. The glycemic index: physiological mechanisms relating to obesity, diabetes, and cardiovascular disease. *JAMA.* 2002;287:2414-2423.

20. Jenkins DJ, Wolever TM, Taylor RH, et al. Glycemic index of foods: a physiological basis for carbohydrate exchange. *Am J Clin Nutr.* 1981;34:362-366.

21. Salmeron J, Ascherio A, Rimm EB, et al. Dietary fiber, glycemic load, and risk of NIDDM in men. *Diabetes Care.* 1997;20:545-550.

22. Hu FB, Willett WC. Optimal diets for prevention of coronary heart disease. *JAMA.* 2002;288:2569-2578.

23. Liese AD, Schulz M, Fang F, et al. Dietary glycemic index and glycemic load, carbohydrate and fiber intake, and measures of insulin sensitivity, secretion, and adiposity in the Insulin Resistance Atherosclerosis Study. *Diabetes Care.* 2005;28:2832-2838.

24. Ma Y, Olendzki B, Chiriboga D, et al. Association between dietary carbohydrates and body weight. *Am J Epidemiol.* 2005;161:359-367.

25. Roberts SB. High-glycemic index foods, hunger, and obesity: is there a connection? *Nutr Rev.* 2000;58:163-169.

26. Sloth B, Krog-Mikkelsen I, Flint A, et al. No difference in body weight decrease between a low-glycemic-index and a high-glycemic-index diet but reduced LDL cholesterol after 10-wk ad libitum intake of the low-glycemic-index diet. *Am J Clin Nutr.* 2004;80:337-347.

27. McMillan-Price J, Petocz P, Atkinson F, et al. Comparison of 4 diets of varying glycemic load on weight loss and cardiovascular risk reduction in overweight and obese young adults: a randomized controlled trial. *Arch Intern Med.* 2006;166:1466-1475.

28. Sichieri R, Moura AS, Genelhu V, Hu FB, Willett WC. An eighteen-month randomized trial of a low-glycemic index diet and weight change among Brazilian women. *Am J Clin Nutr.* 2007;In press.

29. Ebbeling CB, Leidig MM, Feldman HA, Lovesky MM, Ludwig DS. Effects of a low-glycemic load vs low-fat diet in obese young adults: a randomized trial. *JAMA.* 2007;297(19):2092-2102.

30. Halton TL, Hu FB. The effects of high protein diets on thermogenesis, satiety and weight loss: a critical review. *J Am Coll Nutr.* 2004;23:373-385.

31. Skov AR, Toubro S, Ronn B, Holm L, Astrup A. Randomized trial on protein vs carbohydrate in ad libitum fat reduced diet for the treatment of obesity. *Int J Obes Relat Metab Disord.* 1999;23:528-536.

32. Merchant AT, Anand SS, Vuksan V, et al. Protein intake is inversely associated with abdominal obesity in a multi-ethnic population. *J Nutr.* 2005;135:1196-1201.

33. Hu FB. Protein, body weight, and cardiovascular health. *Am J Clin Nutr.* 2005;82:242S-247S.

34. Pereira MA, Jacobs DR J, Slattery ML, et al. The association of whole grain intake and fasting insulin in a biracial cohort of young adults: The CARDIA Study. *CVD Prevention.* 1998;1:231-242.

35. Liu S, Willett WC, Manson JE, Hu FB, Rosner B, Colditz G. Relation between changes in intakes of dietary fiber and grain products and changes in weight and development of obesity among middle-aged women. *Am J Clin Nutr.* 2003;78:920-927.

36. Koh-Banerjee P, Franz M, Sampson L, et al. Changes in whole-grain, bran, and cereal fiber consumption in relation to 8-y weight gain among men. *Am J Clin Nutr.* 2004;80:1237-1245.

37. Slavin JL. Dietary fiber and body weight. *Nutrition.* 2005;21:411-418.

38. Koh-Banerjee P, Rimm EB. Whole grain consumption and weight gain: a review of the epidemiological evidence, potential mechanisms and opportunities for future research. *Proc Nutr Soc.* 2003;62:25-29.

39. Pereira MA, Ludwig DS. Dietary fiber and body-weight regulation. Observations and mechanisms. *Pediatr Clin North Am.* 2001;48:969-980.

40. Pereira MA, Jacobs DR Jr, Pins JJ, et al. Effect of whole grains on insulin sensitivity in overweight hyperinsulinemic adults. *Am J Clin Nutr.* 2002;75:848-855.

41. Ludwig DS, Pereira MA, Kroenke CH, et al. Dietary fiber, weight gain, and cardiovascular disease risk factors in young adults. *JAMA.* 1999;282:1539-1546.

42. Pittler MH, Ernst E. Guar gum for body weight reduction: meta-analysis of randomized trials. *Am J Med.* 2001;110:724-730.

43. He K, Hu FB, Colditz GA, Manson JE, Willett WC, Liu S. Changes in intake of fruits and vegetables in relation to risk of obesity and weight gain among middle-aged women. *Int J Obes Relat Metab Disord.* 2004;28:1569-1574.

44. Fraser GE, Sabate J, Beeson WL, Strahan TM. A possible protective effect of nut consumption on risk of coronary heart disease. The Adventist Health Study. *Arch Intern Med.* 1992;152:1416-1424.

45. Hu FB, Stampfer MJ, Manson JE, et al. Frequent nut consumption and risk of coronary heart disease in women: prospective cohort study. *BMJ.* 1998;317:1341-1345.

46. Bes-Rastrollo M, Sabate J, Gomez-Garcia E, Alonso A, Martinez JA, Martinez-Gonzalez MA. Nut consumption and weight gain in a Mediterranean cohort: the SUN Study. *Obesity.* 2007;15(1):107-116.

47. Jiang R, Manson JE, Stampfer MJ, Liu S, Willett WC, Hu FB. Nut and peanut butter consumption and risk of type 2 diabetes in women. *JAMA.* 2002;288:2554-2560.

48. Sabate J. Nut consumption and body weight. *Am J Clin Nutr.* 2003;78(3 Suppl): 647S-650S.

49. Estruch R, Martinez-Gonzalez MA, Corella D, et al. Effects of a Mediterranean-style diet on cardiovascular risk factors: a randomized trial. *Ann Intern Med.* 2006;145:1-11.

50. Wien MA, Sabate JM, Ikle DN, Cole SE, Kandeel FR. Almonds vs complex carbohydrates in a weight reduction program. *Int J Obes Relat Metab Disord.* 2003; 27:1365-1372.

51. Alper CM, Mattes RD. Effects of chronic peanut consumption on energy balance and hedonics. *Int J Obes Relat Metab Disord.* 2002;26:1129-1137.

52. Fraser GE, Bennett HW, Jaceldo KB, Sabate J. Effect on body weight of a free 76 Kilojoule (320 calorie) daily supplement of almonds for six months. *J Am Coll Nutr.* 2002;21:275-283.

53. Zemel MB. The role of dairy foods in weight management. *J Am Coll Nutr.* 2005;24 (6 Suppl):537S-546S.
54. Zemel MB, Shi H, Greer B, Dirienzo D, Zemel PC. Regulation of adiposity by dietary calcium. *FASEB J.* 2000;14:1132-1138.
55. Barr SI. Increased dairy product or calcium intake: is body weight or composition affected in humans? *J Nutr.* 2003;245S-248S.
56. Zemel MB, Thompson W, Milstead A, Morris K, Campbell P. Calcium and dairy acceleration of weight and fat loss during energy restriction in obese adults. *Obes Res.* 2004;12:582-590.
57. Shapses SA, Heshka S, Heymsfield SB. Effect of calcium supplementation on weight and fat loss in women. *J Clin Endocrinol Metab.* 2004;89:632-637.
58. Lorenzen JK, Molgaard C, Michaelsen KF, Astrup A. Calcium supplementation for 1 y does not reduce body weight or fat mass in young girls. *Am J Clin Nutr.* 2006;83:18-23.
59. Gunther CW, Legowski PA, Lyle RM, et al. Dairy products do not lead to alterations in body weight or fat mass in young women in a 1-y intervention. *Am J Clin Nutr.* 2005;81:751-756.
60. Gonzalez AJ, White E, Kristal A, Littman AJ. Calcium intake and 10-year weight change in middle-aged adults. *J Am Diet Assoc.* 2006;106:1066-1073.
61. Macdonald HM, New SA, Campbell MK, Reid DM. Longitudinal changes in weight in perimenopausal and early postmenopausal women: effects of dietary energy intake, energy expenditure, dietary calcium intake and hormone replacement therapy. *Int J Obes Relat Metab Disord.* 2003;27:669-676.
62. Rajpathak SN, Rimm EB, Rosner B, Willett WC, Hu FB. Calcium and dairy intakes in relation to long-term weight gain in US men. *Am J Clin Nutr.* 2006;83:559-566.
63. Berkey CS, Rockett HR, Willett WC, Colditz GA. Milk, dairy fat, dietary calcium, and weight gain: a longitudinal study of adolescents. *Arch Pediatr Adolesc Med.* 2005;159:543-550.
64. Pereira MA, Jacobs DR Jr, Van Horn L, Slattery ML, Kartashov AI, Ludwig DS. Dairy consumption, obesity, and the insulin resistance syndrome in young adults: the CARDIA Study. *JAMA.* 2002;287:2081-2089.
65. Choi HK, Willett WC, Stampfer MJ, Rimm E, Hu FB. Dairy consumption and risk of type 2 diabetes mellitus in men: a prospective study. *Arch Intern Med.* 2005; 165:997-1003.
66. Bray GA, Nielsen SJ, Popkin BM. Consumption of high-fructose corn syrup in beverages may play a role in the epidemic of obesity. *Am J Clin Nutr.* 2004;79:537-543.
67. Malik VS, Schulze MB, Hu FB. Intake of sugar-sweetened beverages and weight gain: a systematic review. *Am J Clin Nutr.* 2006;84:274-288.
68. Berkey CS, Rockett HR, Field AE, Gillman MW, Colditz GA. Sugar-added beverages and adolescent weight change. *Obes Res.* 2004;12:778-788.
69. Ludwig DS, Peterson KE, Gortmaker SL. Relation between consumption of sugar-sweetened drinks and childhood obesity: a prospective, observational analysis. *Lancet.* 2001;357:505-508.
70. Phillips SM, Bandini LG, Naumova EN, et al. Energy-dense snack food intake in adolescence: longitudinal relationship to weight and fatness. *Obes Res.* 2004;12:461-472.
71. Welsh JA, Cogswell ME, Rogers S, Rockett H, Mei Z, Grummer-Strawn LM. Overweight among low-income preschool children associated with the consumption of sweet drinks: Missouri, 1999-2002. *Pediatrics.* 2005;115:e223-e229.
72. Blum JW, Jacobsen DJ, Donnelly JE. Beverage consumption patterns in elementary school aged children across a two-year period. *J Am Coll Nutr.* 2005;24:93-98.
73. Newby PK, Peterson KE, Berkey CS, Leppert J, Willett WC, Colditz GA. Beverage consumption is not associated with changes in weight and body mass index among low-income preschool children in North Dakota. *J Am Diet Assoc.* 2004;104: 1086-1094.

74. Schulze MB, Manson JE, Ludwig DS, et al. Sugar-sweetened beverages, weight gain, and incidence of type 2 diabetes in young and middle-aged women. *JAMA*. 2004;292:927-934.

75. Bes-Rastrollo M, Sanchez-Villegas A, Gomez-Gracia E, Martinez JA, Pajares RM, Martinez-Gonzalez MA. Predictors of weight gain in a Mediterranean cohort: the Seguimiento Universidad de Navarra Study 1. *Am J Clin Nutr*. 2006;83:362-370.

76. French SA, Jeffery RW, Forster JL, McGovern PG, Kelder SH, Baxter JE. Predictors of weight change over two years among a population of working adults: the Healthy Worker Project. *Int J Obes Relat Metab Disord*. 1994;18:145-154.

77. Kvaavik E, Andersen LF, Klepp KI. The stability of soft drinks intake from adolescence to adult age and the association between long-term consumption of soft drinks and lifestyle factors and body weight. *Public Health Nutr*. 2005;8:149-157.

78. DiMeglio DP, Mattes RD. Liquid versus solid carbohydrate: effects on food intake and body weight. *Int J Obes Relat Metab Disord*. 2000;24:794-800.

79. Raben A, Vasilaras TH, Moller AC, Astrup A. Sucrose compared with artificial sweeteners: different effects on ad libitum food intake and body weight after 10 wk of supplementation in overweight subjects. *Am J Clin Nutr*. 2002;76:721-729.

80. Tordoff MG, Alleva AM. Effect of drinking soda sweetened with aspartame or high-fructose corn syrup on food intake and body weight. *Am J Clin Nutr*. 1990; 51:963-969.

81. James J, Thomas P, Cavan D, Kerr D. Preventing childhood obesity by reducing consumption of carbonated drinks: cluster randomised controlled trial. *BMJ*. 2004;328:12367.

82. Ebbeling CB, Feldman HA, Osganian SK, Chomitz VR, Ellenbogen SJ, Ludwig DS. Effects of decreasing sugar-sweetened beverage consumption on body weight in adolescents: a randomized, controlled pilot study. *Pediatrics*. 2006;117:673-680.

83. Boozer CN, Daly PA, Homel P, et al. Herbal ephedra/caffeine for weight loss: a 6-month randomized safety and efficacy trial. *Int J Obes Relat Metab Disord*. 2002;26:593-604.

84. Boozer CN, Nasser JA, Heymsfield SB, Wang V, Chen G, Solomon JL. An herbal supplement containing Ma Huang-Guarana for weight loss: a randomized, double-blind trial. *Int J Obes Relat Metab Disord*. 2001;25:316-324.

85. Coffey CS, Steiner D, Baker BA, Allison DB. A randomized double-blind placebo-controlled clinical trial of a product containing ephedrine, caffeine, and other ingredients from herbal sources for treatment of overweight and obesity in the absence of lifestyle treatment. *Int J Obes Relat Metab Disord*. 2004;28:1411-1419.

86. Ryan DH. Use of sibutramine and other noradrenergic and serotonergic drugs in the management of obesity. *Endocrine*. 2000;13:193-199.

87. Astrup A, Breum L, Toubro S, Hein P, Quaade F. The effect and safety of an ephedrine/caffeine compound compared to ephedrine, caffeine and placebo in obese subjects on an energy restricted diet. A double blind trial. *Int J Obes Relat Metab Disord*. 1992;16:269-277.

88. Haller CA, Benowitz NL. Adverse cardiovascular and central nervous system events associated with dietary supplements containing ephedra alkaloids. *N Engl J Med*. 2000;343:1833-1838.

89. Clinical Guidelines on the Identification, Evaluation, and Treatment of Overweight and Obesity in Adults. The Evidence Report. *Obes Res*. 1998;6(Suppl):51S-209S.

90. Van Soeren MH, Graham TE. Effect of caffeine on metabolism, exercise endurance, and catecholamine responses after withdrawal. *J Appl Physiol*. 1998;85:1493-1501.

91. Spriet LL, MacLean DA, Dyck DJ, Hultman E, Cederblad G, Graham TE. Caffeine ingestion and muscle metabolism during prolonged exercise in humans. *Am J Physiol*. 1992;262(6 Pt 1):E891-E898.

92. Astrup A, Toubro S, Cannon S, Hein P, Breum L, Madsen J. Caffeine: a double-blind, placebo-controlled study of its thermogenic, metabolic, and cardiovascular effects in healthy volunteers. *Am J Clin Nutr*. 1990;51:759-767.

93. Acheson KJ, Gremaud G, Meirim I, et al. Metabolic effects of caffeine in humans: lipid oxidation or futile cycling? *Am J Clin Nutr.* 2004;79:40-46.

94. Lopez-Garcia E, van Dam RM, Rajpathak S, Willett WC, Manson JE, Hu FB. Changes in caffeine intake and long-term weight change in men and women. *Am J Clin Nutr.* 2006;83:674-680.

95. Johnston KL, Clifford MN, Morgan LM. Coffee acutely modifies gastrointestinal hormone secretion and glucose tolerance in humans: glycemic effects of chlorogenic acid and caffeine. *Am J Clin Nutr.* 2003;78:728-733.

96. van Dam RM, Hu FB. Coffee consumption and risk of type 2 diabetes: a systematic review. *JAMA.* 2005;294:97-104.

97. Westerterp-Plantenga MS, Verwegen CR. The appetizing effect of an aperitif in overweight and normal-weight humans. *Am J Clin Nutr.* 1999;69:205-212.

98. Jequier E. Alcohol intake and body weight: a paradox. *Am J Clin Nutr.* 1999;69: 173-174.

99. Suter PM, Jequier E, Schutz Y. Effect of ethanol on energy expenditure. *Am J Physiol.* 1994;266(4 Pt 2):R1204-R1212.

100. Davies MJ, Baer DJ, Judd JT, Brown ED, Campbell WS, Taylor PR. Effects of moderate alcohol intake on fasting insulin and glucose concentrations and insulin sensitivity in postmenopausal women: a randomized controlled trial. *JAMA.* 2002;287:2559-2562.

101. Hellerstedt WL, Jeffery RW, Murray DM. The association between alcohol intake and adiposity in the general population. *Am J Epidemiol.* 1990;132:594-611.

102. Suter PM. Is alcohol consumption a risk factor for weight gain and obesity? *Crit Rev Clin Lab Sci.* 2005;42:197-227.

103. Liu S, Serdula MK, Williamson DF, Mokdad AH, Byers T. A prospective study of alcohol intake and change in body weight among US adults. *Am J Epidemiol.* 1994;140:912-920.

104. Wannamethee SG, Shaper AG. Alcohol, body weight, and weight gain in middle-aged men. *Am J Clin Nutr.* 2003;77:1312-1317.

105. Lewis CE, Smith DE, Wallace DD, Williams OD, Bild DE, Jacobs DR Jr. Seven-year trends in body weight and associations with lifestyle and behavioral characteristics in black and white young adults: the CARDIA study. *Am J Public Health.* 1997;87: 635-642.

106. Wannamethee SG, Field AE, Colditz GA, Rimm EB. Alcohol intake and 8-year weight gain in women: a prospective study. *Obes Res.* 2004;12:1386-1396.

107. Togo P, Osler M, Sorensen TI, Heitmann BL. Food intake patterns and body mass index in observational studies. *Int J Obes Relat Metab Disord.* 2001;25:1741-1751.

108. Newby PK, Muller D, Hallfrisch J, Andres R, Tucker KL. Food patterns measured by factor analysis and anthropometric changes in adults. *Am J Clin Nutr.* 2004;80:504-513.

109. Newby PK, Muller D, Hallfrisch J, Qiao N, Andres R, Tucker KL. Dietary patterns and changes in body mass index and waist circumference in adults. *Am J Clin Nutr.* 2003;77:1417-1425.

110. Schulz M, Noethlings U, Hoffmann K, Bergmann MM, Boeing H. Identification of a food pattern characterized by high-fiber and low-fat food choices associated with low prospective weight change in the EPIC-Potsdam cohort. *J Nutr.* 2005;135(5): 1183-1189.

111. Schulze MB, Fung TT, Manson JE, Willett WC, Hu FB. Dietary patterns and changes in body weight in women. *Obesity (Silver Spring).* 2006;14:1444-1453.

112. Cummings DE, Purnell JQ, Frayo RS, Schmidova K, Wisse BE, Weigle DS. A preprandial rise in plasma ghrelin levels suggests a role in meal initiation in humans. *Diabetes.* 2001;50:1714-1719.

113. Boyle PJ, Shah SD, Cryer PE. Insulin, glucagon, and catecholamines in prevention of hypoglycemia during fasting. *Am J Physiol.* 1989;256(5 Pt 1):E651-E661.

114. Nakazato M, Murakami N, Date Y, et al. A role for ghrelin in the central regulation of feeding. *Nature.* 2001;409:194-198.
115. Wren AM, Seal LJ, Cohen MA, et al. Ghrelin enhances appetite and increases food intake in humans. *J Clin Endocrinol Metab.* 2001;86:5992.
116. Farshchi HR, Taylor MA, Macdonald IA. Deleterious effects of omitting breakfast on insulin sensitivity and fasting lipid profiles in healthy lean women. *Am J Clin Nutr.* 2005;81:388-396.
117. Melanson KJ, Westerterp-Plantenga MS, Saris WH, Smith FJ, Campfield LA. Blood glucose patterns and appetite in time-blinded humans: carbohydrate versus fat. *Am J Physiol.* 1999;277(2 Pt 2):R337-R345.
118. Cho S, Dietrich M, Brown CJ, Clark CA, Block G. The effect of breakfast type on total daily energy intake and body mass index: results from the Third National Health and Nutrition Examination Survey (NHANES III). *J Am Coll Nutr.* 2003;22:296-302.
119. Ma Y, Bertone ER, Stanek EJ III, et al. Association between eating patterns and obesity in a free-living US adult population. *Am J Epidemiol.* 2003;158:85-92.
120. Song WO, Chun OK, Obayashi S, Cho S, Chung CE. Is consumption of breakfast associated with body mass index in US adults? *J Am Diet Assoc.* 2005;1373:82.
121. Ortega RM, Requejo AM, Lopez-Sobaler AM, et al. Difference in the breakfast habits of overweight/obese and normal weight schoolchildren. *Int J Vitam Nutr Res.* 1998;68:125-132.
122. Barton BA, Eldridge AL, Thompson D, et al. The relationship of breakfast and cereal consumption to nutrient intake and body mass index: the National Heart, Lung, and Blood Institute Growth and Health Study. *J Am Diet Assoc.* 2005;105:1383-1389.
123. Berkey CS, Rockett HR, Gillman MW, Field AE, Colditz GA. Longitudinal study of skipping breakfast and weight change in adolescents. *Int J Obes Relat Metab Disord.* 2003;27:1258-1266.
124. Bazzano LA, Song Y, Bubes V, Good CK, Manson JE, Liu S. Dietary intake of whole and refined grain breakfast cereals and weight gain in men. *Obes Res.* 2005;13:1952-1960.
125. Nooyens AC, Visscher TL, Schuit AJ, et al. Effects of retirement on lifestyle in relation to changes in weight and waist circumference in Dutch men: a prospective study. *Public Health Nutr.* 2005;8:1266-1274.
126. van der Heijden AA, Hu FB, Rimm EB, van Dam RM. A prospective study of breakfast consumption and weight gain among U.S. men. *Obesity (Silver Spring).* 2007;15:2463-2469.
127. Bowman SA, Gortmaker SL, Ebbeling CB, Pereira MA, Ludwig DS. Effects of fast-food consumption on energy intake and diet quality among children in a national household survey. *Pediatrics.* 2004;113(1 Pt 1):112-118.
128. Ebbeling CB, Sinclair KB, Pereira MA, Garcia-Lago E, Feldman HA, Ludwig DS. Compensation for energy intake from fast food among overweight and lean adolescents. *JAMA.* 2004;291:2828-2833.
129. Taveras EM, Berkey CS, Rifas-Shiman SL, et al. Association of consumption of fried food away from home with body mass index and diet quality in older children and adolescents. *Pediatrics.* 2005;116:e518-e524.
130. Pereira MA, Kartashov AI, Ebbeling CB, et al. Fast-food habits, weight gain, and insulin resistance (the CARDIA study): 15-year prospective analysis. *Lancet.* 2005;365:36-42.
131. French SA, Harnack L, Jeffery RW. Fast food restaurant use among women in the Pound of Prevention study: dietary, behavioral and demographic correlates. *Int J Obes Relat Metab Disord.* 2000;24:1353-1359.
132. Duffey KJ, Gordon-Larsen P, Jacobs DR Jr, Williams OD, Popkin BM. Differential associations of fast food and restaurant food consumption with 3-y change in body

mass index: the Coronary Artery Risk Development in Young Adults Study. *Am J Clin Nutr.* 2007;85:201-208.

133. Nielsen SJ, Popkin BM. Patterns and trends in food portion sizes, 1977-1998. *JAMA.* 2003;289:450-453.

134. Rolls BJ, Morris EL, Roe LS. Portion size of food affects energy intake in normal-weight and overweight men and women. *Am J Clin Nutr.* 2002;76:1207-1213.

135. Diliberti N, Bordi PL, Conklin MT, Roe LS, Rolls BJ. Increased portion size leads to increased energy intake in a restaurant meal. *Obes Res.* 2004;12:562-568.

136. McConahy KL, Smiciklas-Wright H, Birch LL, Mitchell DC, Picciano MF. Food portions are positively related to energy intake and body weight in early childhood. *J Pediatr.* 2002;140:340-347.

137. Ello-Martin JA, Ledikwe JH, Rolls BJ. The influence of food portion size and energy density on energy intake: implications for weight management. *Am J Clin Nutr.* 2005;82(1 Suppl):236S-241S.

138. Bes-Rastrollo M, van Dam RM, Li TY, Sampson L, Hu FB. A prospective study of dietary energy density and weight gain in women. Submitted 2007.

139. Rolls BJ, Roe LS, Meengs JS. Reductions in portion size and energy density of foods are additive and lead to sustained decreases in energy intake. *Am J Clin Nutr.* 2006;83:11-17.

140. Drewnowski A, Darmon N. The economics of obesity: dietary energy density and energy cost. *Am J Clin Nutr.* 2005;82(1 Suppl):265S-273S.

141. Howarth NC, Murphy SP, Wilkens LR, Hankin JH, Kolonel LN. Dietary energy density is associated with overweight status among 5 ethnic groups in the multiethnic cohort study. *J Nutr.* 2006;136:2243-2248.

142. Ledikwe JH, Blanck HM, Kettel Khan L, et al. Dietary energy density is associated with energy intake and weight status in US adults. *Am J Clin Nutr.* 2006;83: 1362-1368.

143. Kant AK, Graubard BI. Energy density of diets reported by American adults: association with food group intake, nutrient intake, and body weight. *Int J Obes (London).* 2005;29:950-956.

144. de Castro JM. Dietary energy density is associated with increased intake in free-living humans. *J Nutr.* 2004;134:335-341.

145. Iqbal SI, Helge JW, Heitmann BL. Do energy density and dietary fiber influence subsequent 5-year weight changes in adult men and women? *Obesity (Silver Spring).* 2006;14:106-114.

15

Physical Activity, Sedentary Behaviors, and Obesity

Frank B. Hu

The role of physical activity in body weight regulation has long been recognized. In 1940, Bruch[1] observed much lower physical activity and energy expenditure among obese children than among those of normal body weight. In 1956, Johnson et al.[2] suggested that physical inactivity was more important than overeating in the development of obesity in high school girls. Since the 1950s, Morris and colleagues conducted a series of landmark epidemiologic investigations[3-5] on the relationship between physical activity and coronary heart disease that spurred great interest in physical activity and prevention of chronic diseases (many of which are caused by obesity). In the past several decades, extensive research has been devoted to the role of physical activity in weight control. However, most randomized trials have focused on the effects of exercise on weight loss among overweight and obese persons rather than on the prevention of weight gain in the general population.

Because primary prevention of weight gain is more effective than weight loss in reducing obesity rates, it is critical to understand the role of physical activity in reducing age-related weight gain. Most evidence on weight gain prevention is derived from epidemiologic studies. As with studies of dietary factors and obesity (see Chapter 14), many methodological issues can complicate epidemiologic studies of physical activity and obesity, including inaccurate and imprecise measurements of physical activity and adiposity, reverse causation (i.e., physical inactivity caused by weight gain and obesity), confounding by diet and other lifestyle factors, and different analytic strategies for longitudinal data. Nonetheless, cumulative evidence from prospective cohort studies and randomized clinical trials indicates that physical activity and active lifestyle play an important role in weight control, probably mediated through multiple pathways including increasing total energy expenditure, reducing fat mass, maintaining lean body mass and basal metabolic rate, and increasing psychosocial well-being and thus compliance to physical activity regimens (Fig. 15.1).

In this chapter, we review epidemiologic studies on the relationship between physical activity, sedentary behaviors, and obesity, focusing on the role of increasing physical activity in preventing age-related increases in overall adiposity (reflected by weight gain) and abdominal obesity (reflected by waist gain). Although weight loss is not a main focus of this chapter, we briefly review randomized controlled studies of exercise training and weight loss and maintenance among overweight and obese subjects. Finally, we discuss methodological issues in epidemiologic studies of physical activity and obesity. Issues related to validity of various physical activity assessment methods are discussed in detail in Chapter 7 and will not be repeated here.

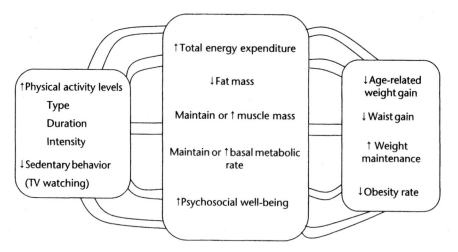

Figure 15.1 Potential pathways through which physical activity and sedentary behavior influence obesity rate and weight gain.

Patterns and Time Trends of Physical Activity

Brownson et al.[6] conducted a comprehensive review of time trends of physical activity in the United States. The study showed that leisure-time physical activity (LTPA) has been relatively stable, or slightly increasing, but activities related to work, transportation, and household chores have all declined substantially. In contrast, sedentary behaviors (e.g., watching television and computer use) have increased dramatically. These changes have led to an overall decline in total physical activity.

In the United States, research on national LTPA levels has been conducted primarily through the Behavioral Risk Factor Surveillance System (BRFSS). In the 1990-2000 BRFSS questionnaire, participants were asked to respond to the following question: "During the past month, did you participate in any physical activities, such as running, calisthenics, golf, gardening, or walking for exercise?" If the response was "yes," the participant was asked about the most common activities and their frequency and duration. These data were used to calculate the percentage of people meeting levels of physical activity recommended by the CDC (30 minutes of moderate physical activity at least five times per week or 20 consecutive minutes of vigorous activity at least three times per week). After year 2000, the physical activity question has been modified to ask about both moderate- and vigorous-intensity activities "in a usual week."[7]

In 2000, 26.2% of U.S. adults were engaged in recommended levels of LTPA. Men (27.1%) were slightly more active than women (25.5%), and non-Hispanic whites (27.5%) were more likely to meet the recommendations than non-Hispanic blacks (21.9%) and Hispanics (21.1%). College-educated individuals were more likely to meet the recommendations (34.2%) than those with less than 12 years of education (14.5%). LTPA was the highest in Hawaii (34.8%) and the Western states (e.g., Washington [32.4%] and Oregon [32.4%]). It was lowest in Southern states, such as Kentucky (17.7%), Louisiana (18.3%), and Mississippi (21.3%).

Between 1990 and 2000, there was a modest increase in the number of men and women who met recommended levels of LTPA (Fig. 15.2). The relative improvement during the 10-year period was greater for men (9.7%) than women (5.8%). Time trends showed a pattern that varied according to education level: while there was a relative increase of 8.9% for people with a college education, the percentage of those meeting the recommended LTPA decreased by 7.6% for those with less than 12 years of education. LTPA had increased slightly for whites and blacks, but decreased for Hispanic adults.

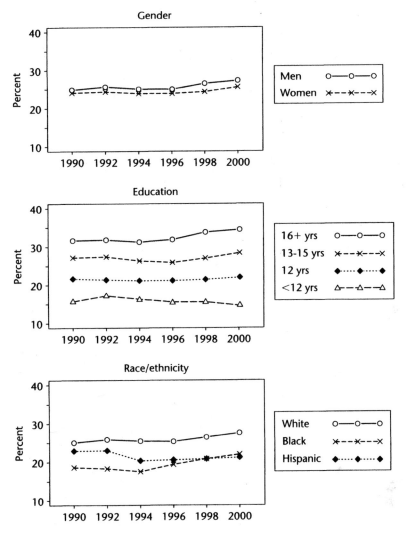

Figure 15.2 Trends in recommended physical activity, United States, 1990-2000. From Brownson, Boehmer, and Luke. *Annu Rev Public Health.* 2005;26:421-443.[6]

The BRFSS is useful in monitoring LTPA trends because of the consistency of questionnaires over time, the large and representative sample, and the availability of data for different states and various ethnic groups.[6] However, the survey is based on telephone interviews, and, thus, the slight increasing trend in LTPA may reflect self-reported bias due to the growing social desirability of physical activity. Low-income individuals are also underrepresented in the survey because they are less likely to have a telephone. Another problem is the change in physical activity questionnaires after the year 2000, making the time trend data difficult to interpret. According to more recent BRFSS data (2001-2005), nearly half of the U.S. adult population reported to be engaging in recommended levels of LTPA in 2005 (http://www.cdc.gov/nccdphp/dupa/physical/stats/index.htm). It is unlikely that LTPA had increased dramatically within a short period of time. Instead, this increase may be largely artificial owing to changes in physical activity questionnaires after the year 2000. Nonetheless, from 2001 to 2005, the prevalence of regular physical activity (defined as at least 30 minutes a day of moderate-intensity activity on 5 or more days a week, or at least 20 minutes a day of vigorous-intensity activity on 3 or more days a week, or both) increased 8.6% among women (from 43.0% to 46.7%) and 3.5% among men (from 48.0% to 49.7%). The increase was greatest for non-Hispanic black women (a 15.0% increase; from 31.4% to 36.1%) and non-Hispanic black men (a 12.4% increase; from 40.3% to 45.3%).[7]

According to data from BRFSS, the proportion of the U.S. population that reported no LTPA (such as running, calisthenics, golf, gardening, or walking) in the previous month decreased from about 31% in 1989 to about 25% in 2005 (http://www.cdc.gov/nccdphp/dupa/physical/stats/index.htm).

As discussed in Chapter 7, LTPA accounts for only a small part of total physical activity energy expenditure. Thus, it is important to examine time trends of other types of physical activity, including occupational, household, and transportation activity. Estimates—based on data from the Bureau of Labor Statistics, the U.S. Census Bureau, and job classifications in a study by King et al.[8]—show that in the past 50 years, the percentage of the labor force in high-activity occupations (e.g., farm workers, waiters and waitresses, construction laborers, and cleaning-service workers) declined from approximately 30% in 1950 to 23% in 2000.[7] Conversely, the percentage of the labor force in low-activity occupations (e.g., executives, administrators, managers, teachers, researchers, clerks, and motor vehicle operators) rose from 23% in 1950 to 42% in 2000.

The shift in job categories, combined with increasing automation and computer use, has led to a substantial decline in occupational physical activity energy expenditure. Another major contributor to the decline in overall physical activity is the dramatic increase in the use of automobiles for both work- and nonwork-related travels, a trend accompanied by a decline in walking or use of public transportation. The proportion of the population living in suburbs or "urban sprawl" has more than doubled in the past several decades to nearly 50% in 2000, contributing to increased driving and decreased walking or use of other means of transportation.[6]

Concurrent with the declines in overall physical activity energy expenditure, sedentary behavior has increased dramatically. TV watching is a major sedentary behavior in the United States; an adult male spends an average of 29 hours/week watching TV and an adult female, 34 hours/week.[9] In parallel with increasing obesity, the past five decades have seen a steady increase in the number of hours spent watching TV and using computers.

To sum up, although time trend data show that LTPA has not decreased, and may have even increased moderately, this increase has not compensated for the substantial declines in occupational, household, and transportation activities. Thus, overall physical activity in the population has decreased considerably.

Ecological and Cross-Sectional Studies of Physical Activity and Obesity

Prentice and Jebb[10] examined the relationship between physical activity and time trends of obesity in Britain. Similar to the secular trends in the United States, increased car ownership and TV viewing were closely related to the growing prevalence of obesity over time. A strong inverse association between social class and prevalence of obesity appeared to be explained by patterns of physical inactivity rather than by changes in dietary fat. Such analyses, however, are affected by simultaneous changes in other dietary and lifestyle factors and should, therefore, be kept in perspective. Nonetheless, the secular decline in physical activity that coincides with increasing obesity rates has been observed in many societies.

Ewing et al.[11] conducted an ecological analysis of the relationship between urban sprawl and physical activity and obesity using data from BRFSS (including 448 counties and 83 metropolitan areas). Sprawl indices derived through principal components analysis from census and other data reflected low residential density in suburban areas. In a multilevel analysis controlling for demographic and behavioral covariates, a higher county sprawl index was associated with decreased time spent walking ($P = .004$) and increased prevalence of obesity ($P < .001$) and hypertension ($P = .018$). These ecological data support the notion that physical environment impacts obesity rates by influencing physical activity (see Chapter 17 for more detailed discussions on urban sprawl and obesity).

At the individual level, numerous cross-sectional studies have examined the relationship between physical activity and obesity. Most have shown an association between higher levels of physical activity and lower body weight. In general, higher-intensity activity was more strongly associated with body weight than moderate- or low-intensity activity. For example, Bernstein et al.[12] demonstrated a clear dose-response relationship between high-intensity activities and lower odds of being obese, but the relationship for moderate-intensity activities was not as clear. Other data, however, have shown an inverse association between walking distance or steps and body weight.[13] Several cross-sectional analyses also found an inverse association between physical activity and waist circumference or waist-to-hip ratio.[14,15] Most studies have focused on LTPA. In one cross-sectional analysis of an NHANES III sample, King et al.[8] found that both LTPA and occupational activity were associated with a lower prevalence of obesity, but the association was stronger for LTPA than for occupational activity.

Several studies have reported a correlation between objectively measured physical activity and adiposity. Chan et al.[16] found an inverse association between pedometer-determined steps per day and body mass index (BMI) ($r = -.40$, $P < .0001$) in all participants and waist circumference in females only ($r = -.43$, $P < .0001$). Accelerometer-measured physical activity has also been associated with lower BMI[17,18] and body fatness.[19]

Several cross-sectional analyses found a strong positive association between time spent watching TV and prevalence of obesity.[20,21] In the Health Professionals' Follow-up Study (HPFS), men who watched 41 or more hours of TV/VCR per week were four times more likely to be overweight than were those who watched no more than 1 hour/week.[22] A strong positive association between time spent watching TV and BMI was also found among middle-aged and older women in the Nurses' Health Study (NHS).[23]

Despite a consistent relationship between physical activity and adiposity in cross-sectional studies, interpretation of these data is hampered because of the temporal relationship, and thus direction of the association cannot be determined. One obvious problem is reverse causation; that is, lower physical activity and increased sedentary behaviors among the obese may be the consequence of carrying too much weight. Obese people are also more likely to be socially stigmatized and thus excluded from sports activities because they are less physically fit. In many studies, the cross-sectional associations between physical activity and obesity are substantially stronger than those in prospective studies (discussed below). The cross-sectional associations may thus reflect a combination of the true effects of physical activity as well as artificial effects due to reverse causation and confounding by diet and other lifestyle factors.

Prospective Studies of Physical Activity and Obesity

Physical Activity and Prevention of Age-Related Weight Gain

Midlife weight gain is a widespread phenomenon in most populations. Hill et al.[24] estimated that U.S. adults have been gaining an average of 0.45 to 0.90 kg/year over the past decades since the start of the obesity epidemic. Similarly, Brown et al.[25]

estimated that middle-aged Australian women add an average of 0.5 kg/year. For most people, midlife weight gain reflects increased body fat, sometimes accompanied by loss of lean body mass with aging. Because weight loss and maintenance are very difficult for obese individuals, finding ways to prevent age-related weight gain is of critical importance.

In the past two to three decades, many prospective cohort studies have examined the relationship between physical activity and weight gain. In 2000, Fogelholm and Kukkonen-Harjula[26] conducted a systematic review of 16 cohort studies on physical activity and weight gain. The follow-up of these studies ranged from 2 to 21 years. Most of the studies have focused on LTPA measured by various physical activity questionnaires. Several studies found that higher physical activity at baseline predicted less weight gain,[27-33] but this finding was not seen in other studies.[34-36] Interestingly, several studies reported a significant inverse association between physical activity at follow-up (rather than at baseline) and long-term weight gain,[37,38] suggesting that weight gain led to changes in physical activity.

In 2005, Wareham et al.[39] conducted a systematic review of 14 cohort studies on physical activity and weight gain published since 2000. The follow-up periods ranged from 3 to 10 years. Twelve studies examined physical activity by means of self-report;[23,40-50] two included an objective measure to assess physical activity.[51,52]

This systematic review found that the more recent studies showed more consistent findings on physical activity and weight gain than the studies reviewed by Fogelholm and Kukkonen-Harjula,[26] although the effects were, in general, modest. Two factors may have contributed to the positive findings in more recent studies. First, the studies were much larger than the earlier ones and thus had more power to detect relatively small effects. Second, the more recent studies were better designed because investigators were able to examine the association between longitudinal changes in physical activity and body weight rather than simply the association between baseline physical activity and subsequent weight gain. Another possibility is related to improvement in physical activity assessment instruments; recent studies have used more detailed and validated physical activity questionnaires to assess activity levels.

Since the review by Wareham et al.,[39] five additional prospective studies have been published. Four of these identified a significant inverse association between physical activity and weight or waist gain;[25,50,53,54] one did not.[55] As with earlier studies, the observed associations were generally modest. The changes in physical activity and weight gain since adolescence were examined by two additional studies.[56,57] In one study, Parsons et al.[56] found that physical activity at 11 years of age had no relationship with BMI trajectories. However, there was an inverse association between physical activity at 16 years of age and weight gain between 16 and 45 years of age in females but not in males. In another study,[57] physical activity reported by children 9 to 18 years old was not directly associated with waist circumference in adulthood during 21 years of follow-up. However, youth physical activity had an indirect effect on adult waist circumference through its correlation with adult physical activity.

Heterogeneity among study designs—particularly with respect to age groups of participants, analytic strategies, and outcome assessment—makes it a challenge to summarize all the studies quantitatively. Thus, we review here several recent large reports with data on repeated measures of physical activity and weight. In 1998, Coakley et al.[32] examined longitudinal predictors of weight change among 19,478 men aged 40 to 75 years in the HPFS from 1988 to 1992. In this cohort of middle-aged and older men, vigorous activity was associated with weight reduction, while TV/VCR viewing and eating between meals were associated with weight gain. Quitting smoking and a history of voluntary

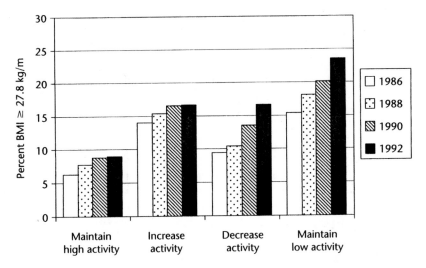

Figure 15.3 Prevalence of obesity (BMI ≥ 27.8) over time for different patterns of recreational vigorous physical activity. This figure is based on 3,666 nonsmoking, nonhypertensive, and nonhypercholesterolemic men aged 45 to 54 years (in 1986). From Coakley EH, Rimm EB, Colditz G, Kawachi I, Willett W. Predictors of weight change in men: results from the Health Professionals Follow-up Study. *Int J Obes Relat Metab Disord.* 1998;22:89-96.[32]

weight loss prior to the study period were consistently related to greater weight gain. The association between vigorous activity and TV watching and weight gain was stronger for younger men than older men.

Over the 4-year follow-up period, men who increased vigorous exercise (including jogging, running, lap swimming, bicycling and rowing, calisthenics and racquet sports) to 1.5 hour/week, decreased TV viewing, and stopped eating between meals, lost an average of 1.4 kg, compared with a weight gain of 1.4 kg in the overall cohort. Those who maintained a relatively high level of vigorous physical activity over time (at least 1.5 hour/week) had the lowest prevalence of obesity as well as the smallest increase in body weight (Fig. 15.3). These data suggest that both maintaining vigorous activity and decreasing TV use are important to prevent weight gain over 4 years.

Schmitz et al.[58] examined the longitudinal relationship between changes in physical activity and weight gain during 10 years of follow-up among 5115 black and white men and women aged 18-30 years at baseline in the Coronary Artery Risk Development in Young Adults (CARDIA) Study. After adjustment for secular trends, age, and other covariates, increasing physical activity was significantly associated with less weight gain in the entire four race and sex subgroups. Specifically, increasing high-intensity activity (requiring 6 MET hours) by 2 hours/week offset the expected weight gain with age for all groups but black men. The benefits of exercise in preventing weight gain were much greater for obese subjects than for those of normal weight at baseline. In addition, an increase in physical activity in the first 2 to 3 years of follow-up was associated with a slowing of weight gain during the subsequent 5-year follow-up.

Wagner et al.[44] examined LTPA and regular walking or cycling to work and 5-year weight gain in a cohort of 8865 men aged 50 to 59 years. After adjustment for age, smoking, alcohol use, education level, and other potential confounders, high-intensity (≥ MET hours) but not low-intensity LTPA was significantly associated with reduced weight gain. In addition, men who regularly spent more than 10 MET hours/week walking or cycling to work had significantly lower BMI at baseline and less weight gain during follow-up than those who did not walk or cycle to work.

Kawachi et al.[59] examined whether exercise could modify weight gain after smoking cessation in women during a 2-year follow-up period (1986-1988) in the NHS. Among those who smoked 1 to 24 cigarettes per day in 1986, quitting smoking was associated with an average of 2.3 kg of additional weight gain. However, women who quit smoking and increased exercise had attenuated weight gain: increasing exercise by 8 to 16 MET hours/week reduced average weight gain by 0.5 kg; increasing it by more than 16 MET hours/week reduced average weight gain by 1.0 kg. Among heavy smokers in 1986 ($\geq$25 cigarettes/day), higher levels of exercise reduced weight gain by 1.6 kg during the 2-year follow-up. This study suggests that increasing exercise can substantially attenuate weight gain associated with stopping smoking.

In a subsequent analysis of data from the NHS,[23] we examined the relationship between walking, sedentary behavior (especially prolonged TV watching), and risk of obesity and type 2 diabetes among 50,277 healthy nonobese women at baseline in 1992. In multivariate analyses adjusting for age, smoking, exercise level, dietary factors, and other covariates, each 1 hour/day increment in brisk walking was associated with a 24% (95% CI: 19% to 29%) reduction in incidence of obesity. Standing or walking around at home (2 hours/day) were associated with a 9% (6% to 12%) reduction in obesity. In contrast, each 2 hours/day increment in TV watching was associated with a 23% (17% to 30%) increase in obesity; and each 2 hours/day increment in sitting at work was associated with a 5% (0% to 10%) increase in obesity.

Droyvold et al.[48] examined the association between self-reported LTPA at baseline and change in BMI among 8305 normal-weight men aged 20 to 69 years during an 11-year follow-up period. Men who were physically active were less likely to gain weight than sedentary men. Among those who were active, self-reported higher intensity of physical activity was associated with less weight gain than lower intensity (weight gain attenuation was about 0.27 BMI unit or 0.86 kg at a height of 178 cm). Among normal-weight women in the same cohort,[50] those with higher levels of physical activity at baseline gained 0.18 BMI units less than women with low levels of physical activity.

Several prospective studies have used objectively measured physical activity or fitness to predict weight gain over time. DiPietro et al.[54] examined the relationship between changes in cardiorespiratory fitness and weight gain in the Aerobics Center Longitudinal Study. Change in fitness, calculated as the difference in maximal treadmill time between the first and second examination (mean interval, 1.8 years), was used to predict body weight change between the first and last examination (mean follow-up, 7.5 years). In multivariate analyses, each 1-minute improvement in treadmill time significantly reduced the risk of a major weight gain of 10 kg or greater by 21% in both men and women.

Ekelund et al.[52] examined the association between physical activity energy expenditure measured by heart rate monitoring and changes in body composition assessed by bioimpedance among 311 men and 428 women (median age, 53.8 years). Among younger participants (<54 years old) followed for 5.6 years, higher physical activity energy expenditure at baseline was associated with a smaller increase in body fat; in older participants, there was a significant positive association between baseline physical activity and increased body fat, lean body mass, and body weight. These results suggest that physical activity reduces gain in body fat in middle-aged people and also preserves fat-free mass in older adults.

In a small study of adult Pima Indians ($n = 94$),[51] weight gain was positively associated with total energy intake assessed by doubly labeled water and inversely associated with resting metabolic rate (RMR) assessed by indirect calorimetry. However, baseline physical activity energy expenditure was not significantly associated with changes in body weight.

Physical Activity and Prevention of Waist Gain

Weight gain in middle-aged adults often results from accumulation of abdominal adiposity, reflected by increased waist circumference. This phenomenon is more common in males than females, who tend to deposit fat in the hips and thighs. Abdominal adiposity has been strongly associated with metabolic diseases, cardiovascular diseases, and mortality (see Chapters 7 to 9 and 11). Thus, prevention of waist gain in middle-aged adults is critical to reduce risk of chronic diseases and premature mortality.

Although many cross-sectional studies have shown an inverse association between physical activity and waist circumference, few prospective cohort studies have examined the impact of physical activity on waist gain. Koh-Banerjee et al.[46] conducted a prospective study of the association between changes in physical activity and diet and 9-year gain in waist circumference among 16,587 men in the HPFS. During the 9-year follow-up period, the mean ($\pm$SD) waist circumference increased 3.3 $\pm$ 6.2 cm. After control for baseline BMI, waist circumference, and other covariates, increases of 25-MET hours/week in vigorous physical activity and $\geq$0.5 hours/week in weight training were associated with 0.38 and 0.91 cm decreases in waist circumference, respectively ($P < .001$). Reduction of TV watching by 20 hours/week was associated with a 0.59 cm decrease in waist circumference. These results suggest that increasing physical activity (especially weight training) and reducing sedentary behavior can offset age-related waist gain.

Sternfeld et al.[53] examined the relationship between physical activity and changes in body weight and waist circumference among 3,064 healthy women aged 42 to 52 years. Over 3 years of follow-up, mean weight increased by 2.1 kg (SD $\pm$ 4.8) and mean waist circumference increased by 2.2 cm (SD $\pm$ 5.4). Increases in both sports/exercise and daily routine physical activity, such as walking or biking, were associated with smaller gains in weight and waist circumference over time.

Physical Activity and Weight Maintenance after Weight Loss

Weight regain following cessation of a weight loss program is a common phenomenon. Wing and Hill[60] estimated that only 20% of overweight or obese people experienced successful weight maintenance (defined as an intentional weight loss of $\geq$10% of initial body weight that is maintained for $\geq$1 year). Short-term clinical trials have shown that physical activity intervention can improve the success of weight maintenance,[60] but long-term observational data are limited. van Baak et al.[61] examined the role of LTPA in long-term weight maintenance after weight loss in the Sibutramine Trial on Obesity Reduction and Maintenance (STORM trial) ($n = 261$). The STORM trial included a 6-month, open-label, run-in, weight loss phase, followed by an 18-month, double-blind, randomized, placebo-controlled, weight maintenance phase. During the 18-month weight maintenance period (among subjects who completed the trial), 43% of those in the sibutramine-treated group maintained $\geq$80% of their original weight loss compared with only 16% of those in the placebo-treated group. However, there were large interindividual variations in weight maintenance in both groups. Thus, an observational analysis was conducted to examine predictors of weight loss maintenance.

In multivariate analyses, three factors were identified as significant determinants of weight maintenance: treatment group (sibutramine vs. placebo), the percentage of the initial body weight lost during the 6-month weight loss phase, and the LTPA index measured at 12 to 24 months. Higher LTPA reflected increased walking and cycling and less TV watching. During the course of the study, LTPA and total physical activity increased, perhaps due to exercise advice given to all participants at baseline. However, it is also possible that greater weight loss caused by sibutramine led to an increase in subsequent physical activity. Thus, this analysis was unable to tease out the direction of the association between physical activity and weight maintenance success.

Physical Activity and Attenuation of Weight Loss in Older People

Weight loss in older people often results from a loss in lean body mass, including muscle mass and bone. Although it is well-known that decline in physical activity contributes to muscle loss in the elderly, whether increasing physical activity can attenuate aging-related weight loss in older persons is unclear. Dziura et al.[62] examined the longitudinal association between physical activity and 12-year weight change in an older cohort ($\geq$65 years of age). The multivariate analyses showed that an increasing baseline total activity score was associated with smaller weight loss over time, especially among those with chronic disease at baseline. These results suggest that physical activity can attenuate weight loss caused by chronic disease in older people. However, higher physical activity may also reflect better functional status at baseline, which could confound the analysis between baseline physical activity and subsequent weight loss.

Controlled Trials of Exercise Training and Weight Loss and Weight Gain Prevention

Numerous randomized clinical trials have been conducted to examine the effects of physical activity on weight loss and maintenance among overweight and obese subjects. Several comprehensive reviews or meta-analyses have summarized the published studies. Miller et al.[63] reviewed 493 intervention studies of diet, exercise, or diet plus exercise on weight loss among overweight and obese subjects. Overall, exercise had a small effect on weight loss. Average weight lost through diet, exercise, and diet plus exercise was 10.7 $\pm$ 0.5, 2.9 $\pm$ 0.4, and 11.0 $\pm$ 0.6 kg, respectively. At 1-year follow-up, diet plus exercise tended to be superior to dietary intervention alone. A recent meta-analysis of longer-term weight loss[64] also found that the combined intervention of diet and exercise resulted in a greater sustained weight loss after 1 year than diet alone (6.7 vs. 4.5 kg).

Wing[65] conducted a narrative review of controlled studies on physical activity and weight loss. Most randomized studies (6 out of 10) found significantly greater weight loss in exercise-alone groups versus controls, but the magnitude of the effect was small (1 to 2 kg average weight loss). Diet plus exercise produced greater initial weight loss compared to diet only, but the difference reached statistical significance in only 2 of 13 studies. All six studies on long-term weight maintenance of 1 year or more showed greater weight loss for diet plus exercise versus diet alone, but only two studies reached statistical significance. Most trials suffered from methodological problems (e.g., small sample sizes, short study duration, and poor adherence to the exercise prescriptions).

Although exercise alone has only a small effect on weight loss, it may preserve lean body mass. In a meta-analysis of 28 trials, Garrow and Summerbell[66] found that aerobic exercise attenuated the amount of weight lost as lean body mass compared with dietary restriction. With the same amount of total weight loss, exercise reduced lean body mass loss by 41% in men and 23% in women. In addition, although resistance training had little effect on weight loss, it increased lean body mass by about 2 kg in men and 1 kg in women.

Controlled trials on the effects of exercise on preventing weight gain in middle-aged or younger adults are limited. A narrative review of seven trials using physical activity and lifestyle intervention programs found inconsistent results (four of the studies showed significantly less weight gain), but most of the studies were small and had multicomponent intervention programs.[39] In the Midwest Exercise Trial,[67] moderate-intensity exercise (45 minutes/day, 5 days/week) prevented weight gain in young overweight women and induced significant weight loss in young overweight men (5.2 kg over 16 months). These results support the benefits of moderate-intensity exercise for weight control in young adults. However, a major limitation of this study was a low completion rate of only 54%.

Methodological Issues in Epidemiologic Studies of Physical Activity and Obesity

Several authors have discussed the methodological issues in epidemiologic studies of physical activity and obesity.[26,39] In cross-sectional studies, an obvious problem is that the direction of the association is unclear. Other problems include confounding and measurement errors. However, even with prospective cohort studies, these challenges remain. Here we discuss several common methodological problems in cohort studies of physical activity and obesity.

Measurement Errors

Imperfect measurements of physical activity and body composition can obscure the association between these variables. Most studies use questionnaires to measure physical activity. While some questionnaires have been rigorously validated, others have unknown validity. As discussed in Chapter 7, self-reported physical activity is prone to errors from day-to-day variations, inaccurate memory and estimation, and biased recall associated with obesity status. In most studies, measurement errors resulting from such problems lessen the ability to observe a true association between physical activity and obesity, especially when it is only modest. Body weight is also self-reported in many studies, but with much greater accuracy and precision. However, changes in body weight or BMI do not distinguish changes in body fat from lean body mass, and thus, the commonly used outcome variable, weight gain, has a different meaning for younger and older people.

Multiple methods can help alleviate the impact of measurement errors on studies of physical activity and adiposity. As with diet, repeated measures of physical activity can reduce misclassifications of long-term physical activity that result from within-person variation. In a subsample of the HPFS, the association between physical activity and high-density lipoprotein (HDL) cholesterol levels was stronger when the average of activity from five questionnaires was used than that when only a single assessment of activity was used.[68] In addition, using the cumulative updating approach we observed a stronger inverse association between physical activity and risk of type 2 diabetes[69] and risk of coronary disease[70] compared to the analyses using only the baseline physical activity measurement.

Objectively measured physical activity may also improve the validity and precision of the measurement. However, objective measures (e.g., activity monitors, doubly labeled water [DLW] indirect calorimetry, fitness tests, and heart rate monitors) are expensive, and none of them capture all dimensions of physical activity (see Chapter 7). Several studies using objective measurements have not yielded stronger associations than those using validated questionnaires. Accelerometers enable the collection of real-time data on the frequency, duration, and intensity of all activities in free-living populations; but large day-to-day variations require recording over multiple days and weeks. To date, none of the large prospective studies of physical activity and obesity have used accelerometers to assess physical activity.

Lastly, measurement error correction methods can be used to correct for both random and systematic errors associated with physical activity measurements (see Chapter 7). However, such methods have rarely been used in epidemiologic studies of physical activity.

Reverse Causation

Body weight is an outcome that study participants can observe. As such, it can have a reciprocal influence on weight control behaviors (e.g., diet and physical activity). It is well-known that obese subjects tend to reduce physical activity and increase sedentary behaviors. Thus, a cross-sectional relationship between physical activity and obesity reflects a combination of the true relationship as well as an artificial one due to reverse causation. It is difficult to disentangle the true and artificial relationships. Prospective studies of physical activity and obesity can decrease the problem of reverse causation by measuring baseline physical activity before assessment of outcome (e.g., weight change). Nonetheless, reverse causation is not eliminated, especially in concurrent analyses of changes in physical activity and body weight, because people who are gaining weight may subsequently reduce physical activity during follow-up.

Several studies have suggested that current physical activity is more predictive of weight change than baseline physical activity. In the NHANES I Epidemiologic Follow-Up Study, Williamson et al.[38] found no relationship between baseline physical activity and subsequent weight gain. However, low recreational physical activity reported at the follow-up survey was strongly related to weight gain that had occurred during the study. Similarly, Petersen et al.[49] found no significant relation between physical activity at baseline and subsequent weight gain. In contrast, overweight at baseline significantly increased the odds ratio of later physical inactivity. These analyses indicate a reciprocal relationship between physical activity and obesity, making it difficult to tease out the direction of the association, even in longitudinal studies. Lagged analyses of changes in physical activity and weight gain can help minimize this problem. For example, in the CARDIA study, Schmitz et al.[58] found that an increase in physical activity in the early follow-up period was associated with attenuation of weight gain during subsequent follow-up.

Confounding

Longitudinal studies of physical activity and obesity are better able to control for confounding than cross-sectional studies, but they are still prone to confounding by diet and lifestyle factors associated with greater physical activity. Typically, people who are physically active tend to eat a healthier diet and be more health conscious. Thus, the benefits of increasing physical activity on body weight may reflect changes in other weight control behaviors, such as increasing fiber intake. Few epidemiologic studies have measured or controlled for dietary factors, and the possibility of residual confounding remains even with adjustments for dietary and lifestyle factors. In longitudinal analyses of changes in physical activity and weight gain, it is therefore important to control for both baseline covariates and changes in covariates over time to minimize residual confounding.

Because chronic diseases can lead to a decline in physical activity as well as weight loss, confounding by existing chronic diseases may distort a relationship between physical activity and obesity. It is therefore desirable to analyze the relationship between physical activity and weight gain in a healthy cohort that excludes those who report a diagnosis of chronic conditions (especially heart disease and cancer) at baseline or during follow-up. This often requires a very large initial sample. Another strategy is to conduct stratified analyses by the presence or absence of chronic diseases at baseline, especially in a cohort of older individuals. In this way, one can specifically examine whether physical activity attenuates weight loss among those who are fragile.

Longitudinal Data Analysis Strategies

The repeated measurements of physical activity and weight that are available in longitudinal studies provide opportunities to test various hypotheses regarding short-term and long-term effects of physical activity on obesity. Several common strategies have been employed to analyze the relationship between physical activity and body weight. First, baseline physical activity can be used to predict subsequent weight gain or onset of obesity during follow-up. For example, using data from the NHS, we examined whether walking and sedentary behaviors assessed in 1992 predicted incident obesity between 1992 and 1998 in women who were not obese at baseline.[23] This classic method clearly establishes the temporal relationship between the exposure (i.e., physical activity at baseline) and the outcome (weight gain or onset of obesity).

A second strategy, concurrent analyses of changes in physical activity and body weight over time, is also commonly used. Many studies reviewed above examined whether changes in physical activity predicted weight gain during follow-up. Such analyses mimic an intervention study by looking at the associations between changes in an exposure variable and changes in outcome. As discussed earlier, the reciprocal relationship between physical activity and body weight often makes it difficult to distinguish cause from effect. However, if more than two repeated measures are collected, a lagged analysis can be conducted to examine whether changes in physical activity in the early follow-up period predict subsequent weight change. With multiple time points, one can also compare weight trajectories of those who are consistently active with those who are consistently sedentary. For example, Coakley et al.[32] found that those who maintained high-activity levels had the lowest BMI at baseline and the smallest incremental increase in BMI over time, whereas those who maintained low-activity levels were not only heavier at baseline, but also experienced the greatest weight gain during follow-up.

The third strategy, random effects or mixed models, has become increasingly popular in analyzing the longitudinal relationship between physical activity and weight changes. This method has the advantage of examining both cross-sectional and longitudinal associations simultaneously while taking into account correlations among the repeated measures of the dependent variable.[71] It also offers flexibility in handling missing data with the assumption of missing at random (MAR).[72] In a typical longitudinal analysis, repeated measures of BMI or body weight are modeled as the dependent variable, while repeated measures of physical activity are entered as an independent variable along with repeated measures of other covariates. A random intercept is typically used to take into account correlations among repeated measures of weight. Two-way interactions of follow-up time with baseline physical activity can be used to estimate whether the trajectory of body weight varies with baseline physical activity levels. If repeated measures of weight change and physical activity are modeled, the interaction between follow-up time and changes in physical activity estimates the impact of changes in physical activity on trajectories of weight gain over time. To establish a clear temporal relationship, a time lag (e.g., 2 to 4 years) can be specified between changes in physical activity and changes in body weight.

Structural equation modeling (SEM), a statistical method used in testing prespecified conceptual models or pathways regarding multiple exposure and outcome variables,[73,74] has recently been used to analyze the relationship between physical activity in youth and adiposity in adulthood in a Finnish cohort.[57] In this study, youth physical activity was hypothesized to influence adult BMI both directly and indirectly through its impact on adult physical activity. The structural equation analysis indicated that both physical activity and obesity tracked from youth to adulthood. Adult physical activity, but not youth physical activity, was directly associated with adiposity in adulthood. These analyses suggest that the impact of physical activity in youth on adulthood obesity is primarily mediated through the maintenance of physical activity in adulthood. SEM is useful for testing specific pathways regarding how exposures such as physical activity influence body weight. The model fit can be evaluated by commonly accepted goodness of fit indices.[73,74] However, SEM is not flexible in controlling for a large number of covariates. Nonetheless, SEM technique has become increasingly popular in modeling psychosocial determinants of obesity (see Chapter 17 for more details).

Summary

As with diet, physical activity plays a critical role in maintaining energy balance and weight control. However, today's obesogenic food environment and sedentary lifestyles can easily tip the energy balance towards weight gain. For most overweight people, it is difficult to lose weight permanently through diet or exercise. Thus, prevention of weight gain is thought to be more effective than weight loss in reducing obesity rates. A key question is whether increasing physical activity can mitigate age-related weight gain in adults. Many epidemiologic studies have addressed this issue. Cross-sectional studies have shown a strong inverse association between physical activity and body weight, but the direction of causality is unclear in such studies. More than 30 prospective cohort studies have examined the association between physical activity and weight change over time. Even though the results are not entirely consistent, most studies have found that increasing physical activity attenuates gain in weight or waist circumference during midlife.

However, the effects of physical activity are generally modest, and increasing physical activity alone does not appear to completely prevent weight or waist gain. Most epidemiologic studies have focused on vigorous exercise or high-intensity activities. An important reason is that these activities are measured more accurately by questionnaires than light- to moderate-intensity activities. Nonetheless, several recent studies have demonstrated that regular walking or cycling can be effective in preventing obesity, especially in middle-aged and older women.

The biological mechanisms by which physical activity prevents weight gain are multiple, and may depend on the type and intensity of physical activity. Increasing energy expenditure by physical activity may help maintain energy balance, but most activities consume small amounts of energy, and it is not clear whether the added exercise is compensated by a later decline in physical activity. In addition, physical activity tends to increase appetite and overall energy intake. Thus, exercise training without dietary intervention has a relatively small effect on weight control. Aerobic exercise helps to maintain lean body mass but does not appear to increase RMR.[75] On the other hand, resistance training increases muscle mass and RMR, although it has little effect on weight loss. The positive effects of exercise on mood and psychosocial well-being may enhance adherence to exercise programs.

The optimal amount of exercise needed to prevent weight gain in adults is unclear, but appears to vary by age, sex, and energy intake.[76] Among male participants 40 to 75 years of age in the HPFS, increasing vigorous exercise to 1.5 hours/week attenuated weight gain but was insufficient to offset it completely.[32] However, increasing exercise, combined with reduced TV watching appeared to be sufficient to offset the expected weight gain during the 4 years of follow-up. In the CARDIA study, increasing high-intensity exercise (requiring 6 MET hours) by 2 hours/week above baseline physical activity was needed to offset observed weight gain for young adults aged 18 to 30 years.[58] Overall, the young adults needed to exercise an average of 4 to 5 hours/week to completely prevent weight gain.

These estimates are in broad agreement with those from the Aerobics Center Longitudinal Study,[77] which suggests that a daily physical activity level (PAL) at least 60% above the RMR (which can be achieved by 45 to 60 min/day of exercise) is necessary to maintain body weight in middle-aged adults. Thus, the amount of physical activity required to maintain a healthy weight may be higher than that recommended in current physical activity guidelines for prevention of chronic diseases; that is, 30 minutes or more of moderate-level activity on most days of the week.[78] Although this moderate level of physical activity can substantially lower risk of morbidity and mortality, most people need more activity (approximately 45 to 60 min/day) to prevent the transition from normal weight to overweight.[76,79] In addition, there is increasing evidence that reducing sedentary behaviors such as prolonged TV watching is beneficial for weight control independent of the amount of exercise. Therefore, public health recommendations for prevention of obesity and chronic disease should encourage not only increasing LPTA but also reducing sedentary behaviors.

Two reasons may explain why greater physical activity is required to maintain body weight. First, the current food environment encourages excess caloric intake and positive energy balance. Second, the lifestyle during non-LTPA time has become increasingly sedentary, a trend that will continue. Thus, in addition to encouraging individual behavioral changes, the physical environment needs to be changed in ways that are conducive to physical activity. For example, residential areas, workplaces, shopping areas, and schools should be made more activity-friendly through innovative architectural design and land use development.[7] In addition, sidewalks, bicycle trails, and recreational parks should be made readily available to foster walking, cycling, and other types of physical activity as part of daily routine (see Chapter 17 for more discussions of research on physical environmental factors).

References

1. Bruch H. Obesity in children. *Am J Dis Child.* 1940;60:1082.
2. Johnson ML, Burke BS, Mayer J. The prevalence and incidence of obesity in a cross-section of elementary and secondary school children. *Am J Clin Nutr.* 1956;4:231-238.
3. Morris JN, Heady JA, Raffle PA, Roberts CG, Parks JW. Coronary heart-disease and physical activity of work. *Lancet.* 1953;265:1111-1120.
4. Morris JN, Clayton DG, Everitt MG, Semmence AM, Burgess EH. Exercise in leisure time: coronary attack and death rates. *Br Heart J.* 1990;63:325-334.
5. Morris JN, Crawford MD. Coronary heart disease and physical activity of work; evidence of a national necropsy survey. *BMJ.* 1958;2:1485-1496.
6. Brownson R, Boehmer TK, Luke DA. Declining rates of physical activity in the United States: what are the contributors? *Annu Rev Public Health.* 2005;26:421-443.
7. Centers for Disease Control and Prevention (CDC). Prevalence of regular physical activity among adults—United States, 2001 and 2005. *MMWR Morb Mortal Wkly Rep.* 2007 Nov 23;56(46):1209-1212.
8. King GA, Fitzhugh EC, Bassett DR Jr, et al. Relationship of leisure-time physical activity and occupational activity to the prevalence of obesity. *Int J Obes Relat Metab Disord.* 2001;25:606-612.

9. *Nielsen Report on Television*. Northbrook, IL: AC Nielsen Co., Media Research Division; 1998.

10. Prentice AM, Jebb SA. Obesity in Britain: gluttony or sloth? *BMJ*. 1995;311:437-439.

11. Ewing R, Schmid T, Killingsworth R, Zlot A, Raudenbush S. Relationship between urban sprawl and physical activity, obesity, and morbidity. *Am J Health Promot*. 2003;18:47-57.

12. Bernstein MS, Costanza MC, Morabia A. Association of physical activity intensity levels with overweight and obesity in a population-based sample of adults. *Prev Med*. 2004;38:94-104.

13. Williams PT. Nonlinear relationships between weekly walking distance and adiposity in 27,596 women. *Med Sci Sports Exerc*. 2005;37:1893-1901.

14. Seidell JC, Cigolini M, Deslypere JP, Charzewska J, Ellsinger BM, Cruz A. Body fat distribution in relation to physical activity and smoking habits in 38-year-old European men. The European Fat Distribution Study. *Am J Epidemiol*. 1991;133:257-265.

15. Visser M, Launer LJ, Deurenberg P, Deeg DJ. Total and sports activity in older men and women: relation with body fat distribution. *Am J Epidemiol*. 1997;145:752-761.

16. Chan CB, Spangler E, Valcour J, Tudor-Locke C. Cross-sectional relationship of pedometer-determined ambulatory activity to indicators of health. *Obes Res*. 2003;11:1563-1570.

17. Cooper AR, Page A, Fox KR, Misson J. Physical activity patterns in normal, overweight and obese individuals using minute-by-minute accelerometry. *Eur J Clin Nutr*. 2000;54:887-894.

18. Yoshioka M, Ayabe M, Yahiro T, et al. Long-period accelerometer monitoring shows the role of physical activity in overweight and obesity. *Int J Obes (London)*. 2005;29:502-508.

19. Tucker LA, Peterson TR. Objectively measured intensity of physical activity and adiposity in middle-aged women. *Obes Res*. 2003;11:1581-1587.

20. Tucker LA, Friedman GM. Television viewing and obesity in adult males. *Am J Public Health*. 1989;79:516-518.

21. Tucker LA, Bagwell M. Television viewing and obesity in adult females. *Am J Public Health*. 1991;8:908-911.

22. Ching PL, Willett WC, Rimm EB, Colditz GA, Gortmaker SL, Stampfer MJ. Activity level and risk of overweight in male health professionals. *Am J Public Health*. 1996;86:25-30.

23. Hu FB, Li TY, Colditz GA, Willett WC, Manson JE. Television watching and other sedentary behaviors in relation to risk of obesity and type 2 diabetes mellitus in women. *JAMA*. 2003;289:1785-1791.

24. Hill JO, Wyatt HR, Reed GW, Peters JC. Obesity and the environment: where do we go from here? *Science*. 2003;299:853-855.

25. Brown WJ, Williams L, Ford JH, Ball K, Dobson AJ. Identifying the energy gap: magnitude and determinants of 5-year weight gain in midage women. *Obes Res*. 2005;13:1431-1441.

26. Fogelholm M, Kukkonen-Harjula K. Does physical activity prevent weight gain—a systematic review. *Obes Rev*. 2000;1:95-111.

27. Klesges RC, Klesges LM, Haddock CK, Eck LH. A longitudinal analysis of the impact of dietary intake and physical activity on weight change in adults. *Am J Clin Nutr*. 1992;55:818-822.

28. Owens JF, Matthews KA, Wing RR, Kuller LH. Can physical activity mitigate the effects of aging in middle-aged women? *Circulation*. 1992;85:1265-1270.

29. Taylor CB, Jatulis DE, Winkleby MA, Rockhill BJ, Kraemer HC. Effects of life-style on body mass index change. *Epidemiology*. 1994;5:599-603.

30. Kahn HS, Tatham LM, Rodriguez C, Calle EE, Thun MJ, Heath CW Jr. Stable behaviors associated with adults' 10-year change in body mass index and likelihood of gain at the waist. *Am J Public Health*. 1997;87:747-754.

31. Barefoot JC, Heitmann BL, Helms MJ, Williams RB, Surwit RS, Siegler IC. Symptoms of depression and changes in body weight from adolescence to mid-life. *Int J Obes Relat Metab Disord.* 1998;22:688-694.

32. Coakley EH, Rimm EB, Colditz G, Kawachi I, Willett W. Predictors of weight change in men: results from the Health Professionals Follow-up Study. *Int J Obes Relat Metab Disord.* 1998;22:89-96.

33. Fogelholm M, Kujala U, Kaprio J, Sarna S. Predictors of weight change in middle-aged and old men. *Obes Res.* 2000;8:367-373.

34. Heitmann BL, Kaprio J, Harris JR, Rissanen A, Korkeila M, Koskenvuo M. Are genetic determinants of weight gain modified by leisure-time physical activity? A prospective study of Finnish twins. *Am J Clin Nutr.* 1997;66:672-678.

35. Parker DR, Gonzalez S, Derby CA, Gans KM, Lasater TM, Carleton RA. Dietary factors in relation to weight change among men and women from two southeastern New England communities. *Int J Obes Relat Metab Disord.* 1997;21:103-109.

36. French SA, Jeffery RW, Murray D. Is dieting good for you?: Prevalence, duration and associated weight and behaviour changes for specific weight loss strategies over four years in US adults. *Int J Obes Relat Metab Disord.* 1999;23:320-327.

37. Rissanen AM, Heliovaara M, Knekt P, Reunanen A, Aromaa A. Determinants of weight gain and overweight in adult Finns. *Eur J Clin Nutr.* 1991;45:419-430.

38. Williamson DF, Madans J, Anda RF, Kleinman JC, Kahn HS, Byers T. Recreational physical activity and ten-year weight change in a US national cohort. *Int J Obes Relat Metab Disord.* 1993;17:279-286.

39. Wareham NJ, van Sluijs EM, Ekelund U. Physical activity and obesity prevention: a review of the current evidence. *Proc Nutr Soc.* 2005;64:229-247.

40. Rainwater DL, Mitchell BD, Comuzzie AG, VandeBerg JL, Stern MP, MacCluer JW. Association among 5-year changes in weight, physical activity, and cardiovascular disease risk factors in Mexican Americans. *Am J Epidemiol.* 2000;152:974-982.

41. Ainsworth BE, Haskell WL, Whitt MC, et al. Compendium of physical activities: an update of activity codes and MET intensities. *Med Sci Sports Exerc.* 2000;32(9 Suppl):S498-S504.

42. Sherwood NE, Jeffery RW, French SA, Hannan PJ, Murray DM. Predictors of weight gain in the Pound of Prevention study. *Int J Obes Relat Metab Disord.* 2000;24:395-403.

43. Bell AC, Ge K, Popkin BM. Weight gain and its predictors in Chinese adults. *Int J Obes Relat Metab Disord.* 2001;25:1079-1086.

44. Wagner A, Simon C, Ducimetiere P, et al. Leisure-time physical activity and regular walking or cycling to work are associated with adiposity and 5 y weight gain in middle-aged men: the PRIME Study. *Int J Obes Relat Metab Disord.* 2001;25:940-948.

45. Ball K, Brown W, Crawford D. Who does not gain weight? Prevalence and predictors of weight maintenance in young women. *Int J Obes Relat Metab Disord.* 2002;26:1570-1578.

46. Koh-Banerjee P, Chu NF, Spiegelman D, et al. Prospective study of the association of changes in dietary intake, physical activity, alcohol consumption, and smoking with 9-y gain in waist circumference among 16 587 US men. *Am J Clin Nutr.* 2003;78:719-727.

47. Macdonald HM, New SA, Campbell MK, Reid DM. Longitudinal changes in weight in perimenopausal and early postmenopausal women: effects of dietary energy intake, energy expenditure, dietary calcium intake and hormone replacement therapy. *Int J Obes Relat Metab Disord.* 2003;27:669-676.

48. Droyvold WB, Holmen J, Midthjell K, Lydersen S. BMI change and leisure time physical activity (LTPA): an 11-y follow-up study in apparently healthy men aged 20-69 y with normal weight at baseline. *Int J Obes Relat Metab Disord.* 2004;28:410-417.

49. Petersen L, Schnohr P, Sorensen TI. Longitudinal study of the long-term relation between physical activity and obesity in adults. *Int J Obes Relat Metab Disord.* 2004;28:105-112.

50. Wenche DB, Holmen J, Kruger O, Midthjell K. Leisure time physical activity and change in body mass index: an 11-year follow-up study of 9357 normal weight health women 20-49 years old. *J Womens Health (Larchmt).* 2004;13:55-62.

51. Tataranni PA, Harper IT, Snitker S, et al. Body weight gain in free-living Pima Indians: effect of energy intake vs expenditure. *Int J Obes Relat Metab Disord.* 2003;27:1578-1583.

52. Ekelund U, Brage S, Franks PW, et al. Physical activity energy expenditure predicts changes in body composition in middle-aged healthy whites: effect modification by age. *Am J Clin Nutr.* 2005;81:964-969.

53. Sternfeld B, Wang H, Quesenberry CP Jr, et al. Physical activity and changes in weight and waist circumference in midlife women: findings from the Study of Women's Health Across the Nation. *Am J Epidemiol.* 2004;160:912-922.

54. DiPietro L, Kohl HW III, Barlow CE, Blair SN. Improvements in cardiorespiratory fitness attenuate age-related weight gain in healthy men and women: the Aerobics Center Longitudinal Study. *Int J Obes Relat Metab Disord.* 1998;22:55-62.

55. Bak H, Petersen L, Sorensen TI. Physical activity in relation to development and maintenance of obesity in men with and without juvenile onset obesity. *Int J Obes Relat Metab Disord.* 2004;28:99-104.

56. Parsons TJ, Manor O, Power C. Physical activity and change in body mass index from adolescence to mid-adulthood in the 1958 British cohort. *Int J Epidemiol.* 2006; 35:197-204.

57. Yang X, Telama R, Leskinen E, Mansikkaniemi K, Viikari J, Raitakari OT. Testing a model of physical activity and obesity tracking from youth to adulthood: the cardiovascular risk in young Finns study. *Int J Obes (Lond).* 2007;31(3):521-527

58. Schmitz KH, Jacobs DR Jr, Leon AS, Schreiner PJ, Sternfeld B. Physical activity and body weight: associations over ten years in the CARDIA study. Coronary Artery Risk Development in Young Adults. *Int J Obes Relat Metab Disord.* 2000;24:1475-1487.

59. Kawachi I, Troisi RJ, Rotnitzky AG, Coakley EH, Colditz GA. Can physical activity minimize weight gain in women after smoking cessation? *Am J Public Health.* 1996;86:999-1004.

60. Wing RR, Hill JO. Successful weight loss maintenance. *Annu Rev Nutr.* 2001;21: 323-341.

61. van Baak MA, van Mil E, Astrup AV, et al. Leisure-time activity is an important determinant of long-term weight maintenance after weight loss in the Sibutramine Trial on Obesity Reduction and Maintenance (STORM trial). *Am J Clin Nutr.* 2003;78:209-214.

62. Dziura J, Mendes de Leon C, Kasl S, DiPietro L. Can physical activity attenuate aging-related weight loss in older people? The Yale Health and Aging Study, 1982-1994. *Am J Epidemiol.* 2004;159:759-767.

63. Miller WC, Koceja DM, Hamilton EJ. A meta-analysis of the past 25 years of weight loss research using diet, exercise or diet plus exercise intervention. *Int J Obes Relat Metab Disord.* 1997;21:941-947.

64. Curioni CC, Lourenco PM. Long-term weight loss after diet and exercise: a systematic review. *Int J Obes (London).* 2005;10:1168-1174.

65. Wing RR. Physical activity in the treatment of the adulthood overweight and obesity: current evidence and research issues. *Med Sci Sports Exerc.* 1999;31(11 Suppl): S547-S552.

66. Garrow JS, Summerbell CD. Meta-analysis: effect of exercise, with or without dieting, on the body composition of overweight subjects. *Eur J Clin Nutr.* 1995;49:1-10.

67. Donnelly JE, Hill JO, Jacobsen DJ, et al. Effects of a 16-month randomized controlled exercise trial on body weight and composition in young, overweight men and women: the Midwest Exercise Trial. *Arch Intern Med.* 2003;163:1343-1350.

68. Fung TT, Hu FB, Yu J, et al. Leisure-time physical activity, television watching, and plasma biomarkers of obesity and cardiovascular disease risk. *Am J Epidemiol.* 2000;152:1171-1178.

69. Hu FB, Sigal RJ, Rich-Edwards JW, et al. Walking compared with vigorous physical activity and risk of type 2 diabetes in women: a prospective study. *JAMA*. 1999;282:1433-1439.

70. Tanasescu M, Leitzmann MF, Rimm, EB, Willett WC, Stampfer MJ, Hu FB. Exercise type and intensity in relation to coronary heart disease in men. *JAMA*. 2002;288: 1994-2000.

71. Hedeker D, Gibbons RD. *Longitudinal Data Analysis*. Hoboken, NJ: John Wiley & Sons, Inc.; 2006.

72. Little RJA, Rubin DB. *Statistical Analysis with Missing Data*. New York, NY: John Wiley & Sons; 1987.

73. Jöreskog K, Sörbom D. LISREL 8: Structural equation modeling with the SIMPLIS command language: Scientific Software International/Lawrence Erlbaum Associates, 1993.

74. Bryne BM. Structural Equation Modeling with EQS and EQS/WINDOWS. Basic Concepts, Applications, and Programming. London, England: SAGE Publications London, 1994.

75. Dishman RK, Washburn RA, Heath GW. Physical activity and obesity (Chapter 8). *Physical Activity Epidemiology*. Champaign, IL: Human Kinetics, 2004:165-188.

76. Blair SN, LaMonte MJ, Nichaman MZ. The evolution of physical activity recommendations: how much is enough? *Am J Clin Nutr*. 2004;79:913S-920S.

77. Di Pietro L, Dziura J, Blair SN. Estimated change in physical activity level (PAL) and prediction of 5-year weight change in men: the Aerobics Center Longitudinal Study. *Int J Obes Relat Metab Disord*. 2004;28:1541-1547.

78. Pate RR, Pratt M, Blair SN, et al. Physical activity and public health. A recommendation from the Centers for Disease Control and Prevention and the American College of Sports Medicine. *JAMA*. 1995;273:402-407.

79. Saris WH, Blair SN, van Baak MA, et al. How much physical activity is enough to prevent unhealthy weight gain? Outcome of the IASO 1st Stock Conference and consensus statement. *Obes Rev*. 2003;4:101-114.

16

Sleep Deprivation
and Obesity

Sanjay R. Patel and Frank B. Hu

Introduction

Evidence has steadily grown over the past decade supporting a role for sleep curtailment as a risk factor for weight gain and obesity. Recent advancements in neurobiology have identified neural pathways such as the orexin system that contribute to the regulation of both sleep and weight. In addition, the rising obesity epidemic has been paralleled by a similar epidemic in sleep deprivation. The development of electricity and indoor lighting began a steady reduction in human sleep durations and the development of a 24-hour society with the increased prevalence of both rotating and night-shift work as well as the widespread use of cable television, and the Internet has further accelerated the decline in time reserved for sleep. At the beginning of the 20th century, young adults were obtaining close to 9 hours of sleep per night.[1] By the late 1960s, adult sleep duration had been reduced to 7.7 hours.[2] In the past 20 years, the prevalence and severity of sleep curtailment has grown even further. According to annual surveys done by the National Sleep Foundation, by 1998 only 35% of American adults were obtaining 8 hours of sleep on weekdays and that number had fallen to 26% by 2005.[3] Conversely, the percentage of American adults obtaining less than 6 hours of sleep per night has increased from 12% in 1998 to 16% in 2005. Because of this rising prevalence in short sleep durations, any causal association between reduced sleep and obesity would have substantial importance from a public health standpoint. In this chapter, we review potential mechanisms by which sleep duration may impact weight regulation, summarize the epidemiologic data supporting an association between sleep and obesity, and discuss the challenges and limitations facing epidemiologic researchers in defining the causal relationship between sleep duration and weight.

Postulated Mechanisms Linking Sleep with Weight Regulation

A number of causal pathways linking reduced sleep with obesity have been posited based on experimental studies of sleep deprivation (Fig. 16.1). Although much work has been performed in both animal models as well as humans on the physiologic effects of acute total sleep deprivation, the relevance of these studies where the exposure of sleep deprivation can only be maintained for a few days to the situation of an individual obtaining 5 or 6 hours of sleep per night over decades is unclear. In fact, data from studies of growth

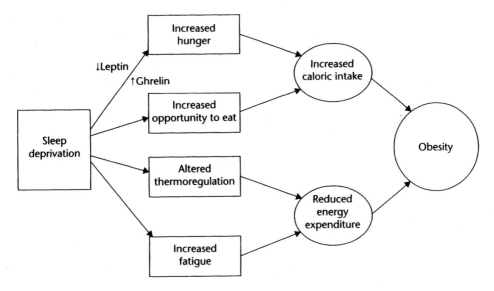

Figure 16.1 Potential mechanisms by which sleep deprivation may predispose to obesity. Reproduced with permission from Patel SR, Hu FB. Short sleep duration and weight gain: a systematic review. *Obesity*. In Press.[26]

hormone and thyroid stimulating hormone (TSH) secretion suggest that the effects of acute total and chronic partial sleep deprivation are substantially different in both magnitude and pattern.[4] Nevertheless, acute sleep deprivation studies can provide insight into the homeostatic systems that may be affected by alterations in sleep habits.

One such system is thermoregulation. Studies of acute sleep deprivation in humans have consistently found a drop in core body temperature in response to sleep loss.[5] Increased complaints of cold and earlier onset of shivering with sleep deprivation suggest that this is not due to a change in the temperature set point.[6] Although some studies suggest this is due to increased heat loss, exercise data suggest sleep deprivation leads to an increase in heat conservation.[7-9] These studies suggest that alterations in sleep may affect energy expenditure through changes in thermoregulation.

Chronic partial sleep deprivation also clearly leads to feelings of fatigue.[10] This tiredness may lead to reductions in physical activity. In fact, cross-sectional studies in children have found short sleep durations to be associated with increased television viewing and reduced participation in organized sports.[11,12] In both the Nurses' Health Study 1 and Nurses' Health Study 2, short habitual sleep durations were associated with reduced reported physical activity.[13,14] However, a recent study found no association between reported sleep duration and energy expenditure measured using doubly labeled water.[15]

Sleep deprivation may also predispose to weight gain by increasing caloric intake. Acute total sleep deprivation paradigms in animals have consistently found that sleep deprivation produces hyperphagia.[16] In humans, total sleep deprivation reduces the amplitude of diurnal leptin rhythms.[17] Recent partial sleep deprivation experiments suggest a similar effect. Comparing 4 hours of sleep opportunity per night to 10 hours over a period of 2 days, both hunger and appetite scores on a visual analog scale were elevated by sleep deprivation.[18] In secondary analyses, the increases were particularly notable for high-fat and high-carbohydrate foods. These changes corresponded with elevations in serum ghrelin levels and reductions in leptin levels, suggesting sleep deprivation may impact peripheral regulators of hunger. A study restricting sleep for 6 consecutive days found a similar reduction in serum leptin levels that persisted throughout the 24-hour day.[19] Chronic partial sleep deprivation has been found to also affect levels of a number of other hormones including cortisol, TSH, and growth hormone that may impact weight regulation through changes in appetite, metabolic rate, and lipogenesis.[20,21] Alternatively, some have argued that in an environment where food is readily available, caloric consumption may be directly proportional to time awake especially if most of wake-time is spent in sedentary activities such as watching television where snacking is common.[22] If this is true, then a curtailed sleep duration simply leads to more time available for eating.

Short-term partial sleep deprivation has also been found to increase insulin resistance as well as sympathovagal balance and epidemiologic studies suggest an association between reduced sleep and both diabetes and hypertension independent of effects on weight.[21,23-25] These data suggest sleep restriction may have a more global effect acting on multiple aspects of the metabolic syndrome.

Studies in Children

Cross-sectional/Case-Control Studies

A recent literature search using standardized criteria identified 13 cross-sectional or case-control studies of the relationship between sleep duration and weight in children (Table 16.1).[26] All of these studies reported a positive association between reduced sleep and obesity. For the most part, obesity was defined by age-adjusted thresholds of body mass index (BMI) measured directly while sleep duration was typically obtained from questionnaires completed by parents. Because sleep requirements change with age through childhood, definitions of short sleep have varied greatly across studies.

Several studies analyzed data from children undergoing health screens on entry to grade school. Locard et al.[11] found the odds of obesity were 40% greater among French schoolchildren sleeping less than 11 hours. A similar study of 6645 German children found the odds ratios (ORs) for obesity were 1.18 and 2.22 for those sleeping 10.5 to 11.0 hours and less than 10.5 hours, respectively, compared to children sleeping 11.5 hours or more.[12] Both studies adjusted for important potential confounders such as parental obesity and time spent watching television.

The largest pediatric study to date has been in a Japanese birth cohort of 8274 children where sleep and weight were compared when participants were aged 6 to 7.[27] Compared to those sleeping 10 hours or more, the ORs for obesity were 1.49, 1.89, and 2.89 for those sleeping 9 to 10 hours, 8 to 9 hours, or fewer than 8 hours, respectively, even after controlling for parental obesity, physical activity, time spent watching television, regularity of eating breakfast, and snacking behaviors. A study of 4,511 Portuguese schoolchildren aged 7 to 9 reported similar findings.[28] Relative to 11 hours or more sleep, the ORs for obesity were 2.27 and 2.56 among those sleeping 9 to 10 hours and 8 hours, respectively.

Three smaller studies have examined a broader range of grade school children. A Canadian study of children aged 5 to 10 reported ORs for obesity were 1.42 and 3.45 in those sleeping 10.5 to 11.5 hours and 10 hours or fewer respectively relative to those sleeping at least 12 hours per night.[29] A Brazilian case-control study of children aged 6 to 11 found obese children slept 31 minutes less per night than normal weight children.[30] A small Tunisian study found the odds for obesity were 11-fold greater in children who slept less than 8 hours.[31]

Four studies have examined the relationship between sleep and weight in adolescent populations. Two are notable for using objective measures of sleep. Gupta et al.[32] measured sleep time using wrist actigraphy over a 24-hour period in 383 children aged 11 to 16.

Table 16.1 Studies of Sleep and Weight in Children

Author/Year/Country	Sample Size	Age Range or Mean	Population Source	Weight Measure	Sleep Measure	Pattern of Association
Locard et al. (1992)[11] France	1031	5	202 schools	Measured BMI	One question to parents	Low ST associated with increased obesity risk OR = 1.4 (1.0, 2.0) for ST < 11 h
Ben Slama et al. (2002)[31] Tunisia	167	6-10	Primary schools in Ariana district	Measured BMI, body fat mass	One question to parents	Low ST associated with increased obesity risk OR = 11 (4.5, 28) for ST < 8 h
Von Kries et al. (2002)[12] Germany	6862	5-6	School entry physicals	Measured BMI	Bedtime/wake-time questions to parents	Low ST associated with increased obesity risk OR = 2.2 (1.3, 3.6) for ST ≤ 10 h compared to > 11 h
Sekine et al. (2002)[27] Japan	8274	6-7	Birth cohort in Toyama	Measured BMI	One question to parents	Low ST associated with increased obesity risk OR = 1.5 (1.1, 2.1) with ST 9 to 10 h, OR = 1.9 (1.3, 2.7) with ST 8 to 9 h, and OR = 2.9 (1.6, 5.1) with ST < 8 h compared to ≥ 10 h
Gupta et al. (2002)[32] USA	383	11-16	Heartfelt Study	Measured BMI, percent body fat	24 h actigraphy	Low ST associated with increased obesity risk OR = 5.0 (2.9, 9.1) for every 1-h drop in ST
Agras et al. (2004)[36] USA	150	3	Birth cohort from San Francisco	Measured BMI	One question to parents each year over 3 years	Cross-sectional relationship not assessed Longitudinally, low ST associated with increased overweight risk 6.5 y later $r = -.21$ ($P < .05$)
Benefice et al. (2004)[33] Senegal	40	13-14	Niakhar district	Measured BMI, triceps skinfold	72 h to 96 h accelerometry	Inverse association between ST and BMI In linear regression, $\beta = -0.11$ h/kg/m^2 (−0.18, −0.05)

(continued)

Table 16.1 continued

Author/Year/Country	Sample Size	Age Range or Mean	Population Source	Weight Measure	Sleep Measure	Pattern of Association
Giugliano and Carneiro (2004)[30] Brazil	165	6-10	Private school	Measured BMI, percent body fat	One question to parents	Inverse association between ST and percent body fat. In linear regression, $r = -.28$ ($P < .02$)
Knutson et al. (2005)[34] USA	4486	17	NLSAH	Measured BMI	One question to child	Low ST associated with increased overweight risk in boys but not girls OR = 1.1 (1.0, 1.2) in boys and 0.9 (0.8, 1.0) in girls for every 1-h drop in ST
Padez et al. (2005)[28] Portugal	4511	7-9	Primary schools	Measured BMI	Weekday/weekend questions to parents	Low ST associated with increased obesity risk OR = 2.6 (2.4, 2.9) for ST = 8 h compared to ≥ 11 h
Reilly et al. (2005)[37] UK	8234	3	ALSPAC	Measured BMI	One question to parents	Cross-sectional relationship not assessed Longitudinally, low ST associated with increased obesity risk 4 y later OR = 1.5 (1.1, 1.9) for ST < 10.5 h compared to > 12 h
Chaput et al. (2006)[29] Canada	422	5-10	14 schools	Measured BMI	One question to parents	Low ST associated with increased overweight risk OR = 3.5 (2.6, 4.7) for ST ≤ 10 h compared to 12 to 13 h
Chen et al. (2006)[35] Taiwan	656	13-18	7 schools	Measured BMI	One question to child (frequency of adequate sleep—sleeping at least 6 to 8 h on weekdays)	Low frequency of adequate sleep associated with increased obesity risk OR = 1.7 (1.3, 2.4) for ≤3d/wk adequate sleep compared to 5 d/wk

Estimates provided with 95% confidence intervals in parentheses. BMI: body mass index; ST: sleep time; OR: odds ratio; ALSPAC: Avon Longitudinal Study of Parents and Children; NLSAH: National Longitudinal Study of Adolescent Health.

Adapted from Patel SR, Hu FB. Short sleep duration and weight gain: a systematic review. *Obesity.* In Press.[26]

The authors reported the odds of obesity increased fivefold for every 1 hour reduction in total sleep time. Using accelerometers worn near the hip to assess sleep over 3 to 4 days in 40 Senegalese girls, Benefice et al.[33] found sleep time was reduced 6.85 minutes for every 1 kg/m² increase in BMI. This work was notable for identifying a sleep-weight relationship in a nonobese population (mean BMI was 16.9 kg/m²). The other two studies in teenagers used reported sleep time as obtained from the children. A study of nearly 4500 American teens found each hour reduction in sleep time was associated with a 0.08% increase in BMI Z-score and an 11% increased risk of overweight in boys.[34] No relationship between sleep and weight measures was identified in girls. Chen et al.[35] surveyed 656 Taiwanese teenagers and found the frequency of obtaining at least 6 to 8 hours of sleep was inversely correlated with obesity risk.

Cohort Studies

Only two longitudinal studies have examined the relationship between sleep and weight in children. On the basis of the data from a birth cohort of 150 children in San Francisco, Agras et al.[36] used a recursive partitioning technique to identify independent risk factors for obesity. Sleep duration data were obtained from parents at yearly intervals from ages 2 to 5. Because of stability of these data from ages 3, 4, and 5, information from these 3 years were averaged. This mean sleep duration was found to independently predict obesity at age 9.5. Reilly et al.[37] studied 8,234 children in a British birth cohort. They found a monotonic relationship between sleep duration reported by parents at 38 months of age and obesity at age 7 with ORs of 1.45, 1.35, and 1.04 for children sleeping less than 10.5 hours, 10.5 to 10.9 hours, and 11.0 to 11.9 hours compared to those sleeping 12 hours or more. Although both studies adjusted for birth weight and weight gain over the first year of life, weight at the time of sleep assessment was not included in the modeling.

Summary

All 13 pediatric studies have identified a positive association between sleep loss and excess weight with a monotonic effect such that increasing levels of sleep restriction are associated with increased risk of obesity. The consistent findings from studies spanning five continents suggest the association is independent of ethnicity though no formal assessment of effect modification by race has been reported. Several studies suggest boys may be more susceptible to sleep loss than girls. Comparing less than 8 hours to more than 10 hours of sleep, Sekine et al.[27] found the OR for obesity was 5.5 in boys compared to 2.1 in girls. Similarly, Chaput et al.[29] found the OR for obesity in those sleeping 10 hours or fewer as opposed to 12 hours or more was 5.7 in boys and 3.2 in girls. Finally, Knutson et al.[34] found a significant association between short sleep and increased weight in boys but not girls.

A few studies have attempted to isolate the causal pathway linking curtailed sleep to obesity but without success. von Kries et al.[12] found no relationship between sleep habits and caloric intake obtained from a food-frequency questionnaire. The two prospective studies also assessed caloric intake—the British study used food-frequency questionnaires while the San Francisco study directly measured food consumption over 24 hours.[36,37] Neither study found differences in dietary intake could explain the sleep-weight relationship. Similarly, little evidence has been found that the association between sleep and obesity is explained by differences in physical activity. Neither Gupta et al.[32] using daytime actigraphic data nor Benefice et al.[33] using accelerometric data found a relationship between sleep duration and activity levels. Agras et al.[36] found sleep duration was negatively correlated with physical activity as measured by actigraphy but this relationship did not explain the sleep-obesity association. On the other hand, Chen et al.[35] found reduced sleep was associated with poorer health-related behaviors in general, including lower scores on measures of nutrition, exercise, stress management, and social supports. Short sleep has been consistently associated with increased television watching but none of the six studies that assessed television viewing found the sleep-obesity relationship was explained by this variable.[11,27,29,35-37]

Studies in Adults

Cross-sectional/Case-Control Studies

A literature search identified 23 cross-sectional studies of sleep and weight in adults (Table 16.2).[26] Results have been less consistent than the pediatric studies. Eleven studies found an association between reduced sleep and increased weight and two studies found mixed results with an association in one gender but not the other. Five studies found no association between sleep and weight while one study found short sleep duration was associated with reduced weight. In addition, four studies found long sleep durations are also associated with increased weight resulting in a U-shaped curve between sleep duration and weight. In general, obesity has been defined as a BMI $\geq$ 30 kg/m^2 based on either direct measurement or self-report, while sleep duration has been typically obtained through questionnaire.

The largest studies examining the relationship between sleep and weight were designed as prospective cohort studies to assess the effect of sleep duration on mortality.[38-41] In these studies, the relationship between sleep and weight was presented simply to consider the potential of weight to confound sleep-mortality relationships and therefore only marginal associations are reported. The largest study was a survey by the American Cancer Society enrolling over 1.1 million participants.[38] A U-shaped association was found between sleep and BMI among women with those sleeping 7 hours being the leanest while a more monotonic trend was observed in men such that longer sleep was associated with a lower BMI. Using 7 hours as the reference, BMI in 4-hour sleepers was 1.39 kg/m^2 greater in women and 0.57 kg/m^2 greater in men. In contrast, BMI in those sleeping 10 hours or more was 1.10 kg/m^2 greater in women but 0.11 kg/m^2 less in men. The next largest study was in a cohort of over 100,000 Japanese individuals. This study is the only one to find reduced sleep was associated with decreased weight. Compared to 7-hour sleepers, mean BMI in those sleeping 4 hours or fewer was 0.3 kg/m^2 less in women and 0.5 kg/m^2 less in men.[40] A Japanese study of 11,000 individuals found no relationship between sleep duration and BMI.[39] On the other hand, a Scottish study of nearly 7000 people found mean BMI was 0.3 kg/m^2 greater among men sleeping less than 7 hours compared to those sleeping 7 to 8 hours.[41] Among women, no relationship between sleep and BMI was found. Two other studies have considered weight as a secondary outcome. The Sleep Heart Health Study found a U-shaped association with BMI 0.7 and 0.2 kg/m^2 greater in those sleeping less than 6 and 9 hours or more, respectively compared to 7- to 8-hour sleepers.[42] A study of Swedish women found sleep duration to be inversely correlated with both BMI ($r = -.06$) and waist-hip ratio ($r = -.08$).[43]

Two studies using population-based sampling techniques have directly assessed the relationship between sleep and obesity in middle-aged populations. Vioque et al.[44] analyzed data from 1,772 Spanish adults and found a monotonic negative association between sleep duration and obesity. Relative to 7-hour sleepers, the OR for obesity was 1.39 in those sleeping 6 hours or less and 0.79 and 0.60 in those sleeping 8 hours and 9 hours

Table 16.2 Studies of Sleep and Weight in Adults

Author/Year/Country	Sample Size	Age Range or Mean	Population Source	Weight Measure	Sleep Measure	Pattern of Association
Gortmaker et al. (1990)[55] USA	712	—	Harvard School of Public Health	Reported BMI	One sleep question	No association between ST and BMI In linear regression, $r = -.02$ with $P > .05$
Vioque et al. (2000)[44] Spain	1,772	≥15	Health and Nutritional Survey of Valencia	Measured BMI	One sleep question	Low ST associated with increased obesity risk OR = 2.1 (1.4, 3.3) for those with ST ≤ 6 h compared to ≥ 9 h
Shigeta et al. (2001)[52] Japan	453	53	Hospital clinic	Measured BMI	One sleep question	Low ST associated with increased obesity risk OR = 2.0 (1.0, 3.8) for those with ST < 6 h
Heslop et al. (2002)[41] UK	6,797	35-64	Work places in Scotland	Measured BMI	One sleep question	Low ST associated with higher BMI in men but not women Among men, BMI 0.30 kg/m^2 (0.05, 0.55) greater in those with ST < 7 h compared to 7-8 h
Kripke et al. (2002)[38] USA	1,116,936	33-102	American Cancer Society volunteers	Reported BMI	One sleep question	Inverse linear association between ST and BMI in men, U-shaped association in women BMI 0.57 kg/m^2 (0.46, 0.68) greater in men and 1.39 kg/m^2 (1.25, 1.53) greater in women for ST 4 h compared to 7 h
Tamakoshi and Ohno (2004)[40] Japan	104,010	40-79	Japan Collaborative Cohort Study	Reported BMI	One sleep question	Low ST associated with lower BMI BMI 0.50 kg/m^2 (0.15, 0.85) lower in men and 0.30 kg/m^2 (0.03, 0.57) lower in women with ST < 4.5 h compared to 6.5 to 7.5 h
Amagai et al. (2004)[39] Japan	11,325	19-93	Jichi Medical School Cohort Study	Measured BMI	Bedtime/wake-time questions	No association between ST and BMI BMI 0.20 kg/m^2 (−0.71, 0.31) lower in men and 0.20 kg/m^2 (−0.19, 0.59) greater in women with ST < 6 h compared to 7 to 8 h

(continued)

Table 16.2 continued

Author/Year/Country	Sample Size	Age Range or Mean	Population Source	Weight Measure	Sleep Measure	Pattern of Association
Cournot et al. (2004)[46] France	3127	32-62	VISAT study	Measured BMI	Bedtime/wake-time questions	Low ST associated with higher BMI in women but not men. BMI 0.20 kg/m² (−0.19, 0.59) greater among men with ST ≤ 6 h in unadjusted analysis and 0.63 kg/m² (0.17, 1.09) greater among women
Hasler et al. (2004)[58] Switzerland	496	27	Zurich Cohort Study	Reported BMI	Three sleep questions (bedtime, wake-time, and sleep latency) at four time points	Cross-sectionally, low ST associated with increased obesity risk. OR = 7.4 (1.3, 43.1) at age 27, 8.1 (1.6, 37.4) at age 29, 4.7 (1.5, 14.8) at age 34 and 1.1 (0.3, 4.0) at age 40 for those with ST < 6 h compared to ≥ 6 h. Longitudinally, low ST associated with increased obesity risk. OR = 8.2 (1.9, 36.3) at age 27 and 2-y follow-up, 4.6 (1.3, 16.5) at age 29 and 5-y follow-up, 3.5 (1.0, 12.2) at age 34 and 6-y follow-up for those with ST < 6 h compared to ≥ 6 h
Ohayon (2004)[57] Europe	8091	55-101	Random sampling in seven European countries	Reported BMI	Nighttime/daytime sleep questions	No association between short nighttime ST and BMI but positive association between long nighttime ST and underweight. OR = 1.9 (1.1, 3.1) for ST > 95th percentile and BMI < 19 kg/m²
Taheri et al. (2004)[47] USA	1024	53	Wisconsin Sleep Cohort Study	Measured BMI	6 d Sleep Diary	U-shaped association between ST and BMI. In quadratic model, minimum BMI at ST = 7.7 h. BMI is 1.1 kg/m² greater for those with ST = 5 h compared to 8 h
Bjorkelund et al. (2005)[43] Sweden	1462	38-60	Population-based cohort of Gothenburg	Measured BMI, WHR	One sleep question	Inverse association between ST and BMI. In linear regression, r = −.06 for BMI (P = .03)

Study	N	Age	Population	BMI	Sleep measure	Results
Gangwisch et al. (2005)[59] USA	9,588	32-86	NHANES	Measured and reported BMI	One sleep question	Cross-sectionally, U-shaped association between ST and obesity risk $OR = 2.4$ (1.4, 4.0) at age 32-49, 1.9 at age 50-67, and 1.7 at age 68-86 for those with ST < 5 h compared to 7 h Longitudinally, low ST associated with increased obesity risk Among those aged 32-49, $OR = 1.8$ (1.0, 3.3) after 4 y and $OR = 2.0$ (1.1, 3.6) after 9 y for those with ST < 5 h compared to 7 h
Ohayon and Vecchierini (2005)[56] France	1,026	≥60	Population-based cohort of Paris	Reported BMI	Nighttime/daytime sleep questions	Low nighttime ST associated with increased BMI category OR for BMI > 27 kg/m^2 relative to BMI 20-25 kg/m^2 is 3.6 (1.0-13.1) with ST ≤ 4.5 h and 1.9 (0.7, 5.6) with ST 4.5-6.0 h relative to 6.0-8.0 h No association between total ST and BMI category
Singh et al. (2005)[45] USA	3,158	18-65	Population-based cohort of Detroit	Reported BMI	Weekday/weekend sleep questions	Low ST associated with increased obesity risk $OR = 1.7$ (1.3, 2.3) for ≤5 h and $OR = 1.4$ (1.1, 1.8) for 5-6 h relative to 7-8 h
Vorona et al. (2005)[53] USA	924	18-91	Four Primary Care Clinics	Measured BMI	Weekday/weekend sleep questions	Low ST associated with increased BMI category ST is 16 min shorter with BMI > 25 kg/m^2
Gottlieb et al. (2006)[42] USA	5,910	40-100	Sleep Heart Health Study	Measured BMI	Weekday/weekend sleep questions	U-shaped association between ST and BMI BMI 0.7 kg/m^2 (0.2, 1.2) greater with ST < 6 h compared to 7-8 h
Kohatsu et al. (2006)[50] USA	990	48	Employed adults in rural Iowa	Measured BMI	One sleep question	Inverse association between ST and BMI In linear regression, $\beta = -0.42$ kg/m^2 per h (-0.77, -0.07)
Lauderdale et al. (2006)[54] USA	669	35-49	CARDIA Study	Measured BMI (3 y prior to sleep assessment)	72-h actigraphy	No association between ST and BMI In linear regression, $\beta = -0.01$ $h/kg/m^2$ (-0.02, 0.01)

(continued)

Table 16.2 continued

Author Year Country	Sample Size	Age Range or Mean	Population Source	Weight Measure	Sleep Measure	Pattern of Association
Moreno et al. (2006)[48] Brazil	4,878	40	Male truck drivers in São Paulo	Measured BMI	One sleep question	Low ST associated with increased obesity risk OR = 1.2 (1.1-1.4) for ST < 8 h compared to ≥ 8 h
Patel et al. (2006)[14] USA	68,183	45-65	Nurses Health Study	Reported BMI	One sleep question	Cross-sectionally, U-shaped association between ST and obesity risk OR = 1.5 (1.4, 1.7) for ST ≤ 5 h compared to 7 h Longitudinally, low ST associated with increased obesity and weight gain risk Over 16 y, HR = 1.2 (1.0, 1.3) for developing obesity and 1.3 (1.2, 1.4) for 15 kg weight gain for ST ≤ 5 h compared to 7 h
Chaput et al. (2007)[51] Canada	740	21-64	Quebec Family Study	Measured BMI, WHR, skinfold thicknesses, body fat mass	One sleep question	U-shaped association between ST and obesity risk OR = 1.7 (1.2-2.4) for ST 5-6 h compared to 7-8 h
Ko et al. (2007)[49] China	4,793	17-83	Hong Kong union members	Measured BMI, waist circumference	One sleep question	Inverse association between ST and both BMI and waist circumference In age-adjusted regression, r = −.04 for BMI (P = .02) and r = −.05 for waist (P = .004)

Estimates provided with 95% confidence intervals or P values in parentheses if available. BMI: body mass index; WHR: waist-hip ratio; ST: sleep time; OR: odds ratio (unless otherwise specified, all odds ratios are for obesity); HR: hazard ratio; NHANES: National Health and Nutrition Examination Survey; CARDIA: Coronary Artery Risk Development in Young Adults. Adapted from Patel SR, Hu FB. Short sleep duration and weight gain: a systematic review. *Obesity*. In Press.[26]

or more, respectively. A study of 3158 Americans also reported a negative association between sleep and obesity with the minimum risk in those sleeping 8 to 9 hours.[45]

Several studies have examined the sleep-weight relationship in working populations. A French study of 3,127 workers found that while no association between sleep duration and weight was found in men, among women, those sleeping 6 hours or fewer had a BMI 0.63 kg/m^2 greater than women who slept more.[46] Among 1,024 Wisconsin government workers, a U-shaped relationship was found between sleep time obtained from sleep diaries and BMI with minimum BMI corresponding to a sleep duration of 7.7 hours.[47] A survey of 4,878 Brazilian truck drivers found sleeping less than 8 hours/day was associated with a 24% greater odds of obesity while a survey of 4,793 Hong Kong union members found sleep time and BMI were inversely correlated ($r = -.037$, $P = .02$).[48,49] Similarly, a study of 990 Iowans found BMI was 0.42 kg/m^2 greater for each hour less of sleep per night.[50]

Data from a Canadian family-based study support the presence of a U-shaped relationship between sleep and obesity.[51] Compared to 7- to 8-hour sleepers, the ORs for obesity were 1.63 and 1.72 in women and men sleeping 5 to 6 hours, respectively and 1.51 and 1.18 in women and men sleeping 9-10 hours. Two studies examined the association between sleep and weight in clinic populations. A Japanese study found the odds of obesity was nearly double in patients who slept less than 6 hours.[52] Among 924 Americans attending a primary care clinic, sleep duration was longest in those with BMI < 25 kg/m^2.[53] Among men, a U-shaped relationship existed such that the least sleep was reported by overweight men (BMI 25 to 29 kg/m^2). Total sleep time was 19 minutes less than that in normal weight men. In women, a larger effect was seen such that those with a BMI of 30 to 40 kg/m^2 slept 49 minutes less than those with BMI < 25 kg/m^2.

Only one study of adults has examined the sleep-weight relationship using an objective measure of sleep duration. Lauderdale et al.[54] used 3 days of wrist actigraphy to investigate predictors of sleep duration in 669 middle-aged adults. Using linear regression methods, a weak negative correlation was found between sleep duration and BMI that was not statistically significant. A study of 712 individuals also used linear regression analysis and found a weak negative correlation between self-reported sleep and weight that was not statistically significant.[55]

Two reports have focused on examining the relationship between sleep and weight in geriatric populations. Both studies were designed to define normative sleep habits in the elderly and considered weight as a predictor of sleep. A study of 1026 French individuals over age 60 found those with a BMI > 27 kg/m^2 were 3.6 times more likely to report a nocturnal sleep duration in the lowest fifth percentile than those with a BMI of 20 to 25 kg/m^2.[56] However, those who weighed more were also more likely to report daytime naps so that no association between total sleep duration and BMI was found. A survey of 8091 individuals over age 55 from across western Europe found obesity did not predict being in the bottom fifth percentile of nocturnal sleep duration but a BMI < 19 kg/m^2 did predict being in the top fifth percentile.[57] Again, however, daytime napping was greater in those who were overweight.

Cohort Studies

Three studies have examined the longitudinal relationship between sleep and weight in adults. Hasler et al.[58] followed 496 adults in the Zurich Cohort Study from age 27 to 40. Height and weight were self-reported while sleep duration was calculated from questions regarding bedtime, wake-time, and sleep latency. These questions were asked at four separate times. In cross-sectional analyses, the association between sleeping less than 6 hours and obesity was found to weaken with increasing age. The ORs were 7.4, 8.1, 4.7, and 1.1 at ages 27, 29, 34, and 40. The rate of change of BMI had a monotonic relationship with sleep duration averaged across the 13 years. Those sleeping less than 5 hours gained weight at a rate of nearly 0.4 kg/m²/year while those sleeping more than 9 hours lost weight. Interestingly, sleep duration appeared to be more strongly associated with previous weight than concurrent or future weight. For example at age 29, the ORs for less than 6 hours of sleep was 11.8 with obesity at age 27, 8.1 with obesity at age 29, and 4.6 with obesity at age 34.

Gangwisch et al.[59] analyzed data from 9588 participants of the National Health and Nutrition Examination Survey (NHANES) study. Heights and weights were measured at baseline but at subsequent timepoints, self-reported weight was utilized. Sleep duration was obtained from a question asking about only nocturnal sleep. At baseline, a U-shaped association was found with minimum obesity risk in 7-hour sleepers. The strength of the sleep-obesity relationship waned with age such that the ORs for obesity in those sleeping 4 hours or fewer relative to 7-hour sleepers were 3.21, 1.81, and 1.71 among those aged 32 to 49, 50 to 67, and 68 to 86. Because the strongest cross-sectional association between sleep and weight was found in the youngest tertile, longitudinal analysis was only performed in this subgroup. Over 9 years, a linear relationship between sleep and weight gain was found with those sleeping 4 hours or fewer gaining 1.46 kg/m² and those sleeping 10 hours or more gaining only 0.08 kg/m². After adjusting for potential confounders such as alcohol and tobacco habits, sleep-related complaints, depression, and physical activity, mean BMI was found to increase only 0.05 kg/m² for every hour decrease in sleep duration. This difference was not statistically significant.

Patel et al.[14] followed 68,183 American women in the Nurses Health Study aged 45-65 for up to 16 years. Questionnaire response to habitual sleep duration over a 24-hour period was obtained at baseline and self-reported weights were obtained at baseline and every 2 years. Cross-sectionally, a U-shaped association was found with minimum weight in those sleeping 7 hours. Adjusting for differences in baseline weight, weight gain was 1.14 and 0.71 kg greater over the 16 years among 5- and 6-hour sleepers, respectively compared to 7-hour sleepers. No significant difference was observed among those sleeping 7 hours or more. The hazard ratios for developing obesity and a 15-kg weight gain were 1.15 and 1.28, respectively, in 5-hour sleepers.

Summary

Overall, research in adults suggest short sleepers are heavier than those who sleep 7-8 hours with supportive findings from the majority of cross-sectional analyses as well as all three prospective studies. Results regarding a positive association between obesity and longer sleep durations are more mixed but this is in part due to the fact that many studies did not specifically separate long sleepers from normal sleepers. Interestingly, both the NHANES and Nurses Health Study found a positive association between long sleep and obesity assessed simultaneously but no association with future obesity, suggesting the cross-sectional relationship might be due to reverse causation or residual confounding.[14,59] Potential mechanisms for an association between long sleep duration and obesity, whether causal or not, include depression, low socioeconomic status, and societal isolation.[13] If the cross-sectional relationship between sleep and weight truly is U-shaped, the effect of short sleep would be underestimated in studies that conducted linear regression analyses since this forces a linear relationship between the two variables. This could explain the negative findings in two studies.[54,55]

Several groups have explored whether the sleep-weight association differs across important subgroups. Two studies have suggested the effect of reduced sleep on weight regulation may wane with age. In the NHANES study, the short sleep-obesity association was strongest in those aged 32 to 49 and weakest in those over 67.[59] The Zurich study found the cross-sectional association between short sleep and obesity diminished as their cohort aged from an OR of 7.4 at age 27 to 1.1 at age 40.[58] The negative findings in the two geriatric studies further support the hypothesis that the effect of sleep deprivation on weight regulation wanes with age.[56,57]

Findings on differences between genders have been mixed. While several studies suggest a greater vulnerability in women,[38,46,51,53] at least two studies have reported curtailed sleep is associated with obesity only in men.[41,49] No study has directly examined whether the metabolic effects of sleep vary by ethnicity. However, Singh et al.[45] did find that both reduced sleep and obesity were much more common in African Americans.

Several studies have attempted to identify pathways linking sleep and weight. Physical activity was assessed by questionnaire in six studies reporting an association between reduced sleep and obesity; in none of these studies did adjusting for differences in activity explain the association.[14,44,46,51,58,59] Similarly, the short sleep-obesity association was independent of television viewing in the two studies that assessed this behavior.[44,46]

Short sleep has been associated with reduced leptin levels independent of obesity in two studies.[47,51] In the Quebec Family Study, the sleep-weight association disappeared after adjusting for leptin, suggesting this hormone may be the causal intermediate.[51] Short sleep was also associated with BMI-adjusted ghrelin levels in the Wisconsin Sleep Cohort Study.[47] However, the Nurses Health Study found the sleep-weight relationship could not be explained by differences in dietary intake; in that study, caloric intake measured through a food-frequency questionnaire was least in short sleepers.[14]

Reverse Causation

While the short-term physiology studies provide biologic plausibility to the belief that sleep duration can affect weight regulation, increased weight may influence sleep patterns as well. Obesity increases the risk of such medical conditions as osteoarthritis, gastroesophageal reflux, asthma, and congestive heart failure that can all commonly disrupt sleep and lead to insomnia.[60-63] Obesity is the strongest risk factor for obstructive sleep apnea, which has as its hallmark disruption of sleep.[64] Several studies have attempted to control for these comorbidities by including the presence of these diseases as covariates in multivariate modeling.[14,45,48,50,53,54] Questionnaires about snoring and related symptoms have typically been used as a surrogate for sleep apnea in these studies. Another argument against reverse causation comes from the positive findings in the pediatric studies where the prevalence of comorbid disorders related to obesity is rare. Although sleep apnea exists in childhood, obesity is a less important risk factor in this age group.

Whether obesity has an effect on sleep independent of its medical complications is unclear, but the data that exist suggest that any effect might be in the opposite direction. Inflammation associated with obesity may lead to the release of soporific cytokines producing longer sleep times.[65] A mouse model of diet-induced obesity has recently supported this notion that obesity increases sleep duration.[66]

Confounding

The relationship between sleep duration and obesity may be confounded through the presence of one or more common causes. Potential conditions that have been associated with both reduced sleep and obesity include coexisting medical disorders such as chronic pain syndromes as well as psychiatric disorders such as depression that may limit an individual's ability to be physically active as well as interfere with sleep continuity. Impaired sleep is a defining criterion for clinical depression.[67] In addition, medications commonly used for treating many of these conditions can have effects on weight and sleep. Several studies have attempted to measure and control for comorbid medical and psychiatric disorders as well as medication use through multivariate analysis.[14,48,50,53,58,59] Because the Zurich Cohort Study was designed to investigate psychiatric outcomes, detailed assessments of depressive symptoms were performed and the sleep-weight association was found to be independent of depression.[58] The Nurses' Health Study restricted analyses to individuals without significant comorbidity such as cancer, heart disease, and diabetes.[14] The positive results from the pediatric cohorts where comorbidity is rare also argues against the sleep-weight relationship being secondary to confounding due to medical or psychiatric disease.

Differences in socioeconomic status may also importantly confound the relationship between sleep and weight. People of lower socioeconomic status may have less favorable sleep environments, work longer hours, and work less desirable hours such as rotating or overnight shifts resulting in poor sleep. Low income has been associated with reduced sleep durations.[54] Many studies have attempted to prevent confounding by socioeconomic status by including covariates regarding income, educational level, and/or occupation in multivariate analyses.[11,12,28,29,34,36,37,44-46,50,54,58,59] Many pediatric studies controlled for family structure including living with a single parent and the presence of siblings.[11,12,28,29,37] Two studies limited recruitment to a single profession thereby limiting variability in socioeconomic status.[14,48]

Another mechanism by which confounding may exist is through genetic pleiotropy. Many of the neural systems in the hypothalamus important in sleep/wake regulation also play a key role in systems integral to weight homeostasis.[68] For example, orexin plays an important role in both maintaining wakefulness and increasing appetite. Both sleep habits and weight have been found to be highly heritable traits.[69,70] A recent study in twins found significant shared genetic variance between insomnia and obesity.[71] Thus, it is possible that polymorphisms in genes that regulate pathways such as orexin have pleiotropic effects influencing both sleep and obesity phenotypes simultaneously. Genes regulating circadian rhythm may represent another shared pathway. Homozygous mutation of one of the key circadian genes, CLOCK, in the mouse has been found to produce a phenotype of obesity.[72] Many pediatric studies have attempted to minimize bias from this effect by controlling for parental obesity.[11,12,27-29,36,37]

Measurement Error

Measuring habitual sleep duration is problematic in epidemiologic studies. Few studies have utilized objective measures of sleep duration. The gold standard for documenting sleep is polysomnography (PSG). The expense and burden of this testing limits its utility for epidemiologic studies. The well-documented first night effect found with laboratory PSG suggests the reason total sleep time measured in this manner is substantially less than sleep time in the home is in part due to requiring the subject to sleep in an unfamiliar environment. However, even home PSG may reduce sleep duration due to discomfort related to the placement of electrodes and other recording instruments. In the Wisconsin Sleep Cohort Study, mean sleep time from PSG was 6.2 hours as opposed to 7.2 hours from a weighted average of responses about weekday and weekend sleep and 7.7 hours from sleep diaries.[47] In a nonobese subgroup of the Sleep Heart Health Study free of comorbidity, sleep duration on PSG conducted in the home was 1 hour less than habitual sleep time reported on questionnaire.[73]

Actigraphy has been developed as a less intrusive method to measure sleep duration. This measurement method assesses motion using an accelerometer placed on an arm or leg. These devices are typically the size of a wristwatch and so have little effect on one's ability to sleep. In healthy adults, the correlation in sleep duration measured using PSG has been reported as high as 0.97 with no first night effect.[74,75] Wrist actigraphy tends to overestimate sleep duration slightly in healthy individuals as quiet wakefulness can be interpreted as sleep. This effect is relatively small, with a mean difference of 12 minutes in one study.[74] Owing to these performance characteristics as well as the lower expense and ability to easily record over an extended period of time, actigraphy is likely the optimal method of assessing sleep time in epidemiologic studies. Unfortunately, only two studies of sleep and obesity to date have utilized actigraphy and both used recording times that were too short to incorporate variability across the week.[32,54] Interestingly, one of these studies used actigraph data to not only measure total sleep time but also estimate the level of physical activity, a key variable required to understand how sleep habits can lead to changes in weight.[32] Another study used an accelerometer placed at the hip to measure both sleep and activity.[33] While measurements from this location have been validated for assessing physical activity, adequate validation for sleep measurements is lacking.

Owing to cost and patient burden issues, most epidemiologic studies have relied on subjective assessments of sleep duration using questionnaires. The response to a question about average nocturnal sleep duration is often much greater than the time calculated by asking subjects their usual bedtime and wake-time, suggesting individuals overestimate their sleep time in order to be closer to the accepted norm of 8 hours. Many questionnaires only ask about sleep at night. This can result in substantial underestimation of time spent asleep since it excludes daytime napping. In addition, an increasing part of the population works nightshifts so that their major sleep period is during daytime hours. The importance of considering daytime sleep is seen in the study by Ohayon et al.[56] where obesity was associated with reduced nighttime sleep and increased daytime sleep resulting in no association with total sleep time. The magnitude of error in questionnaire-derived measures of sleep duration is unclear. In the study by Lauderdale et al.,[54] reported habitual sleep duration was 0.7 hour greater than average sleep duration obtained from 72 hours of actigraphy, suggesting substantial bias may exist.

Another issue in assessing sleep habits is the substantial night-to-night variability. In the Toyama birth cohort study, 3-month reproducibility was found to be moderate (kappas ranging from 0.48 to 0.64) for questions asked to parents about their child's sleep habits.[27] Of particular concern is the fact that among students and the employed, sleep duration is typically longer on weekends compared to weekdays. In the 2005 Sleep in America Poll, reported sleep duration was 0.6 hour shorter on weekdays than weekends.[3] Lauderdale et al.[54] also reported a difference between weekday and weekend sleep of 0.6 hour. In a subgroup of the Sleep Heart Health Study, weekday sleep was 0.8 hour shorter than weekend sleep in those aged 40 to 54, while the difference was only 0.2 hour in those aged 70 to 91, who were presumably retired.[73] It is unclear how accurately individuals are able to average their sleep times over weekends and weekdays. To combat this, several studies have asked separate questions regarding sleep duration for work days and nonwork days and then computed a weighted average.[28,42,45,47,53]

Some studies have used daily sleep diaries over a period of a week or more to overcome night-to-night fluctuations in sleep habits. These diaries ask the subject to record bedtime and wake-time each night as well as time spent napping during the day. Daily sleep duration is then averaged over the time period of the diaries. The Nurses Health Study conducted a validation study of their one question on sleep duration against one week of sleep diaries in an elderly population (mean age 68 years) and found good correlation ($r = .79$).[76] In general, short sleepers tended to underestimate their sleep durations while long sleepers overestimated their sleep. Thus, those reporting a typical sleep duration of 5 hours or fewer, slept 5.2 hours on average by sleep diaries, while those reporting 9 hours or more slept 8.5 hours on average.

Sleep diaries, themselves, are associated with a fair amount of error. Correlations between sleep time estimated by actigraphy and by sleep diaries have been moderate ($r = .57$ for nocturnal sleep and $r = .48$ for daytime sleep).[77] As with other subjective measures of sleep duration, sleep diaries are prone to inaccuracy due to sleep-state misperception. Because individuals are only aware of the time they are awake, they may overestimate their time awake in bed and underestimate the time slept. This underestimation is more common among those with insomnia who tend to spend a substantial time in bed awake.[78,79] This can magnify the apparent difference in sleep time between short- and normal-duration sleepers.

With the exception of the works by Agras et al.[36] and Hasler et al.,[58] epidemiologic studies to date have only assessed sleep duration at one point in time. Sleep patterns clearly change in individuals over time and there are known changes in sleep requirements over the lifespan. Thus, the use of a sleep assessment at only one point in time can result in substantial misclassification bias in measures of association between short sleep and weight. The Nurses Health Study found the kappa statistic for 2-year reproducibility of habitual sleep duration to be .39.[76] This increased to .81 when deviation of 1 hour in either direction was allowed.

Sleep Biology

Sleep is not a homogeneous state—several distinct stages exist with the clearest distinction being between nonrapid eye movement (non-REM) and REM sleep. Autonomic tone is substantially different between these two conditions suggesting that the relationship between these different phases of sleep with metabolism and weight regulation may be very different.[80] The effects of selective REM deprivation on thermoregulation differ in pattern compared to total sleep deprivation.[81] Within non-REM sleep, slow wave sleep or delta power EEG activity appears to have important differences from lighter periods of non-REM sleep in terms of neurohormonal effects. In particular, growth hormone secretion is closely tied to slow wave sleep.[82] To date, most epidemiologic studies of obesity have not distinguished between these various sleep states. Data from the Sleep Heart Health Study suggest that increased weight is associated with an increase in the proportion of light non-REM sleep and a corresponding reduction in slow wave sleep while the proportion of REM sleep does not differ across weight class categories.[83] Further research on which components of sleep are most closely associated with weight regulation is needed.

No study to date has assessed whether the association between short sleep and obesity is affected by the cause of the short sleep. At least three common causes of short sleep exist—individuals who feel fully rested with less than 7 hours of sleep; those who voluntarily curtail their sleep to spend more time on other things such as jobs, childcare or recreation (e.g., watching television, using the Internet) despite neurocognitive effects from this sleep restriction; and those who want to sleep longer because of daytime symptoms but cannot because of insomnia. The biologic effects of chronic sleep restriction may be very different in these three populations. It is clear that psychiatric comorbidity is much more common among those with insomnia and these individuals have increased adrenocorticotropic hormone (ACTH) and cortisol secretion that does not appear to exist in the other groups.[84,85] On the other hand, a study of the association between short sleep duration and diabetes found an elevated risk of similar magnitude among short sleepers with and without insomnia.[24] Clearly, a better understanding of differential susceptibility to obesity is required to design public health initiatives that improve sleep habits as well as to understand the biological link between short sleep and excess weight.

Another important problem to consider when comparing individuals with different sleep patterns is that there may be important phase differences in their circadian rhythms either as a cause of the reduced sleep or as a consequence. This becomes particularly important in the study of biomarkers that exhibit a circadian rhythmicity. Examples of hormones with known circadian rhythms include cortisol, TSH, growth hormone, and leptin.[4] Thus, in comparing individuals with differing sleep durations, it may become more important to compare biomarker levels at the same point in circadian phase rather than the same absolute time. Unfortunately, thus far, this effect has not been considered in epidemiologic studies of sleep and obesity.

Future Directions

Better measurements of sleep habits are sorely needed in this field. Actigraphy appears to represent a useful tool in this regard though measurements of at least a week in duration are needed to compensate for the night-to-night variability present in sleep habits. Investigation into potential mechanisms linking short sleep with weight regulation should also be a priority as such research will help define whether the association with weight gain is causal in nature and may provide important insights into the evolutionary rationale for sleep. Thus, future epidemiologic studies need to consider more closely the associations between sleep duration and potential intermediate factors such as dietary choices, levels of physical activity, and energy expenditure.

Subgroup differences need to be investigated more closely as well. The effects of reduced sleep may be very different in those who sleep less due to insomnia or comorbid medical or psychiatric disorders as compared to those who sleep less due to personal preference. A better understanding of the potential for age to modify the effect of short sleep is also needed. Current data suggest that the association between short sleep and obesity is much stronger in younger populations, which may reflect a greater susceptibility to the biologic effects of sleep loss in younger individuals.

In the end, interventional trials that alter sleep patterns will be needed to definitively establish a causal relationship between sleep and weight regulation. For such studies to occur, behavioral interventions that can effectively improve sleep habits in the general population need to be developed and tested.

References

1. Terman L, Hocking A. The sleep of school children, its distribution according to age, and its relationship to physical and mental efficiency. *J Educ Psychol.* 1913;4:269-282.
2. Tune GS. Sleep and wakefulness in normal human adults. *BMJ.* 1968;2:269-271.

3. *2005 Sleep in America Poll*. Washington: National Sleep Foundation, 2005.

4. Spiegel K, Leproult R, Van Cauter E. Metabolic and endocrine changes. In: Kushida CA, ed. *Sleep Deprivation: Basic Science, Physiology, and Behavior*. New York: Marcel Dekker; 2005:293-318.

5. Shaw PJ. Thermoregulatory changes. In: Kushida CA, ed. *Sleep Deprivation: Basic Science, Physiology, and Behavior*. New York: Marcel Dekker; 2005:319-338.

6. Savourey G, Bittel J. Cold thermoregulatory changes induced by sleep deprivation in men. *Eur J Appl Physiol Occup Physiol*. 1994;69:216-220.

7. Rechtschaffen A, Bergmann BM. Sleep deprivation in the rat: an update of the 1989 paper. *Sleep*. 2002;25:18-24.

8. Sawka MN, Gonzalez RR, Pandolf KB. Effects of sleep deprivation on thermoregulation during exercise. *Am J Physiol*. 1984;246:R72-R77.

9. Kolka MA, Martin BJ, Elizondo RS. Exercise in a cold environment after sleep deprivation. *Eur J Appl Physiol Occup Physiol*. 1984;53:282-285.

10. Dinges DF, Pack F, Williams K, et al. Cumulative sleepiness, mood disturbance, and psychomotor vigilance performance decrements during a week of sleep restricted to 4-5 hours per night. *Sleep*. 1997;20:267-277.

11. Locard E, Mamelle N, Billette A, Miginiac M, Munoz F, Rey S. Risk factors of obesity in a five year old population. Parental versus environmental factors. *Int J Obes Relat Metab Disord*. 1992;16:721-729.

12. von Kries R, Toschke AM, Wurmser H, Sauerwald T, Koletzko B. Reduced risk for overweight and obesity in 5- and 6-y-old children by duration of sleep—a cross-sectional study. *Int J Obes Relat Metab Disord*. 2002;26:710-716.

13. Patel SR, Malhotra A, Gottlieb DJ, White DP, Hu FB. Correlates of long sleep duration. *Sleep*. 2006;29:881-889.

14. Patel SR, Malhotra A, White DP, Gottlieb DJ, Hu FB. Association between reduced sleep and weight gain in women. *Am J Epidemiol*. 2006;164:947-954.

15. Manini TM, Everhart JE, Patel KV, et al. Daily activity energy expenditure and mortality among older adults. *JAMA*. 2006;296:171-179.

16. Rechtschaffen A, Bergmann BM. Sleep deprivation in the rat by the disk-over-water method. *Behav Brain Res*. 1995;69:55-63.

17. Mullington JM, Chan JL, Van Dongen HP, et al. Sleep loss reduces diurnal rhythm amplitude of leptin in healthy men. *J Neuroendocrinol*. 2003;15:851-854.

18. Spiegel K, Tasali E, Penev P, Van Cauter E. Sleep curtailment in healthy young men is associated with decreased leptin levels, elevated ghrelin levels, and increased hunger and appetite. *Ann Intern Med*. 2004;141:846-850.

19. Spiegel K, Leproult R, L'Hermite-Baleriaux M, Copinschi G, Penev PD, Van Cauter E. Leptin levels are dependent on sleep duration: relationships with sympathovagal balance, carbohydrate regulation, cortisol, and thyrotropin. *J Clin Endocrinol Metab*. 2004;89:5762-5771.

20. Spiegel K, Leproult R, Colecchia EF, et al. Adaptation of the 24-h growth hormone profile to a state of sleep debt. *Am J Physiol Regul Integr Comp Physiol*. 2000;279:R874-R883.

21. Spiegel K, Leproult R, Van Cauter E. Impact of sleep debt on metabolic and endocrine function. *Lancet*. 1999;354:1435-1439.

22. Sivak M. Sleeping more as a way to lose weight. *Obes Rev*. 2006;7:295-296.

23. Ayas NT, White DP, Al-Delaimy WK, et al. A prospective study of self-reported sleep duration and incident diabetes in women. *Diabetes Care*. 2003;26:380-384.

24. Gottlieb DJ, Punjabi NM, Newman AB, et al. Association of sleep time with diabetes mellitus and impaired glucose tolerance. *Arch Intern Med*. 2005;165:863-867.

25. Gangwisch JE, Heymsfield SB, Boden-Albala B, et al. Short sleep duration as a risk factor for hypertension: analyses of the first National Health and Nutrition Examination Survey. *Hypertension*. 2006;47:833-839.

26. Patel SR, Hu FB. Short sleep duration and weight gain: a systematic review. *Obesity*. In Press.

27. Sekine M, Yamagami T, Handa K, et al. A dose-response relationship between short sleeping hours and childhood obesity: results of the Toyama Birth Cohort Study. *Child Care Health Dev.* 2002;28:163-170.

28. Padez C, Mourao I, Moreira P, Rosado V. Prevalence and risk factors for overweight and obesity in Portuguese children. *Acta Paediatr.* 2005;94:1550-1557.

29. Chaput JP, Brunet M, Tremblay A. Relationship between short sleeping hours and childhood overweight/obesity: results from the 'Quebec en Forme' Project. *Int J Obes (London).* 2006;30:1080-1085.

30. Giugliano R, Carneiro EC. Factors associated with obesity in school children. *J Pediatr (Rio J).* 2004;80:17-22.

31. Ben Slama F, Achour A, Belhadj O, Hsairi M, Oueslati M, Achour N. [Obesity and life style in a population of male school children aged 6 to 10 years in Ariana (Tunisia)]. *Tunis Med.* 2002;80:542-547.

32. Gupta NK, Mueller WH, Chan W, Meininger JC. Is obesity associated with poor sleep quality in adolescents? *Am J Hum Biol.* 2002;14:762-768.

33. Benefice E, Garnier D, Ndiaye G. Nutritional status, growth and sleep habits among Senegalese adolescent girls. *Eur J Clin Nutr.* 2004;58:292-301.

34. Knutson KL. Sex differences in the association between sleep and body mass index in adolescents. *J Pediatr.* 2005;147:830-834.

35. Chen MY, Wang EK, Jeng YJ. Adequate sleep among adolescents is positively associated with health status and health-related behaviors. *BMC Public Health.* 2006;6:59.

36. Agras WS, Hammer LD, McNicholas F, Kraemer HC. Risk factors for childhood overweight: a prospective study from birth to 9.5 years. *J Pediatr.* 2004;145:20-25.

37. Reilly JJ, Armstrong J, Dorosty AR, et al. Early life risk factors for obesity in childhood: cohort study. *BMJ.* 2005;330:1357.

38. Kripke DF, Garfinkel L, Wingard DL, Klauber MR, Marler MR. Mortality associated with sleep duration and insomnia. *Arch Gen Psychiatr.* 2002;59:131-136.

39. Amagai Y, Ishikawa S, Gotoh T, et al. Sleep duration and mortality in Japan: the Jichi Medical School Cohort Study. *J Epidemiol.* 2004;14:124-128.

40. Tamakoshi A, Ohno Y. Self-reported sleep duration as a predictor of all-cause mortality: results from the JACC study, Japan. *Sleep.* 2004;27:51-54.

41. Heslop P, Smith GD, Metcalfe C, Macleod J, Hart C. Sleep duration and mortality: the effect of short or long sleep duration on cardiovascular and all-cause mortality in working men and women. *Sleep Med.* 2002;3:305-314.

42. Gottlieb DJ, Redline S, Nieto FJ, et al. Association of usual sleep duration with hypertension: the Sleep Heart Health Study. *Sleep.* 2006;29:1009-1014.

43. Bjorkelund C, Bondyr-Carlsson D, Lapidus L, et al. Sleep disturbances in midlife unrelated to 32-year diabetes incidence: the prospective population study of women in Gothenburg. *Diabetes Care.* 2005;28:2739-2744.

44. Vioque J, Torres A, Quiles J. Time spent watching television, sleep duration and obesity in adults living in Valencia, Spain. *Int J Obes Relat Metab Disord.* 2000; 24:1683-1688.

45. Singh M, Drake CL, Roehrs T, Hudgel DW, Roth T. The association between obesity and short sleep duration: a population-based study. *J Clin Sleep Med.* 2005;1:357-363.

46. Cournot M, Ruidavets JB, Marquie JC, Esquirol Y, Baracat B, Ferrieres J. Environmental factors associated with body mass index in a population of Southern France. *Eur J Cardiovasc Prev Rehabil.* 2004;11:291-297.

47. Taheri S, Lin L, Austin D, Young T, Mignot E. Short sleep duration is associated with reduced leptin, elevated ghrelin, and increased body mass index. *PLoS Med.* 2004;1:e62.

48. Moreno CR, Louzada FM, Teixeira LR, Borges F, Lorenzi-Filho G. Short sleep is associated with obesity among truck drivers. *Chronobiol Int.* 2006;23:1295-1303.

49. Ko GT, Chan JC, Chan AW, et al. Association between sleeping hours, working hours and obesity in Hong Kong Chinese: the 'better health for better Hong Kong' health promotion campaign. *Int J Obes (London).* 2007;31:254-260.

50. Kohatsu ND, Tsai R, Young T, et al. Sleep duration and body mass index in a rural population. *Arch Intern Med.* 2006;166:1701-1705.

51. Chaput JP, Després JP, Bouchard C, Tremblay A. Short sleep duration is associated with reduced leptin levels and increased adiposity: results from the Québec Family Study. *Obesity.* 2007;15:253-261.

52. Shigeta H, Shigeta M, Nakazawa A, Nakamura N, Yoshikawa T. Lifestyle, obesity, and insulin resistance. *Diabetes Care.* 2001;24:608.

53. Vorona RD, Winn MP, Babineau TW, Eng BP, Feldman HR, Ware JC. Overweight and obese patients in a primary care population report less sleep than patients with a normal body mass index. *Arch Intern Med.* 2005;165:25-30.

54. Lauderdale DS, Knutson KL, Yan LL, et al. Objectively measured sleep characteristics among early-middle-aged adults: the CARDIA study. *Am J Epidemiol.* 2006;164:5-16.

55. Gortmaker SL, Dietz WH Jr, Cheung LW. Inactivity, diet, and the fattening of America. *J Am Diet Assoc.* 1990;90:1247-1252, 1255.

56. Ohayon MM, Vecchierini MF. Normative sleep data, cognitive function and daily living activities in older adults in the community. *Sleep.* 2005;28:981-989.

57. Ohayon MM. Interactions between sleep normative data and sociocultural characteristics in the elderly. *J Psychosom Res.* 2004;56:479-486.

58. Hasler G, Buysse DJ, Klaghofer R, et al. The association between short sleep duration and obesity in young adults: a 13-year prospective study. *Sleep.* 2004;27:661-666.

59. Gangwisch JE, Malaspina D, Boden-Albala B, Heymsfield SB. Inadequate sleep as a risk factor for obesity: analyses of the NHANES I. *Sleep.* 2005;28:1289-1296.

60. Felson DT, Anderson JJ, Naimark A, Walker AM, Meenan RF. Obesity and knee osteoarthritis. The Framingham Study. *Ann Intern Med.* 1988;109:18-24.

61. Jacobson BC, Somers SC, Fuchs CS, Kelly CP, Camargo CA Jr. Body-mass index and symptoms of gastroesophageal reflux in women. *N Engl J Med.* 2006;354:2340-2348.

62. Kenchaiah S, Evans JC, Levy D, et al. Obesity and the risk of heart failure. *N Engl J Med.* 2002;347:305-313.

63. Camargo CA Jr, Weiss ST, Zhang S, Willett WC, Speizer FE. Prospective study of body mass index, weight change, and risk of adult-onset asthma in women. *Arch Intern Med.* 1999;159:2582-2588.

64. Young T, Peppard PE, Gottlieb DJ. Epidemiology of obstructive sleep apnea: a population health perspective. *Am J Respir Crit Care Med.* 2002;165:1217-1239.

65. Vgontzas AN, Papanicolaou DA, Bixler EO, Kales A, Tyson K, Chrousos GP. Elevation of plasma cytokines in disorders of excessive daytime sleepiness: role of sleep disturbance and obesity. *J Clin Endocrinol Metab.* 1997;82:1313-1316.

66. Jenkins JB, Omori T, Guan Z, Vgontzas AN, Bixler EO, Fang J. Sleep is increased in mice with obesity induced by high-fat food. *Physiol Behav.* 2006;87:255-262.

67. *Diagnostic and Statistical Manual of Mental Disorders, DSM-IV-TR: Text Revision.* Washington: American Psychiatric Publishing, Inc.; 2000.

68. Flier JS, Elmquist JK. A good night's sleep: future antidote to the obesity epidemic? *Ann Intern Med.* 2004;141:885-886.

69. Partinen M, Kaprio J, Koskenvuo M, Putkonen P, Langinvainio H. Genetic and environmental determination of human sleep. *Sleep.* 1983;6:179-185.

70. Stunkard AJ, Foch TT, Hrubec Z. A twin study of human obesity. *JAMA.* 1986;256:51-54.

71. Watson NF, Goldberg J, Arguelles L, Buchwald D. Genetic and environmental influences on insomnia, daytime sleepiness, and obesity in twins. *Sleep.* 2006;29:645-649.

72. Turek FW, Joshu C, Kohsaka A, et al. Obesity and metabolic syndrome in circadian Clock mutant mice. *Science.* 2005;308:1043-1045.

73. Walsleben JA, Kapur VK, Newman AB, et al. Sleep and reported daytime sleepiness in normal subjects: the Sleep Heart Health Study. *Sleep.* 2004;27:293-298.

74. Jean-Louis G, von Gizycki H, Zizi F, et al. Determination of sleep and wakefulness with the actigraph data analysis software (ADAS). *Sleep.* 1996;19:739-743.

75. Jean-Louis G, von Gizycki H, Zizi F, Spielman A, Hauri P, Taub H. The actigraph data analysis software: I. A novel approach to scoring and interpreting sleep-wake activity. *Percept Mot Skills*. 1997;85:207-216.
76. Patel SR, Ayas NT, Malhotra MR, et al. A prospective study of sleep duration and mortality risk in women. *Sleep*. 2004;27:440-444.
77. Lockley SW, Skene DJ, Arendt J. Comparison between subjective and actigraphic measurement of sleep and sleep rhythms. *J Sleep Res*. 1999;8:175-183.
78. Carskadon MA, Dement WC, Mitler MM, Guilleminault C, Zarcone VP, Spiegel R. Self-reports versus sleep laboratory findings in 122 drug-free subjects with complaints of chronic insomnia. *Am J Psychiatr*. 1976;133:1382-1388.
79. Means MK, Edinger JD, Glenn DM, Fins AI. Accuracy of sleep perceptions among insomnia sufferers and normal sleepers. *Sleep Med*. 2003;4:285-296.
80. Somers VK, Dyken ME, Mark AL, Abboud FM. Sympathetic-nerve activity during sleep in normal subjects. *N Engl J Med*. 1993;328:303-307.
81. Shaw PJ, Bergmann BM, Rechtschaffen A. Effects of paradoxical sleep deprivation on thermoregulation in the rat. *Sleep*. 1998;21:7-17.
82. Van Cauter E, Latta F, Nedeltcheva A, et al. Reciprocal interactions between the GH axis and sleep. *Growth Horm IGF Res*. 2004;14 (Suppl A):S10-S17.
83. Redline S, Kirchner HL, Quan SF, Gottlieb DJ, Kapur V, Newman A. The effects of age, sex, ethnicity, and sleep-disordered breathing on sleep architecture. *Arch Intern Med*. 2004;164:406-418.
84. Ford DE, Kamerow DB. Epidemiologic study of sleep disturbances and psychiatric disorders. An opportunity for prevention? *JAMA*. 1989;262:1479-1484.
85. Vgontzas AN, Bixler EO, Lin HM, et al. Chronic insomnia is associated with nyctohemeral activation of the hypothalamic-pituitary-adrenal axis: clinical implications. *J Clin Endocrinol Metab*. 2001;86:3787-3794.

17

Social Determinants of Obesity

Gary G. Bennett, Kathleen Y. Wolin, and Dustin T. Duncan

Introduction

Over 2000 years ago, the philosopher Aristotle issued a simple, yet prescient thesis, writing, "Society is something in nature that precedes the individual." Aristotle's notion is one that is particularly salient today. In an era characterized by an explosion of research into fundamental biological systems, we are seeing a parallel surge of interest in understanding the social determinants of health. Myriad recent reports from the Institute of Medicine, World Health Organization, United Nations, and other organizations have emphasized the importance of more frequently considering social determinants as fundamental influences on health and disease. The reader is directed to reviews providing the theoretical bases of the social determinants perspective.[1] Briefly, however, the social determinants approach requires attention to "the causes of the causes," moving beyond the individual to explore potential determinants occurring at multiple levels. While social determinants clearly include factors reflecting sociodemographic (e.g., gender, nativity, race/ethnicity, socioeconomic position [SEP]) and psychosocial (e.g., stress, occupational demands, purely psychological constructs such as depression and anxiety) characteristics, they also include more upstream factors, including neighborhood characteristics, social structures, and the social environment. Certainly, one of the more important social determinants of health in most societies is the level of economic development; in most societies, greater development is associated with increased longevity, and reductions in the prevalence of infectious disease. For most conditions, patterns of disease distribution cannot be fully explained by focusing solely on individual behaviors and health practices; health behaviors, rather, are heavily influenced by the broader social context in which they occur. The challenge of the social determinants perspective then, both for epidemiological investigation and ultimately for intervention, is that while the more upstream social determinants undeniably pattern individual-level behavior, the ubiquity in and variability of social determinants challenges their empirical assessment. This is particularly the case when one considers social determinants in a global context, as many such determinants are influenced by globalization, and the increasing inequities between industrialized and nonindustrialized nations.

The social determinants perspective is one that is particularly well suited to obesity research, conducted both in the United States and in most of the industrialized world.

Obesity is a condition whose primary and most proximate determinants (diet and physical activity) are not elusive; however, we are increasingly learning that to promote a shift in population distribution of obesity requires attention to the full range of social factors that impact dietary and physical activity practices. Indeed, embedded within the social context are myriad determinants of obesity; these factors are tightly interrelated with the condition at multiple levels. It is well known, for example, that dietary choices and opportunities for physical activity are heavily patterned by socioeconomic resources. Chronic exposure to psychosocial stress may increase the likelihood of "comfort eating." Depression might diminish one's interest in a physical activity regimen. Together, a range of social determinants are implicated in the epidemic rates of obesity both in the United States and abroad. However, research attention to the social determinants of obesity is in its infancy; it is critical to both identify determinants with putative relations to obesity, while continuing to investigate their assessment better.

The purpose of this chapter is to review the empirical evidence, in a range of populations, detailing associations between selected social determinants and obesity. Secondary aims include discussing measurement strategies for the various social determinants reviewed and introducing methodological approaches that might be useful when conducting social determinants research. We primarily focus on obesity outcomes, although we will discuss associations that are mediated by diet or physical activity when appropriate. There are a wide range of potential constructs that might potentially fall under the umbrella of social determinants research. In selecting the social determinants reviewed here, we have attempted to identify factors for which there is sufficient evidence to draw meaningful conclusions and for which there is some consensus regarding appropriate measurement strategies. As the literature in this area is extensive, our discussion is limited to (a) studies examining obesity outcomes (including body mass index [BMI] and weight data) rather than dietary and/or physical activity end points; (b) general, nonclinical, and adult populations; and (c) data collected outside of intervention trials.

Sociodemographic Characteristics

Sociodemographic variation in obesity is considerable. Individuals generally gain weight as they age (with the most substantial weight gains occurring during middle age). Over the last quarter-century, obesity prevalence among those aged 65 to 74 has been particularly striking; rates of obesity in this age group have doubled from 1976-1980 to 1999-2002. In nearly all industrialized nations, women are found to have the highest levels of obesity. In the United States, women's higher rates of obesity have been shown nearly consistently for the past 40 years, as demonstrated in the nationally representative National Health and Nutrition Examination Survey (NHANES) studies (see Chapter 2). Sociocultural factors among some populations, high rates of childhood overweight in girls, midlife weight gain, and postpartum weight retention may be implicated in these gender differences. In addition to age and gender, ranges of other sociodemographic characteristics are closely related with obesity, particularly for race/ethnicity and nativity.

Race/Ethnicity

The 1985 Heckler report brought widespread popular attention in the United States to the problem of racial/ethnic disparities in health. By 1998, public health attention to the issue was rising and in a radio address that year, President William J. Clinton challenged researchers to eliminate racial/ethnic disparities by the year 2010. In response, the National Institutes of Health (NIH) integrated disparities research into its strategic plan. Since then research investigating the social determinants of disparities in a range of health conditions has increased considerably. While obesity has received comparatively less attention, racial/ethnic variation in obesity has nevertheless been observed.

The United States Census Bureau projects that by the year 2100, America will be majority-minority, with non-Hispanic whites occupying only 40% of the U.S. population. At present however, obesity is disproportionately prevalent in several racial/ethnic minority populations, which becomes all the more concerning when one considers the expected increase in the proportion of racial/ethnic minority groups in the U.S. population in years to come.

According to the 2000 U.S. Census, approximately 30% of the U.S. population belongs to a defined racial/ethnic minority group, which includes those who self-identify as black or African American (those with origins in any of the black racial groups of Africa), Asian Americans (those with origins in the Far East, Southeast Asia, or the Indian subcontinent), American Indian or Alaska Native (those descended from the original peoples of North, Central, and South America), native Hawaiian or Pacific Islander (those with origins in any of the original peoples of Hawaii, Guam, Samoa, or other Pacific Islands), and Hispanic or Latino populations (those with Cuban, Mexican, Puerto Rican, South or Central American, or other Spanish culture or origin). Individuals who self-identify as Hispanic or Latino may be of any racial category, including white. In addition, beginning with the 2000 U.S. Census, individuals were permitted to indicate two or more federally designated racial categories—such individuals are generally referred to as multiracial. The most recent data from the NHANES study show that in 2003-2004, the prevalence of obesity among non-Hispanic blacks was 45%, compared to 37% among Mexican Americans and 30% for non-Hispanic whites.

Most studies generally agree that obesity is less prevalent among the Asian Americans, compared to whites and other U.S. racial/ethnic minority populations. Self-reported BMI data from the National Health Interview Survey (NHIS) show, however, that there is sizeable ethnic variation within the Asian population, such that BMI is highest among Japanese and Filipino men and Filipino and Indian women (Vietnamese men and women have the lowest BMI among Asian Americans). As is discussed shortly, nativity is highly related to obesity in the United States; the prevalence of obesity among Asian Americans is highest among those who are native-born. Among the foreign-born, obesity increases proportionately with duration of residence. Very little data exists to capture accurately the obesity prevalence in native Hawaiian/Pacific Islander populations; however, the available evidence suggests that the group has slightly higher obesity prevalence compared to non-Hispanic whites.[2]

Racial/ethnic disparities in obesity are particularly striking when examined by gender; presently, nearly 54% of black women are obese, and non-Hispanic black women are more than twice as likely to be obese, compared to non-Hispanic white women. Compared to whites, the prevalence of obesity is higher among non-Hispanic black and Hispanic men,[3] though most data indicate that the differences are not statistically significant.[3-5] Indeed, this pattern of minimal (and not statistically significant) differences in obesity between black and white U.S. men has persisted during most of the second half of the 20th century. In contrast, odds of obesity are nearly twice as high among black and Hispanic women than among white women in most,[3-6] but not all,[7] studies.

Numerous hypotheses have been offered to explain racial/ethnic differences in obesity. As a higher proportion of racial/ethnic minorities in the United States are of lower SEP, some have argued that race/ethnicity might be a proxy for differences influenced by SEP. More recent evidence among U.S. blacks, showing limited SEP variation in obesity, contradicts this notion. Some but not all evidence[8] suggests that racial/ethnic minorities, compared to whites, may have a more rapid onset of obesity. Most frequently however, sociocultural factors that affect social norms for dietary patterns and physical activity have been cited as primary determinants of race/ethnicity differences in obesity.

U.S. blacks, for example, appear to have a greater social acceptance of overweight, less body weight dissatisfaction, and higher body weight ideals compared to whites.[9-15] In addition, emerging evidence in nationally representative cohorts suggest that blacks, and to a lesser extent Hispanics, may have lower rates of perceived overweight compared to whites.[16-17] Bennett et al.[17] reported that overweight blacks and Hispanics are more likely to perceive themselves to be at average weight compared to whites. Misperception of weight status may drive obesity-related behaviors, including dietary patterns and intentional physical activity.[16-17]

While racial/ethnic differences in health are robust and consistent, it is perhaps surprising that the most commonly used measure of self-identified race/ethnicity in the United States is adapted from federal criteria established by the Office of Management and Budget (OMB). These OMB racial/ethnic designations are widely used in large population-based health surveillance studies and in the U.S. census. Despite their ubiquity, the designations present considerable interpretive difficulties in epidemiologic research.

Race/ethnicity has been commonly used as a proxy for unmeasured confounders, including those social, cultural, and environmental factors that are often more proximately associated with health-related outcomes. Although, for example, a higher proportion of U.S. blacks are in poverty when compared to whites, variability within the population makes race/ethnicity a poor proxy for socioeconomic deprivation. Similarly, the experience of immigration and acculturation may result in foreign-born Hispanics having drastically different health behavior practices than their native-born Hispanic counterparts, despite their collective membership in a single ethnic category.

There is widespread consensus that "race" reflects a socially determined construct and not one that is necessarily biologically based or particularly scientific in nature. Nevertheless, racial/ethnic variation in health has also been used as a proxy for genetic differences. The traditional analytic approach that attributes residual "racial" effects (those remaining after adjustment for identifiable confounders) to genetic differences has been criticized by a number of authors. Cooper[18] has argued that as a fixed attribute, race/ethnicity is unsuitable for causal modeling because of the counterfactual challenge; that is, one is unable to answer what the health of those with race X would be if they developed as race Y. However, given the emergent data suggesting the importance of genetic variation in obesity risk, it may be increasingly important to understand the extent to which variation occurs by group. There is consensus, however, that the use of stratified (within-race) designs is most suitable for the exploration of racial/ethnic variation in genetic susceptibility to obesity.

Over the past decade, there has been substantial debate regarding the most appropriate measurement strategy for capturing racial/ethnic data. There is consensus that self-identified race/ethnicity is preferable in comparison to external ratings (e.g., those performed by a physician or researcher). While self-identified race/ethnicity has value in allowing individuals to select a designation that most closely matches their social and cultural backgrounds and experiences, nearly all commonly used measures of race/ethnicity lack precision. The OMB designated racial/ethnic categories, for example, will almost certainly mask important within-group variation. For example, they designate only one ethnic category (Hispanic or Latino), despite the sizable ethnic variation in other racial categories (e.g., among Asian Americans and blacks). An additional challenge concerns misclassification of those who designate multiracial heritage. At present, such individuals are assigned to a single *multiracial* category, or to a single *dominant* racial/ethnic category, or are removed from analysis. There are scant data in the adult obesity literature regarding appropriate strategies for treating multiracial U.S. population data; this remains an important area of future study.

In summary, though racial/ethnic categories are useful in defining populations with disproportionate prevalence of obesity, the existing categorizations are generally regarded as nonspecific and may lead to incorrect assumptions about biological, social, cultural, and socioeconomic homogeneity. In the United States, studies funded by the NIH are required to report accrual data by race and ethnicity; the availability of these data may promote interest in exploring racial/ethnic differences. However, given the inherent challenges in extrapolating meaningful interpretations when racial/ethnic differences are identified, researchers should be advised to carefully consider their rationale for exploring racial/ethnic variation, whether their study design supports such examinations, and perhaps most importantly, whether additional data have been collected to determine whether racial/ethnic variation is attributable to other factors that are more proximately associated with the outcome.

Nativity

Immigration to the Unites States has increased by over 16% in the past 5 years and has been accompanied by increasing popular attention paid to the issue. Such interest has been mirrored in the research literature, in which a number of studies (primarily conducted in developed nations) have explored associations between nativity and obesity, with a particular focus on the immigrants' duration of residence in the host country.

Most U.S. data indicate lower obesity prevalence among immigrants, compared to native-born residents.[19,20] These findings likely reflect the migration of individuals from nonindustrialized countries (where the prevalence of obesity is ostensibly low) to industrialized nations. The acculturative process has been associated with rapid gains in obesity, such that in a relatively short period, immigrant's obesity prevalence "catches up" with that of the host country. Several U.S. and Canadian studies show that the prevalence of obesity among immigrants increases with longer duration of residence.[21,22] Mostly independent of ethnic background (with the exception of black immigrants to the United States, among whom no such association is found);[23] some evidence suggests that the increase in obesity (associated with the duration of residence) occurs more rapidly among women than men.[24] In contrast to other data from industrialized nations, studies from Sweden and the United Kingdom indicate that immigrants are more likely to be obese.[25,26]

Together, these findings may suggest that it is not the migration process itself that contributes to obesity differences, but the obesity prevalence and/or lifestyle practices in the country of emigration. However, most U.S. research suggests that some characteristics of the acculturative process are associated with increasing rates of obesity among immigrants. The term acculturation is used in reference to many different things, including, but not limited to, dimensions of language usage, migration status, generational status, duration of time spent in the United States, ethnicity of social networks, and cultural pride. Several acculturation scales have been created and validated across a variety of populations.[27-30] Many studies use a single measure of language acculturation[31,32] along with the birthplace of the one's parents.[33,34] Language acculturation is most commonly measured by asking participants about their language preference, often in specific settings. For example, study participants might be asked to report their preferred language for reading, speaking, thinking, conversing with friends, and watching television or listening to the radio.[27,35] Despite the limitations of the language acculturation measure, language acculturation has frequently been positively associated with obesity.

Finally, other measures of acculturation have been employed. These often include questions on knowledge of U.S. (or dominant culture) values, familiarity with country of origin cultural practices and the value placed on preserving them, attitude toward traditional family structure, and the ethnicity of the participants social network.[27,36] In black immigrants, Tull et al.[37] found the adoption of U.S. values was positively associated with BMI.

The majority of research demonstrating an association between acculturation and obesity has been conducted in Hispanic populations;[35,38-41] although studies in non-Hispanic populations reveal more mixed findings, they still demonstrate an inverse association between immigration status and obesity.[42,43]

Together, the available data suggests that nativity is a powerful predictor of obesity and with increasing duration of residence and perhaps through acculturation, immigrants' obesity eventually reaches that of their native-born counterparts. Therefore, following immigrant populations prospectively might provide additional insight into the impact of social determinants on obesity.

Socioeconomic Position

SEP is a multidimensional construct that incorporates a range of potential indicators reflecting one's status/position in the social hierarchy, wealth, power/prestige, ownership of material resources, and the associated social standing. Throughout, we use the term *socioeconomic position*, which has been defined as "an aggregate concept that includes both resource- and prestige-based measures as linked to both childhood and adult social class position."[44] This is in contrast to the term *socioeconomic status*, which refers exclusively to the prestige associated with one's standing in the social hierarchy.

Although it is a multidimensional construct, SEP is frequently indexed using single indicators, and without sufficient attention to the interpretive difficulties inherent with that approach. At the individual level, a variety of SEP indicators are frequently found in the empirical literature. Educational attainment is commonly assessed using the number of years of formal schooling and/or by capturing data on educational credentialing. Income is captured by requesting wages (at the annual, monthly, weekly, or hourly level) in continuous dollars or categories. Using a categorical response scale (best determined by the expected range among study participants) is more common because individuals are notoriously reticent about providing their precise income (relative to reporting education or occupation). Income can also be examined by incorporating data on income from all sources and/or at the household level (requiring knowledge of the household size), though one must consider that income may not be equally available to all household members. There has been increasing interest in measuring wealth assessed using household assets, home/car ownership, and so on. Poverty status often incorporates data on family/household income, adjusted for family/household size and can be compared to a given poverty threshold (provided at the state or federal level) for that year. Occupational status can be measured by capturing data on one's level of current employment, occupational prestige, job history, occupational title, managerial status, number of hours worked, and/or full-time/part-time status. Some studies also assess participation in government financial assistance programs (e.g., WIC, food stamps, AFDC, Medicare, Medicaid, SCHIP), and some studies use indices that combine multiple sources of data.

At the area level, numerous SEP indicators are accessible, including variables like wealth, poverty, occupational class, education, and indices such as the Townsend index (which combines unemployment, the proportion of households without a car, proportion of those who do not own their homes, and overcrowding). We discuss methodological issues related to the collection and utilization of neighborhood SEP and area-based socioeconomic measures (ABSMs) in the following sections.

Non-Western and Developing Countries

Generally speaking, the literature investigating on non-Western and developing countries reports a positive association between SEP and obesity in many,[45,46] but not all, studies.[47,48] Given the great variation in the design of these studies, it is challenging to draw conclusions, but the data here are striking; one study showed that being impoverished in a poor country (per capita gross national product [GNP] less than $800 per year) was associated with a decreased obesity risk and malnutrition, while the poor in more affluent countries have an increased obesity risk.[49] For example, Subramanian and Smith[45] measured the standard of living, caste, education level, occupation, and living environment of Indians and found that each of the SEP measures were positively associated with obesity.

That we would observe a positive relation between SEP and obesity among those in the developing world is perhaps not surprising. We have begun to see rapidly increasing rates of obesity in developing nations over the past 20 years, as characteristics of the Western lifestyle (decreasing physical activity and increased consumption of energy-dense foods) have become more prevalent, starting among the affluent. As developing nations become more economically prosperous, urbanized, and industrialized, conditions such as obesity (which are sensitive to the lifestyle changes promoted by economic development) can be expected to increase.

United States, Western Europe, Canada, and Australia

Studies conducted in developed countries have similarly employed a range of socioeconomic indicators; however, in developed countries, particularly in the United States (where the bulk of this work has been conducted), associations between SEP and obesity are complex and vary by both gender and race/ethnicity. The accumulated evidence suggests an inverse association between SEP and obesity among women in developed societies; among all racial and ethnic groups combined, women of lower income are approximately 50% more likely to be obese than those with higher income levels. Evidence of the inverse association is less consistent among men.[50,51] As noted, however, the association varies by race/ethnicity.

Using data from the Atherosclerosis Risk in Communities (ARIC) study, Mujahid et al.[52] found high levels of obesity for women with low income and low-education levels, independent of race or ethnicity.[52] Among men, however, the association varied by race; in white men, obesity was inversely associated with income, while for black men obesity and income were positively associated. Similarly, Zhang and Wang,[53] using NHANES III data, found that among non-Hispanic black and Mexican American men, SEP and BMI were positively associated, but among non-Hispanic white men, an inverse association existed. In contrast with the ARIC data, only non-Hispanic white women in NHANES III demonstrated an association between SEP and obesity. Most European studies generally report an inverse association with obesity across several SEP indicators.[54] The vast majority of studies thus far have used cross-sectional designs. Ball and Crawford,[51] however, reviewed the existing longitudinal evidence examining associations between SEP and weight change. They found that in nonblack research samples, there were strong inverse associations with obesity of occupational status among men and women, with less evidence for educational attainment (particularly for men). Data were inconsistent among both women and men in studies examining income as a SEP indicator of weight gain. The authors found little evidence for an association between SEP and weight gain among blacks (though they noted having limited studies). The latter finding is consistent with other evidence showing limited socioeconomic variation in obesity among blacks, particularly women.[55]

Among the areas of emerging interest, some have begun to create indices of lifecourse SEP to better capture the impact of early life adversity and socioeconomic mobility on obesity in adulthood.[56-58] Most commonly, attempts to capture lifecourse SEP used indicators of parental education (particularly father's education), parental occupation, measures of the early life household context (e.g., food sufficiency, receipt of governmental assistance during childhood), or similarly crude summary indices reflecting socioeconomic mobility from childhood to adulthood. For example, James et al.[58] have examined lifecourse SEP effects on obesity by first creating a four-level SEP exposure that categorizes socioeconomic mobility as low childhood SEP-low adulthood SEP, low childhood SEP-high adulthood SEP, high childhood SEP-low adulthood SEP, or high childhood SEP-high adulthood SEP. Each of these strategies is subject to recall bias and presents some interpretive challenges; for example, use of parental education as a surrogate for early life adversity must be carefully interpreted given the potential for noncomparability between participants, due to their parent's age, geographic residence, gender, occupational status, and race/ethnicity (to name but a few). James et al.[58] found, in a sample of African American women, that low childhood SEP doubled the likelihood of adulthood obesity, as compared to women of high childhood SEP. In addition, the authors found that women who were of low SEP in both childhood and adulthood had a 2-fold greater obesity risk compared to women who were of high SEP at both times. Suggesting the importance of early life circumstances, the odds of obesity were 55% higher in women who had low childhood SEP but high adulthood SEP (compared to women of high SEP during both periods).

A number of considerations should be noted when drawing conclusions from studies examining SEP. In general, most SEP indicators are subject to reverse causality when examined in association with obesity outcomes. Individuals may experience decreases in income, wealth, occupational status, and increased poverty status with elevated BMI, owing to health difficulties, disability, and stigmatization. Although education, occupational status, and income are among the most widely used measures of SEP, they are not interchangeable, and maybe differentially predictive by population. Further, each of these three widely used variables has distinct qualities that should be considered. Unlike income or occupation, educational attainment is stable, can be assessed for all individuals, is useful across the age spectrum (including among those who are retired, or disabled), and is less subject to reverse causality when adulthood health outcomes are studied. Educational attainment, however, is subject to cohort biases and generational effects. Further, the economic return/occupational prestige associated with a given level of education may vary by race/ethnicity, gender, and nativity.

Occupational status has many benefits as a measure, given that it reflects the gains produced by educational attainment, and it is more stable than income over time. Occupational status can also reflect exposure to environmental and occupational conditions. Despite these benefits, there are challenges in selecting appropriate occupational status measures. A common strategy is to link job titles to the U.S. Census Standard Occupational Classification, a federal system used to classify workers into occupational categories; the huge variation in present day job titles can make this a challenging endeavor. Most approaches to linking job titles promote the possibility of misclassification, and the noncomparability of jobs across populations and geographic regions challenges the utility of the measures. Income (in comparison to education and occupation) is unstable, yet is sensitive to life circumstances. Income is also age dependent and may be less useful among those of retirement age. There are a number of challenges interpreting such data, as purchasing power associated with income may be noncomparable across geographic regions or sociodemographically diverse groups; for example, it is well known that fruits and vegetables as well as dairy foods are more expensive in low-income urban neighborhoods than in middle-class suburban environments. All economic measures (including income, wealth, and poverty status) may not be sensitive to informal financial transactions and assets (e.g., inheritances, savings, and benefits).

Neighborhood Characteristics

Where you live is undeniably linked to health. Living in a neighborhood with access to multiple full-service supermarkets, plentiful safe options for physical activity, and options for walking for transportation (rather than using an automobile) may decrease one's likelihood for becoming obese. While recognition of the importance of the local neighborhood context is not new, such research has surged in popularity in recent years as the limitations of focusing only on individual-level determinants have been increasingly acknowledged. Particularly in industrialized nations, recent research has explored the myriad potential connections between obesity and aspects of the neighborhood context (including the built environment). Although epidemiological attention to these issues is relatively new, and evidence is still accumulating, the importance of considering neighborhood characteristics as fundamental determinants of obesity is nevertheless becoming increasingly apparent. In this section, we review the accumulating body of empirical evidence on selected obesogenic neighborhood characteristics. We begin with an overview of neighborhood SEP and then discuss specific neighborhood characteristics that primarily act through dietary pathways (supermarkets and other food stores, fast food restaurants), followed by those that are primarily associated with physical activity (urban sprawl, neighborhood safety).

Neighborhood Socioeconomic Position

As has been discussed, there is abundant evidence that individual SEP is strongly associated with obesity risk and related behaviors across a wide range of populations. Arguably, the bulk of evidence in the neighborhood effects literature pertains to neighborhood SEP. It generally shows that residing in a socioeconomically disadvantaged neighborhood is also associated with poorer health in general, and increased odds of obesity more specifically (largely independent of individual SEP). Both individual-level and neighborhood SEP independently (and perhaps differentially) affect health status,[59] with neighborhood SEP serving as a strong predictor of sociostructural determinants of obesity. For example, neighborhood deprivation may influence obesity risk by restricting access to healthy food and opportunities for physical activity, while also impacting cultural characteristics (e.g., social norms).

A number of cross-sectional investigations (conducted in the United States, United Kingdom, Australia, and Sweden) show that living in a more socioeconomically disadvantaged neighborhood is associated with higher odds of obesity.[52,60-65] For example, Cubbin et al.[62] linked socioeconomic indicators of neighborhood-level deprivation with individual-level data from the Swedish Annual Level of Living Survey. They found that living in a neighborhood characterized by low socioeconomic deprivation was associated (after adjusting for a range of individual-level indicators) with lower odds of obesity, compared to residing in a neighborhood with moderate socioeconomic deprivation.

Opposing findings have been documented and relatively few prospective studies have been conducted. In one of the very few longitudinal studies in this area, Mujahid et al.[52] linked data from the ARIC (a prospective investigation in four U.S. communities of varying socioeconomic and racial/ethnic composition) with data on neighborhood socioeconomic characteristics taken from the 1990 U.S. census. Over time, they found no association between neighborhood SEP and BMI; however, there was some evidence of a positive association between neighborhood SEP and BMI among black men and women. This finding is largely consistent with the bulk of prospective evidence, which has generally been mixed with respect to its prediction of significant differences in BMI change associated with various dimensions of neighborhood SEP. Why cross-sectional evidence is more consistent than prospective data linking neighborhood SEP with BMI is largely unclear. Certainly, methodological issues could be implicated (e.g., loss to follow-up, selection of analytic strategies), but strong secular trends for weight gain in the general population may also be responsible. In addition, if socioeconomic differences strongly impact BMI at baseline, variation over time may be less apparent.

Ultimately, however, the randomized controlled trial design provides the best evidence for an association between neighborhood-level factors and obesity; such trials are generally not feasible, given their logistic, political, and financial implications. However, between 1994 and 1998, 4600 low-income families were recruited from five cities (Baltimore, Boston, Chicago, Los Angeles, and New York) and recruited to participate in the Moving to Opportunity for Fair Housing (MTO) demonstration program. Individuals randomly assigned to the experimental group were offered housing vouchers that could be used in exchange for residence in low-poverty neighborhoods (<10% poor); others were randomly assigned either to receive standard Section 8 benefits or to a control group, in which they continue to live in public housing or receive other housing assistance. Interim effects of the MTO project were published in 2003 and among the positive mental and physical health changes documented in the experimental group; study planners described the reduction in obesity as *substantial*.[66]

Some empirical evidence indicates that neighborhood SEP has a differing effect by gender, age, income, and race/ethnicity.[52,60,63,64,67-69] For example, several studies have found that neighborhood SEP is associated with greater BMI among women, but not men.[52,60,64,65] Although the effects of neighborhood SEP are often independent of individual SEP, some studies have shown a moderating effect of individual socioeconomic indicators. One study showed that among those living in high poverty areas, blacks and those with the lowest incomes had the lowest levels of physical activity.[69] Another study showed that in low SEP neighborhoods, low-income blacks were the most likely to have unhealthy diets (compared with their low-income white, higher-income white, and higher-income black counterparts).[68]

Tightly interwoven with neighborhood disadvantage is residential segregation, a complex, multidimensional construct that also may drive the emergence of other obesity risk exposures in the neighborhood context.[70,71] Put simply, residential segregation is physical separation in residential contexts.[71] Residential segregation is pervasive in the United States, particularly in major metropolitan areas. Neighborhoods in the United States are often highly segregated across racial/ethnic and socioeconomic lines; the situation may result from institutional discrimination (e.g., housing discrimination and mortgage-lending discrimination)[70,71] and residential preferences (particularly among immigrants), and may be reinforced by a concentrated socioeconomic disadvantage found in many areas where such segregation is rampant. Research investigating residential segregation and obesity risk is extremely limited.

One study[72] found that higher racial isolation among non-Hispanic blacks was positively associated with BMI, even after adjustment for several individual-level factors, including SEP. No significant association was found between racial isolation and BMI among whites.[72]

The effects of residential segregation (and neighborhood SEP for that matter) are most likely mediated through its influence on obesity-related neighborhood characteristics.[55,73,74] Illustratively, a number of studies have showed that racial/ethnic minorities and persons of lower SEP have restricted access to supermarkets,[75-78] fewer fruit and vegetable markets,[75] lower quality of fresh products in neighborhood stores,[79] and limited access to stores with fresh produce.[80] Furthermore, U.S.-based research shows that predominantly black neighborhoods have more fast food restaurants compared to predominantly white neighborhoods,[81] and a study in the United Kingdom found positive associations between neighborhood deprivation and the presence of McDonald's restaurants.[82] In addition, research demonstrates that low SEP neighborhoods have significantly fewer physical activity resources than areas of higher SEP.[83-85] These obesogenic neighborhood characteristics are a concerning byproduct of neighborhood disadvantage and residential segregation. Deleterious obesity-related neighborhood characteristics do not exist only in poor and predominantly racial/ethnic minority communities; however, overwhelming evidence suggests that they are more prevalent in such neighborhoods and individuals in these settings may be more susceptible to their influence.[71,86]

Area-Based Socioeconomic Measures

The use of ABSMs has emerged as extremely useful tools for probing socioeconomic differentials in a range of health conditions. Use of ABSMs allows for the assessment of socioeconomic variation occurring beyond the individual-level (e.g., variation occurring at the neighborhood, city, state, and national levels). Given the growing evidence showing that obesity can be influenced by one's place in society (whether framed in terms of socioeconomic standing, neighborhood, occupation, etc.), ABSMs can be used to further explore this variation when their application along with the appropriate statistical strategy (to be discussed below) allow one to model these socioeconomic exposures. Use of ABSMs is not new; though the approach has existed for almost a century, there has been very little empirical consensus regarding a selection of the most appropriate measures for analysis. These considerations are not trivial, given the sheer volume of ABSM data that can be examined. One needs to be concerned with the selection of appropriate socioeconomic indicators—income, for example, can be expressed as median household income, percentage low-income, percentage high income, as a Gini coefficient (a measure of income inequality), or a composite measure. One also must select the most appropriate geographical level for analysis.

ABSMs can be linked to a number of geographic levels, including the census block group, census tract, and zip code. The seminal work of Krieger et al.[87-92] was designed to investigate which of 18 specific ABSMs (11 single variables and 7 composite) and geographical levels were the most useful and sensitive to predict socioeconomic gradients in a range of health outcomes. They found that the census tract poverty measure consistently demonstrated socioeconomic variation in the expected directions and had widespread availability and straightforward interpretability. The work of Krieger et al.[87-92] provides guidance in the selection of ABSMs that might be used to further understand how such socioeconomic variation is manifest in the United States.

However, geocoding can be used to link data emerging from a range of other sources. The process of geocoding simply refers to the assignment of a code representing geographic location;[87] common geocodes include latitude and longitude. These can be used to link one's source data to other external data with geographic identifiers (e.g., police precinct, postal area, supermarket vicinity). In this way, one can link individual-level data with any number of available area-level indicators; as more data sources emerge with such identifiers, this process will greatly enhance our ability to understand the associations of area-level variables with obesity.[88-92]

Most studies in the neighborhood effects literature have used aggregate data (e.g., neighborhood SEP, racial segregation), with very little attention paid to whether these variables are indeed appropriate proxies for the specific features of the neighborhood environment that are believed to directly impact health behavior practices. For example, if one is specifically interested in making causal arguments regarding neighborhood-level features that are associated with obesity, modeling those exposures (number of fast food restaurants for full-service supermarkets in a given census tract) is a preferable approach to using aggregate data (e.g., neighborhood SEP), which likely reflect a different source of influence. A major limitation in the existing neighborhood effects literature has been the failure to adequately discuss the potential mechanisms linking neighborhood characteristics (particularly neighborhood SEP) with obesity outcomes.

Neighborhood Influences on Diet

Supermarkets and Other Food Stores

Though evidence in this area is still emerging, it is becoming clear that access to food stores (that offer healthful options) may be associated with reduced obesity risk. Studies in this area have investigated a range of food store types, including supermarkets, grocery stores, convenience stores, and specialty stores.[77] Most studies have investigated access (or proximity) to specific food stores as determinants of obesity and dietary practices. To illustrate, Morland et al.[93] found that the presence of supermarkets in one's census tract was associated with lower obesity prevalence, and that the presence of convenience stores was associated with higher obesity rates. Importantly, the study also found that people living in areas with grocery and/or convenience stores but no supermarkets had the highest prevalence of obesity. Fruit and vegetable intake, however, was found to be positively associated with the number of supermarkets in a census tract. Another study, utilizing structural equation modeling, found that women shopping at supermarkets and specialty stores consumed fruits and vegetables more often than those who shopped at independent grocery stores.[76]

While the relation between food store availability and obesity seems mostly consistent in the United States, in the United Kingdom, findings have been mixed.[94,95] In the United States, however, there is some evidence of effect modification by race/ethnicity in the association between food store availability and dietary outcomes, but less with regard to obesity outcomes.[93] Research on food store access, availability, and quality as contributors to obesity is an important area for future study.

Much of the most compelling existing research on food stores exists at the area level; studies that combine measures of access (in a given census tract for example) with original assessments of food store quality are needed. No standard definitions exist at present to describe the various food store types (i.e., grocery, supermarkets, full-service supermarkets, bodegas)—most categorizations differ by study. Many related studies have failed to consider important effect modifiers, such as individual shopping patterns, transportation patterns, and sociodemographic characteristics. Factors including price, freshness, and health considerations have been shown to influence food-purchasing decisions; these practices may vary between populations, and may influence the decision to seek food sources outside of one's neighborhood. While studies examining area-level food store penetration on individual-level obesity are an important first step, multilevel strategies that incorporate individual behavioral patterns as effect modifiers are needed. Finally, the temporal direction of the association may seem straightforward; however, obese individuals may select neighborhoods with certain types of stores, or market research may locate stores in areas where individuals prefer certain foods (i.e., where demand for their products is high) and/or by obesity prevalence.

Fast Food Restaurants

Eating away from home has increased dramatically in the United States over the past 25 years, which is of concern given that food prepared at home is of a higher quality than that consumed while eating out.[96] Fast food restaurants (which often have limited and unhealthy food options) are a popular source of food consumed away from home, but the high energy density of many foods available in these settings constitutes a significant risk factor for obesity.[97] Most Americans do not eat fast food daily, but nearly 40% report eating it one to two times/week. A number of U.S. studies have shown positive cross-sectional (and some longitudinal) associations between fast food consumption and poorer dietary practices, including higher total energy intake and higher percentage fat energy; there is somewhat less evidence for decreased consumption of fiber and fruits and vegetables[98-100] and obesity.[98,99,101] For example, one study[102] found an association between the concentration of residents per fast food restaurant and state-level obesity prevalence.

There is other evidence demonstrating effect modification in the relation between fast food restaurants and obesity, in sometimes-unexpected directions. For instance, Jeffery and French[99] found that the number of fast food meals eaten per week was positively associated with BMI among high-income women, but not among low-income women and men. Another study found that change in the frequency of fast food consumption over 15 years was directly associated with changes in body weight in whites, but more weakly in blacks.[101] Given area-level variation in access to fast food as well as individual variation in purchasing power and food preferences, examining the full range of effect modifiers in the association between fast food and obesity is necessary.

How to best define what constitutes fast food is not clear—it is almost certain that both misclassification and undercounting have occurred. For example, should ethnic food stores (e.g., Chinese, Indian), pizzerias, and coffee shops that sell baked goods be included? Methodological work is necessary to both define food store types and establish appropriate categorization strategies. Finally, as with other food stores, the direction of the association may seem mostly uncontroversial, but it is unclear whether fast food store placement (which can also be based on neighborhood characteristics) may affect interpretations drawn regarding the direction of the fast food-obesity association.

We should remember that regular fast food consumption is a reality for many Americans; it may also be a functional strategy for those in low SEP groups, who benefit from widely available, inexpensive, and highly palatable food (despite its energy density). Public health strategies are already shifting to recommend that individuals purchase the more *healthful* fast food options that are becoming increasingly available.

Neighborhood Influences on Physical Activity

Urban Sprawl

Over the last quarter century, we have observed a secular shift towards greater urban sprawl in the United States. With increasing longevity and the steady increase in population, urban sprawl has become widespread, particularly in areas with rapid population growth (e.g., Atlanta, Houston). The term "urban sprawl" is somewhat loosely defined, but generally is characterized by the confluence of several land use patterns, including (but not limited to) low-density land use, single-use zoning, employment dispersion, reductions in pedestrian-friendly thoroughfares, architectural homogeneity, and limited options for walking or biking. Urban sprawl is believed to heighten rates of obesity by spurring increased automobile use and decreasing the time and contexts available for safe, routine physical activity (as areas with greater sprawl may have more distant parks and fitness facilities, fewer sidewalks, and more heavily trafficked thoroughfares).

It is beyond the scope of this chapter to present a comprehensive overview of the myriad aspects of urban sprawl, but readers are referred to more detailed reports.[103,104]

Although the evidence base is limited, there is emerging evidence suggesting that people who live in more mixed-use neighborhoods are less likely to be obese and are more physically active. Urban sprawl is assessed in a variety of ways and consensus has not emerged for the most effective assessment strategy for use in obesity studies examining obesity outcomes. Most assessment strategies utilize either single/multiple proxy indicators (e.g., residential density, walkability, intersection density/street connectivity, car ownership, land use mix) or summary indices. Lopez[105] developed such an index, using data from the 2000 U.S. Census that, assessed residential density and its compactness (or how residential density is distributed across a metropolitan area). Using a multilevel design, combining individual-level variables from the 2000 Behavioral Risk Factor Surveillance System (BRFSS) with the urban sprawl index (measured at the metropolitan level), Lopez found an increased risk of obesity associated with urban sprawl, after adjusting for individual-level characteristics (including age, race/ethnicity, household income, and education).

In studies using urban sprawl proxy indicators, similar results have been shown; the available evidence indicates that greater urban sprawl is negatively associated with physical activity,[106-109] and positively associated with BMI[108] and obesity.[105,108,110] More specifically, positive relations with obesity have been found for a range of sprawl indicators, including less land use mix,[111] residential density,[111] intersection density/street connectivity,[111] greater time spent in cars,[111] and car ownership.[112]

Similarly, increased physical activity has been found to be associated with several proxy sprawl indicators: greater land mix,[103,106,113] residential density,[103,106,111,114,115] and intersection density/street connectivity.[103,106,111]

Urban sprawl research investigating connections with obesity is still in its infancy. Some null results have been shown for both physical activity and obesity outcomes, although the wide range of urban sprawl assessment strategies limits the comparability of studies and by extension, interpretations that can be drawn from the empirical inconsistency. The bulk of research has been conducted in the United States, with emerging work from India and Australia; studies in these areas have generally shown the expected pattern of results.

Some work has found that race/ethnicity and gender may each modify the association of urban sprawl indicators with both physical activity and obesity, suggesting that urban sprawl is particularly predictive among whites (vs. blacks) and men (vs. women).[111] For example, Frank et al.[111] showed used travel survey data collected among 10 878 residents in 13 counties throughout the Atlanta region. They found a general effect of urban sprawl indicators on the likelihood of being obese; there was a 12.2% decrease in obesity odds for each quartile of increased mixed use, and an increase of 6% for each additional hour spent in a car. However, the authors also observed significant associations with BMI of numerous indicators (including mixed use, street connectivity, residential density, walking distance, and time spent in cars) among whites (particularly white men), but not blacks. Some have suggested that the impact of urban design on transportation patterns, particularly the decision to engage in physical activity for transportation purposes, may vary by race/ethnicity. It may also be the case that sprawl affects some racial/ethnic populations less because they have a higher likelihood of remaining concentrated in mixed use areas.

There are several methodological considerations for research in this area. Different methodologies for assessing the effect of community design on physical activity and obesity are used across studies;[103,116] this may in part explain the differing results, and varying magnitudes of association. A number of studies have assessed urban design using an aggregate measurement, increasing the potential for ecologic bias. In addition, there are different definitions of *neighborhood*. Unmeasured confounding is also possible, as several aspects of the built environment are not frequently examined (including light posts, benches, sidewalk quality).

Neighborhood Safety

Concerns about neighborhood safety may influence willingness to engage in outdoor physical activity. Particularly in urban settings, neighborhood safety concerns may also promote utilization of nonambulatory transportation options (e.g., use of buses, subways, and automobiles). Many have hypothesized an inverse association between perceived neighborhood safety and physical activity, but empirical investigations of the association have yielded mixed findings.[117] Some,[118-120] but not all,[84,103,121-123] studies have found an inverse relation between perceived neighborhood safety and physical activity. Furthermore, there is some evidence that perceived neighborhood safety is related to overweight[124] and obesity.[125] This research has primarily been conducted in the United States although some work has emerged from both Europe and Australia.

Sociodemographic variation (including racial/ethnic, gender, and age) may exist in the association between neighborhood safety and physical activity. One study found an inverse association between perceived neighborhood safety and physical activity in whites, while a null association was found in blacks,[126] but it is necessary to note that other studies have found a positive relation between perceived neighborhood safety and physical activity among blacks,[127] and other evidence indicates that neighborhood safety may be a stronger physical activity predictor for nonwhites than for whites.[128] Furthermore, research indicates that concerns of neighborhood safety seem to be more important for women.[129,130]

Several methodological considerations are significant to note. There is considerable variation in the measurement strategies used to ascertain *safety* in most research on the topic. For example, some have assessed safety related to crime, and others have assessed safety related to traffic, dogs, or used perceived safety measures; this variation may explain, in part, the inconsistent findings. Few of the studies in this area have directly examined obesity outcomes despite the clear potential for perceived neighborhood safety to increase obesity risk, particularly among those in low income and urban environments. Effect modification is essential to understanding the effects of neighborhood safety. Given the relevance of this experience for those of low SEP (who have a disproportionately high obesity prevalence), much more work in this area is necessary.

Neighborhood Measurement Considerations

In summary, considerable empirical evidence demonstrates that obesogenic neighborhood characteristics impact diet, physical activity, and obesity. However, a number of considerations affect interpretations that can be drawn from these literatures.

While the science of individual measurement has been well established over the past 5 decades, we are only beginning to explore the possible strategies for assessing neighborhood-level influences and how they might be best integrated with individual-level data. The potential threats to validity using the current arsenal of neighborhood assessment techniques are considerable and a complete review of the challenges inherent in using these approaches is beyond our scope; there are, however, a number of major issues that should be considered.

There is no precise and universally accepted definition of what constitutes a neighborhood. As has been described, Krieger et al.[88] have demonstrated the utility of the census tract unit, which is widely utilized in the United States. Little attention has been paid to whether census tracts and similar geographic units are consistent with individual's perceptions of what constitutes a neighborhood. While the convenience of using these geographic units has enabled the neighborhood effects literature to grow rapidly and produce compelling early results, misclassification remains a major threat to validity. And, as Messer[131] notes, "the geographic unit that maximizes predictive utility may not be the one that best corresponds to one's theory of causation." Theory is particularly important because it drives the a priori identification of potential causal mechanisms that can be empirically investigated. There is little utility in exploring patterns of association without seeking to uncover causal processes.

A variety of measurement approaches have been employed to capture neighborhood-level features. A common strategy is to incorporate data available in administrative, commercial, municipal, or online corporate databases (e.g., locations of food stores, fast food restaurants, parks) using geographic information systems.[132] Original data collection can also be used, employing human raters to identify neighborhood characteristics using standardized inventories. For example, in the past 5 years, a number of standardized rating scales have become available to identify neighborhood characteristics that might serve as barriers/facilitators to regular physical activity. These inventories permit (often multiple) raters to capture neighborhood data in a predefined catchment area; when used, inter-rater reliability estimates should be presented when using these strategies given the inherent biases. These observational approaches can prove a powerful tool for identifying neighborhood-level features that are inaccessible through other means; however, logistical challenges prohibit the use of original data collection in large geographically dispersed epidemiological samples.

Self-report remains a widely used strategy for capturing neighborhood-level data and a number of measures exist to assess various dimensions of the neighborhood environment that might be associated with obesity. The challenges associated with self-report assessment strategies are widely noted, but a particularly pressing concern in the area of neighborhood effects is the potential for source bias. Social desirability, lifestyle behaviors, and personality characteristics might increase the likelihood of systematic biases in participant reporting. Perceptions of neighborhood characteristics may vary widely and it is inappropriate to consider self-reports as consistent with objective reality. Mujahid et al.[133] presented an intriguing strategy for overcoming these biases. Interested in studying neighborhood actors associated with cardiovascular disease (CVD) risk, the authors collected data on neighborhood conditions from a separate sample of individuals who resided in the same neighborhoods as the primary study participants. Data from those who rated neighborhood characteristics were aggregated and linked with the study sample to examine the hypothesized associations.

It is likely that the major challenge in the neighborhood effects literature is the issue of structural confounding.[131] In most cases, individuals are not randomly distributed into neighborhoods; rather, a variety of macro-level forces (e.g., policy, history, economic trends) as well as personal preferences, cultural traditions, and occupational considerations drive individuals into some neighborhoods and not others. Structural confounding occurs because, even after adjusting for traditional covariates (e.g., age, income, race/ethnicity, occupational status, lifestyle behaviors), individuals still differ with regard to the unmeasured confounders that influenced their differential distribution into specific neighborhoods. As a result, even after statistical adjustment, individuals are noncomparable, rendering causal inferences inappropriate.[132]

Ultimately, the emerging data on neighborhood effects are both exciting and compelling. Methodological challenges are increasingly being addressed, enhancing the potential for these data to substantively inform future intervention and prevention efforts. However, to maximize the utility of neighborhood-level data, researchers need to not only describe those factors correlated with obesity and its related risk behaviors but also identify the mechanisms that may ultimately lead to individuals adopting more healthful behaviors.[131]

Psychosocial Factors

The term *psychosocial* has been used widely without explicit definition to describe primary individual-level influences on health and disease. Martikainen et al.[134] suggest that psychosocial factors are those that (a) mediate effects of social structural factors on individual health outcomes, and/or (b) are conditioned and modified by the social context in which they exist.[134] They view psychosocial factors as meso-level influences; as such, they serve as crucial links that mediate the impact of macro-level exposures on micro-level processes occurring at the individual level. Thus, in some cases these psychosocial factors may serve as mediators, making them appropriate targets for intervention; in others, they may serve to modify the impact of more distal exposures on obesity outcomes. Here we review several common psychosocial factors with demonstrated associations with obesity: stress, social support, and depression.

Stress

The notion that chronic stress may exert a deleterious effect on health is not a new one. For generations, investigators have sought to discern the etiological contributions of chronic stress to the development of many chronic health conditions. Most have pursued the hypothesis that physiological dysregulation results from increased levels of perceived stress and/or the utilization of a coping disposition that fails to adequately buffer the impact of exposure to chronic stress. The investigation of stress as a determinant of health has been complicated by its numerous conceptualizations. Stress is a rather loosely defined term that has often been used empirically as a general descriptor of a latent (or unobservable) force that disturbs homeostasis or allostasis.

It is widely believed in popular circles that stress is associated with obesity—so much so, that a cottage nutritional supplements industry has emerged to help individuals prevent stress-induced weight gain. Despite this, the literature detailing relations between stress and obesity is much more limited than might be expected (though studies investigating dietary end points are much more common).[135-137] Nevertheless, positive findings have been reported. In a prospective investigation, Korkeila et al.[138] found that high levels of psychosocial stress at baseline were associated with greater weight gain at 6 and up to 15 years post-baseline. Similarly, compared to those with healthy children, Smith et al.[139] showed that parents of child cancer patients had significantly greater weight gain over a 3-month period. Interestingly, the effect was proportional to the amount of stress reported and the weight gain was more tightly related to reductions in physical activity than diet.

Many have posited mechanistic links to explain the association between stress and obesity.[140-143] Among the range of biological responses to stress, activation of the hypothalamic-pituitary-adrenal (HPA) axis is associated with a range of resulting processes, including dysregulation in the glucocorticoid hormone cortisol (also see Chapter 18). A number of observational studies have demonstrated associations of cortisol dysregulation with visceral adiposity, and obesity.[140,143-145] Marniemi et al.[146] showed, in a sample of monozygotic twins, discordant for obesity, that visceral fat accumulation was associated with higher levels of psychosocial stress and the consequent elevations in cortisol and noradrenaline. More recent evidence suggests that the association between cortisol secretion and obesity may be mediated by sex steroid and growth hormone secretion, and potentially, polymorphisms in a number of key genetic markers.[140]

Increased food intake has also been posited as a possible link between stress and obesity; stress may drive the consumption of highly caloric *comfort foods*. For example, in a prospective study of 5,150 Finnish men and women, Laitinen et al.[147] found that by age 31, BMI was highest among those who were rated "stress-driven eaters and drinkers"; such individuals experienced numerous stressful life events and were more likely to consume energy-dense foods, compared to other participants. Biological processes may also drive stress-induced comfort food consumption.[148] A number of studies have shown that elevations in glucocorticoid secretion increase the likelihood of one consuming energy-dense foods.[149] In addition to weight gain (particularly in the abdominal region), comfort food consumption may stimulate pleasure centers in the brain, thus regulating stress-induced systemic arousal.[149]

Occupational Stress

The workplace is a context that provides almost routine exposure to chronic psychosocial stressors. Occupational demands account for a large proportion of the daily stressors encountered by individuals,[150,151] primarily because of the extended amount of time (30% to 40% of one's waking hours) and effort expended there.[152] Unlike other stressors that can be more easily avoided, most are continuously subjected to the demands of the occupational arena.

The demand/control or *job strain* model[153] is the dominant theoretical construct of occupational stress.[152] The model posits that risk is influenced "from the joint effects of the demands of a work situation and the range of decision-making freedom (discretion) available to the workers facing those demands." Jobs with high demands require an excessive amount of work output, usually under a variety of constraints (i.e., time pressures, performance expectations, layoff possibilities). Those in jobs with low decision latitude have little control over their assigned tasks, work that is often characterized by its simplicity and repetitive nature. The job strain condition is characterized by jobs with high demands and low perceived control. The accumulated evidence supports an association between job strain and CVD incidence and mortality,[152,154-157] as well as all-cause mortality[158,159] (though there have been several negative studies as well).

The literature on job strain and obesity is also mixed;[160-162] some studies have shown elevated BMI among those with high job strain.[163-165] Higher BMI has also been observed among those high job demands[163,166] and low levels of decision latitude.[165,167,168] In the Whitehall II study, Kivimaki et al.[169] hypothesized that the association between job strain and elevated BMI may be particularly evident among the overweight, who (in contrast to normal-weight individuals) might be disposed to overeating when experiencing occupational stress. They found that the effects of both job strain and low job control were dependent on baseline BMI; participants in the highest BMI quintile had the greatest weight gain over 5 years of follow-up. In addition, there is some evidence that gender may moderate the effects of occupational stress on obesity;[165,170] this is not surprising as gender is correlated both with perceived stress and choice of coping response. As such, researchers interested in better understanding the stress-obesity relation are advised to consider the potential for effect moderation by gender.[169]

Measurement Issues

Although it has been somewhat loosely defined, a number of strategies in the measurement of stress are apparent. The first has attempted to measure characteristics of the social environment that are believed to be particularly demanding (either objectively or normatively). Checklist measures of stressful life events have often been used in this regard. Such measures invite the participant to indicate which of a number of stressful events (e.g., death of a spouse or child, divorce, job loss) have occurred to them within a specific time period. Generally speaking, these measures are scored by summing the number of stressful life events, with higher scores indicating elevated stress; some measures, however, weigh the intensity of particular events. A number of other measures have been widely used to measure stressful life events,[171] though they are not particularly well suited to population-based epidemiological investigations; these include semistructured personal interviews and stressful event measures (that are completed daily by a participant over a given time period).[172]

The other broad stress measurement approach has been to examine perceived stress, or an individual's subjective ratings of their ability to manage (or cope with) the demands of their social environment.[173] While there are comparatively fewer of these measures, Cohen's Perceived Stress Scale[174,175] has been very widely used (in 4-, 10-, and 14-item versions) to assess the degree to which individuals believe that their stress outweighs their ability to cope. As exposure to stress can be associated with negative affect, adjective checklist measures can be used to assess participant's mood. A number of such measures exist,[176] although the number of items (which can exceed one hundred) may be too large for routine epidemiologic use.

Regardless of approach, stress measures have numerous limitations. Clearly, stress is a subjective construct and whether the existing stress measures are appropriate for use across populations remains to be determined. Many suggest that there is a social class gradient in exposure to chronic stress, such that individuals of lower SEP are more likely to encounter adverse stressors and less likely to be adequately prepared to manage these demands; racial/ethnic minority groups and women may similarly be at risk for higher stress levels.[177] Researchers should therefore be careful to ensure that the chosen measure has been tested and is appropriate for administration in the target population. Further, investigators should be clear that the measure effectively distinguishes between stressors that are acute (which may be highly intense but resolve or become manageable over time) and those that are chronic (which may or may not be highly intense, but are unremitting over time). Ultimately, investigators should be clear regarding their research questions when selecting stress measures, as measures are not interchangeable and in some cases, use of multiple measures may be indicated.

Social Support

There is a vast literature that explores the benefits of interpersonal relationships for health-related outcomes.[178-185] These studies are based on the premise that greater connectedness with other individuals and one's social context at large are beneficial for health and well-being. Perhaps surprisingly, there are correspondingly fewer studies demonstrating independent associations with obesity outcomes. The vast majority of studies in this area concern the importance of social connections for intervention processes/outcomes[186-190] and maintenance of weight loss.[191-193]

Social support, which can be thought of simply as resources provided by others,[194] has arguably received the bulk of research attention; there are at least two major types of social support that are frequently investigated. Emotional support generally refers to things that others do to demonstrate love, caring, and encouragement; this type of support is thought to be nontangible in nature. Instrumental support, on the other hand, refers to more tangible assistance (e.g., providing money, transportation, and childcare). Most work investigating social support has been performed in the intervention context and evidence suggests that receiving social support is at least moderately associated with better weight reduction outcomes, regardless of whether that support comes from a friend/family member[195] or a counselor/coach.[196-198]

There is evidence suggesting that individuals with lower levels of social support may be at risk for obesity. Raikkonen et al.[199] found that low overall social support was inversely associated with waist circumference among postmenopausal women. Similarly, in a cross-sectional study of 1967 Swedish women aged 18 to 34 years, Ali and Lindstrom[200] found that individuals with low emotional support were almost 70% more likely to be obese, while those with low instrumental support had a 2-fold higher obesity risk. Gender differences may also be present; Lallukka et al.[201] found that low social support was associated with 12-month weight gain only among women, in their sample of 8,892 Helsinki residents, aged 40 to 60 years. In addition, among women, low levels of emotional support have been associated with stress-related food consumption and obesity.[202]

The association between social support and obesity is a challenging one because of the clear plausibility of reverse causation driving any positive findings. Social isolation, perhaps resulting from stigmatization, is a well-established consequence of obesity for many individuals. Social support is likely best thought of as an effect modifier and may be used to identify the proportion of individuals who are at elevated obesity risk associated given exposure to adverse circumstances. The benefits of social support may vary by sociodemographic characteristics, and specific dimensions of social support (e.g., type, source, consistency of support) may also be differentially associated with obesity-related outcomes.

Although a wide range of measures are currently available to assess social support, consensus does not exist for the use of any single measure—this is one of the primary limitations of social support as a construct. Measures range from simple checklists detailing the availability of various support types to more elaborate inventories that delve into type, source, and availability of support.

Depression

Depression is a serious clinical disorder with considerable psychiatric and somatic consequences. It also constitutes an independent risk factor for several major medical conditions, including CVD. The extent to which depression serves as a determinant of obesity has intrigued many researchers over numerous decades, as the two conditions are heavily comorbid, given 15% prevalence of depression in the general population.[203] Thus, evidence supporting the supposition is complex.

There are a number of challenges when investigating the relation between depression and obesity. First, one must draw distinction in the literature between studies that have examined patient populations with major depressive disorder, from those who have investigated individuals in the general population. Given the intent of this chapter, we have primarily focused on the latter in the forthcoming discussion. Next, one must be particularly careful about terminology and measurement in this area. The term depression has been used widely to describe general negative affect, the presence of depressive symptoms (without a diagnosis), and major depressive disorder. Assessment strategies have been similarly varied, from short self-report scales of negative affect and mood to structured interviews, designed with the express purpose of making a psychiatric diagnosis.

The overwhelming majority of studies investigating this question have focused on depression or the negative effect experienced as a consequence of obesity.[204-206] Despite this intent, many of these studies have also been cross-sectional in nature, which has allowed the question of causality to linger. There have been a number of cross-sectional, general population studies showing a significant positive association between obesity and depression.[207-217] Kress et al.,[210] for example, found in cross-sectional data collected from 10,400 active duty U.S. service personnel, a significant positive relation between obesity and depression symptoms among both men and women; women, however, had a 3-fold increased odds of depressive symptoms. Similarly, Jorm et al.[218] showed, in a cross-sectional investigation among Australian residents, that depressive symptoms and obesity were positively associated among women, but weakly among men. However, after adjusting for potential mediators (e.g., physical health, physical activity, social support, and socioeconomic resources) the association weakened considerably. Haukkala and Uutela[219] administered the widely used Beck Depression Inventory (BDI) among 3,361 men and women, aged 25 to 64 years, and found a significantly positive relation between higher BDI scores, waist-hip ratio and BMI, though only among women. Carpenter et al.[214] measured major depression in the last year (as well as suicidal ideation and suicide attempts), diagnosed using the *Diagnostic and Statistical Manual of Mental Disorders* (DSM-IV) guidelines. They found that the pattern of results differed by gender, such that there was a positive association of increased BMI with both a major depression diagnosis and suicidal ideation among women. However, among men, major depression, suicide attempts, and suicidal ideation were associated with lower BMI. Together, the assembled studies are quite varied in approach[220] and the magnitude of these associations has generally been small;[220] some studies have shown an inverse relation,[221] and others have shown null results.[222,223] This has highlighted the need for prospective studies to investigate the association between depression and obesity, with particular attention to temporal ordering.

Only a handful of prospective investigations in this area have been conducted.[224,225] In one of the earliest, Pine et al.[226] administered psychiatric interviews to a sample of 776 adolescents in 1983 (aged 9 to 18 years) and followed them again in 1992, when they were aged 17 to 28 years. They found a positive relation between baseline depression levels and BMI; however, the association did not persist after adjustment for covariates. These findings were consistent with a smaller clinical study,[227] conducted by the same research group, which followed children aged 6 to 17 years who had either a depression diagnosis or no diagnosis. Over 10 to 15 years of follow-up, participants with a childhood depression diagnosis had significantly greater adulthood BMI. Most recently, the research group[228] studied a prospective cohort of 591 individuals (followed between ages of 19 and 40 years), who were administered clinical interviews to assess depression. After adjustment for multiple covariates, findings suggested that a diagnosis of depression before age 17 was associated with increased weight gain during adulthood and obesity among women, but not men. These findings were consistent with another prospective study conducted among a birth cohort of New Zealand residents, which found that at 26 years of follow-up, adolescent depression was associated with a significantly greater likelihood of obesity among adult women, but not men. In one of the more well-designed studies on the topic, Roberts et al.[229] examined depression (assessed using DSM-IV criteria) among 2,123 participants (aged 50 and older) in two waves of the Alameda County Study. This allowed the investigators to discern the temporal relation between the two constructs. After adjustment for relevant covariates, investigators found support for an association between obesity at baseline predicting depression after 5 years. Depression, however, was not found to increase the risk of obesity. Despite the strength of the design, only 5-year (self-reported) follow-up data were available; this was a major limitation, given the sample's higher age range.[50-94]

Both obesity and depression appear to have shared biological origins; the HPA-axis plays a major role in the development of both conditions.[230] Many have speculated on condition's shared determinants.[220,230] Briefly, excess production of, or external administration of glucocorticoids, such as cortisol, can lead to metabolic changes, indicative of visceral fat accumulation and obesity.[230-232] HPA-axis activity is similarly involved in depression.[233,234] Together, the available evidence clearly identifies the dysregulation of many HPA-axis components (with hypercortisolemia) as integral to both depression and obesity, leading to speculation of their shared origins and highlighting the importance of continuing to investigate their co-occurrence and potential roles as determinants of one another.

In addition to these biological processes, behavioral pathways may also be involved. Depression has been associated with increased comfort food consumption (which has been speculated to activate pleasure centers that regulate mood). Weight gain is also listed as a symptom of depression in the DSM-IV. Depression has also been associated with reductions in physical activity; similarly, physical activity interventions have been shown to improve mood.[235]

Widely regarded as a gold standard for depression assessment, the Structured Clinical Interview for DSM-IV Axis I Disorders (SCID) is a semistructured interview that allows for the diagnosis of the major DSM-IV Axis I disorders. The SCID is a modular assessment device that can be used to assess depression solely. An indicator reflecting the presence/absence of the condition of a current episode or for the lifetime occurrence is provided. Despite its utility, the time and expense associated with administering the SCID make it less useful for population-based epidemiologic investigations. As noted, the BDI is often used in clinical and epidemiologic investigations; the 21-item measure assesses major affective and somatic symptoms associated with depression. Similarly, the 20-item Center for Epidemiologic Studies of Depression Scale (CES-D) also assesses the presence of depressive symptomatology. Both the CES-D and BDI measures can distinguish between clinical populations and community samples; they can be scored continuously or can be used with thresholds associated with clinical diagnoses (that vary by population). A wide range of additional depression measures have been used in the literature; many of these scales are primarily measures of depressive symptomatology (rather than clinical depression). If a clinical diagnosis is needed, a structured interview with clinician administration is preferable. Key concerns when selecting a depression measure are both time and expense of administration, whether one needs to establish a clinical diagnosis, and the dimensions of depression that are hypothesized to be implicated.

In summary, there is sufficient evidence of an association between obesity and depression, although the direction and precise nature of the association are unclear.[220] The bulk of studies have been focused on the consequences of obesity for depression and even here, results are mixed.[220] While some prospective evidence suggests that early life depression predicts later weight gain and in some cases, obesity; other, well-designed studies counter these findings.[204,229] Gender also appears to be an important moderator of the association between depression and obesity and should be investigated in future work. The precise explanations for this finding are not clear, but both conditions are disproportionately prevalent among women; in addition, the social expression and consequences of both conditions may differentially affect women as well. Similarly, though admittedly with less evidence, SEP may be an important moderator as well; some studies have shown that the positive relation between obesity and depression holds for those with greater access to economic resources, while not consistently for those who are less well off. Future prospective studies are desperately needed on this topic, particularly those like the Alameda studies that have the ability to test the direction of the association.

Emerging Methodologies

A number of exciting new social and behavioral methodologies and analytical approaches are beginning to permeate the scientific literature. Structural equation modeling (SEM) is one such strategy that is particularly relevant to the study of social determinants of obesity. SEM is a technique that is particularly useful in theory-driven hypothesis testing.

Structural Equation Modeling

In most cases, social determinants do not maintain univariate associations with obesity-related outcomes, that is, for example, education likely has no direct relation with obesity; rather, it may increase the likelihood of experiencing psychosocial stress, which in turn leads to increased comfort food consumption and decreased physical activity. Stress might also increase the likelihood of experiencing depressive symptoms, both of which might be mediated through dysregulated cortisol secretion. Unlike most other areas, traditional analytic methods do not allow for easy investigation of these complex theoretical associations. As a result, the importance of using multivariate statistical methods in the social and behavioral sciences is increasingly being recognized.

SEM is one such multivariate solution that has been discussed widely. Briefly, SEM is a hypothesis-testing strategy that allows for examination of the structure (or underlying relations) in a theoretical model; it can be distinguished from other multivariate techniques because it utilizes a confirmatory rather than an exploratory approach. SEM (also referred to as causal, path, latent variable, or covariance structure models) is an important contribution to the study of social determinants for several reasons. First, as discussed, SEM allows for the investigation of dynamic relations occurring among multiple social predictors and their correspondingly numerous outcomes. Next, it controls for spurious inflation of type 1 error, which is a risk experienced when using multiple univariate analyses to test complex theoretical models. Unlike other multivariate methods, SEM allows the researcher to specify hypothesized relations among the studied variables. Most modern SEM software allow this to be done visually: the researcher literally draws the hypothesized theoretical model. SEM model specifications can include both nondirectional and unidirectional associations. For example, one might specify that depression and obesity are related (correlated), without specifying a precise direction; however, one could also specify a temporal ordering of the association. SEM also allows the researcher to specify latent variables and to specify relations among latent variables using observed measures. Finally, most SEM analysis packages allow for advanced strategies to manage missing data.

The most fundamental steps of SEM analysis involve building and testing of both measurement and structural models. To specify the measurement model, the researcher identifies constructs (both observable and latent), based on his/her a priori expectations. In the measurement-modeling step, model fit is tested in a process roughly equivalent to performing a confirmatory factor analysis. Once the measurement model fit has been determined, the structural model is specified, which involves examining the underlying relations between constructs specified in the measurement model, accounting for direct, indirect, and total effects of the factors. Although SEM is a sophisticated analytic strategy, it does have a number of limitations. Although often referred to as causal modeling, SEM is actually a corelational strategy that requires attention to temporality for causality to be inferred. Finally, though it allows for the building of sophisticated models, SEM is most effective with parsimonious models and large sample sizes.[236] Finally, the quality of SEM analyses is largely dependent on the quality of one's theoretical approach.

This is a key differentiator for SEM; most other multivariate strategies are primarily useful for describing patterns of association, while SEM's real strength is in testing theoretical models.[237] The utility of the strategy has increased, as scientists are increasingly interested in making sense of the wide range of seemingly disconnected associations demonstrated in the social epidemiological literatures.

Conclusion

Our aim in the present chapter was to provide the reader with a description of the evidence linking social determinants with obesity in a range of populations, while introducing some of the measurement considerations inherent in this line of work. As discussed, there is considerable empirical evidence demonstrating that social factors impact obesity, although there is great need for additional studies to reconcile areas with mixed evidence. A critical examination of this literature reveals that social determinants do not influence obesity in a uniform manner; rather, they are frequently modified by a range of variables, particularly sociodemographic characteristics. Further exploring the impact of effect modification on social determinants is an important area of future study.

The rapid secular rise in rates of obesity, both in the United States and abroad, strongly suggests the importance of devoting more systematic investigation into the influence of social determinants of the condition. Future research should consider addressing the methodological limitations noted and elucidating the mechanisms by which social factors may influence individual obesity risk. Although some hypotheses have been offered, the mechanisms linking social determinants (particularly the more upstream factors) and obesity have not been fully identified. A clearer understanding of these mechanisms will be essential to the development of effective intervention solutions. It is becoming increasingly well accepted that the epidemic rise in rates of obesity is reflective of the condition's social origins. This highlights the importance of adopting a societal orientation to identifying obesity's determinants and, ultimately, strategies to eradicate the condition.

References

1. Kawachi I, Berkman L. *Neighborhoods and Health*. Oxford: Oxford University Press; 2003.
2. Howarth NC, Murphy SP, Wilkens LR, Hankin JH, Kolonel LN. Dietary energy density is associated with overweight status among 5 ethnic groups in the multiethnic cohort study. *J Nutr*. 2006;136:2243-2248.
3. Ogden CL, Carroll MD, Curtin LR, McDowell MA, Tabak CJ, Flegal KM. Prevalence of overweight and obesity in the United States, 1999-2004. *JAMA*. 2006;295:1549-1555.

4. Flegal KM, Carroll MD, Ogden CL, Johnson CL. Prevalence and trends in obesity among US adults, 1999-2000. *JAMA*. 2002;288:1723-1727.

5. Dustan HP. Obesity and hypertension in blacks. *Cardiovasc Drugs Ther*. 1990;4 (Suppl 2):395-402.

6. Koutoubi S, Huffman FG. Body composition assessment and coronary heart disease risk factors among college students of three ethnic groups. *J Natl Med Assoc*. 2005;97:784-791.

7. Hemiup JT, Carter CA, Fox CH, Mahoney MC. Correlates of obesity among patients attending an urban family medical center. *J Natl Med Assoc*. 2005;97:1642-1648.

8. Sheehan TJ, DuBrava S, DeChello LM, Fang Z. Rates of weight change for black and white Americans over a twenty year period. *Int J Obes Relat Metab Disord*. 2003;27:498-504.

9. Flynn KJ, Fitzgibbon M. Body images and obesity risk among black females: a review of the literature. *Ann Behav Med*. 1998;20:13-24.

10. Kumanyika S, Wilson JF, Guilford-Davenport M. Weight-related attitudes and behaviors of black women. *J Am Diet Assoc*. 1993;93:416-422.

11. Striegel-Moore RH, Wilfley DE, Caldwell MB, Needham ML, Brownell KD. Weight-related attitudes and behaviors of women who diet to lose weight: a comparison of black dieters and white dieters. *Obes Res*. 1996;4:109-116.

12. Stevens J, Kumanyika SK, Keil JE. Attitudes toward body size and dieting: differences between elderly black and white women. *Am J Public Health*. 1994;84:1322-1325.

13. Smith DE, Thompson JK, Raczynski JM, Hilner JE. Body image among men and women in a biracial cohort: the CARDIA Study. *Int J Eat Disord*. 1999;25:71-82.

14. Powell AD, Kahn AS. Racial differences in women's desires to be thin. *Int J Eat Disord*. 1995;17:191-195.

15. Altabe M. Ethnicity and body image: quantitative and qualitative analysis. *Int J Eat Disord*. 1998;23:153-159.

16. Paeratakul S, White MA, Williamson DA, Ryan DH, Bray GA. Sex, race/ethnicity, socioeconomic status, and BMI in relation to self-perception of overweight. *Obes Res*. 2002;10:345-350.

17. Bennett GG, Wolin KY, Goodman M, et al. Attitudes regarding overweight, exercise, and health among Blacks (United States). *Cancer Causes Control*. 2006;17:95-101.

18. Cooper RS. Race, genes, and health—New wine in old bottles? *Int J Epidemiol*. 2003;32:23-25.

19. Singh GK, Siahpush M. Ethnic-immigrant differentials in health behaviors, morbidity, and cause-specific mortality in the United States: an analysis of two national data bases. *Hum Biol*. 2002;74:83-109.

20. Park SY, Murphy SP, Sharma S, Kolonel LN. Dietary intakes and health-related behaviours of Korean American women born in the USA and Korea: the Multiethnic Cohort Study. *Public Health Nutr*. 2005;8:904-911.

21. McDonald JT, Kennedy S. Is migration to Canada associated with unhealthy weight gain? Overweight and obesity among Canada's immigrants. *Soc Sci Med*. 2005;61:2469-2481.

22. Tremblay MS, Perez CE, Ardern CI, Bryan SN, Katzmarzyk PT. Obesity, overweight and ethnicity. *Health Rep*. 2005;16:23-34.

23. Goel MS, McCarthy EP, Phillips RS, Wee CC. Obesity among US immigrant subgroups by duration of residence. *JAMA*. 2004;292:2860-2867.

24. Antecol H, Bedard K. Unhealthy assimilation: Why do immigrants converge to American health status levels? *Demography*. 2006;43:337-360.

25. Lindstrom M, Sundquist K. The impact of country of birth and time in Sweden on overweight and obesity: a population-based study. *Scand J Public Health*. 2005;33:276-284.

26. Lean ME, Han TS, Bush H, Anderson AS, Bradby H, Williams R. Ethnic differences in anthropometric and lifestyle measures related to coronary heart disease risk between South Asian, Italian and general-population British women living in the west of Scotland. *Int J Obes Relat Metab Disord*. 2001;25:1800-1805.

27. Marin G, Sabogal F, Marin BV, Otero-Sabogal R, Perez-Stable EJ. Development of a short acculturation scale for Hispanics. *Hisp J Behav Sci.* 1987;9:183-205.

28. Elder JP, Castro FG, de Moor C, et al. Differences in cancer-risk-related behaviors in Latino and Anglo adults. *Prev Med.* 1991;20:751-763.

29. Marin G, Perez-Stable EJ, Marin BV. Cigarette smoking among San Francisco Hispanics: the role of acculturation and gender. *Am J Public Health.* 1989;79:196-198.

30. Marin G, Gamba RJ. A new measurement of acculturation for Hispanics: The Bidimensional Acculturation Scale for Hispanics (BAS). *Hisp J Behav Sci.* 1996;18:297-316.

31. Wallen GR, Feldman RH, Anliker J. Measuring acculturation among Central American women with the use of a brief language scale. *J Immig Health.* 2002;4:95-102.

32. Sundquist J, Winkleby M. Country of birth, acculturation status and abdominal obesity in a national sample of Mexican-American women and men. *Int J Epidemiol.* 2000;29:470-477.

33. Khan LK, Sobal J, Martorell R. Country of birth, acculturation status and abdominal obesity in a national sample of Mexican-American women and men. *Int J Epidemiol.* 1997;21:91-96.

34. Crespo CJ, Smit E, Carter-Pokras O, Andersen R. Acculturation and leisure-time physical inactivity in Mexican American adults: results from NHANES III, 1988-1994. *Am J Public Health.* 2001;91:1254-1257.

35. Cantero PJ, Richardson JL, Baezconde-Garbanati L, Marks G. The association between acculturation and health practices among middle-aged and elderly Latinas. *Ethn Dis.* 1999;9:166-180.

36. Hazuda HP, Haffner SM, Stern MP, Eifler CW. Effects of acculturation and socioeconomic status on obesity and diabetes in Mexican Americans. The San Antonio Heart Study. *Am J Epidemiol.* 1988;128:1289-1301.

37. Tull ES, Thurland A, LaPorte RE, Chambers EC. Acculturation and psychosocial stress show differential relationships to insulin resistance (HOMA) and body fat distribution in two groups of blacks living in the US Virgin Islands. *J Natl Med Assoc.* 2003;95:560-569.

38. Hubert HB, Snider J, Winkleby MA. Acculturation and overweight-related behaviors among Hispanic immigrants to the US: the National Longitudinal Study of Adolescent Health. *Soc Sci Med.* 2003;57:2023-2034.

39. Lin H, Bermudez OI, Tucker KL. Dietary patterns of Hispanic elders are associated with acculturation and obesity. *J Nutr.* 2003;133(11):3651-3657.

40. Khan LK, Sobal J, Martorell R. Acculturation, socioeconomic status, and obesity in Mexican Americans, Cuban Americans, and Puerto Ricans. *Int J Obes Relat Metab Disord.* 1997;21:91-96.

41. Hazuda HP, Haffner SM, Stern MP, Eifler CW. Effects of acculturation and socioeconomic status on obesity and diabetes in Mexican Americans. The San Antonio Heart Study. *Am J Epidemiol.* 1998;128(6):1289-1301.

42. Song YJ, Hofstetter CR, Hovell MF, et al. Acculturation and health risk behaviors among Californians of Korean descent. *Prev Med.* 2004;39:147-156.

43. Lee SK, Sobal J, Frongillo EA Jr. Acculturation and health in Korean Americans. *Soc Sci Med.* 2000;51:159-173.

44. Krieger N. A glossary for social epidemiology. *J Epidemiol Community Health.* 2001;55:693-700.

45. Subramanian SV, Smith GD. Patterns, distribution, and determinants of under- and overnutrition: a population-based study of women in India. *Am J Clin Nutr.* 2006;84:633-640.

46. Fezeu L, Minkoulou E, Balkau B, et al. Association between socioeconomic status and adiposity in urban Cameroon. *Int J Epidemiol.* 2006;35:105-111.

47. Al-Kandari YY. Prevalence of obesity in Kuwait and its relation to sociocultural variables. *Obes Rev.* 2006;7:147-154.

48. Ersoy C, Imamoglu S, Tuncel E, Erturk E, Ercan I. Comparison of the factors that influence obesity prevalence in three district municipalities of the same city with

different socioeconomical status: a survey analysis in an urban Turkish population. *Prev Med.* 2005;40:181-188.

49. Hossain P, Kawar B, El Nahas M. Obesity and diabetes in the developing world—a growing challenge. *N Engl J Med.* 2007;356:213-215.

50. Sobal J, Stunkard AJ. Socioeconomic status and obesity: a review of the literature. *Psychol Bull.* 1989;105:260-275.

51. Ball K, Crawford D. Socioeconomic status and weight change in adults: a review. *Soc Sci Med.* 2005;60:1987-2010.

52. Mujahid MS, Diez Roux AV, Borrell LN, Nieto FJ. Cross-sectional and longitudinal associations of BMI with socioeconomic characteristics. *Obes Res.* 2005;13:1412-1421.

53. Zhang Q, Wang Y. Trends in the association between obesity and socioeconomic status in U.S. adults: 1971 to 2000. *Obes Res.* 2004;12:1622-1632.

54. Manios Y, Panagiotakos DB, Pitsavos C, Polychronopoulos E, Stefanadis C. Implication of socio-economic status on the prevalence of overweight and obesity in Greek adults: the ATTICA study. *Health Policy.* 2005;74:224-232.

55. Lewis TT, Everson-Rose SA, Sternfeld B, Karavolos K, Wesley D, Powell LH. Race, education, and weight change in a biracial sample of women at midlife. *Arch Intern Med.* 2005;165:545-551.

56. Ball K, Mishra GD. Whose socioeconomic status influences a woman's obesity risk: her mother's, her father's, or her own? *Int J Epidemiol.* 2006;35:131-138.

57. Bennett GG, Wolin KY, James SA. Lifecourse socioeconomic position and weight change among blacks: The Pitt County study. *Obesity (Silver Spring).* 2007;15:172-181.

58. James SA, Fowler-Brown A, Raghunathan TE, Van Hoewyk J. Life-course socio-economic position and obesity in African American Women: the Pitt County Study. *Am J Public Health.* 2006;96:554-560.

59. Robert S. Community-level socioeconomic status effects on adult health. *J Health Soc Behav.* 1998;39:18-37.

60. Robert SA, Reither EN. A multilevel analysis of race, community disadvantage, and body mass index among adults in the US. *Soc Sci Med.* 2004;59:2421-2434.

61. Sundquist J, Malmstrom M, Johansson SE. Cardiovascular risk factors and the neighbourhood environment: a multilevel analysis. *Int J Epidemiol.* 1999;28:841-845.

62. Cubbin C, Sundquist K, Ahlen H, Johansson S, Winkleby M, Sundquist J. Neighborhood deprivation and cardiovascular disease risk factors: protective and harmful effects. *Scand J Public Health.* 2006;34:228-237.

63. Cubbin C, Hadden W, Winkleby M. Neighborhood context and cardiovascular disease risk factors: the contribution of material deprivation. *Ethn Dis.* 2001;11:687-700.

64. Smith G, Hart C, Watt G, Hole D, Hawthorne V. Individual social class, area-based deprivation, cardiovascular disease risk factors, and mortality: the Renfrew and Paisley Study. *J Epidemiol Community Health.* 1998;52:399-405.

65. Ellaway A, Anderson A, Macintyre S. Does area of residence affect body size and shape? *Int J Obes Relat Metab Disord.* 1997;21:304-308.

66. Orr L, Feins J, Jacob R, et al. *Moving to Opportunity for Fair Housing Demonstration: Interim Impacts Evaluation.* U.S. Department of Housing and Urban Development; 2003.

67. Ecob R, Macintyre S. Small area variations in health related behaviors; do these depend on the behaviour itself, its measurement, or on personal characteristics? *Health Place.* 2000;6:261-274.

68. Diez-Roux A, Nieto F, Caulfield L, Tyroler H, Watson R, Szklo M. Neighbourhood differences in diet: the Atherosclerosis Risk in Communities (ARIC) Study. *J Epidemiol Community Health.* 1999;53:55-63.

69. Yen I, Kaplan G. Poverty area residence and changes in physical activity level: evidence from the Alameda County Study. *Am J Public Health.* 1998;88:1709-1712.

70. Acevedo-Garcia D, Lochner KA, Osypuk TL, Subramanian SV. Future directions in residential segregation and health research: a multilevel approach. *Am J Public Health.* 2003;93:215-221.

71. Williams D, Collins C. Racial residential segregation: a fundamental cause of racial disparities in health. *Public Health Reports.* 2001;116:404-416.

72. Chang V. Racial residential segregation and weight status among US adults. *Soc Sci Med.* 2006;63:1289-1303.

73. Baker E, Schootman M, Barnidge E, Kelly C. The role of race and poverty in access to foods that enable individuals to adhere to dietary guidelines. *Prev Chronic Dis.* 2006;3:A76.

74. Horowitz CR, Colson KA, Hebert PL, Lancaster K. Barriers to buying healthy foods for people with diabetes: evidence of environmental disparities. *Am J Public Health.* 2004;94:1549-1554.

75. Moore LV, Diez Roux AV. Associations of neighborhood characteristics with the location and type of food stores. *Am J Public Health.* 2006;96:325-331.

76. Zenk SN, Schulz AJ, Hollis-Neely T, et al. Fruit and vegetable intake in African Americans income and store characteristics. *Am J Prev Med.* 2005;29:1-9.

77. Morland K, Wing S, Diez Roux A. The contextual effect of the local food environment on residents' diets: the atherosclerosis risk in communities study. *Am J Public Health.* 2002;92:1761-1767.

78. Powell L, Slater S, Mirtcheva D, Bao Y, Chaloupka F. Food store availability and neighborhood characteristics in the United States. *Prev Med.* 2007;E-pub ahead of print.

79. Zenk S, Schulz A, Israel B, James S, Bao S, Wilson M. Fruit and vegetable access differs by community racial composition and socioeconomic position in Detroit, Michigan. *Ethn Dis.* 2006;16:275-280.

80. Algert SJ, Agrawal A, Lewis DS. Disparities in access to fresh produce in low-income neighborhoods in los angeles. *Am J Prev Med.* 2006;30:365-370.

81. Block JP, Scribner RA, DeSalvo KB. Fast food, race/ethnicity, and income: a geographic analysis. *Am J Prev Med.* 2004;27:211-217.

82. Cummins S, Petticrew M, Higgins C, Findlay A, Sparks L. Large scale food retailing as an intervention for diet and health: quasi-experimental evaluation of a natural experiment. *J Epidemiol Community Health.* 2005;59:1035-1040.

83. Estabrooks PA, Lee RE, Gyurcsik NC. Resources for physical activity participation: does availability and accessibility differ by neighborhood socioeconomic status? *Ann Behav Med.* 2003;25:100-104.

84. Parks SE, Housemann RA, Brownson RC. Differential correlates of physical activity in urban and rural adults of various socioeconomic backgrounds in the United States. *J Epidemiol Community Health.* 2003;57:29-35.

85. McCormack G, Giles-Corti B, Bulsara M, Pikora T. Correlates of distances traveled to use recreational facilities for physical activity behaviors. *Int J Behav Nutr Phys Act.* 2006;3:18.

86. Schulz, AJ, Williams D, Israel B, Lempert L. Racial and spatial relations as fundamental determinants of health in Detroit. *Milbank Q.* 2002;80:677-707, iv.

87. Geocodes. Available at: http://www.hsph.harvard.edu/thegeocodingproject/webpage/monograph/introduction.htm#introref3. Last accessed 2/5/2007.

88. Krieger N, Chen J, Waterman P, Soobader M-J, Subramanian S, Carson R. Choosing area-based socioeconomic measures to monitor social inequalities in low birthweight and childhood lead poisoning—The Public Health Disparities Geocoding Project (US). *J Epidemiol Community Health.* 2003;57:186-199.

89. Krieger N, Chen J, Waterman P, Soobader M-J, Subramanian S. Monitoring socioeconomic inequalities in sexually transmitted infections, tuberculosis, and violence: geocoding and choice of area-based socioeconomic measures—The Public Health Disparities Geocoding Project (US). *Public Health Reports.* 2003; 118:240-260.

90. Krieger N, Chen J, Waterman P, Rehkopf D, Subramanian S. Race/ethnicity, gender, and monitoring socioeconomic gradients in health: a comparison of area-based socioeconomic measures—the Public Health Disparities Geocoding Project. *Am J Public Health.* 2003;93:1655-1671.

91. Krieger N, Waterman P, Lemieux K, Zierler S, Hogan JW. On the wrong side of the tracts? Evaluating the accuracy of geocoding in public health research. *Am J Public Health.* 2001;91:1114-1116.

92. Krieger N, Waterman P, Chen J, Soobader M-J, Subramanian S, Carson R. ZIP Code caveat: bias due to spatiotemporal mismatches between ZIP Codes and US census-defined areas—The Public Health Disparities Geocoding Project. *Am J Public Health.* 2002;92:1100-1102.

93. Morland K, Diez Roux A, Wing S. Supermarkets, other food stores, and obesity: the atherosclerosis risk in communities study. *Am J Prev Med.* 2006;30:333-339.

94. Wrigley N, Warm D, Margetts B, Whelan A. Assessing the impact of improved retail access on diet in a "food desert": a preliminary report. *Urban Stud.* 2002;39:2061-2082.

95. Pearson T, Russell J, Campbell M, Barker M. Do "food deserts" influence fruit and vegetable consumption?—A cross-sectional study. *Appetite.* 2005;45:195-197.

96. Guthrie JF, Lin BH, Frazao E. Role of food prepared away from home in the American diet, 1977-78 versus 1994-96: changes and consequences. *J Nutr Educ Behav.* 2002;34:140-150.

97. Prentice A, Jebb S. Fast foods, energy density and obesity: a possible mechanistic link. *Obes Rev.* 2003;4:187-194.

98. Satia JA, Galanko JA, Siega-Riz AM. Eating at fast-food restaurants is associated with dietary intake, demographic, psychosocial and behavioural factors among African Americans in North Carolina. *Public Health Nutr.* 2004;7:1089-1096.

99. Jeffery RW, French SA. Epidemic obesity in the United States: are fast foods and television viewing contributing? *Am J Public Health.* 1998;88:277-280.

100. Jeffery R, Baxter J, McGuire M, Linde J. Are fast food restaurants an environmental risk factor for obesity? *Int J Behav Nutr Phys Act.* 2006;3:2.

101. Pereira MA, Kartashov AI, Ebbeling CB, et al. Fast-food habits, weight gain, and insulin resistance (the CARDIA study): 15-year prospective analysis. *Lancet.* 2005;365:36-42.

102. Maddock J. The relationship between obesity and the prevalence of fast food restaurants: state-level analysis. *Am J Health Promot.* 2004;19:137-143.

103. Saelens BE, Sallis JF, Black JB, Chen D. Neighborhood-based differences in physical activity: an environment scale evaluation. *Am J Public Health.* 2003;93:1552-1558.

104. Frumkin H. Urban sprawl and public health. *Public Health Rep.* 2002;117:201-217.

105. Lopez R. Urban sprawl and risk for being overweight or obese. *Am J Public Health.* 2004;94:1574-1579.

106. Frank L, Schmid T, Sallis J, Chapman J, Saelens B. Linking objectively measured physical activity with objectively measured urban form: findings from SMARTRAQ. *Am J Prev Med.* 2005;28:117-125.

107. King W, Belle S, Brach J, Simkin-Silverman L, Soska T, Kriska A. Objective measures of neighborhood environment and physical activity in older women. *Am J Prev Med.* 2005;28:461-469.

108. Ewing R, Schmid T, Killingsworth R, Zlot A, Raudenbush S. Relationship between urban sprawl and physical activity, obesity, and morbidity. *Am J Health Promot.* 2003;18:47-57.

109. Berrigan D, Troiano R. The association between urban form and physical activity in U.S. adults. *Am J Prev Med.* 2002;23:74-79.

110. Vandegrift D, Yoked T. Obesity rates, income, and suburban sprawl: an analysis of US states. *Health Place.* 2004;10:221-229.

111. Frank L, Andresen M, Schmid T. Obesity relationships with community design, physical activity, and time spent in cars. *Am J Prev Med.* 2004;27:87-96.

112. Bell A, Ge K, Popkin B. The road to obesity or the path to prevention: motorized transportation and obesity in China. *Obes Res.* 2002;10:277-283.

113. Rhodes R, Brown S, McIntyre C. Integrating the perceived neighborhood environment and the theory of planned behavior when predicting walking in a Canadian adult sample. *Am J Health Promot.* 2006;21:110-118.

114. Atkinson J, Sallis J, Saelens B, Cain K, Black J. The association of neighborhood design and recreational environments with physical activity. *Am J Health Promot.* 2005;19:304-309.

115. De Bourdeaudhuij I, Sallis J, Saelens B. Environmental correlates of physical activity in a sample of Belgian adults. *Am J Health Promot.* 2003;18:83-92.

116. Booth K, Pinkston M, Poston W. Obesity and the built environment. *J Am Diet Assoc.* 2005;105:S110-S117.

117. Humpel N, Owen N, Leslie E. Environmental factors associated with adults' participation in physical activity: a review. *Am J Prev Med.* 2002;22:188-199.

118. Li F, Fisher KJ, Bauman A, et al. Neighborhood influences on physical activity in middle-aged and older adults: a multilevel perspective. *J Aging Phys Act.* 2005;13:87-114.

119. Suminski RR, Poston WS, Petosa RL, Stevens E, Katzenmoyer LM. Features of the neighborhood environment and walking by U.S. adults. *Am J Prev Med.* 2005;28:149-155.

120. Heesch KC, Brown DR, Blanton CJ. Perceived barriers to exercise and stage of exercise adoption in older women of different racial/ethnic groups. *Women's Health (Hillsdale, NJ).* 2000;30:61-76.

121. Eyler AA, Matson-Koffman D, Young DR, et al. Quantitative study of correlates of physical activity in women from diverse racial/ethnic groups: The Women's Cardiovascular Health Network Project—summary and conclusions. *Am J Prev Med.* 2003;25:93-103.

122. Thompson PD, Buchner D, Pina IL, et al. Exercise and physical activity in the prevention and treatment of atherosclerotic cardiovascular disease: a statement from the Council on Clinical Cardiology (Subcommittee on Exercise, Rehabilitation, and Prevention) and the Council on Nutrition, Physical Activity, and Metabolism (Subcommittee on Physical Activity). *Circulation.* 2003;107:3109-3116.

123. Brownson RC, Baker EA, Housemann RA, Brennan LK, Bacak SJ. Environmental and policy determinants of physical activity in the United States. *Am J Public Health.* 2001;91:1995-2003.

124. Catlin T, Simoes E, Brownson R. Environmental and policy factors associated with overweight among adults in Missouri. *Am J Health Promot.* 2003;17:249-258.

125. Burdette H, Wadden T, Whitaker R. Neighborhood safety, collective efficacy, and obesity in women with young children. *Obesity (Silver Spring).* 2006;14:518-525.

126. Hooker S, Wilson D, Griffin S, Ainsworth B. Perceptions of environmental supports for physical activity in African American and white adults in a rural county in South Carolina. *Prev Chronic Dis.* 2005;2:A11.

127. Wilbur J, Chandler P, Dancy B, Lee H. Correlates of physical activity in urban Midwestern African-American women. *Am J Prev Med.* 2003;25:45-52.

128. Centers for Disease Control and Prevention (CDC), National Center for Health Statistics (NCHS). *National Health and Nutrition Examination Survey Data.* Hyattsville, MD; 1999-2000.

129. Shenassa E, Liebhaber A, Ezeamama A. Perceived safety of area of residence and exercise: a pan-European study. *Am J Epidemiol.* 2006;163:1012-1017.

130. Foster C, Hillsdon M, Thorogood M. Environmental perceptions and walking in English adults. *J Epidemiol Community Health.* 2004;58:924-928.

131. Messer LC. Invited commentary: beyond the metrics for measuring neighborhood effects. *Am J Epidemiol.* 2007;165:868-871.

132. Morland K, Wing S, Diez Roux A, Poole C. Neighborhood characteristics associated with the location of food stores and food service places. *Am J Prev Med.* 2002;22:23-29.

133. Mujahid MS, Diez Roux AV, Morenoff JD, Raghunathan T. Assessing the measurement properties of neighborhood scales: from psychometrics to ecometrics. *Am J Epidemiol.* 2007;165:858-867.

134. Martikainen P, Bartley M, Lahelma E. Psychosocial determinants of health in social epidemiology. *Int J Epidemiol.* 2002;31:1091-1093.

135. Ganley R. Emotion and eating in obesity: a review of the literature. *Int J Eat Disord.* 1989;8:343-361.
136. Macht M, Simons G. Emotions and eating in everyday life. *Appetite.* 2000;35:65-71.
137. Greeno C, Wing R. Stress-induced eating. *Psychol Bull.* 1994;115:444-464.
138. Korkeila M, Kaprio J, Rissanen A, Koshenvuo M, Sorensen TI. Predictors of major weight gain in adult Finns: stress, life satisfaction and personality traits. *Int J Obes Relat Metab Disord.* 1998;22:949-957.
139. Smith AW, Baum A, Wing RR. Stress and weight gain in parents of cancer patients. *Int J Obes (London).* 2005;29:244-250.
140. Bjorntorp P. Do stress reactions cause abdominal obesity and comorbidities? *Obes Rev.* 2001;2:73-86.
141. Dallman MF, Pecoraro NC, La Fleur SE, et al. Glucocorticoids, chronic stress, and obesity. *Prog Brain Res.* 2006;153:75-105.
142. Kral JG. The pathogenesis of obesity: stress and the brain-gut axis. *Surg Obes Relat Dis.* 2005;1:25-34.
143. Steinman L, Conlon P, Maki R, Foster A. The intricate interplay among body weight, stress, and the immune response to friend or foe. *J Clin Invest.* 2003; 111:183-185.
144. Drapeau V, Therrien F, Richard D, Tremblay A. Is visceral obesity a physiological adaptation to stress? *Panminerva Med.* 2003;45:189-195.
145. Gluck ME, Geliebter A, Lorence M. Cortisol stress response is positively correlated with central obesity in obese women with binge eating disorder (BED) before and after cognitive-behavioral treatment. *Ann NY Acad Sci.* 2004;1032:202-207.
146. Marniemi J, Kronholm E, Aunola S, et al. Visceral fat and psychosocial stress in identical twins discordant for obesity. *J Intern Med.* 2002;251:35-43.
147. Laitinen J, Ek E, Sovio U. Stress-related eating and drinking behavior and body mass index and predictors of this behavior. *Prev Med.* 2002;34:29-39.
148. Dallman MF, Pecoraro N, Akana SF, et al. Chronic stress and obesity: a new view of "comfort food." *Proc Natl Acad Sci USA.* 2003;100:11696-11701.
149. Dallman MF, Pecoraro NC, la Fleur SE. Chronic stress and comfort foods: self-medication and abdominal obesity. *Brain Behav Immun.* 2005;19:275-280.
150. Oxman TE, Freeman DH, Manheimer ED. Lack of social participation or religious strength and comfort as risk factors for death after cardiac surgery in the elderly. *Psychosom Med.* 1995;57:5-15.
151. Farmer I, Meyer PS, Ramsey DJ, et al. Higher levels of social support predict greater survival following acute myocardial infarction: The Corpus Christi Heart Project. *Behav Med.* 1996;22:59-66.
152. Krumholz HM, Butler J, Miller J, et al. The prognostic importance of emotional support for elderly patients hospitalized with heart failure. *Circulation.* 1998;97:958-964.
153. Berkman LF, Breslow L. *Health and Ways of Living: The Alameda County Study.* New York, NY:Oxford University Press; 1983.
154. Morris PL, Robinson RG, Andrzejewski P, Samuels J, Price TR. Association of depression with 10-year poststroke mortality. *Am J Psychiatr.* 1993;150:124-129.
155. Siegist J. Adverse health effects of high-effort/low-reward conditions. *J Occup Health Psychol.* 1996;1:27-41.
156. Repetti RL. Short-term effects of occupational stressors on daily mood and health complaints. *Health Psychol.* 1993;12:125-131.
157. Schwartz JE, Pickering TG, Landsbergis PA. Work-related stress and blood pressure: current theoretical models and considerations from a behavioral medicine perspective. *J Occup Health Psychol.* 1996;1:287-310.
158. Karasek RA. Job demands, job decision latitude, and mental strain: implications for job redesign. *Administrative Science Quarterly.* 1979;24:285-307.
159. Karasek R, Theorell T. *Healthy Work: Stress, Productivity, and the Reconstruction of Working Life.* New York: Basic Books; 1990.

160. Brisson C, Larocque B, Moisan J, Vezina M, Dagenais GR. Psychosocial factors at work, smoking, sedentary behavior, and body mass index: a prevalence study among 6995 white collar workers. *J Occup Environ Med.* 2000;42:40-46.

161. Landsbergis PA, Schnall PL, Deitz DK, Warren K, Pickering TG, Schwartz JE. Job strain and health behaviors: results of a prospective study. *Am J Health Promot.* 1998;12:237-245.

162. Jonsson D, Rosengren A, Dotevall A, Lappas G, Wilhelmsen L. Job control, job demands and social support at work in relation to cardiovascular risk factors in MONICA 1995, Goteborg. *J Cardiovasc Risk.* 1999;6:379-385.

163. Hellerstedt WL, Jeffery RW. The association of job strain and health behaviours in men and women. *Int J Epidemiol.* 1997;26:575-583.

164. Wamala SP, Wolk A, Orth-Gomer K. Determinants of obesity in relation to socioeconomic status among middle-aged Swedish women. *Prev Med.* 1997;26:734-744.

165. Kouvonen A, Kivimaki M, Cox SJ, Cox T, Vahtera J. Relationship between work stress and body mass index among 45,810 female and male employees. *Psychosom Med.* 2005;67:577-583.

166. Niedhammer I, Goldberg M, Leclerc A, David S, Bugel I, Landre MF. Psychosocial work environment and cardiovascular risk factors in an occupational cohort in France. *J Epidemiol Community Health.* 1998;52:93-100.

167. Kivimaki M, Leino-Arjas P, Luukkonen R, Riihimaki H, Vahtera J, Kirjonen J. Work stress and risk of cardiovascular mortality: prospective cohort study of industrial employees. *BMJ.* 2002;325:857.

168. Steptoe A, Cropley M, Griffith J, Joekes K. The influence of abdominal obesity and chronic work stress on ambulatory blood pressure in men and women. *Int J Obes Relat Metab Disord.* 1999;23:1184-1191.

169. Kivimaki M, Head J, Ferrie JE, et al. Work stress, weight gain and weight loss: evidence for bidirectional effects of job strain on body mass index in the Whitehall II study. *Int J Obes (London).* 2006;30:982-987.

170. Overgaard D, Gyntelberg F, Heitmann BL. Psychological workload and body weight: is there an association? A review of the literature. *Occup Med (London).* 2004;54:35-41.

171. Wethington E, Brown G, Kessler R. *Interview Measurement of Stressful Life Events.* New York: Oxford University Press; 1995:59-79.

172. Lepore S. *Measurement of Chronic Stressors.* New York: Oxford University Press; 1995:102-121.

173. Monroe S, Kelley J. *Measurement of Stress Appraisal.* New York: Oxford University Press; 1995:122-147.

174. Cohen S, Kamarck T, Mermelstein R. A global measure of perceived stress. *J Health Soc Behav.* 1983;24:385-396.

175. Cohen S, Williamson G. Perceived stress in a probability sample of the United States. Newbury Park, CA: Sage; 1988.

176. Stone A. *Measurement of Affective Response.* New York: Oxford University Press; 1995:148-174.

177. Williams DR. Race/ethnicity and socioeconomic status: measurement and methodological issues. *Int J Health Serv.* 1996;26:483-505.

178. Moller J, Hallqvist J, Diderichsen F, Theorell T, Reuterwall C, Ahlbom A. Do episodes of anger trigger myocardial infarction? A case-crossover analysis in the Stockholm Heart Epidemiology Program (SHEEP). *Psychosom Med.* 1999;61:842-849.

179. Gabbay FH, Krantz DS, Kop WJ, et al. Triggers of myocardial ischemia during daily life in patients with coronary artery disease: physical and mental activities, anger and smoking. *J Am Coll Cardiol.* 1996;27:585-592.

180. Ironson G, Taylor CB, Boltwood M, et al. Effects of anger on left ventricular ejection fraction in coronary artery disease. *Am J Cardiol.* 1992;70:281-285.

181. Miller TQ, Smith TW, Turner CW, Guijarro ML, Hallet AJ. A meta-analytic review of research on hostility and physical health. *Psychol Bull.* 1996;119:322-348.

182. Gump BB, Matthews KA, Raikkonen K. Modeling relationships among socioeconomic status, hostility, cardiovascular reactivity, and left ventricular mass in African American and White children. *Health Psychol.* 1999;18:140-150.

183. Smith TW. Hostility and health: current status of a psychosomatic hypothesis. *Health Psychol.* 1992;11:139-150.

184. Anderson D, Deshaies G, Jobin J. Social support, social networks and coronary artery disease rehabilitation: a review. *Can J Cardiol.* 1996;12:739-744.

185. Berkman LF. The role of social relations in health promotion. *Psychosom Med.* 1995;57:245-254.

186. Verheijden M, Bakx J, van Weel C, Koelen M, van Staveren W. Role of social support in lifestyle-focused weight management interventions. *Eur J Clin Nutr.* 2005;59 (suppl 1):179-186.

187. Wolfe WA. A review: maximizing social support—a neglected strategy for improving weight management with African-American women. *Ethn Dis.* 2004;14:212-218.

188. Parham ES. Enhancing social support in weight loss management groups. *J Am Diet Assoc.* 1993;93:1152-1156; quiz 1157-1158.

189. Brownell KD. Behavioral, psychological, and environmental predictors of obesity and success at weight reduction. *Int J Obes.* 1984;8:543-550.

190. Wing RR, Jeffery RW. Benefits of recruiting participants with friends and increasing social support for weight loss and maintenance. *J Consult Clin Psychol.* 1999;67:132-138.

191. Quartetti HR. Shedding pounds for life. Been there done that. Successful weight losers share their secrets for keeping weight off for good. *Diabetes Forecast.* 2003;56:83-84.

192. Elfhag K, Rossner S. Who succeeds in maintaining weight loss? A conceptual review of factors associated with weight loss maintenance and weight regain. *Obes Rev.* 2005;6:67-85.

193. Jeffery R, Bjornson-Benson W, Rosenthal B, et al. Correlates of weight loss and its maintenance over two years of follow-up among middle-aged men. *Prev Med.* 1984;13:155-168.

194. Cohen S, Syme S. *Social Support and Health.* Orlando, FL: Academic Press; 1984.

195. Gallagher KI, Jakicic JM, Napolitano MA, Marcus BH. Psychosocial factors related to physical activity and weight loss in overweight women. *Med Sci Sports Exerc.* 2006;38:971-980.

196. Wing RR, Tate DF, Gorin AA, Raynor HA, Fava JL. A self-regulation program for maintenance of weight loss. *N Engl J Med.* 2006;355:1563-1571.

197. Harvey-Berino J, Pintauro S, Buzzell P, Gold EC. Effect of internet support on the long-term maintenance of weight loss. *Obes Res.* 2004;12:320-329.

198. Foreyt JP, Poston WS II. The role of the behavioral counselor in obesity treatment. *J Am Diet Assoc.* 1998;98:S27-S30.

199. Raikkonen K, Matthews KA, Kuller LH. Anthropometric and psychosocial determinants of visceral obesity in healthy postmenopausal women. *Int J Obes Relat Metab Disord.* 1999;23:775-782.

200. Ali SM, Lindstrom M. Socioeconomic, psychosocial, behavioural, and psychological determinants of BMI among young women: differing patterns for underweight and overweight/obesity. *Eur J Public Health.* 2006;16:325-331.

201. Lallukka T, Laaksonen M, Martikainen P, Sarlio-Lahteenkorva S, Lahelma E. Psychosocial working conditions and weight gain among employees. *Int J Obes (London).* 2005;29:909-915.

202. Laitinen J, Nayha S, Kujala V. Body mass index and weight change from adolescence into adulthood, waist-to-hip ratio and perceived work ability among young adults. *Int J Obes (London).* 2005;29:697-702.

203. Kessler RC, McGonagle KA, Zhao S, Nelson CB. Lifetime and 12-month prevalence of DSM-III-R psychiatric disorders in the United States: Results from the National Comorbidity Study. *Arch General Psychiatr.* 1994;51:8-19.

204. Roberts RE, Kaplan GA, Shema SJ, Strawbridge WJ. Are the obese at greater risk for depression? *Am J Epidemiol.* 2000;152:163-170.
205. Palinkas LA, Wingard DL, Barrett-Connor E. Depressive symptoms in overweight and obese older adults: a test of the "jolly fat" hypothesis. *J Psychosom Res.* 1996;40:59-66.
206. Rothschild M, Peterson HR, Pfeifer MA. Depression in obese men. *Int J Obes.* 1989;13:479-485.
207. Wing RR, Matthews KA, Kuller LH, Meilahn EN, Plantinga P. Waist to hip ratio in middle-aged women. Associations with behavioral and psychosocial factors and with changes in cardiovascular risk factors. *Arterioscler Thromb.* 1991;11:1250-1257.
208. Istvan J, Zavela K, Weidner G. Body weight and psychological distress in NHANES I. *Int J Obes Relat Metab Disord.* 1992;16:999-1003.
209. Sullivan M, Karlsson J, Sjostrom L, et al. Swedish obese subjects (SOS)—an intervention study of obesity. Baseline evaluation of health and psychosocial functioning in the first 1743 subjects examined. *Int J Obes Relat Metab Disord.* 1993;17:503-512.
210. Kress AM, Peterson MR, Hartzell MC. Association between obesity and depressive symptoms among U.S. Military active duty service personnel, 2002. *J Psychosom Res.* 2006;60:263-271.
211. Roberts R, Strawbridge W, Deleger S, Kaplan G. Are the fat more jolly? *Ann Behav Med.* 2002;24:169-180.
212. Dong C, Sanchez L, Price R. Relationship of obesity to depression: a family-based study. *Int J Obes.* 2004;28:1-6.
213. Blazer D, Moody-Ayers S, Craft-Morgan J, Burchett B. Depression in diabetes and obesity, racial/ethnic/gender issues in older adults. *J Psychosom Res.* 2002;53:913-916.
214. Carpenter K, Hasin D, Allison D, Faith M. Relationship between obesity and DSM-IV major depressive disorder, suicide ideation and suicide attempts: results from a general population study. *Am J Public Health.* 2000;90:251-257.
215. Siegel J, Yancey A, McCarthy W. Overweight and depressive symptoms among African-American women. *Prev Med.* 2000;31:232-240.
216. Onyike C, Crum R, Lee H, Lyketsos C, Eaton W. Is obesity associated with major depression? Results from the Third National Health and Nutrition Examination Survey. *Am J Epidemiol.* 2003;158:1139-1147.
217. Noppa H, Hallstrom T. Weight gain in adulthood in relation to socioeconomic factors, mental illness and personality traits: a prospective study of middle-aged women. *J Psychosom Res.* 1981;25:83-89.
218. Jorm AF, Korten AE, Christensen H, Jacomb PA, Rodgers B, Parslow RA. Association of obesity with anxiety, depression and emotional well-being: a community survey. *Aust NZ J Public Health.* 2003;27:434-440.
219. Haukkala A, Uutela A. Cynical hostility, depression, and obesity: the moderating role of education and gender. *Int J Eat Disord.* 2000;27:106-109.
220. Faith MS, Matz PE, Jorge MA. Obesity-depression associations in the population. *J Psychosom Res.* 2002;53:935-942.
221. Crisp AH, McGuiness B. Jolly fat: relation between obesity and psychoneurosis in general population. *BMJ.* 1976;1:7-9.
222. Friedman MA, Brownell KD. Psychological correlates of obesity: moving to the next research generation. *Psychol Bull.* 1995;117:3-20.
223. Kittel F, Rustin RM, Dramaix M, de Backer G, Kornitzer M. Psycho-socio-biological correlates of moderate overweight in an industrial population. *J Psychosom Res.* 1978;22:145-158.
224. Juarbe TC, Gutierrez Y, Gilliss C, Lee KA. Depressive symptoms, physical activity, and weight gain in premenopausal Latina and White women. *Maturitas.* 2006;55:116-125.
225. Barefoot JC, Heitmann BL, Helms MJ, Williams RB, Surwit RS, Siegler IC. Symptoms of depression and changes in body weight from adolescence to mid-life. *Int J Obes Relat Metab Disord.* 1998;22:688-694.

226. Pine D, Cohen P, Brook J, Coplan J. Psychiatric symptoms in adolescence as predictors of obesity in early adulthood: a longitudinal study. *Am J Public Health.* 1997;87:1303-1310.
227. Pine DS, Goldstein RB, Wolk S, Weissman MM. The association between childhood depression and adulthood body mass index. *Pediatrics.* 2001;107:1049-1056.
228. Hasler G, Pine DS, Kleinbaum DG, et al. Depressive symptoms during childhood and adult obesity: the Zurich Cohort Study. *Mol Psychiatr.* 2005;10:842-850.
229. Roberts RE, Deleger S, Strawbridge WJ, Kaplan GA. Prospective association between obesity and depression: evidence from the Alameda County Study. *Int J Obes Relat Metab Disord.* 2003;27:514-521.
230. Bornstein SR, Schuppenies A, Wong ML, Licinio J. Approaching the shared biology of obesity and depression: the stress axis as the locus of gene-environment interactions. *Mol Psychiatr.* 2006;11:892-902.
231. McMahon M, Gerich J, Rizza R. Effects of glucocorticoids on carbohydrate metabolism. *Diabetes Metab Rev.* 1988;4:17-30.
232. Hauner H, Entenmann G, Wabitsch M, et al. Promoting effect of glucocorticoids on the differentiation of human adipocyte precursor cells cultured in a chemically defined medium. *J Clin Invest.* 1989;84:1663-1670.
233. Amsterdam J, Maislin G, Winokur A, Berwish N, Kling M, Gold P. The oCRH stimulation test before and after clinical recovery from depression. *J Affect Disord.* 1988;14:213-222.
234. Nemeroff C, Bissette G, Akil H, Fink M. Neuropeptide concentrations in the cerebrospinal fluid of depressed patients treated with electroconvulsive therapy. Corticotrophin-releasing factor, beta-endorphin and somatostatin. *Br J Psychiatr.* 1991;158:59-63.
235. Brosse AL, Sheets ES, Lett HS, Blumenthal JA. Exercise and the treatment of clinical depression in adults: recent findings and future directions. *Sports Med.* 2002;32:741-760.
236. Buhi ER, Goodson P, Neilands TB. Structural equation modeling: a primer for health behavior researchers. *Am J Health Behav.* 2007;31:74-85.
237. Crowley S, Fan X. Structural equation modeling: basic concepts and applications in personality assessment research. *J Pers Assess.* 1997;68:508-531.

18

Metabolic and Hormonal Predictors of Obesity

Frank B. Hu

Whether obesity is behaviorally or biologically driven has long been debated. Most dietary and lifestyle factors have a relatively small impact on the prevention of weight gain (see Chapters 14 and 15), and weight regain following weight loss in initially overweight people is highly common. It is therefore believed that inherent metabolic factors play a critical role in determining an individual's susceptibility to obesity, and that there is strong biological pressure to regain lost weight. In the past several decades, extensive research has been conducted to search for metabolic predictors of weight gain and obesity. These studies have focused on resting metabolic rate (RMR), fat oxidation reflected by respiratory quotient (RQ), and insulin sensitivity. If a relatively low RMR predicts weight gain, it would support the popular idea that metabolically efficient individuals are prone to obesity in an energy-abundant environment.[1] For this reason, research on RMR is of particular interest.

Seminal longitudinal studies conducted in Pima Indians have identified several predictors of subsequent weight gain: a lower RMR, a higher RQ (reflecting reduced fat oxidation), increased insulin sensitivity, and lower leptin levels (Table 18.1).[1] Interestingly, the direction of these associations was reversed in cross-sectional analyses, reflecting adaptive metabolic changes in obese subjects. These metabolic predictors have been investigated in prospective analyses of other populations, but the results have been mixed.

Recent studies have shifted attention to the role of gut hormones, such as ghrelin, in weight gain and obesity. It is well established that ghrelin is critical for regulating hunger and appetite. However, it is not clear whether plasma levels of ghrelin predict future risk of weight gain. In addition, although obesity is now widely accepted as an inflammatory condition, it is also unknown whether chronic inflammation contributes to the development of obesity in apparently healthy individuals.

In this chapter, we conduct a critical review of epidemiologic studies on metabolic and hormonal predictors of obesity. As with earlier chapters, we focus primarily on prospective cohort studies, first discussing metabolic predictors, including RMR, RQ, and insulin sensitivity, then examining studies of hormonal predictors (such as ghrelin, leptin, and adiponectin) of obesity. For inflammatory cytokines, we review recent prospective studies on C-reactive protein (CRP) and fibrinogen. Finally, we discuss the relationship between the stress hormone cortisol and adiposity.

Table 18.1 Metabolic Factors Related to Obesity: Cross-sectional versus Longitudinal Studies in Pima Indian Adults

	Cross-sectional (Associated with Obesity)	Longitudinal (Predicts Weight Gain)
Resting metabolic rate	Normal or high	Low
Fat oxidation	Normal or high	Low
Insulin sensitivity	Low	High
Sympathetic nervous system activity	High	Low
Plasma leptin concentration	High	Low

Adapted from Ravussin E, Gautier JF. Metabolic predictors of weight gain. *Int J Obes Relat Metab Disord.* 1999;23(Suppl 1):37-41.[1]

Resting Metabolic Rate

As discussed in Chapter 6, total energy expenditure consists of three components: RMR, the thermic effect of food, and the energy expended by physical activity. RMR, which accounts for 60% to 75% of total daily energy expenditure, is primarily determined by fat-free mass, but is also related to fat mass, age, and sex.[2] In the obese state, RMR is increased to adapt to larger body size; during weight loss, RMR is typically decreased. It has been suggested that at the same levels of energy intake and physical activity expenditure, individuals with a relatively low RMR are more likely to gain weight than those with a relatively high RMR. This hypothesis is conceptually appealing, but the epidemiologic evidence to support it is mixed.

So far, nine prospective studies have examined the association between RMR and weight gain (Table 18.2). Three showed that a relatively low RMR predicted greater weight gain.[3-5] Three others, however, did not.[6-8] One study found a positive association between RMR and future weight gain.[9] The other two examined the relationship between RMR and regain after weight loss. One reported that a higher RMR predicted less weight regain,[10] while the other found no relationship between RMR and weight regain over time.[11]

In the first of the nine prospective studies, Ravussin et al.[3] found a significant association between low resting and 24-hour metabolic rates and weight gain in two small cohorts of Pima Indians. The study also demonstrated a family aggregation of RMR values in Pima Indian siblings, suggesting that RMR is partially genetically determined. A subsequent study in another cohort of Pima Indians also found an inverse association between RMR and changes in body weight over time.[5] Although Buscemi et al.[5] confirmed this association in a small study conducted in Italy, this finding has not been replicated in other studies. The Baltimore Longitudinal Study of Aging[6] found a significant positive association between RQ and weight gain, but no association between baseline RMR and subsequent weight change. Similarly, the Quebec Family Study[7] reported no association between RMR and changes in body weight, waist circumference, or skinfold thickness over 5.5 years of follow-up. Conversely, Luke et al.[9] found a positive association between weight gain and RMR adjusted for body size and composition in lean Nigerian adults.

It is difficult to reconcile these contradictory results. One possible explanation is that most studies cannot detect what might be a very weak association between RMR and

Table 18.2 Prospective Epidemiologic Studies on Resting Metabolic Rate and Weight Gain

Study	Population	Years of Follow-up	Adjusted Covariates	Main Results
Ravussin (1988)[3]	The first study included 95 Pima Indians; the second, 126 Pima Indians	The first study lasted 2 y; the second, 4 y	Age, sex, fat-free mass, fat mass	In both studies, a low baseline RMR significantly predicted weight gain during the follow-up. After the weight gain, the adjusted RMR during follow-up significantly increased. In addition, family aggregation of RMR values was observed.
Seidell (1992)[6]	775 men aged 18-98 y in the Baltimore Longitudinal Study of Aging	10 y	Age, RQ, BMI, fat-free mass, duration of follow-up	RMR was not significantly associated with weight change. A significant positive association was observed between RQ and weight gain.
Weinsier (1995)[8]	24 post-obese women and 24 never-obese controls	4 y	Age, fat mass, and fat-free mass	No significant associations observed between RMR or RQ and weight change over time.
Katzmarzyk (2000)[7]	76 males and 71 females aged 16-68 y in the Quebec Family Study	5.5 y	Age, sex, body mass, and sum of skinfolds	No significant association between RMR or RQ and weight gain or change in waist circumference or skinfolds.
Tataranni (2003)[12]	92 nondiabetic Pima Indians	4 ± 3 y of follow-up in 74 subjects	Age, sex, body composition, and duration of follow-up	The correlation between change in weight and RMR was −.28 ($P = .016$). Calculated total energy intake was also associated with weight gain ($r = .25, P = .028$).
Weinsier (2003)[11]	49 formerly overweight women and 49 never-overweight controls	87% of the women were re-evaluated after 1 year of follow-up and 38% after 2 y	Age, race, lean body mass	No significant correlation between baseline resting or sleeping energy expenditure and 1- or 2-year weight change. No difference in RMR or RQ between formerly overweight women and the controls.
Buscemi (2005)[5]	72 males and 83 females aged 18-55 y from Italy	10-12 y	Fat-free mass	Baseline RMR was significantly and inversely associated with gain in body weight ($r = -.57$) and fat mass ($r = -.44$).

(continued)

379

Table 18.2 continued

Study	Population	Years of Follow-up	Adjusted Covariates	Main Results
Vogels (2005)[10]	29 men and 62 women aged 18-65 y	At least 2 y after completing a weight loss program	Fat-free mass	Baseline RMR was associated with percent weight regain ($r = -.38$, $P = .01$). Other predictors of weight maintenance after weight loss were an increase in dietary restraint during weight loss and a relatively high baseline fat mass.
Luke (2006)[9]	352 men and 392 women aged 45.9 ± 16.1 y from Nigeria	5.5 y	Age, sex, fat-free mass, and fat mass	A significant positive association was observed between baseline RMR and weight change. In stratified analyses, the association was seen among those who gained weight but not among those who lost weight.

RMR: resting metabolic rate; RQ: respiratory quotient.

weight change. Another might be that the biological relationship between RMR and weight gain is ethnically specific, as indicated by greater susceptibility to obesity in Pima Indians compared with other ethnic groups. The Pima Indian results are consistent with the *thrifty gene* hypothesis: that metabolic efficiency confers a survival advantage by conserving energy during times of famine but becomes a liability for obesity in an energy-abundant environment.[12] However, it is unclear why such a biological mechanism would operate in Pima Indians but not in the Nigerian population. Although both populations have historically experienced periods of energy scarcity, the majority of the Nigerian population has never been exposed to an energy-abundant environment, which may potentially explain divergent findings.

Studies comparing RMR in formerly obese subjects with never-obese subjects have also yielded mixed results. In a meta-analysis of 121 formerly obese and 121 control subjects, Astrup et al.[13] found that RMR adjusted for differences in fat-free mass and fat mass was 2.9% lower in formerly obese subjects than in matched controls ($P = .09$). Leibel et al.[14] reported a significant reduction in total energy expenditure and RMR in formerly overweight subjects after loss of 10% of initial body weight compared with weight-maintainers who had never been obese. However, in a study among participants in the National Weight Control Registry, Wyatt et al.[15] found no significant difference in RMR between 40 formerly obese subjects who had maintained weight loss for more than 1 year and 46 weight-matched controls. Weinsier et al.[16] also demonstrated that in energy-balanced conditions, there was no significant difference in RMR between weight-reduced women and never-overweight controls. These findings cast doubt on the *set-point theory*, which postulates that those who have lost weight are prone to weight regain because of adaptive downregulation in RMR.[17]

Several cross-sectional studies have reported lower RMR in African Americans than in Caucasians. For example, Forman et al.[18] found that after adjusting for body weight and lean body mass, African American women had 12% lower RMR than Caucasian women. After adjusting for age, Tanner stage, fat mass, and lean body mass, Sun et al.[19] likewise found a significantly lower RMR in African American children than in white children. These findings could explain a higher prevalence of obesity in African Americans than Whites. However, no prospective study has examined whether ethnic differences in RMR predict differences in weight gain. Interestingly, in a cross-sectional comparative study of 58 Nigerian and 34 African Americans, Luke et al.[20] observed no significant difference in RMR between the two genetically related groups despite a much higher prevalence of obesity among African Americans than Nigerians.

Fox et al.[21] observed similar RMR and leptin concentrations (discussed later) in lean Pima Indians living a traditional lifestyle in Mexico and non-Pima Mexicans matched for age, sex, and body composition. These findings indicate that low RMR or leptin levels (both thought to suggest expression of the *thrifty genotype*) do not explain increased susceptibility to obesity among Pima Indians. In contrast, physical activity levels were substantially higher in lean Pima Indians living in Mexico than in their genetically similar relatives living in Arizona,[22] underscoring the importance of *environmental* causes of obesity.

Respiratory Quotient

Low rates of fat oxidation have been suggested to be an important factor in weight gain and obesity.[1] The oxidation of fuels is assessed by RQ, the ratio of carbon dioxide production to oxygen uptake. RQ is typically measured through indirect calorimetry. Its values range from 0.70 (pure fat oxidation) to 1.0 (pure carbohydrate oxidation), with a typical value of approximately 0.8. Thus, increased RQ reflects decreased fat oxidation, which has been hypothesized to increase fat accumulation and weight gain.[1] RQ is influenced by dietary composition (a high-carbohydrate meal induces higher RQ), gender (females tend to have lower fat oxidation and higher RQ), age (RQ is higher in older people), body fat mass (higher adiposity causes greater fat oxidation and lower RQ), and genetic factors.[1]

Several prospective studies have examined the relationship between 24-hour or fasting RQ and weight gain and obesity, and the results have been largely inconsistent. Zurlo et al.[23] found a significant correlation between baseline 24-hour RQ and subsequent changes in body weight and fat mass ($r = .27$, $P < .01$ and $r = .19$, $P < .05$, respectively) in Pima Indians. Independent of energy expenditure, subjects in the 90th percentile of 24-hour RQ were 2.5 times more likely to gain 5 kg or more of body weight than those in the bottom 10th percentile. In the Baltimore Longitudinal Study of Aging, Seidell et al.[6] found a significant association between baseline fasting RQ and weight gain in nonobese men during 10 years of follow-up. Those with a fasting RQ of 0.85 were nearly 2.5 times more likely to gain 5 kg or more than men with a fasting RQ less than 0.76. During a 3-year follow-up in an Italian study, Marra et al.[24] demonstrated a significant association between a relatively high fasting RQ and subsequent weight gain. A low RQ has also been associated with reduced weight regain after rapid weight loss.[25]

Several other studies, however, found no significant association between low RQ and reduced weight regain.[7,8] In the Quebec Family Study,[7] there was no significant association between fasting RQ measured by indirect calorimetry and changes in weight or body fatness during 5.5 years of follow-up. Weinsier et al.[8] also found no difference in RQ between post-obese women and never-obese controls. In addition, baseline RQ did not predict 4-year weight change in post-obese women, although self-reported physical inactivity was associated with greater weight gain.

Overall, the existing literature does not provide convincing evidence that fat oxidation plays a major role in subsequent body weight gain. Similar to the studies on RMR and body weight, most studies on RQ have been relatively small and of short duration. In addition, substantial errors in RQ measurement could have attenuated the effects.

The interpretation of RQ is complex, because it is influenced by many factors, including age, sex, energy balance, and body fatness. Thus, differences in characteristics of the study populations can lead to heterogeneity in study results.

Insulin Resistance

Numerous cross-sectional analyses have shown a close relationship between obesity and insulin resistance. In addition, prospective epidemiologic studies and randomized clinical trials have shown that weight gain increases insulin resistance while weight loss improves insulin sensitivity. However, the impact of insulin resistance on subsequent weight gain remains unclear. The *thrifty gene* hypothesis suggests that populations with certain genetic traits—that is, those that promote metabolic efficiency and insulin resistance in peripheral tissues—are more likely to survive famine and starvation because of more efficient food utilization and greater fat accumulation.[26] From this perspective, insulin resistance can be seen as a cause of fat and weight gain.

Because insulin resistance suppresses insulin-sensitive lipolysis in the adipose tissue, Arner[27] hypothesized that hyperinsulinemia resulting from insulin resistance promotes weight gain. Eckel,[28] on the other hand, proposed that insulin resistance is "a necessary adaptation for preventing further weight gain in the obese subject." This suggests that an insulin-resistant state, although metabolically detrimental, may prevent future weight gain. Conversely, improved insulin sensitivity may induce subsequent weight gain or regain. This hypothesis is partly supported by the observation that treatment with thiazolidinediones (TZDs), an insulin-sensitizer, causes weight gain.[29]

To date, 16 prospective cohort studies (14 in adults and 2 in children) have examined the relationship between insulin resistance and subsequent weight change (Table 18.3). The results from these studies are mixed. In a prospective study among 192 nondiabetic Pima Indians, Swinburn et al.[30] measured insulin resistance by euglycemic clamp and followed subjects for approximately 3.5 years. Those with insulin resistance gained less weight than subjects who were insulin-sensitive (3.1 vs. 7.6 kg, $P < .0001$). There was a significant correlation between increasing glucose disposal at maximum-stimulating insulin concentration and percent weight change per year ($r = .34$, $P < .0001$). The San Antonio Heart Study[31] found a significant association between fasting insulin and lower weight gain among obese subjects, but not leaner ones. The San Luis Valley Diabetes Study[33] found an association between higher fasting insulin concentration and reduced risk of weight gain. In a linear regression model adjusting for age, sex, ethnicity, and body mass index (BMI), a doubling of baseline fasting insulin concentration was associated with an average of 6.3 kg less weight gain ($P = .006$). Wedick et al.[41] examined the relationship between insulin resistance and weight change among 725 nondiabetic men and women aged 50 to 89 years in the Rancho Bernardo Study. They found that insulin-resistant individuals were three times more likely to lose 10 kg or more compared to those without insulin resistance.

Results from other studies have been inconsistent. Folsom et al.[37] examined the relationship between fasting insulin concentration and weight gain in two cohort studies: the Coronary Artery Risk Development in Young Adults (CARDIA) study and the Atherosclerosis Risk in Communities (ARIC) study. In the CARDIA cohort, there was no association between fasting insulin and weight gain after adjusting for baseline weight. However, in the ARIC cohort, there was an inverse association between fasting insulin and weight gain, even after adjusting for baseline BMI. Different age groups and baseline BMI may have accounted for the discrepant outcomes; participants in the ARIC cohort were older and heavier than those in the CARDIA cohort.

Table 18.3 Prospective Epidemiologic Studies on Insulin Resistance and Weight Gain

First Author (Year)	Study Population	Exposure	Outcome	Associations
Swinburn et al. (1991)[30]	Arizona Pima Indians FU = 3.5 y Age = 25 y BMI = 34 192 nondiabetic men (n = 104) and women (n = 88)	Hyperinsulinemic, euglycemic clamp insulin resistance (IR = below regression line for glucose disposal regressed on weight)	Percent weight change	Increased IR associated with reduced rate of weight gain ($P < .0001$)
Valdez (1994)[31]	San Antonio Heart Study (Mexican American/non-Hispanic white) FU = 8 y Age = 25-64 y BMI = 24-28 1493 nondiabetic men and women	Fasting insulin	Weight change	Increased fasting insulin associated with a lower likelihood of gaining weight among obese subjects ($P < .001$)
Schwartz (1995)[32]	Arizona Pima Indians FU = 3 y Age = 25 y BMI = 34 97 nondiabetic men (n = 64) and women (n = 33)	Insulin secretion: MTT_{AUC} $OGTT_{AUC}$ AIRg (acute insulin response to glucose) IR: Submax M Max M	Percentage of weight change Percentage of fat mass change	All three measures of reduced insulin secretion significantly predicted increased percent weight change in multivariate linear regression analyses ($P < .05$). Measures of IR predictive of weight gain in univariate analyses, but not multivariate analyses
Hoag (1995)[33]	San Luis Valley Diabetes Study (Hispanic/non-Hispanic white) FU = 4 y Age = 53 y BMI = 26 789 nondiabetic men and women	Fasting insulin	Weight change	Higher initial fasting insulin related to lower subsequent rates of weight gain in nonglucose tolerant (NGT) persons ($P = .006$)

(continued)

Table 18.3 continued

First Author (Year)	Study Population	Exposure	Outcome	Associations
Hodge (1996)[34]	Mauritians (Asian Indian, Creole, and Chinese) FU = 5 y Age = 25 to 74 y BMI = 22 to 27 3156 nondiabetic men and women	Fasting insulin HOMA-IR Fasting insulin/glucose	Percent weight change WHR	IR predicted increased weight gain in Chinese men only—multivariate (fasting insulin: $P = .004$), (HOMA: $P = .002$), (fasting I/G: $P = .02$)
Boyko (1996)[35]	Japanese-American Community Diabetes Study FU = 5 y Age = 61 y BMI = 25.5 137 nondiabetic men (48% impaired glucose tolerant)	Fasting insulin Insulin secretion ratio: (30-0 min insulin/30-0 min glucose) Insulin AUC	Weight change BMI change IAF Subcutaneous abdominal fat	Increased fasting insulin and decreased insulin secretion ratio predicted IAF accumulation in multivariate linear regression analyses ($P = .048$ and .027, respectively) In logistic regression models for categorical IAF and tertiles of either fasting insulin or insulin secretion ratio; no significant associations were observed No other significant associations observed for other outcomes, or the exposure insulin AUC
Sigal (1997)[36]	Joslin Diabetes Center offspring of couple with type 2 diabetes mellitus (T2DM) FU = 16.7 y Age = 32.9 y BMI = 25.5 (calculated from mean height and weight) 107 nondiabetic men and women	Insulin sensitivity (S_I) from Bergman's minimal model Acute insulin secretion: 0-10 min insulin AUC 10-120 min insulin AUC	Weight gain rate (regression slope of subject's weight over time, g/y)	Both increased insulin sensitivity and increased acute insulin secretion significantly predicted subsequent weight gain ($P < .05$ in multivariate models)

Study	Exposure	Outcome	Results
Folsom (1998)[37]	Fasting insulin	Weight change	ARIC: Higher baseline fasting insulin associated with a lower rate of weight gain for whites and black women ($P < .05$)
ARIC (Caucasian/African American) FU = 6 y Age = 54 y BMI = 27 11 197 nondiabetic men and women			CARDIA: Positive association between fasting insulin and weight change was eliminated after adjusting for baseline weight
CARDIA (Caucasian/African American) FU = 7 y Age = 25 y BMI = 24 3636 nondiabetic men and women			
Lazarus (1998)[38] Normative Aging Study (Caucasian) FU = 3 y Age = 62 y BMI = 26.9 376 nondiabetic men	Fasting insulin	Weight change	Baseline insulin correlated with subsequent weight loss (unadjusted, $r = -.12$, $P < .05$) Increase of fasting insulin over time predicted subsequent weight increase ($P = .026$)
Zavaroni (1998)[39] Italian factory workers FU = 14 y Age = 40 y BMI = 25.0-27.3 647 nondiabetic men and women	2 h postchallenge insulin Fasting insulin	Weight change	IR not associated with weight change over follow-up
Gould (1999)[40] Isle of Ely Diabetes Study, UK FU = 4.4 y Age = 40-65 y BMI = 25 883 nondiabetic men and women	Fasting insulin	Weight change	Fasting hyperinsulinemia associated with increased WHR over time in women over 50 y ($P = .007$); no association in men
	Postchallenge insulin response	WHR	Reduced first-phase insulin secretion associated with weight gain (age-adjusted $r = -.13$, $P = .01$) in women; no association in men

(continued)

Table 18.3 continued

First Author (Year)	Study Population	Exposure	Outcome	Associations
Wedick (2001)[41]	Rancho Bernardo Study (Caucasian) FU = 8 y Age = 50-89 y BMI = 24.7 725 nondiabetic men and women	Fasting insulin HOMA	Weight change	IR associated with weight loss (multivariate, $\beta = -1.3$, $P = .01$). Similar results for HOMA
Mayer-Davis (2003)[42]	IRAS (Hispanic/non-Hispanic white/African American) FU = 5 y Age = 69-69 BMI = 29.2 1194 (only 554 were normal glucose tolerant)	Fasting insulin S_I from Bergman's minimal model Acute insulin response Disposition index	Weight change Waist BMI	Among NGT, no measures of insulin metabolism significantly predictive of weight change
Howard (2004)[43]	Women's Health Initiative (White 60%, Black 30%, Hispanic 12%, Asian: Pacific Islander 8%) FU = 3 y Age = 62 y BMI = 27 3389 nondiabetic, postmenopausal women	Fasting insulin HOMA-IR	Weight change	Fasting insulin levels significantly predicted weight gain in white women (multivariate, $\beta = 11.5$, $P = .004$) and the total cohort (multivariate, $\beta = 6.5$, $P = .039$), but not in black or Asian women
Odeleye (1997)[44]	Arizona Pima Indians FU = 9 y Age = 5-9 y BMI = 19 328 nondiabetic boys and girls	Fasting insulin	Weight change	Fasting insulin positively correlated with rate of weight gain per year in boys ($r = .42$, $P < .0001$) and girls ($r = .20$, $P < .01$)
Travers (2002)[45]	Caucasian (3 African Americans) FU = 3 y Age = 9.7-14.5 BMI = 19-22	S_I from Bergman's minimal model	Body composition (via skinfold thickness, BMI, hydrodensitometry, bioimpedance)	IR associated with decreased body fat

FU: Follow-up; IAF: intra-abdominal fat; IR: Insulin resistance; HOMA-IR: homeostasis model assessment of insulin resistance; MTT: meal tolerance test; AUC: area under the curve; WHR: waist-to-hip ratio; OGTT: Oral glucose tolerance test.

While several studies reported no association between insulin resistance and weight gain,[39,42] others found a positive relationship. Hodge et al.[34] observed that in Chinese men, insulin resistance predicted greater weight gain during follow-up. However, there were no associations between insulin resistance and changes in weight and waist-hip ratio (WHR) in Asian Indian and Creole men and women. Gould et al.[40] found that in middle-aged women, fasting insulin was associated with increased WHR during 4.4 years of follow-up. In addition, there was an association between reduced first-phase insulin secretion and greater weight gain. The Normative Aging Study[38] showed that increased fasting insulin predicted future weight gain. During a 3-year follow-up in the Women's Health Initiative observational cohort, Howard et al.[43] reported an independent association between higher insulin resistance and weight gain, especially among women with a lower BMI at baseline. In Japanese Americans, Boyko et al.[35] examined the relationship between insulin resistance and changes in intra-abdominal fat (IAF) measured by CT scan during 5.5 years of follow-up. After adjusting for baseline IAF, they found that baseline fasting insulin and C-peptide were significantly associated with increased IAF over time. Schwartz et al.[32] observed that reduced insulin secretion rather than insulin resistance was an independent predictor of weight gain in Pima Indian adults. In addition, Sigal et al.[36] found that insulin resistance measured by Bergman's minimal model predicted a lower risk of weight gain only among those with higher insulin secretion.

Studies conducted among children have also produced contradictory results. Odeleye et al.[44] examined the association between fasting insulin concentration measured in 328 Pima Indian children 5 to 9 years old and the rate of weight gain during 9.3 years of follow-up. After adjusting for initial relative weight, sex, and changes in height and age over time, there was a significant association between higher fasting plasma insulin concentration and weight gain per year in both boys and girls. The authors concluded that increased insulin resistance may predict greater weight gain in Pima Indian children. On the other hand, Travers et al.[45] found that lower insulin resistance was associated with increased body fat among 111 healthy children aged 9.7 to 14.5 years. The authors suggested that during puberty, increased insulin resistance may prevent fat accumulation.

Whether insulin sensitivity predicts weight regain after weight loss remains controversial. Yost et al.[46] followed 10 obese women who had undergone a 3-month weight loss program followed by 3 months of weight maintenance. Improved insulin sensitivity, measured by a euglycemic clamp before weight loss and at the end of the weight maintenance phase, significantly predicted the amount of weight regain at both 12 and 18 months. Wing et al.,[47] however, found no significant association between changes in fasting insulin from baseline to 6 months and weight regain in either nondiabetic or diabetic subjects who had been through a weight loss program.

On the whole, the literature does not provide clear evidence supporting the hypothesis that insulin resistance is an adaptive mechanism that prevents further weight gain among the obese. In other words, an increase in insulin sensitivity does not necessarily lead to weight gain. In contrast, there appears to be more evidence that insulin resistance may lead to subsequent weight gain in some populations. The interpretation of the literature, however, is complicated by a number of factors. First, population characteristics (e.g., ethnicity, sex, and age groups) differ across and within studies. Because insulin sensitivity is affected by these variables, the relationship between insulin sensitivity and weight change trajectories may differ across different age, sex, and ethnic groups. Second, some studies have focused on obese subjects, while others have evaluated weight changes among relatively lean subjects. Initially obese subjects who already have high insulin resistance at baseline tend to not gain weight or even lose weight during follow-up. Therefore, the observation that baseline insulin resistance promotes subsequent weight maintenance or even weight loss may reflect the fact that initially obese subjects tend to gain less weight than those who are initially lean. Thus, the relationship between baseline insulin resistance and weight gain during follow-up can be confounded by baseline weight. Although many studies have adjusted for baseline weight, residual confounding remains a concern. In several studies, the relationship between insulin sensitivity and weight gain became nonsignificant after adjusting for baseline weight. Third, measurements of insulin resistance differ across studies. Several studies used euglycemic clamp, the gold standard for measurement of insulin resistance, but most used homeostasis model assessment (HOMA) insulin resistance index or fasting insulin, which is a good surrogate measure of insulin resistance in nondiabetic populations, but its validity in diabetic populations and in children and the elderly is less established. Finally, most studies assessed insulin resistance only once at baseline. Longitudinal studies are needed to examine whether change in insulin resistance predicts subsequent weight change.

Leptin

Leptin, one of the first identified adipocyte-secreted hormones,[48] stimulates energy expenditure and reduces appetite, thus decreasing food intake. In *ob/ob* mice, leptin deficiency caused by mutations of the *ob* gene leads to hyperphagia and extreme obesity, while administration of recombinant leptin reduced body weight and obesity.[48-50] Unlike mice, overweight and obese humans typically have elevated leptin levels.[51,52] Resistance to leptin's activity, which is analogous to insulin resistance, is thought to be a mechanism underlying the direct relationship between obesity and plasma leptin levels.[53]

In cross-sectional studies, plasma leptin levels have been strongly associated with BMI and measures of fat distribution (e.g., skinfold and waist circumference).[54-56] Several prospective cohort studies have evaluated the relationship between plasma leptin concentrations and subsequent weight change. Ravussin et al.[57] measured fasting plasma leptin concentrations in two groups of weight-matched nondiabetic Pima Indians followed for approximately 3 years. After adjusting for initial percent body fat, low leptin concentrations at baseline were associated with greater weight gain.

As in studies on other metabolic predictors of obesity in Pima Indians, initial results on low leptin and weight gain have not been consistently replicated in other populations. Lindroos et al.[58] found that during a 4-year follow-up, high baseline leptin levels predicted less weight gain (or more weight loss) in women without an obese parent. Among those with at least one obese parent, it had no predictive capability. In an 8-year study, Folsom et al.[59] reported no relationship between initial leptin levels and weight change in a biracial sample (whites and blacks) ($P = .47$). However, there was a strong correlation between increases in leptin levels and body weight over time ($r = .62$). Similarly, in the Mauritius Non-communicable Disease Study, Hodge et al.[60] found no difference in 5-year changes in BMI, WHR, or waist circumference among men with low, normal, or high leptin levels at baseline. Among women, the largest increase in WHR was found in the low leptin group. In the Rancho Bernardo cohort,[61] there was a positive association between leptin levels and attained body weight, but leptin levels did not predict subsequent weight change. In the Mexico City Diabetes Study,[62] baseline leptin levels did not predict weight gain during 3.25 years of follow-up in nondiabetic subjects. In addition, relatively low leptin levels did not appear to predict 4-year weight regain after weight loss in postmenopausal women.[63] Furthermore, Niskanen et al.[64] reported that baseline leptin levels did not predict response to weight loss intervention in obese men and women.

Several prospective studies have identified a positive association between baseline leptin levels and subsequent weight gain. Among Japanese-Americans, Chessler et al.[65] found a positive association between leptin levels and increased body weight, BMI, and body fat after adjusting for baseline adiposity, age, and fasting insulin. In the Health Professionals' Follow-up Study,[66] higher baseline leptin levels predicted 4-year weight gain among overweight men but not among normal-weight men. In a Dutch study with 6.8 years of follow-up, van Rossum et al.[67] compared baseline leptin in 259 subjects who had gained substantial weight (an average of 12.6 kg) to baseline leptin in 277 subjects with stable weight. Those who gained weight had significantly elevated leptin levels compared with weight maintainers.

Several studies have also suggested that higher plasma leptin levels predict future weight gain in children. Savoye et al.[68] measured baseline fasting leptin levels in a biracial cohort of 68 obese children aged 7 to 18 years. After adjusting for baseline BMI, Tanner stage, years of follow-up, and fasting insulin, there was a positive association between higher leptin levels and a greater increase in BMI Z-scores in girls ($P = .006$) (but not boys) during 2.5 years of follow-up. Johnson et al.[69] studied the relationship between initial leptin levels and body fat mass in 85 children (42 white, 43 African American) and found a positive association between initial leptin levels and increase in body fat mass (measured by dual energy x-ray absorptiometry [DXA]) over time, suggesting that higher leptin levels may promote fat gain in children. These results could also imply that children on a trajectory towards obesity have already developed leptin resistance.

In contrast to earlier findings that relatively low leptin levels predicted future weight gain in Pima Indian adults, most subsequent studies found either no relationship between leptin and weight gain or that higher leptin levels predicted increased weight gain in adults and children. There is little evidence that leptin levels predict response to weight loss interventions. Although leptin is known to have a strong cross-sectional relationship with obesity and to play a critical role in energy homeostasis, it does not appear to have a major role in predicting future weight trajectories.

Adiponectin

Adiponectin (also known as APM1) is a protein synthesized and secreted exclusively by adipose tissue.[70,71] In humans, adiponectin is one of the most abundant plasma proteins, with a concentration of about 5-10 μg/mL.[72] These levels are reduced in obese adults, but increase with weight loss.[73] Adiponectin is inversely correlated with fasting glucose, insulin, and insulin resistance independent of BMI.[72] Several studies have reported that subjects with lower adiponectin levels are more likely to develop type 2 diabetes independent of adiposity.[74-76]

Despite a clear relationship between adiponectin levels and improved insulin sensitivity, there is no evidence that low plasma adiponectin levels predict subsequent weight gain. Vozarova et al.[77] examined plasma adiponectin concentrations and weight change in 219 nondiabetic Pima Indians and found no significant association between plasma adiponectin concentrations at baseline and changes in weight or BMI during the follow-up. Similarly, the Rancho Bernardo cohort[61] showed no relationship between baseline adiponectin levels and subsequent changes in body weight in men or women 60 to 91 years of age. These results suggest that low adiponectin levels are a consequence of obesity rather than a cause. They also suggest that the beneficial effects of adiponectin on risk of type 2 diabetes may be mediated through mechanisms that are independent of body weight.

Ghrelin

Ghrelin, a hormone secreted primarily by the stomach and duodenum, plays an important role in regulating appetite and weight control.[78] Ghrelin acts as the endogenous ligand for the growth hormone secretagogue receptor (GHS-R). In humans, plasma ghrelin levels increase shortly before a meal and fall shortly after, suggesting meal-initiation effects of this hormone.[79] In rodents, administration of ghrelin caused weight gain by increasing food intake.[80] Ghrelin administration also stimulated food intake and growth hormone secretion in human experiments.[81]

Paradoxically, plasma ghrelin levels are significantly reduced in obese subjects compared with lean ones. In cross-sectional studies, fasting ghrelin was inversely correlated with BMI, percent body fat, and leptin levels in both children and adults.[82,83] Other studies have shown an inverse association between plasma ghrelin and prevalence of metabolic syndrome.[84,85] In humans, diet-induced weight loss leads to an increase in 24-hour plasma ghrelin levels, whereas gastric bypass surgery results in markedly suppressed ghrelin levels.[86]

Only two prospective studies have examined whether fasting ghrelin predicts future weight gain. Bunt et al.[87] found that fasting plasma ghrelin concentrations were lower in taller and heavier Pima Indian children but did not independently predict subsequent weight, BMI, or future growth rates. In the Rancho Bernardo Cohort,[61] baseline ghrelin concentration did not predict weight gain among older men and women during 4.7 years of follow-up. These results suggest that lower ghrelin levels are a consequence rather than a cause of obesity. It has been suggested that ghrelin suppression in obesity is another manifestation of insulin resistance, although the precise mechanism explaining this relationship remains to be elucidated.[83]

Inflammatory Markers

In that adipose tissue is a major secretive organ for proinflammatory cytokines (see Chapter 8), obesity is considered a state of low-level inflammation. In cross-sectional studies, obesity is associated with increased plasma concentrations of interleukin-6 (IL-6), tumor necrosis factor-alpha (TNF-α), CRP, and fibrinogen.[88] Elevated serum CRP concentrations are a significant predictor of future risk of metabolic syndrome,[89] type 2 diabetes,[90-92] and coronary heart disease.[93]

Despite a clear cross-sectional relationship between adiposity and inflammatory markers, data on whether inflammatory markers predict subsequent weight gain are limited. These have examined different inflammatory markers in relation to weight gain in various populations. Duncan et al.[94] examined fibrinogen and other inflammatory markers in middle-aged adults in the ARIC Study. During 3 years of follow-up, subjects in the highest quartile of fibrinogen gained on average 0.23 kg/year more than those in the lowest quartile ($P < .001$). In multivariate analyses, the adjusted RR of a large weight gain (greater than the 90th percentile) for the highest quartile of fibrinogen versus the lowest quartile was 1.65 (95% CI: 1.38 to 1.97). The adjusted RRs for large weight gain in those with a high white blood cell count, factor VIII, and von Willebrand factor were 1.38 (1.14 to 1.67), 1.28 (1.08 to 1.53), and 1.28 (1.08 to 1.51), respectively. These results suggest that heightened inflammation may play a role in the development of obesity.

In a subsequent analysis of those participants in the ARIC cohort who quit smoking,[95] elevated inflammatory markers augmented weight gain associated with quitting smoking.

Among new quitters, subjects in the highest quartile of leukocytes gained 0.56 kg/year more than those in the lowest quartile. In multivariate analyses, the RR for a large weight gain after quitting smoking (vs. continuing) was 6.2 for those in the highest quartile of leukocytes and 2.2 for those in the lowest quartile (*P* for interaction between smoking status and leukocytes = .03).

Engstrom et al.[96] evaluated whether elevated levels of inflammation-sensitive plasma proteins (ISPs) (fibrinogen, orosomucoid, alpha-1-antitrypsin, haptoglobin, and ceruloplasmin) were associated with future weight gain in 2,821 nondiabetic healthy men 38 to 50 years of age in the Malmo Preventive Study cohort. During 6.1 years of follow-up, the proportion of subjects with a large weight gain (75th percentile ≥ 3.8 kg) increased with the number of ISPs in the top quartile in a dose-response manner (*P* for trend = .0005). In a subsequent analysis of the Malmo Preventive Study cohort, Engström et al.[97] found an association between plasma concentrations of complement factor 3 (C3) and weight gain. After adjustments for initial weight, age, height, and follow-up time, the RRs of a large weight gain (75th percentile ≥ 3.8 kg) were 1.00 (reference), 0.96 (95% CI: 0.7 to 1.2), 1.1 (0.9 to 1.5), and 1.4 (1.1 to 1.8) across increasing quartiles of C3 levels (*P* for trend = .01). This relationship remained significant after further adjustments for physical inactivity, alcohol intake, smoking, and ISP levels. Because the hepatic production of C3 is stimulated by inflammatory cytokines, this study suggests that the immune response induced by inflammation may lead to increased weight gain.

In the Cardiovascular Health Study, Barzilay et al.[98] examined several inflammatory markers in relation to weight change among 3,254 subjects (≥65 years old) during a 3-year follow-up. They found a significant association between higher baseline concentrations of CRP and weight change (5%, either gained or lost) during the follow-up. Other inflammatory markers (e.g., fibrinogen and factor VIIIc) were also associated with greater weight gain, whereas white blood cell (WBC) count was associated with greater weight loss. These analyses suggest that elevated inflammatory markers may precede both weight loss and gain. The relationship with weight loss may result from elevated inflammation associated with existing and subclinical diseases.

Taken together, these data indicate that inflammatory markers may predict subsequent weight gain, especially in younger subjects who are more prone to age-related weight gain. However, the association is modest and there could be confounding by dietary and lifestyle factors associated with inflammation if adjustment for these factors is inadequate. The biological mechanism for the association between inflammatory markers and subsequent weight change is unclear. There is some evidence from animal studies that infection by pathogens may have a potential etiological role in obesity,[99] and thus, it is conceivable that infection-induced inflammation may predict weight gain. So far, however, the evidence of a link between infection and obesity is largely limited to animal studies. It is also possible that the effects of inflammatory factors on weight gain are mediated through insulin resistance, because these cytokines have been shown to promote insulin resistance in peripheral tissues. However, as discussed above, the relationship between insulin resistance and weight gain is not well characterized.

Cortisol

More than four decades ago, Dunkelman et al.[100] suggested that increased cortisol secretion might play a role in the development of obesity. A relationship between cortisol and obesity, especially central obesity, is well supported by clinical observations.[101] For example, patients treated with corticosteroids tend to gain weight and become centrally obese. Also, patients with Cushing's syndrome or hypercortisolism often develop central obesity, a condition that can be cured by resolution of the hypercortisolism.[101] These observations indicate that variations in cortisol in apparently healthy people may be involved in central obesity.

Elevated cortisol secretion has been found in the obese, especially among those with abdominal adiposity.[102] Wallerius et al.[103] observed positive correlations between rise in morning saliva cortisol levels and BMI ($r = .45$), WHR ($r = .54$), abdominal sagittal diameter ($r = .54$), glucose ($r = .54$), insulin ($r = .57$), and triglycerides ($r = .46$). These findings suggest that the rise of cortisol immediately after awakening, which reflects enhanced hypothalamic-pituitary-adrenal (HPA) drive, may be an indicator of central obesity and metabolic syndrome. However, no prospective studies are available on whether morning cortisol levels predict weight gain or the development of the metabolic syndrome.

Although obese people have elevated cortisol secretion, plasma cortisol levels are normal or low, suggesting that turnover of cortisol is enhanced in the obese. Whether increased production or enhanced peripheral metabolism is involved in the pathophysiology of obesity is still unclear. Bjorntorp[101] hypothesized that elevated cortisol production resulting from the activation of the HPA axis mediated the relationship between psychosocial stress and abdominal obesity. In a cross-sectional study, Rosmond et al.[104] assessed salivary cortisol concentrations and perceived stress on seven occasions over a random working day among 284 men. There was a positive correlation between stress-related cortisol secretion and central obesity measured by sagittal diameter, blood pressure, and total and low-density lipoprotein (LDL) cholesterol. However, due to the cross-sectional nature of the analyses, the direction of these associations is unclear.

Summary

Extensive research has been devoted to the search for metabolic and hormonal predictors of future weight gain. Initial results from studies in Pima Indian adults, one of the populations most prone to obesity, indicated that low RMR adjusted for lean body mass and high RQ (reflecting low fat oxidation) predicted future weight gain. However, subsequent studies in other populations have not confirmed these results. Several methodological issues (heterogeneity across populations, measurement errors, and inadequate power) may have led to divergent findings. Nonetheless, the preponderance of evidence suggests that RMR and RQ may not be as important as initially thought in predicting the trajectory of weight gain or the magnitude of weight regain after weight loss.

The hypothesis that insulin resistance may be an adaptive mechanism that prevents further weight gain among the obese has not found clear support. Although obese people are more resistant to insulin, prospective studies have shown inverse as well as positive associations between baseline insulin resistance and weight gain. In several studies, the relationship between insulin resistance and weight gain was attenuated and became nonsignificant after adjusting for baseline weight, suggesting that baseline weight is a major confounder in these analyses.

Initial results from Pima Indians also indicated that low leptin levels predict greater weight gain, but subsequent studies reported a null or positive association between baseline leptin levels and weight gain. Baseline weight is also an important confounder in these analyses. Ghrelin is a recently discovered gut hormone that regulates appetite and satiety. It has effects on meal initiation and increases food intake. Paradoxically, cross-sectional studies have consistently indicated that plasma ghrelin levels are lower in obese people than in lean people. However, there is no evidence that ghrelin levels predict future weight gain.

It is now widely accepted that obesity is an inflammatory condition. Cross-sectional studies have demonstrated that inflammatory cytokines such as CRP, TNF-α, and IL-6 are significantly elevated in obesity. Several prospective studies have shown that elevated inflammatory markers at baseline predict future weight gain, but the effects are modest. Confounding by lifestyle factors and baseline weight is a concern in these analyses.

Finally, there is extensive literature on the role of cortisol in the development of obesity. Elevated cortisol secretion, through activation of the HPA axis, may underlie the relationship between psychosocial stress and obesity. However, virtually all evidence linking cortisol and obesity is limited to cross-sectional studies. Therefore, prospective studies are needed to confirm the cross-sectional findings.

In summary, although obesity is clearly associated with metabolic and hormonal disturbances, no single metabolic or hormone characteristic strongly predicts future weight gain. The literature underscores the complex pathophysiology of obesity and the methodological challenges facing epidemiologic research on metabolic risk factors and weight gain. Current evidence suggests that for most people, weight gain is probably not the consequence of clinically detectable metabolic defects, but rather the result of many subtle metabolic disturbances caused by a myriad of behavioral and environmental factors, such as unhealthy diet and decreased physical activity, as discussed in earlier chapters. Nonetheless, further research is needed to understand the heterogeneity in metabolic responses to the obesogenic environment.

References

1. Ravussin E, Gautier JF. Metabolic predictors of weight gain. *Int J Obes Relat Metab Disord.* 1999;23(Suppl 1):37-41.
2. Filozof C, Gonzalez C. Predictors of weight gain: the biological-behavioural debate. *Obes Rev.* 2000;1:21-26.
3. Ravussin E, Lillioja S, Knowler WC, et al. Reduced rate of energy expenditure as a risk factor for body-weight gain. *N Engl J Med.* 1988;318:467-472.
4. Buscemi S, Verga S, Caimi G, Cerasola G. Low relative resting metabolic rate and body weight gain in adult Caucasian Italians. *Int J Obes (London).* 2005;29:287-291.
5. Tataranni PA, Harper IT, Snitker S, et al. Body weight gain in free-living Pima Indians: effect of energy intake vs expenditure. *Int J Obes Relat Metab Disord.* 2003;27:1578-1583.
6. Seidell JC, Muller DC, Sorkin JD, Andres R. Fasting respiratory exchange ratio and resting metabolic rate as predictors of weight gain: the Baltimore Longitudinal Study on Aging. *Int J Obes Relat Metab Disord.* 1992;16:667-674.
7. Katzmarzyk PT, Perusse L, Tremblay A, Bouchard C. No association between resting metabolic rate or respiratory exchange ratio and subsequent changes in body mass and fatness: 5-1/2 year follow-up of the Quebec family study. *Eur J Clin Nutr.* 2000;54:610-614.
8. Weinsier RL, Nelson KM, Hensrud DD, Darnell BE, Hunter GR, Schutz Y. Metabolic predictors of obesity. Contribution of resting energy expenditure, thermic effect of food, and fuel utilization to four-year weight gain of post-obese and never-obese women. *J Clin Invest.* 1995;95:980-985.
9. Luke A, Durazo-Arvizu R, Cao G, Adeyemo A, Tayo B, Cooper R. Positive association between resting energy expenditure and weight gain in a lean adult population. *Am J Clin Nutr.* 2006;83:1076-1081.
10. Vogels N, Diepvens K, Westerterp-Plantenga MS. Predictors of long-term weight maintenance. *Obes Res.* 2005;13:2162-2168.

11. Weinsier RL, Hunter GR, Zuckerman PA, Darnell BE. Low resting and sleeping energy expenditure and fat use do not contribute to obesity in women. *Obes Res.* 2003;11:937-944.
12. Neale BM, Sham PC. The future of association studies: gene-based analysis and replication. *Am J Hum Genet.* 2004;75:353-362.
13. Astrup A, Gotzsche PC, van de Werken K, et al. Meta-analysis of resting metabolic rate in formerly obese subjects. *Am J Clin Nutr.* 1999;69:1117-1122.
14. Leibel RL, Rosenbaum M, Hirsch J. Changes in energy expenditure resulting from altered body weight. *N Engl J Med.* 1995;332:621-628.
15. Wyatt HR, Grunwald GK, Seagle HM, et al. Resting energy expenditure in reduced-obese subjects in the National Weight Control Registry. *Am J Clin Nutr.* 1999;69:1189-1193.
16. Weinsier RL, Nagy TR, Hunter GR, Darnell BE, Hensrud DD, Weiss HL. Do adaptive changes in metabolic rate favor weight regain in weight-reduced individuals? An examination of the set-point theory. *Am J Clin Nutr.* 2000;72:1088-1094
17. Harris RB. Role of set-point theory in regulation of body weight. *FASEB J.* 1990;4:3310-3318.
18. Forman JN, Miller WC, Szymanski LM, Fernhall B. Differences in resting metabolic rates of inactive obese African-American and Caucasian women. *Int J Obes Relat Metab Disord.* 1998;22:215-221.
19. Sun M, Gower BA, Bartolucci AA, Hunter GR, Figueroa-Colon R, Goran MI. A longitudinal study of resting energy expenditure relative to body composition during puberty in African American and white children. *Am J Clin Nutr.* 2001;73:308-315.
20. Luke A, Rotimi CN, Adeyemo AA, et al. Comparability of resting energy expenditure in Nigerians and U.S. blacks. *Obes Res.* 2000;8:351-359.
21. Fox CS, Esparza J, Nicolson M, et al. Is a low leptin concentration, a low resting metabolic rate, or both the expression of the "thrifty genotype"? Results from Mexican Pima Indians. *Am J Clin Nutr.* 1998;68:1053-1057.
22. Esparza J, Fox C, Harper IT, et al. Daily energy expenditure in Mexican and USA Pima Indians: low physical activity as a possible cause of obesity. *Int J Obes Relat Metab Disord.* 2000;24:55-59.
23. Zurlo F, Lillioja S, Esposito-Del Puente A, et al. Low ratio of fat to carbohydrate oxidation as predictor of weight gain: study of 24-h RQ. *Am J Physiol.* 1990;259:E650-E657.
24. Marra M, Scalfi L, Covino A, Esposito-Del Puente A, Contaldo F. Fasting respiratory quotient as a predictor of weight changes in non-obese women. *Int J Obes Relat Metab Disord.* 1998;22:601-603.
25. Valtuena S, Salas-Salvado J, Lorda PG. The respiratory quotient as a prognostic factor in weight-loss rebound. *Int J Obes Relat Metab Disord.* 1997;21:811-817.
26. Neel J. Diabetes mellitus: a "thrifty" genotype rendered detrimental by "progress?" *Am J Hum Genet.* 1962;14:353-362.
27. Arner P. Control of lipolysis and its relevance to development of obesity in man. *Diabetes Metab Rev.* 1988;4:507-515.
28. Eckel RH. Insulin resistance: an adaptation for weight maintenance. *Lancet.* 1992;340:1452-1453.
29. Fonseca V. Effect of thiazolidinediones on body weight in patients with diabetes mellitus. *Am J Med.* 2003;115(Suppl 8A):42S-48S.
30. Swinburn BA, Nyomba BL, Saad MF, et al. Insulin resistance associated with lower rates of weight gain in Pima Indians. *J Clin Invest.* 1991;88:168-173.
31. Valdez R, Mitchell BD, Haffner SM, et al. Predictors of weight change in a bi-ethnic population. The San Antonio Heart Study. *Int J Obes Relat Metab Disord.* 1994;18:85-91.

32. Schwartz MW, Boyko EJ, Kahn SE, Ravussin E, Bogardus C. Reduced insulin secretion: an independent predictor of body weight gain. *J Clin Endocrinol Metab*. 1995;80:1571-1576.

33. Hoag S, Marshall JA, Jones RH, Hamman RF. High fasting insulin levels associated with lower rates of weight gain in persons with normal glucose tolerance: the San Luis Valley Diabetes Study. *Int J Obes Relat Metab Disord*. 1995;19:175-180.

34. Hodge AM, Dowse GK, Alberti KG, Tuomilehto J, Gareeboo H, Zimmet PZ. Relationship of insulin resistance to weight gain in nondiabetic Asian Indian, Creole, and Chinese Mauritians. Mauritius Non-communicable Disease Study Group. *Metabolism*. 1996;45:627-633.

35. Boyko EJ, Leonetti DL, Bergstrom RW, Newell-Morris L, Fujimoto WY. Low insulin secretion and high fasting insulin and C-peptide levels predict increased visceral adiposity. 5-year follow-up among initially nondiabetic Japanese-American men. *Diabetes*. 1996;45:1010-1015.

36. Sigal RJ, El-Hashimy M, Martin BC, Soeldner JS, Krolewski AS, Warram JH. Acute postchallenge hyperinsulinemia predicts weight gain: a prospective study. *Diabetes*. 1997;46:1025-1029.

37. Folsom AR, Vitelli LL, Lewis CE, Schreiner PJ, Watson RL, Wagenknecht LE. Is fasting insulin concentration inversely associated with rate of weight gain? Contrasting findings from the CARDIA and ARIC study cohorts. *Int J Obes Relat Metab Disord*. 1998;22:48-54.

38. Lazarus R, Sparrow D, Weiss S. Temporal relations between obesity and insulin: longitudinal data from the Normative Aging Study. *Am J Epidemiol*. 1998;147:173-179.

39. Zavaroni I, Zuccarelli A, Gasparini P, Massironi P, Barilli A, Reaven GM. Can weight gain in healthy, nonobese volunteers be predicted by differences in baseline plasma insulin concentration? *J Clin Endocrinol Metab*. 1998;83:3498-3500.

40. Gould AJ, Williams DE, Byrne CD, Hales CN, Wareham NJ. Prospective cohort study of the relationship of markers of insulin resistance and secretion with weight gain and changes in regional adiposity. *Int J Obes Relat Metab Disord*. 1999;23:1256-1261.

41. Wedick NM, Mayer-Davis EJ, Wingard DL, Addy CL, Barrett-Connor E. Insulin resistance precedes weight loss in adults without diabetes: the Rancho Bernardo Study. *Am J Epidemiol*. 2001;153:1199-1205.

42. Mayer-Davis EJ, Kirkner GJ, Karter AJ, Zaccaro DJ. Metabolic predictors of 5-year change in weight and waist circumference in a triethnic population: the insulin resistance atherosclerosis study. *Am J Epidemiol*. 2003;157:592-601.

43. Howard BV, Adams-Campbell, L, Allen C, et al. Insulin resistance and weight gain in postmenopausal women of diverse ethnic groups. *Int J Obes Relat Metab Disord*. 2004;28:1039-1047.

44. Odeleye OE, de Courten M, Pettitt DJ, Ravussin E. Fasting hyperinsulinemia is a predictor of increased body weight gain and obesity in Pima Indian children. *Diabetes*. 1997;46:1341-1345.

45. Travers SH, Jeffers BW, Eckel RH. Insulin resistance during puberty and future fat accumulation. *J Clin Endocrinol Metab*. 2002;87:3814-3818.

46. Yost TJ, Jensen DR, Eckel RH. Weight regain following sustained weight reduction is predicted by relative insulin sensitivity. *Obes Res*. 1995;3:583-587.

47. Wing RR. Insulin sensitivity as a predictor of weight regain. *Obes Res*. 1997;5:24-29.

48. Zhang Y, Proenca R, Maffei M, Barone M, Leopold L, Friedman JM. Positional cloning of the mouse obese gene and its human homologue. *Nature*. 1994;372:425-432.

49. Campfield LA, Smith FJ, Guisez Y, Devos R, Burn P. Recombinant mouse OB protein: evidence for a peripheral signal linking adiposity and central neural networks. *Science*. 1995;269:546-549.

50. Frederich RC, Hamann A, Anderson S, Lollmann B, Lowell BB, Flier JS. Leptin levels reflect body lipid content in mice: evidence for diet-induced resistance to leptin action. *Nat Med*. 1995;1:1311-1314.

51. Considine RV, Caro JF. Leptin in humans: current progress and future directions. *Clin Chem.* 1996;42(6 Pt 1):843-844.
52. Considine RV, Sinha MK, Heiman ML, et al. Serum immunoreactive-leptin concentrations in normal-weight and obese humans. *N Engl J Med.* 1996;334:292-295.
53. Arch JR, Stock MJ, Trayhurn P. Leptin resistance in obese humans: does it exist and what does it mean? *Int J Obes Relat Metab Disord.* 1998;22:1159-1163.
54. Hu FB, Chen C, Wang B, Stampfer MJ, Xu X. Leptin concentrations in relation to overall adiposity, fat distribution, and blood pressure in a rural Chinese population. *Int J Obes Relat Metab Disord.* 2001;25:121-125.
55. Haffner SM, Gingerich RL, Miettinen H, Stern MP. Leptin concentrations in relation to overall adiposity and regional body fat distribution in Mexican Americans. *Int J Obes Relat Metab Disord.* 1996;20:904-908.
56. Zimmet P, Hodge A, Nicolson M, et al. Serum leptin concentration, obesity, and insulin resistance in Western Samoans: cross sectional study. *BMJ.* 1996;313:965-969.
57. Ravussin E, Pratley RE, Maffei M, et al. Relatively low plasma leptin concentrations precede weight gain in Pima Indians. *Nat Med.* 1997;3:238-240.
58. Lindroos AK, Lissner L, Carlsson B, et al. Familial predisposition for obesity may modify the predictive value of serum leptin concentrations for long-term weight change in obese women. *Am J Clin Nutr.* 1998;67:1119-1123.
59. Folsom AR, Jensen MD, Jacobs DR Jr, Hilner JE, Tsai AW, Schreiner PJ. Serum leptin and weight gain over 8 years in African American and Caucasian young adults. *Obes Res.* 1999;7:1-8.
60. Hodge AM, de Courten MP, Dowse GK, et al. Do leptin levels predict weight gain?—A 5-year follow-up study in Mauritius. Mauritius Non-communicable Disease Study Group. *Obes Res.* 1998;6:319-325.
61. Langenberg C, Bergstrom J, Laughlin GA, Barrett-Connor E. Ghrelin, adiponectin, and leptin do not predict long-term changes in weight and body mass index in older adults: longitudinal analysis of the Rancho Bernardo cohort. *Am J Epidemiol.* 2005;162:1189-1197.
62. Haffner SM, Mykkanen LA, Gonzalez CC, Stern MP. Leptin concentrations do not predict weight gain: the Mexico City Diabetes Study. *Int J Obes Relat Metab Disord.* 1998;22:695-699.
63. Nagy TR, Davies SL, Hunter GR, Darnell B, Weinsier RL. Serum leptin concentrations and weight gain in postobese, postmenopausal women. *Obes Res.* 1998;6:257-261.
64. Niskanen LK, Haffner S, Karhunen LJ, Turpeinen AK, Miettinen H, Uusitupa MI. Serum leptin in obesity is related to gender and body fat topography but does not predict successful weight loss. *Eur J Endocrinol.* 1997;137:61-67.
65. Chessler SD, Fujimoto WY, Shofer JB, Boyko EJ, Weigle DS. Increased plasma leptin levels are associated with fat accumulation in Japanese Americans. *Diabetes.* 1998;47:239-243.
66. Chu NF, Spiegelman D, Yu J, Rifai N, Hotamisligil GS, Rimm EB. Plasma leptin concentrations and four-year weight gain among US men. *Int J Obes Relat Metab Disord.* 2001;25:346-353.
67. van Rossum CT, Hoebee B, van Baak MA, Mars M, Saris WH, Seidell JC. Genetic variation in the leptin receptor gene, leptin, and weight gain in young Dutch adults. *Obes Res.* 2003;11:377-386.
68. Savoye M, Dziura J, Castle J, DiPietro L, Tamborlane WV, Caprio S. Importance of plasma leptin in predicting future weight gain in obese children: a two-and-a-half-year longitudinal study. *Int J Obes Relat Metab Disord.* 2002;26:942-946.
69. Johnson MS, Huang TT, Figueroa-Colon R, Dwyer JH, Goran MI. Influence of leptin on changes in body fat during growth in African American and white children. *Obes Res.* 2001;9:593-598.
70. Scherer PE, Williams S, Fogliano M, Baldini G, Lodish HF. A novel serum protein similar to C1q, produced exclusively in adipocytes. *J Biol Chem.* 1995;270:26746-26749.

71. Hu E, Liang P, Spiegelman BM. AdipoQ is a novel adipose-specific gene dysregulated in obesity. *J Biol Chem*. 1996;271:10697-10703.

72. Havel PJ. Control of energy homeostasis and insulin action by adipocyte hormones: leptin, acylation stimulating protein, and adiponectin. *Curr Opin Lipidol*. 2002;13:51-59.

73. Esposito K, Pontillo A, Di Palo C, Giugliano G, Masella M, Marfella R, Giugliano D. Effect of weight loss and lifestyle changes on vascular inflammatory markers in obese women: a randomized trial. *JAMA*. 2003;289:1799-1804.

74. Lindsay RS, Funahashi T, Hanson RL, et al. Adiponectin and development of type 2 diabetes in the Pima Indian population. *Lancet*. 2002;360:57-58.

75. Spranger J, Kroke A, Mohlig M, et al. Adiponectin and protection against type 2 diabetes mellitus. *Lancet*. 2003;361:226-228.

76. Daimon M, Oizumi T, Saitoh T, et al. Decreased serum levels of adiponectin are a risk factor for the progression to type 2 diabetes in the Japanese Population: the Funagata study. *Diabetes Care*. 2003;26:2015-2020.

77. Vozarova B, Stefan N, Lindsay RS, et al. Low plasma adiponectin concentrations do not predict weight gain in humans. *Diabetes*. 2002;51:2964-2967.

78. Kojima M, Hosoda H, Date Y, Nakazato M, Matsuo H, Kangawa K. Ghrelin is a growth-hormone-releasing acylated peptide from stomach. *Nature*. 1999;402:656-660.

79. Cummings DE, Purnell JQ, Frayo RS, Schmidova K, Wisse BE, Weigle DS. A preprandial rise in plasma ghrelin levels suggests a role in meal initiation in humans. *Diabetes*. 2001;50:1714-1719.

80. Tschop M, Smiley DL, Heiman ML. Ghrelin induces adiposity in rodents. *Nature*. 2000;407:908-913.

81. Wren AM, Small CJ, Ward HL, et al. The novel hypothalamic peptide ghrelin stimulates food intake and growth hormone secretion. *Endocrinology*. 2000;141: 4325-4328.

82. Tschop M, Weyer C, Tataranni PA, Devanarayan V, Ravussin E, Heiman ML. Circulating ghrelin levels are decreased in human obesity. *Diabetes*. 2001;50:707-709.

83. Bacha F, Arslanian SA. Ghrelin suppression in overweight children: a manifestation of insulin resistance? *J Clin Endocrinol Metab*. 2005;90:2725-2730.

84. Fagerberg B, Hulten LM, Hulthe J. Plasma ghrelin, body fat, insulin resistance, and smoking in clinically healthy men: the atherosclerosis and insulin resistance study. *Metabolism*. 2003;52:1460-1463.

85. Langenberg C, Bergstrom J, Laughlin GA, Barrett-Connor E. Ghrelin and the metabolic syndrome in older adults. *J Clin Endocrinol Metab*. 2005;90:6448-6453.

86. Cummings DE, Weigle DS, Frayo RS, et al. Plasma ghrelin levels after diet-induced weight loss or gastric bypass surgery. *N Engl J Med*. 2002;23:1623-1630.

87. Bunt JC, Salbe AD, Tschop MH, DelParigi A, Daychild P, Tataranni PA. Cross-sectional and prospective relationships of fasting plasma ghrelin concentrations with anthropometric measures in pima Indian children. *J Clin Endocrinol Metab*. 2003;88:3756-3761.

88. Das UN. Is obesity an inflammatory condition? *Nutrition*. 2001;17:953-966.

89. Han TS, Sattar N, Williams K, Gonzalez-Villalpando C, Lean ME, Haffner SM. Prospective study of C-reactive protein in relation to the development of diabetes and metabolic syndrome in the Mexico City Diabetes Study. *Diabetes Care*. 2002;25: 2016-2021.

90. Pradhan AD, Manson JE, Rifai N, Buring JE, Ridker PM. C-reactive protein, interleukin 6, and risk of developing type 2 diabetes mellitus. *JAMA*. 2001;286:327-334.

91. Spranger J, Kroke A, Mohlig M, et al. Inflammatory cytokines and the risk to develop type 2 diabetes: results of the prospective population-based European Prospective Investigation into Cancer and Nutrition (EPIC)-Potsdam Study. *Diabetes*. 2003;52:812-817.

92. Hu FB, Meigs JB, Li TY, Rifai N, Manson JE. Inflammatory markers and risk of developing type 2 diabetes in women. *Diabetes*. 2004;53:693-700.

93. Willerson JT, Ridker PM. Inflammation as a cardiovascular risk factor. *Circulation.* 2004;109(Suppl 1):II2-II10.

94. Duncan BB, Schmidt MI, Chambless LE, Folsom AR, Carpenter M, Heiss G. Fibrinogen, other putative markers of inflammation, and weight gain in middle-aged adults—the ARIC study. Atherosclerosis Risk in Communities. *Obes Res.* 2000;8:279-286.

95. Duncan BB, Schmidt MI, Chambless LE, Folsom AR, Heiss G, Atherosclerosis Risk in Communities Study Investigators. Inflammation markers predict increased weight gain in smoking quitters. *Obes Res.* 2003;11:1339-1344.

96. Engstrom G, Hedblad B, Stavenow L, Lind P, Janzon L, Lindgarde F. Inflammation-sensitive plasma proteins are associated with future weight gain. *Diabetes.* 2003;52:2097-2101.

97. Engström G, Hedblad B, Janzon L, Lindgärde F. Weight gain in relation to plasma levels of complement factor 3: results from a population-based cohort study. *Diabetologia.* 2005;48(12):2525-2531.

98. Barzilay JI, Forsberg C, Heckbert SR, Cushman M, Newman AB. The association of markers of inflammation with weight change in older adults: the Cardiovascular Health Study. *Int J Obes (London).* 2006;30:1362-1367.

99. Dhurandhar NV. Infectobesity: obesity of infectious origin. *J Nutr.* 2001;131: 2794S-2797S.

100. Dunkelman SS, Fairhurst B, Plager J, Waterhouse C. Cortisol metabolism in obesity. *J Clin Endocrinol Metab.* 1964;24:832-841.

101. Bjorntorp P. Do stress reactions cause abdominal obesity and comorbidities? *Obes Rev.* 2001;2:73-86.

102. Bjorntorp P, Rosmond R. Obesity and cortisol. *Nutrition.* 2000;16:924-936.

103. Wallerius S, Rosmond R, Ljung T, Holm G, Bjorntorp P. Rise in morning saliva cortisol is associated with abdominal obesity in men: a preliminary report. *J Endocrinol Invest.* 2003;26:616-619.

104. Rosmond R, Dallman MF, Bjorntorp P. Stress-related cortisol secretion in men: relationships with abdominal obesity and endocrine, metabolic and hemodynamic abnormalities. *J Clin Endocrinol Metab.* 1998;83:1853-1859.

19

Developmental Origins of Obesity

Matthew W. Gillman

Obesity Prevention Must Start Early

The obesity epidemic is in full swing in upper- and middle-income countries, and it is emerging through the epidemiologic transition in many developing countries. One of its most remarkable features is that the epidemic has not spared even very young children. Among preschool age children and even among infants, the prevalence of obesity has dramatically increased over the past few decades (Fig. 19.1).[1,2]

While obesity in young children does not predict adult consequences as well as obesity in later childhood does,[3] it nevertheless carries morbidity. Excess weight in children can cause type 2 diabetes mellitus,[4-6] hypertension and hyperlipidemia,[7,8] sleep apnea,[9] early maturation,[10] and psychosocial stress, and is associated with the risk of asthma, the only childhood chronic disease that rivals obesity in prevalence, morbidity, and cost.[11-14]

Once present, obesity is hard to treat, not only because of entrenched behaviors, but also because of evolutionarily conserved thrifty physiology, that is, physiologic mechanisms tend to resist weight loss.[15,16]

For these reasons it is critical to begin preventive efforts as early in human development as possible—even before birth. This chapter focuses therefore on pre- and perinatal factors that determine obesity and its consequences later on in life.

Measurement of Obesity in Young Children Is Tricky

As many studies of pre- and perinatal origins of obesity employ outcomes during childhood, it is important to consider relevant measures of adiposity. From the age of 2 years, the U.S. Centers for Disease Control and Prevention (CDC) and other authoritative organizations recommend using body mass index (BMI, kg/m^2) as the standard measure of adiposity for clinical and public health purposes. As noted in Chapter 5, BMI has the advantage of being relatively easily measured, as long as one obtains accurate measures of height, and the CDC has widely disseminated growth charts using the BMI. In the United States, the recommended ranges for overweight (formerly called *at-risk for overweight*) and obesity (formerly called *overweight*) are age- and sex-specific 85th to 95th percentile and >95th percentile, respectively (also see Chapter 20). The reference population for these percentile calculations is based on nationally representative surveys from primarily

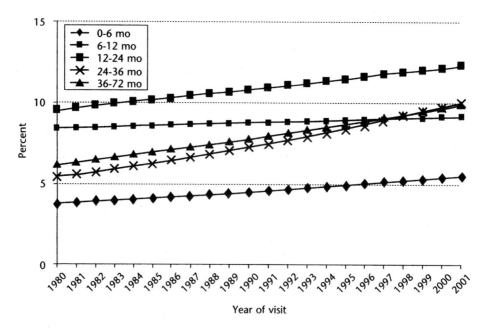

Figure 19.1 Age-specific predicted prevalence of overweight from 1980 to 2001 among 120,680 children 0 to 71.9 months seen at 366,109 well-child care visits at a Massachusetts HMO, according to age group. Reproduced with permission from Kim J, Peterson KE, Scanlon KS, et al. Trends in overweight from 1980 through 2001 among preschool-aged children enrolled in a health maintenance organization. *Obesity (Silver Spring)*. 2006;14:1107-1112.[1]

the 1970s, when the population was much thinner as a whole. Many other countries use growth curves promulgated by the International Obesity Task Force (IOTF).[17]

Instead of using percentiles, the IOTF defines overweight and obesity by age/sex-specific cutpoints that predict the adult cutpoints of 25 and 30 kg/m², respectively. In adolescence, the CDC curves tend to overestimate these adult ranges, so the IOTF standards have advantages. But for young children, the CDC growth curves are adequate. In the future, researchers and clinicians may be using newer WHO charts based on breast-fed infants.[18-21]

For children 0 to 2 years of age, the definitions of overweight and obesity are based on CDC's weight-for-length standards rather than BMI. The major difference is that length is not squared. Similar to the standards for older children, the definitions are based on the 85th and 95th percentile cutpoints. But the definitions are less certain. One reason is that fewer nationally representative data exist to create the reference population. Another is that fewer data exist on the complications of excess weight at these ages.

Further, errors in length measurement in clinical practice are common and nefarious. In a validation study of 160 children aged 0 to 23 months in a primary care practice, Rifas-Shiman et al.[22] showed that clinical length measures overestimate research-standard measures by a reliably predictable amount, an average of over 1 cm across this age range (Fig. 19.2).

This overestimation of length results in weight-for-length measures that wildly underestimate obesity prevalence and actually make typical U.S. populations appear to be in the grip of famine. Thus, clinicians currently under-detect overweight among their very young patients; clinical practices ought to adopt accurate measurement equipment and technique. Researchers using clinical databases to estimate length, and thus weight-for-length,

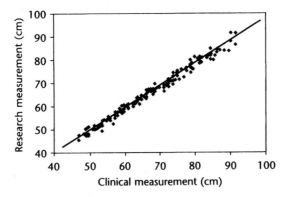

Figure 19.2 Relationship between clinical and research measurements of length among 160 children aged 0 to 23 months. Research measurement = clinical measurement × 0.953 + 1.88 cm. Reproduced with permission from Rifas-Shiman SL, Rich-Edwards JW, Scanlon KS, Kleinman KP, Gillman MW. Misdiagnosis of overweight and underweight children younger than 2 years of age due to length measurement bias. *Medscape General Med.* 2005;7:55.[22]

must be aware of this limitation, and could consider using the regression equation from that study (see Fig. 19.2) to correct length measurements.

The situation in 2- to 3-year-olds is even more confusing. Depending on how well the child can stand, clinicians may measure recumbent length or standing height. Even with research-standard measurement, standing height is about 0.5 to 0.75 cm lower than recumbent length.[23,24] Thus researchers need to know which type of measure applies to an individual, and use the appropriate CDC chart—weight-for-length for 0- to 36-month olds, or BMI (assumes standing height) for 24 months or older.

One of the implications of this discussion is that researchers should directly measure length/height with state-of-the-art technique whenever possible. Even if one can measure length or height accurately, however, both BMI and weight-for-length have the inherent limitation of not measuring body composition directly. While BMI > 95th percentile appears to be a highly valid measure of excess adiposity, the further one gets from that extreme category, the lower the correlation between a weight-for-length measure and fatness.[25]

In a research setting, direct measures of body composition are feasible starting at birth. These include dual-energy x-ray absorptiometry (DXA)[26-28] and the PEAPOD, which uses plethysmographic technique.[29,30] Both DXA and PEAPOD measure total body fat. DXA can also estimate regional fat as well as lean body mass and bone density and content, but it is more expensive. Skinfold thicknesses are a much cheaper alternative, but require strict attention to technique and thus highly skilled training, and they are limited to a relatively small number of measurement sites. Bioimpedance techniques are not reliable in very young children because of divergence from assumptions that underlie the equations to determine fat mass.[31,32]

Whether to use weight/length/height measures or a more direct measure of adiposity in any research study rests not only on feasibility but also purpose. Many current studies of early origins of obesity are limited to simple anthropometric indices, and they contribute substantially to the literature. As reviewed in the remainder of the chapter, however, many questions remain about observed associations of pre- and perinatal factors with later adiposity or obesity, and for these, direct measures of body composition or, indeed, the physiologic/metabolic concomitants of excess adiposity, can be quite helpful.

Lifecourse Approach to Chronic Disease and DOHaD Are Converging Concepts

Two recent paradigms offer useful conceptual frameworks. One, termed the life course approach to chronic disease,[33] invokes two axes. The first is time. Factors may act in the preconceptional through the prenatal period, into infancy, childhood, and beyond to determine risk of chronic disease. The other axis is hierarchical: these factors can range from the social/built/natural environment (macro) through behavior, physiology, and genetics (micro). Factors interact with each other over the life course, with different determinants being more or less important at different life stages.

Under this paradigm, some factors may be more deterministic than others. *Programming* refers to perturbations at critical or sensitive periods of developmental processes that have lifelong, sometimes irreversible consequences. An example from a well-characterized rat model is that a low-protein maternal diet consumed *only* during the few-day embryonic period can cause lifelong hypertension in the offspring.[34] The mechanism underlying this finding appears to involve reduced activity of the placental enzyme that normally protects the fetus from excess exposure to glucocorticoids, which are stress hormones. Other factors may contribute to chronic disease through accumulation of risk. For example, chronic exposure to elevated lipid levels is associated with preatherosclerotic coronary lesions among adolescents.[35]

A second, related, paradigm is called developmental origins of health and disease (DOHaD, formerly fetal origins of adult disease). On the basis of similar principles, DOHaD focuses primarily on the prenatal period and infancy as determinants of long-term health.[36]

Both of these frameworks highlight the primacy of the period of developmental plasticity for determining lifelong trajectories of health. The plastic period is somewhat different for different organs and systems, but is generally complete by birth or the first years of life.[36] Under this perspective, factors that occur later in life, for example, adult risk factors, modify these trajectories. One theory to explain the salience of these interactions relies on the concept of predictive adaptive responses. In brief, under this theory, developmental processes program the organism to "expect" a certain environment through the lifecourse. When the environment in childhood and adulthood matches expectations, disease risk is low. When there is a mismatch, adverse health outcomes occur. While empirical testing of this theory has only begun, the fact that the highest risk of cardiometabolic outcomes occurs among individuals with the combination of lower birth weight and higher BMI later in life—mediated through accelerated weight gain during childhood—provides epidemiologic support.[37-43]

This particular pattern has been termed *thrifty phenotype*, a subset of predictive adaptive responses.[44] Animal models of energy deprivation during pregnancy followed by energy excess in the offspring clearly demonstrate that such patterns are the result of changes in the fetal environment, that is, not due to variation in the fetal genome.[45-47]

Observational Designs to Study DOHaD

Animal experiments provide compelling data that early developmental cues influence lifelong health.[48] Long-term effects on body composition, hypertension, and cardiometabolic outcomes are relatively easy to induce by interventions ranging from nutritional—typically protein or energy restriction—to administration of hormones such as glucocorticoids, mechanical disruption such as uterine artery ligation, and inducing anemia or hypoxia.[36] While these experiments constitute proof of principle, translation to the human condition is not straightforward. First, obtaining physiologic data from the maternal-placental-fetal unit is most often indirect. Second, the majority of animal interventions are infeasible or too extreme for humans. Thus, clinical- and population-based researchers need to make judicious inferences from well-designed epidemiologic studies.

The first generation of epidemiologic studies were historical. They took advantage of serendipitously available administrative or recalled data on birth size. Barker et al.[49] were among the first and most prolific to recognize that birth weight is associated with cardiovascular disease and its risk factors many decades later. Birth weight was the main entry point into DOHaD research. But it is not an etiologic factor itself, and so cannot lead the field toward understanding of mechanism or public health implication. For example, both lower and higher birth weight are associated with later adiposity-related outcomes, probably representing different underlying pathways.[50] DOHaD researchers now recognize that birth weight, or even its components, fetal growth and length of gestation, is a proxy for many determinants of lifelong health, and it is crucial to identify and quantify these determinants themselves.[51] Thus, other types of studies with data on potentially etiologic pre- and postnatal factors are required.

A second type of study "resurrects" cohort studies of pregnant women and their children that were begun decades ago. In the United States, good examples are the National Collaborative Perinatal Project (NCPP) and Child Health and Development Study, both cohort studies with prenatal recruitment in the 1950s-1960s and initial follow-up until school age. Several investigators have now recontacted and followed up subcohorts in adulthood, and publications on obesity as well as other health outcomes are beginning to appear.[52-57] This type of study has the advantages of research-quality data collection during pregnancy and early childhood, but it can lack key data elements in which researchers are now interested. For example, the NCPP collected no maternal dietary data, and blood samples were stored at –20°C, not the current –80°C or lower.

A third type of epidemiologic study is creating new "prebirth" cohorts of pregnant women and their children. These have the advantage of collecting more modern data, especially the opportunity to collect and store biosamples. But one has to wait a long time for hard clinical outcomes—typically longer than the initial investigator's life! Fortunately, obesity and its cardiometabolic sequelae have a relatively large number of accepted surrogate outcomes in childhood. In the United States, the National Children's Study, currently in its "gestational" stage, offers an example of such a design on a large scale.[58]

Investigators Are Beginning to Identify Modifiable Developmental Determinants

Prenatal Determinants: Maternal Smoking during Pregnancy, Gestational Weight Gain, Gestational Diabetes

Because severe protein or energy restriction in pregnant animal species reproducibly causes adverse offspring outcomes, maternal "undernutrition" is a useful construct for experimental physiologists. But it has no direct human counterpart. A more helpful concept is *fetal nutrition*, that is, the entire supply line of nutrients, oxygen, hormones, and so on to the growing embryo and fetus. Under this concept, one considers not only maternal diet, but also other maternal behaviors. Moreover, both downstream influences such as

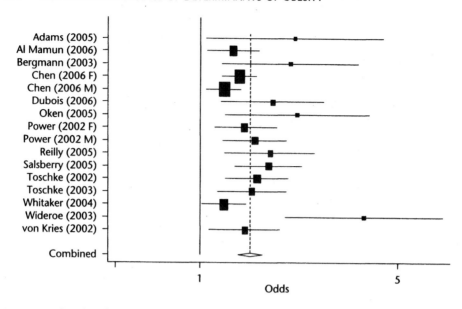

Figure 19.3 Results of meta-analysis of maternal smoking during pregnancy and child overweight. The pooled adjusted odds ratio was 1.50 (95% CI: 1.36 to 1.65). Reproduced with permission from Oken E, Levitan EB, Gillman MW. Maternal smoking during pregnancy and child overweight: systematic review and meta-analysis. *Int J Obes.* Advance online publication, 27 November 2007;doi:10.1038/sj.ijo.0803760.[59]

uteroplacental blood flow and placental and fetal metabolism, and upstream influences, such as maternal preconceptional health and even mother's own intrauterine and early life experiences, come to the fore.

Using this conceptual basis, researchers have begun to investigate modifiable prenatal determinants of offspring obesity and its consequences. Maternal smoking during pregnancy is one example. While maternal smoking causes reduced fetal growth, more than a dozen studies now confirm that it is associated with offspring obesity. In a meta-analysis of 14 studies, Oken et al.[59] estimated that maternal smoking during pregnancy conferred an increased odds of 50% (adjusted odds ratio 1.50 [95% CI: 1.36 to 1.65]) for offspring obesity defined by BMI cutpoints, across an age range of 3 to 33 years (Fig. 19.3). Adjustment for factors related to social and economic position did not markedly affect estimates, but residual confounding is still possible. Animal studies of this phenomenon are few; one in rats indicates that nicotine administration in the puerperium leads to higher weight through early adulthood.[60]

If this relationship is causal, the public health implications could be large in developing countries in which maternal smoking is rising with the obesity epidemic. The small fetus, obese child phenotype of maternal smoking is not only characteristic of the epidemiologic transition from acute to chronic disease,[61] but also confers the highest risk for cardiometabolic health outcomes.[37-42]

Another example is gestational weight gain. As summarized in a recent workshop report from the U.S. National Academy of Sciences,[62] more mothers are entering pregnancy overweight or obese than ever before, and excessive weight gain during pregnancy is also probably more frequent than in earlier decades. In Project Viva, a Boston-area *prebirth* cohort study, Oken et al.[63] showed that excessive gestational weight gain, as defined by the 1990 Institute of Medicine guidelines,[64] was associated with higher BMI

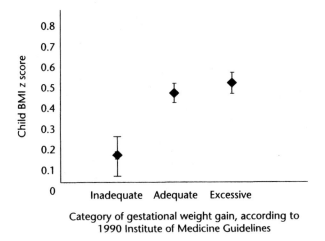

Figure 19.4 Adjusted mean child BMI z-score (95% CI) at age 3 years, according to the maternal gestational weight gain category recommended by the Institute of Medicine.[64] Data from Project Viva. Reproduced with permission from Oken E, Taveras EM, Kleinman K, Rich-Edwards JW, Gillman MW. Gestational weight gain and child adiposity at age 3 years. *Am J Obstet Gynecol.* 2007;196:322e8.[63]

and risk of obesity in the offspring at the age of 3 years (Fig. 19.4). Remarkably little is known about the determinants of gestational weight gain, although wide fluctuations over the past few decades provide hope of modifiability. In the current era of epidemic obesity, more evidence on optimal weight gain during pregnancy is urgently needed, so that new recommendations can be formulated.

Higher maternal BMI at the start of pregnancy is a strong risk factor for many adverse outcomes, including offspring obesity.[65] I do not review it in this chapter, because it is not modifiable once pregnancy begins. Nevertheless, ensuring optimal BMI at the start of pregnancy is one of the most important goals for intergenerational prevention of obesity.

One major outcome of maternal prepregnancy obesity is gestational diabetes (GDM). GDM is associated with higher fetal growth, and thus birth weight, and many studies now show that birth weight is directly related to later BMI.[66-68] Thus it makes sense to investigate GDM as a determinant of offspring obesity. Animal studies of induced GDM suggest that this relationship holds, as do epidemiologic studies—including the methodologically strong within-family (sib-pair) approach—in areas of high GDM prevalence (Fig. 19.5).[69,70]

Some other studies, however, in more general population samples, are equivocal.[66,71] It is important to quantify these relationships: given the anticipated rise in obesity and diabetes around the world,[72] the obesity-GDM-offspring obesity intergenerational vicious cycle could contribute to the spiraling of the obesity epidemic.

In addition, many challenges remain in studying causes and consequences of GDM. While physical activity both before and during pregnancy appears to be protective,[73-75] only dietary factors before—but not during—pregnancy seem to play a preventive role.[76-78] In addition, studies of body composition and cardiometabolic outcomes in childhood and adulthood, not just BMI, are important to understand more fully the intergenerational consequences of GDM.

Maternal dietary intakes during pregnancy represent another potential determinant of offspring obesity. Perhaps surprisingly, the literature reveals no consistent findings. Part

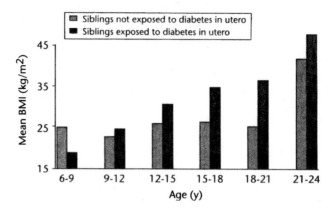

Figure 19.5 Higher mean BMI among siblings exposed versus not exposed to diabetic intrauterine environment. Data from Pima Indians. Reproduced with permission from Dabelea D, Hanson RL, Lindsay RS, et al. Intrauterine exposure to diabetes conveys risks for type 2 diabetes and obesity: a study of discordant sibships. *Diabetes*. 2000;49:2208–2211.[70]

of the issue is methodological; the combination of accurate dietary data collected during pregnancy and offspring follow-up long enough to detect salient outcomes is scarce. Current research focuses on the role of both micronutrients (e.g., vitamin D), macronutrient quantity and quality (e.g., glycemic load), and dietary patterns. Novel work in a mouse model indicates that maternal diet around the time of conception that is replete with methyl donors can lower the risk of offspring obesity and diabetes through epigenetic mechanisms.[79] But analogous studies in humans are yet to surface because of the need for longitudinal studies with accurate periconceptional diet, biomarker, and outcome data, as well as difficulties surrounding tissue and species specificity.

Postnatal Determinants: Infant Weight Gain, Feeding, Sleep

Life *after* birth also counts! In the first year of life, at least three factors play a role in determining later obesity. The first is infant growth. It is critical to distinguish linear growth from weight gain. Further, weight gain accompanies linear growth; weight gain in excess of linear growth is thus more interesting than weight gain alone. As noted earlier in the section "Measurement of Obesity in Young Children Is Tricky," obtaining accurate length measures is crucial. Most studies to date do not have accurate lengths, and therefore resort to examining weight gain alone. Future studies would benefit from having longitudinal measures of body composition in addition to accurate weights and lengths.

Two meta-analyses now show that accelerated weight gain during the first weeks or months of life is associated with higher BMI or obesity later in life.[80,81] For example, Baird et al.[80] reviewed 10 studies that assessed the relation of infant growth with subsequent obesity. Compared with other infants, among infants with more rapid growth odds ratios and relative risks of later obesity ranged from 1.17 to 5.70. Associations were consistent for obesity at different ages and for people born over a period from 1927 to 1994.

One study of formula-fed infants suggests that weight gain even in the first week of life predicts obesity at age 20 to 32 years.[82] After adjustment for confounding factors, each 100 g increase in weight gain during the first week of life was associated with a 28% increased odds of adult overweight (OR, 1.28; 95% CI: 1.08 to 1.52). Follow-up of infants, either premature or small for gestational age, who had experienced higher rates of weight gain in early infancy from being allocated higher-energy infant formula, showed higher BMI, blood pressure, insulin, and leptin levels in later childhood or adolescence.[83,84] In one of the few studies employing accurate length measures, Belfort et al.[85] showed that gain in weight-for-length from birth to 6 months was associated with higher systolic blood pressure among 3-year-old participants in Project Viva.

Despite the seeming consistency of these studies, one must also be aware of counter examples. Among Finnish men, those who eventually developed coronary heart disease, compared with the cohort as a whole, appeared to have experienced declining height, weight, and BMI during the first year of life before increasing dramatically after the age of 2 years.[43] Indian men and women who developed impaired glucose tolerance or type 2 diabetes in young adulthood appeared to follow the same pattern.[42] Disentangling these discrepancies in the role of infant weight (and fat) gain during infancy is critical. Clinicians and parents will be paying close attention.

One determinant of infant weight gain is infant feeding. Having been breast-fed at all, or for a longer duration, may lower risk for subsequent obesity. A meta-analysis of duration of breast-feeding estimated a 4% decreased odds for each additional month of breast-feeding.[86] Two meta-analyses of breast versus bottle feeding showed a 13% to 22% reduction in odds of later obesity.[87,88] However, the two largest U.S. studies with racial/ethnic information indicated that effects were limited to whites.[89,90] One potential explanation is different breast-feeding traditions in different cultural groups, for example, topping off nursing with a bottle, but evidence is lacking. Also, one additional meta-analysis that employed individual-level data, rather than combining published group results, did not show a protective effect of having been breast-fed on mean BMI as a continuous variable.[91] What could explain this finding of no association? One reason could be different outcomes. The studies with dichotomous outcomes appear to show an effect, while the ones with mean BMI do not. Effects at the extreme of the BMI distribution could be larger than those at the mean. An alternative explanation could be better adjustment for social and economic confounding factors in the individual-level meta-analysis. However, in the Growing Up Today Study, Gillman et al.[92] found similar odds ratios for a within-family and an overall cohort analysis of breast-feeding duration, suggesting that residual socioeconomic confounding did not play a major role. In addition, some recent studies have taken into account a range of potentially confounding variables, and still confirm an association.[93] Further follow-up of children in a large randomized trial of breast-feeding promotion in the Republic of Belarus will likely inform this issue.[94]

A third factor during infancy is sleep duration, the bane of many new parents' existence. As reviewed elsewhere in this book (Chapter 16), lack of sleep among adults is associated with excess weight gain and development of obesity. Although the data are still few, the same relationship appears to exist in early childhood. For example, in the Project Viva cohort, Taveras et al.[95] showed that infant sleep of less than 12 hours/day was associated with an odds ratio of 2.04 (95% CI: 1.07 to 3.91) for overweight at age 3 years. Sleep quality and possibly duration appear modifiable in infancy.[96-98]

Combination of Pre- and Postnatal Factors

The life course approach to chronic disease[33] reminds us that combinations of factors at different life stages entrain trajectories toward different health states. Thus, it is important to consider combinations of developmental determinants of obesity that occur before and after birth. Using data from Project Viva, Gillman et al.[99] recently examined predicted probabilities of obesity at age 3 years according to covariate-adjusted levels of four potentially modifiable risk factors. These factors were maternal smoking during pregnancy, gestational weight gain, breast-feeding duration, infant weight gain from birth to 6 months, and infant sleep. Given optimal levels of all four factors, the predicted probability of obesity was 6%, whereas the predicted probability associated with adverse levels of all four was 29%. This wide range of predicted probabilities suggests that interventions to modify these factors during pregnancy and infancy could have a substantial impact on reducing childhood obesity rates.

Applying newer analytic methods may help in disentangling complex pathways. Analyses involving growth in particular are challenging because, for example, weight gain in one period of life typically entrains weight gain in the next. Isolating one or more critical periods of weight gain is difficult,[100] as is combining growth with other parameters in one analysis. De Stavola[101] suggests use of structural equation modeling, a promising but unproven technique for these issues. In addition, for growth analyses, newer studies with serial prenatal ultrasound measurements will allow more direct measures of prenatal growth parameters than merely measuring anthropometry at birth.

Clinical and Public Health Implications, and Future Directions

While much more work is needed on identifying and quantifying pre- and perinatal determinants of obesity and its consequences, some implications are already clear. The first is that intervening to change birth weight is likely to be ineffectual, if not harmful. Birth weight is a proxy for many determinants, not an etiologic factor itself. Efforts should focus on the etiologic factors themselves, as reviewed in this chapter, each of which may or may not affect birth weight.

While having gone down in recent decades in the developed world, rates of maternal smoking during pregnancy are probably rising in developing countries, owing to clever marketing practices by tobacco companies.[102-106] The combination of policy, environmental, and individual behavior change strategies that have been successful in the United States to reduce rates of smoking may be more difficult to plan and implement in other parts of the world.[107-110] Nevertheless, preventing smoking among girls and women of reproductive age is a health priority worldwide, only one reason of which is to potentially prevent offspring obesity.

Prevention of GDM is also a priority. GDM causes many perinatal complications as well as offspring obesity.[66,71] The most important prevention measure is the least attainable at present: to ensure that women enter pregnancy at a normal BMI. However, promotion of light-to-moderate physical activity during pregnancy appears to be a promising strategy.[73]

It is not known whether treatment of GDM will reduce risk of offspring obesity. Following up children whose mothers participated in successful short-term trials of GDM treatment[111] represents a robust study design to answer this question as well as to solidify the causal link between GDM and offspring obesity.

Modifying gestational weight gain appears to be an attractive public health goal at this time. But some caution is warranted, as too little weight gain is associated with reduced fetal growth and neonatal morbidity.[64] Before revising recommendations for women, the National Academy of Sciences and other authoritative groups need more data on the balance of short- and long-term risks and benefits of various amounts of gestational weight gain in general, and according to groups defined by prepregnancy BMI. In addition, the best strategies to modify gestational weight gain are unknown, as its determinants are yet to be clarified. Fortunately, pregnancy appears to be one period of a woman's life during which behavior change may be readily achievable.[112]

Breast-feeding initiation and maintenance benefit many health outcomes in children, including atopy and gastrointestinal illness.[94] While confounding is still an issue, the best evidence to date suggests that having been breast-fed also lowers the risk of later obesity; no studies suggest harm. Therefore, it is reasonable for clinicians and public health officials to include obesity prevention as one of the benefits in programs to increase breast-feeding rates. Breast-feeding behavior is surely modifiable, as both initiation and maintenance rates have increased in the United States substantially in the past 30 to 40 years.[113]

Not enough is known yet about infant weight gain or sleep duration to include them in clinical or public health programs to prevent childhood obesity. Over and above the effects of infant feeding, determinants of infant weight gain that are related to later obesity are obscure. Therefore, it is not known whether (or how) moderating infant weight gain will lower obesity rates later in childhood or adulthood. Further, at least among premature infants, weight gain that is too low is associated with adverse neuropsychological outcomes.[114,115] Therefore, more information is needed about optimal levels of infant weight gain, as well as its modifiability, before anyone should make clinical recommendations.

Similarly, recommendations about sleep duration for obesity prevention are premature. More data are required about the underlying association, its mechanisms, and potential determinants. In the meantime, however, clinicians and parents may wish to employ evidence-based sleep hygiene techniques to improve sleep quality and perhaps increase sleep duration.[116-118]

Future research should take advantage of longitudinal study designs to explore new pre- and perinatal determinants and pathways leading to offspring adiposity and its consequences. For example, analogous to animal models, Gillman et al.[119] reported that maternal second trimester levels of corticotrophin-releasing hormone, a proxy for fetal glucocorticoid exposure, was associated with lower BMI but higher ratio of subscapular:triceps skinfold ratio, a measure of central adiposity, among 3-year-old children. This result raises the possibility that maternal stress, irrespective of any lifestyle behavior choice, may program offspring metabolic dysfunction.

In addition, more refined measurement techniques and new analytic methods, as discussed in this chapter, will provide more insight into underlying pathways. Through these approaches, researchers are becoming more and more likely to find modifiable etiologic factors that lend themselves to judicious clinical and public health interventions. Ultimately, the hope is that interventions during pregnancy and early childhood that are developmentally appropriate, and that employ strategies to change both environmental and behavioral factors, will go a long way toward preventing obesity and its consequences throughout the life course.

References

1. Kim J, Peterson KE, Scanlon KS, et al. Trends in overweight from 1980 through 2001 among preschool-aged children enrolled in a health maintenance organization. *Obesity (Silver Spring)*. 2006;14:1107-1112.
2. Ogden CL, Carroll MD, Curtin LR, McDowell MA, Tabak CJ, Flegal KM. Prevalence of overweight and obesity in the United States, 1999-2004. *JAMA*. 2006;295:1549-1555.
3. Whitaker RC, Wright JA, Pepe MS, Seidel KD, Dietz WH Jr. Predicting obesity in young adulthood from childhood and parental obesity. *N Engl J Med*. 1997;337:869-873.
4. Liese AD, D'Agostino RB Jr, Hamman RF, et al. The burden of diabetes mellitus among US youth: prevalence estimates from the SEARCH for Diabetes in Youth Study. *Pediatrics*. 2006;118:1510-1518.

5. Haines L, Wan KC, Lynn R, Barrett TG, Shield JP. Rising incidence of type 2 diabetes in children in the United Kingdom. *Diabetes Care.* 2007;Epub ahead of print.
6. Molnar D. The prevalence of the metabolic syndrome and type 2 diabetes mellitus in children and adolescents. *Int J Obes Relat Metab Disord.* 2004;28 (Suppl 3):S70-S74.
7. Freedman DS, Serdula MK, Srinivasan SR, Berenson GS. Relation of circumferences and skinfold thicknesses to lipid and insulin concentrations in children and adolescents: the Bogalusa Heart Study. *Am J Clin Nutr.* 1999;69:308-317.
8. Morrison JA, Sprecher DL, Barton BA, Waclawiw MA, Daniels SR. Overweight, fat patterning, and cardiovascular disease risk factors in black and white girls: the National Heart, Lung, and Blood Institute Growth and Health Study. *J Pediatr.* 1999;135:458-464.
9. Daniels SR. The consequences of childhood overweight and obesity. *Future Child.* 2006;16:47-67.
10. Lee JM, Appugliese D, Kaciroti N, Corwyn RF, Bradley RH, Lumeng JC. Weight status in young girls and the onset of puberty. *Pediatrics.* 2007;119:E624-E630.
11. Gold DR, Damokosh AI, Dockery DW, Berkey CS. Body-mass index as a predictor of incident asthma in a prospective cohort of children. *Pediatr Pulmonol.* 2003;36:514-521.
12. Akinbami L. The state of childhood asthma, United States, 1980-2005. Advance data from vital and health statistics (381). 12-12-2006. Hyattsville, MD: National Center for Health Statistics.
13. Lozano P, Sullivan SD, Smith DH, Weiss KB. The economic burden of asthma in US children: estimates from the National Medical Expenditure Survey. *J Allergy Clin Immunol.* 1999;104:957-963.
14. Wang G, Dietz WH. Economic burden of obesity in youths aged 6 to 17 years: 1979-1999. *Pediatrics.* 2002;109:e81.
15. Rosenbaum M, Leibel RL. The physiology of body weight regulation: relevance to the etiology of obesity in children. *Pediatrics.* 1998;101:525-539.
16. Rosenbaum M, Goldsmith R, Bloomfield D, et al. Low-dose leptin reverses skeletal muscle, autonomic, and neuroendocrine adaptations to maintenance of reduced weight. *J Clin Invest.* 2005;115:3579-3586.
17. Cole TJ, Bellizzi MC, Flegal KM, Dietz WH. Establishing a standard definition for child overweight and obesity worldwide: international survey. *BMJ.* 2000;320:1240-1243.
18. World Health Organization. New Growth Charts. Available at: http://www.who.int/nutrition/media_page/en/index.html. 2007. Accessed October 9, 2007.
19. de Onis M, Onyango AW. The Centers for Disease Control and Prevention 2000 growth charts and the growth of breastfed infants. *Acta Paediatr.* 2003;92:413-419.
20. Wright CM. Growth charts for babies. *BMJ.* 2005;330:1399-1400.
21. de Onis M, Garza C, Onyango AW, Borghi E. Comparison of the WHO child growth standards and the CDC 2000 growth charts. *J Nutr.* 2007;137:144-148.
22. Rifas-Shiman SL, Rich-Edwards JW, Scanlon KS, Kleinman KP, Gillman MW. Misdiagnosis of overweight and underweight children younger than 2 years of age due to length measurement bias. *Medscape General Med.* 2005;7:55.
23. WHO. Child Growth Standards based on length/height, weight and age. *Acta Paediatr.* Suppl 2006;450:85.
24. Buyken AE, Hahn S, Kroke A. Differences between recumbent length and stature measurement in groups of 2- and 3-y-old children and its relevance for the use of European body mass index references. *Int J Obes (London).* 2005;29:24-28.
25. Daniels SR, Khoury PR, Morrison JA. The utility of body mass index as a measure of body fatness in children and adolescents: differences by race and gender. *Pediatrics.* 1997;99:804-807.
26. Goran MI. Measurement issues related to studies of childhood obesity: assessment of body composition, body fat distribution, physical activity, and food intake. *Pediatrics.* 1998;101:505-518.

27. Eisenmann JC, Heelan KA, Welk GJ. Assessing body composition among 3- to 8-year-old children: anthropometry, BIA, and DXA. *Obes Res.* 2004;12:1633-1640.

28. Fors H, Gelander L, Bjarnason R, Albertsson-Wikland K, Bosaeus I. Body composition, as assessed by bioelectrical impedance spectroscopy and dual-energy x-ray absorptiometry, in a healthy paediatric population. *Acta Paediatr.* 2002;91:755-760.

29. Ellis KJ, Yao M, Shypailo RJ, Urlando A, Wong WW, Heird WC. Body-composition assessment in infancy: air-displacement plethysmography compared with a reference 4-compartment model. *Am J Clin Nutr.* 2007;85:90-95.

30. Ma G, Yao M, Liu Y, et al. Validation of a new pediatric air-displacement plethysmograph for assessing body composition in infants. *Am J Clin Nutr.* 2004;79:653-660.

31. Dung NQ, Fusch G, Armbrust S, Jochum F, Fusch C. Body composition of preterm infants measured during the first months of life: bioelectrical impedance provides insignificant additional information compared to anthropometry alone. *Eur J Pediatr.* 2007;166:215-222.

32. Mast M, Sonnichsen A, Langnase K, et al. Inconsistencies in bioelectrical impedance and anthropometric measurements of fat mass in a field study of prepubertal children. *Br J Nutr.* 2002;87:163-175.

33. Kuh D, Ben-Shlomo Y. *A Life Course Approach to Chronic Disease Epidemiology: Tracing the Origins of Ill-Health from Early to Adult Life.* 2nd ed. London: Oxford University Press; 2004.

34. Kwong WY, Wild AE, Roberts P, Willis AC, Fleming TP. Maternal undernutrition during the preimplantation period of rat development causes blastocyst abnormalities and programming of postnatal hypertension. *Development.* 2000;127:4195-4202.

35. PDAY Research Group. Relationship of atherosclerosis in young men to serum lipoprotein cholesterol concentrations and smoking. A preliminary report from the Pathobiological Determinants of Atherosclerosis in Youth (PDAY) Research Group. *JAMA.* 1990;264:3018-3024.

36. Gluckman P, Hanson M. *Developmental Origins of Health and Disease.* New York: Cambridge University Press; 2006.

37. Bavdekar A, Yajnik CS, Fall CHD, et al. The insulin resistance syndrome in eight-year-old Indian children; small at birth, big at eight years or both? *Diabetes.* 1999;48:2422-2429.

38. Adair LS, Cole TJ. Rapid child growth raises blood pressure in adolescent boys who were thin at birth. *Hypertension.* 2003;41:451-456.

39. Valdez R, Mitchell BD, Haffner SM, et al. Predictors of weight change in a bi-ethnic population. The San Antonio Heart Study. *Int J Obes Relat Metab Disord.* 1994;18:85-91.

40. Frankel S, Elwood P, Sweetnam P, Yarnell J, Davey-Smith G. Birthweight, body-mass index in middle age, and incident coronary heart disease. *Lancet.* 1996;348:1478-1480.

41. Rich-Edwards JW, Kleinman K, Michels KB, et al. Longitudinal study of birth weight and adult body mass index in predicting risk of coronary heart disease and stroke in women. *BMJ.* 2005;330:1115.

42. Bhargava SK, Sachdev HS, Fall CH, et al. Relation of serial changes in childhood body-mass index to impaired glucose tolerance in young adulthood. *N Engl J Med.* 2004;350:865-875.

43. Barker DJP, Osmond C, Forsen TJ, Kajantie E, Eriksson JG. Trajectories of growth among children who later have coronary events. *N Engl J Med.* 2005;353:1802-1809.

44. Hales CN, Barker DJP. Type 2 (non-insulin-depedent) diabetes mellitus: the thrifty phenotype hypothesis. *Diabetologia.* 1992;35:595-601.

45. Ikenasio-Thorpe BA, Breier BH, Vickers MH, Fraser M. Prenatal influences on susceptibility to diet-induced obesity are mediated by altered neuroendocrine gene expression. *J Endocrinol.* 2007;193:31-37.

46. Vickers MH, Breier BH, McCarthy D, Gluckman PD. Sedentary behavior during postnatal life is determined by the prenatal environment and exacerbated by postnatal hypercaloric nutrition. *Am J Physiol Regul Integr Comp Physiol.* 2003;285:R271-R273.

47. Vickers MH, Gluckman PD, Coveny AH, et al. Neonatal leptin treatment reverses developmental programming. *Endocrinology.* 2005;146:4211-4216.
48. McMillen IC, Robinson JS. Developmental origins of the metabolic syndrome: prediction, plasticity, and programming. *Physiol Rev.* 2005;85:571-633.
49. Barker DJP. *Mothers, Babies, and Disease in Later Life.* London: Harcourt Brace & Co., Limited; 1998.
50. Oken E, Gillman MW. Fetal origins of obesity. *Obes Res.* 2003;11:496-506.
51. Gillman MW. Developmental origins of health and disease. *N Engl J Med.* 2005;353:1848-1850.
52. Stettler N, Kumanyika SK, Katz SH, Zemel BS, Stallings VA. Rapid weight gain during infancy and obesity in young adulthood in a cohort of African Americans. *Am J Clin Nutr.* 2003;77:1374-1378.
53. Monuteaux MC, Blacker D, Biederman J, Fitzmaurice G, Buka SL. Maternal smoking during pregnancy and offspring overt and covert conduct problems: a longitudinal study. *J Child Psychol Psychiatr.* 2006;47:883-890.
54. Martin LT, Fitzmaurice GM, Kindlon DJ, Buka SL. Cognitive performance in childhood and early adult illness: a prospective cohort study. *J Epidemiol Community Health.* 2004;58:674-679.
55. Buka SL, Shenassa ED, Niaura R. Elevated risk of tobacco dependence among offspring of mothers who smoke during pregnancy: a 30-year prospective study. *Am J Psychiatr.* 2003;160:1978-1984.
56. Susser ES, Schaefer CA, Brown AS, Begg MD, Wyatt RJ. The design of the prenatal determinants of schizophrenia study. *Schizophr Bull.* 2000;26:257-273.
57. Insel BJ, Brown AS, Bresnahan MA, Schaefer CA, Susser ES. Maternal-fetal blood incompatibility and the risk of schizophrenia in offspring. *Schizophr Res.* 2005;80:331-342.
58. Landrigan PJ, Trasande L, Thorpe LE, et al. The National Children's Study: a 21-year prospective study of 100,000 American children. *Pediatrics.* 2006;118:2173-2186.
59. Oken E, Levitan EB, Gillman MW. Maternal smoking during pregnancy and child overweight: systematic review and meta-analysis. *Int J Obes.* Advance online publication, 27 November 2007;doi:10.1038/sj.ijo.0803760.
60. Gao YJ, Holloway AC, Zeng ZH, et al. Prenatal exposure to nicotine causes postnatal obesity and altered perivascular adipose tissue function. *Obes Res.* 2005;13:687-692.
61. Rivera JA, Barquera S, Gonzalez-Cossio T, Olaiz G, Sepulveda J. Nutrition transition in Mexico and in other Latin American countries. *Nutr Rev.* 2004;62:S149-S157.
62. Committee on the Impact of Pregnancy Weight on Maternal and Child Health, National Research Council. Influence of Pregnancy Weight on Maternal and Child Health: Workshop Report. The National Academies Press; 2007.
63. Oken E, Taveras EM, Kleinman K, Rich-Edwards JW, Gillman MW. Gestational weight gain and child adiposity at age 3 years. *Am J Obstet Gynecol.* 2007;196:322e8.
64. Institute of Medicine. *Nutrition during Pregnancy.* Washington, DC: National Academy Press; 1990.
65. Whitaker RC, Whitaker RC. Predicting preschooler obesity at birth: the role of maternal obesity in early pregnancy. *Pediatrics.* 2004;114:e29-e36.
66. Gillman MW, Rifas-Shiman SL, Berkey CS, Field AE, Colditz GA. Maternal gestational diabetes, birth weight, and adolescent obesity. *Pediatrics.* 2003;111:e221-e226.
67. Rogers I. The influence of birthweight and intrauterine environment on adiposity and fat distribution in later life. *Int J Obes Relat Metab Disord.* 2003;27:755-777.
68. Parsons TJ, Powers C, Logan S, Summerbell CD. Childhood predictors of adult obesity: a systematic review. *Int J Obes Relat Metab Disord.* 1999;23:S1-S107.
69. Silverman BL, Cho NH, Rizzo TA, Metzger BE. Long-term effects of the intrauterine environment. *Diabetes Care.* 1998;21:B142-B148.
70. Dabelea D, Hanson RL, Lindsay RS, et al. Intrauterine exposure to diabetes conveys risks for type 2 diabetes and obesity: a study of discordant sibships. *Diabetes.* 2000;49:2208-2211.

71. Whitaker RC, Pepe MS, Seidel KD, Wright JA, Knopp RH. Gestational diabetes and the risk of offspring obesity. *Pediatrics.* 1998;101:e9.

72. Wild S, Roglic G, Green A, Sicree R, King H. Global prevalence of diabetes: estimates for the year 2000 and projections for 2030. *Diabetes Care.* 2004;27:1047-1053.

73. Oken E, Ning Y, Rifas-Shiman SL, Radesky JS, Rich-Edwards JW, Gillman MW. Associations of physical activity and inactivity before and during pregnancy with glucose tolerance. *Obstet Gynecol.* 2006;108:1200-1207.

74. Zhang C, Solomon CG, Manson JE, Hu FB. A prospective study of pregravid physical activity and sedentary behaviors in relation to the risk for gestational diabetes mellitus. *Arch Intern Med.* 2006;166:543-548.

75. Dempsey JC, Butler CL, Sorensen TK, et al. A case-control study of maternal recreational physical activity and risk of gestational diabetes mellitus. *Diabetes Res Clin Pract.* 2004;66:203-215.

76. Zhang C, Liu S, Solomon CG, Hu FB. Dietary fiber intake, dietary glycemic load, and the risk for gestational diabetes mellitus. *Diabetes Care.* 2006;29:2223-2230.

77. Zhang C, Schulze MB, Solomon CG, Hu FB. A prospective study of dietary patterns, meat intake and the risk of gestational diabetes mellitus. *Diabetologia.* 2006;49:2604-2613.

78. Radesky JS, Oken E, Rifas-Shiman SL, Kleinman KP, Rich-Edwards JW, Gillman MW. Diet during early pregnancy and development of gestational diabetes. *Paediatr Perinat Epidemiol.* In press.

79. Waterland RA, Jirtle RL. Early nutrition, epigenetic changes at transposons and imprinted genes, and enhanced susceptibility to adult chronic diseases. *Nutrition.* 2004;20:63-68.

80. Baird J, Fisher D, Lucas P, Kleijnen J, Roberts H, Law C. Being big or growing fast: systematic review of size and growth in infancy and later obesity. *BMJ.* 2005;331:929-934.

81. Ong KK, Loos RJ. Rapid infancy weight gain and subsequent obesity: systematic reviews and hopeful suggestions. *Acta Paediatr.* 2006;95:904-908.

82. Stettler N, Stallings VA, Troxel AB, et al. Weight gain in the first week of life and overweight in adulthood: a cohort study of European American subjects fed infant formula. *Circulation.* 2005;111:1897-1903.

83. Singhal A, Lucas A. Early origins of cardiovascular disease: is there a unifying hypothesis? *Lancet.* 2004;363:1642-1645.

84. Singhal A, Cole TJ, Fewtrell M, et al. Promotion of faster weight gain in infants born small for gestational age: is there an adverse effect on later blood pressure? *Circulation.* 2007;115:213-220.

85. Belfort MB, Rifas-Shiman SL, Rich-Edwards JW, Kleinman KP, Gillman MW. Size at birth, infant growth, and blood pressure at 3 years of age. *J Pediatr.* 2007;151:670-4.

86. Harder T, Bergmann R, Kallischnigg G, Plagemann A. Duration of breastfeeding and risk of overweight: a meta-analysis. *Am J Epidemiol.* 2005;162:397-403.

87. Arenz S, Ruckerl R, Koletzko B, von Kries R. Breast-feeding and childhood obesity—a systematic review. *Int J Obes Relat Metab Disord.* 2004;28:1247-1256.

88. Owen CG, Martin RM, Whincup P, Davey-Smith G, Cook DG. Effect of infant feeding on the risk of obesity across the life course: a quantitative review of published evidence. *Pediatrics.* 2005;115:1367-1377.

89. Bogen DL, Hanusa BH, Whitaker RC. The effect of breast-feeding with and without formula use on the risk of obesity at 4 years of age. *Obes Res.* 2004;12:1527-1535.

90. Grummer-Strawn LM, Mei Z. Does breastfeeding protect against pediatric overweight? Analysis of longitudinal data from the Centers for Disease Control and Prevention Pediatric Nutrition Surveillance System. *Pediatrics.* 2004;113:e81-e86.

91. Owen CG, Martin RM, Whincup PH, Davey-Smith G, Gillman MW, Cook DG. The effect of breastfeeding on mean body mass index throughout life: a quantitative review of published and unpublished observational evidence. *Am J Clin Nutr.* 2005;82:1298-1307.

92. Gillman MW, Rifas-Shiman SL, Berkey CS, et al. Breastfeeding and overweight in adolescence: within-family analysis. *Epidemiology.* 2006;17:112-114.

93. Taveras EM, Rifas-Shiman SL, Scanlon KS, Sherry BL, Grummer-Strawn LM, Gillman MW. To what extent is the protective effect of breastfeeding on future overweight explained by decreased maternal feeding restriction? *Pediatrics.* 2006;118:2341-2348.

94. Kramer MS, Chalmers B, Hodnett ED, et al. Promotion of Breastfeeding Intervention Trial (PROBIT): a randomized trial in the Republic of Belarus. *JAMA.* 2001; 285:413-420.

95. Taveras EM, Rifas-Shiman SL, Oken E, Gunderson EP, Gillman MW. A prospective study of sleep duration and adiposity among preschool age children. *Arch Ped Adol Med.* In press.

96. Ferber R. *Solve Your Child's Sleep Problems: New, Revised, and Expanded Edition.* New York: Fireside; 2006.

97. Eckerberg B. Treatment of sleep problems in families with young children: effects of treatment on family well-being. *Acta Paediatr.* 2004;93:126-134.

98. Mindell JA, Kuhn B, Lewin DS, Meltzer LJ, Sadeh A. Behavioral treatment of bedtime problems and night wakings in infants and young children. *Sleep.* 2006;29:1263-1276.

99. Gillman MW, Rifas-Shiman SL, Kleinman KP, Taveras EM, Oken E. Developmental origins of childhood obesity: potential public health impact. Early Hum Dev. 2007;83(Suppl 1):S66.

100. Cole TJ. Modeling postnatal exposures and their interactions with birth size. *J Nutr.* 2004;134:201-204.

101. De Stavola BL, Nitsch D, dos Santos SI, et al. Statistical issues in life course epidemiology. *Am J Epidemiol.* 2006;163:84-96.

102. Mackay J, Amos A. Women and tobacco. *Respirology.* 2003;8:123-130.

103. Tobacco Control State Highlights 2002: Impact and Opportunity. Department of Health and Human Services, Centers for Disease Control and Prevention National Center for Chronic Disease Prevention and Health Promotion Office on Smoking and Health. Atlanta, GA; 2002.

104. Orleans CT, Barker DC, Kaufman NJ, Marx JF. Helping pregnant smokers quit: meeting the challenge in the next decade. *Tob Control.* 2000;9:III6-III11.

105. Taylor T, Lader D, Bryant A, Keyse L, McDuff TJ. *Smoking-Related Behavior and Attitudes, 2005.* London: Office for National Statistics; 2006.

106. *Women and the Tobacco Epidemic: Challenges for the 21st Century.* Samet JM, Young S-Y. London: Office for National Statistics; 2007.

107. Jha P, Chaloupka F. *Tobacco Control in Developing Countries.* Cary, NC: Oxford University Press; 2001.

108. Abdullah AS, Husten CG. Promotion of smoking cessation in developing countries: a framework for urgent public health interventions. *Thorax.* 2004;59:623-630.

109. Mackay J. The tobacco problem: commercial profit versus health—the conflict of interests in developing countries. *Prev Med.* 1994;23:535-538.

110. Lumley J, Oliver SS, Chamberlain C, Oakley L. Interventions for promoting smoking cessation during pregnancy. *Cochrane Database Syst Rev.* 2004;CD001055.

111. Crowther CA, Hiller JE, Moss JR, McPhee AJ, Jeffries WS, Robinson JS. Effect of treatment of gestational diabetes mellitus on pregnancy outcomes. *N Engl J Med.* 2005;352:2477-2486.

112. Oken E, Kleinman KP, Berland WE, Simon S, Rich-Edwards JW, Gillman MW. Decline in fish consumption after a national mercury advisory. *Obstet Gynecol.* 2003;102:346-351.

113. Ryan AS, Wenjun Z, Acosta A. Breastfeeding continues to increase into the new millennium. *Pediatrics.* 2002;110:1103-1109.

114. Casey PH, Whiteside-Mansell L, Barrett K, Bradley RH, Gargus R. Impact of prenatal and/or postnatal growth problems in low birth weight preterm infants on school-age outcomes: an 8-year longitudinal evaluation. *Pediatrics.* 2006;118:1078-1086.

115. Ehrenkranz RA, Dusick AM, Vohr BR, Wright LL, Wrage LA, Poole WK. Growth in the neonatal intensive care unit influences neurodevelopmental and growth outcomes of extremely low birth weight infants. *Pediatrics.* 2006;117:1253-1261.

116. Taheri S. The link between short sleep duration and obesity: we should recommend more sleep to prevent obesity. *Arch Dis Child.* 2006;91:881-884.

117. Stremler R, Hodnett E, Lee K, et al. A behavioral-educational intervention to promote maternal and infant sleep: a pilot randomized, controlled trial. *Sleep.* 2006;29:1609-1615.

118. Hiscock H, Wake M. Randomised controlled trial of behavioural infant sleep intervention to improve infant sleep and maternal mood. *BMJ.* 2002;324:1062-1065.

119. Gillman MW, Rich-Edwards JW, Huh S, et al. Maternal corticotropin-releasing hormone levels during pregnancy and offspring adiposity. *Obesity.* 2006;14:1647-1653.

20

Predictors and Consequences of Childhood Obesity

Alison E. Field

Introduction

Obesity is an important public health problem among children and adolescents in the United States. The 2003-2004 National Health and Nutrition Examination Survey (NHANES) estimates 37% of children and 34% of adolescents are overweight or at risk of overweight (i.e., body mass index [BMI] ≥ U.S. national 85th percentile for age and sex).[1] Moreover, during the past two decades, the prevalence of overweight has more than doubled among children and adolescents.[2] The prevalence of overweight is similar among boys and girls,[3] but large race/ethnic group differences are seen, with Hispanics and African Americans being more likely than Asians or whites to be overweight.[4] Pediatric and adolescent overweight are public health problems in many developed and affluent countries and are now becoming problems in less affluent countries.[5] Genetics may predispose certain individuals to gain more weight than their peers, but the rapid increase in prevalence of obesity among children and adolescents over the past 30 years[1] suggests that additional nonbiological factors are contributing to the current problem.

Definitions

One of the complexities of studying predictors of overweight in youth is that the definitions of "overweight" and "obese" have changed over time and are slightly different in the United States than in other countries. Among pediatric obesity researchers in the United States, the term *obesity* is infrequently used; instead, the terms *at-risk of overweight* and *overweight* are frequently used to define high weight status in childhood and adolescence.[6] In other countries these two groups are referred to as overweight and obese, respectively,[7] which are the same terms used to define degrees of excessive weight among adults both in the United States and elsewhere.

In general, overweight refers to weighing more than a standard level for height and age. People who are overweight are not necessarily overfat. Highly active people who have substantial muscle mass may weigh slightly more than the standard for their height despite low body fat and thus be overweight but have relatively low body fat. Although obesity was once primarily classified based on body fat stores, it is now frequently defined as weighing much more than a standard level for age and height. Because children and adolescents are still growing, there is not one cutoff value to demarcate healthy weight from overweight or obese. Instead, age- and gender-specific percentiles of BMI (kg/m²), a formula that combines weight and height and is commonly used in epidemiologic studies, are used to evaluate a child's weight status. Children who are between the 85th and 95th percentiles of BMI for age and gender are referred to as *at risk for overweight* (in the United States) or overweight (elsewhere), whereas, children at or above the 95th percentile are referred to as *overweight* (United States) or obese (elsewhere). One complication is that in the United States the percentiles used are usually those developed by the Centers for Disease Control and Disease (CDC).[8] These standards were based on several large national datasets, but unlike the International Obesity Task Force (IOTF) cutoffs, the CDC cutoffs for excessive weight were not developed to mesh with the adult BMI cutoffs for overweight and obese as young people become adults. The international pediatric standards developed by Cole et al.,[7] which are based on data from six countries, were developed to map to the adult standards at age 18 and therefore it is clear when the transition should be made. Moreover, they have age- and gender-specific BMI cutoff values to pass through a BMI of 25 kg/m² (overweight) and 30 kg/m² (obesity) at age 18. Although the CDC cutoff values are not extremely different from Cole's international standards, there is a problem with misclassification of overweight among adolescents because some adolescents would be considered overweight (BMI $\geq$ 25 kg/m²) according to the adult standards, but not the CDC pediatric standards (BMI < 95th percentile for age and gender). This misclassification begins to occur at age 13.5 years for boys and age 12 for girls. The problem is much less of an issue when a BMI $\geq$ 85th percentile for age and gender is used to define the excessive weight outcome. In that case, the inconsistent classification does not occur until 17.5 years for boys and 17 years for girls. Thus studies that have relied on the CDC growth standards to define overweight among adolescents may have underestimated the true prevalence of overweight and their analyses focusing on predictors of overweight will be somewhat biased.

Predictors of Obesity

Childhood and Adolescent Weight Status

One of the reasons for the concern with pediatric overweight is that overweight children and adolescents are more likely than their peers to become overweight adults. The risk of an overweight child becoming an obese adult rises with age.[9-11] Obese preschool children are approximately twice as likely as nonobese children to become an obese adult,[12] whereas, overweight adolescents are almost 18 times more likely than their leaner peers to become obese in early adulthood.[13] Not only are overweight youth more likely to be overweight adults, those in the upper end of the *normal* weight range are also at risk. Among 269 children in East Boston, Field et al.[14] observed that being in the upper one-half of the normal weight range (i.e., BMI between the 50th and 84th percentiles for age and gender in childhood) was a predictor of becoming overweight as a young adult. Compared to children with a BMI < 50th percentile, girls and boys between the 50th and 74th percentiles of BMI were approximately five times more likely, and those with a BMI between the 75th and 84th percentiles were up to 20 times more likely, to become overweight by the time they were young adults. Similar results were observed by Freedman et al.[15] in the Bogalusa Heart Study. The strong tracking of childhood overweight into adulthood highlights the need for early intervention to prevent adult obesity.

Diet and Weight Gain

Genetic differences may predispose certain individuals more than others to excessive weight gain; however, weight gain is also a function of energy intake exceeding energy expenditure. The role of fat, protein, carbohydrate, certain food groups, and specific foods in the development of obesity is not well understood. Many obesity-prevention interventions have focused on increasing fruit and vegetable servings per day,[16,17] decreasing consumption of fat,[18-20] and limiting soda intake,[21,22] but whether these changes effectively prevent weight gain remains unclear.

Dietary Factors that Protect Against Weight Gain

Among adults high fiber diets are associated with a decreased risk of many chronic diseases;[23,24] however, the association of fiber, fruit, and vegetable intake to weight gain is not well understood among children and adolescents. Despite a lack of data, several obesity-prevention interventions have included efforts to increase the consumption of fruits and vegetables.[18-20] It is thought that the consumption of fruits and vegetables might lead to greater satiety due to their high dietary fiber and hence decrease total caloric intake. It is also thought they might be consumed as an alternative to more energy-dense food items, such as soda and snack foods, which are popular among children and adolescents, and thus lead to a decrease in total daily caloric intake. Although dietary fiber has been associated with less weight gain among adults,[25,26] the findings among children are conflicting. Among 6,149 girls and 4,620 boys, aged 9 to 15 years, in the Growing Up Today Study (GUTS), no association was observed between fiber intake and weight gain.[27] In contrast, fiber intake was inversely related to weight gain among the African American and white young-adults and adults, aged 18 and older, in the Coronary Artery Risk in Young Adults (CARDIA) study.[28] It is possible that the discrepancy in results reflects the differences in ages between the study populations or it may be that the BMI gains in CARDIA were much larger than those seen in GUTS, thus making it easier to detect predictors of weight gain. One can assume that for the great majority of adults, weight gain is unhealthy, whereas, at younger ages weight gain is healthy and expected for most, therefore making it difficult to differentiate between predictors of normal and healthy weight gain from predictors of excessive weight gain. Further research is necessary to establish whether increasing fiber intake will protect against excessive weight gain.

Although fruit juice is included as a fruit serving in many campaigns to increase fruit and vegetable intake, there has been some concern that fruit juice intake might lead to weight gain among children.[29,30] Among children, fruit juice may account for considerable proportion of total fruit intake, thus it is possible that interventions aimed at increasing fruit intake could promote weight gain since it has been observed that total caloric intake is positively related to intake of 100% fruit juice and fruit drinks, as well as soda.[31] In contrast to fruit juice, fruit (other than juice) and vegetable intake is believed to protect against the development of overweight; however, the results have been inconsistent. In a 3-year follow-up among 8,203 girls and 6,715 boys in GUTS, only a weak inverse association between vegetable intake and BMI z-score change among the boys and no association among the girls were observed.[32] One explanation for the lack of effect could be that fruit and vegetable consumption among children and adolescents were in addition to high calorie-dense foods, rather than being a replacement for unhealthy food choices.

Several intervention trials have incorporated components that focus on increasing fruit and vegetable intake; however, distinguishing the effect of increased fruit and vegetable consumption on weight change from the other lifestyle changes that interventions often include is not possible. It should also be noted that only one of these trials reported significant effects on weight on follow-up.[17] Together, these results suggest that unless fruits and vegetables are consumed as a substitute for unhealthy energy-dense foods, promotion of fruit and vegetable consumption for weight control would have little impact on overweight and obesity among children and adolescents.

Dietary Fat

The association between dietary fat and weight gain has been widely studied but is still highly controversial. Dietary fat is more energy-dense per gram than carbohydrates and protein. Furthermore, high fat foods are often very palatable; therefore, some individuals may consume larger amounts of them, and in turn, a large number of calories. Thus, dietary fat could be related to weight gain owing to either a true effect of overall fat consumption or the larger number of calories in high fat foods. One difficulty in reviewing the literature on dietary fat and weight gain is that some studies statistically control for total caloric intake, but others do not. This methodological difference may explain the conflicting results that have been observed.

Cross-sectional studies are particularly difficult to interpret. For example, in a cross-sectional study of 95 four-year old Swedish children, Garemo et al.[33] found that high BMI was associated with a low percentage of energy from fat. The inverse association could be due to reverse causation, namely, that some overweight children may be trying to lose weight and, therefore, eating a low-fat diet. Thus, the association is that high weight causes a lower intake of dietary fat, not that a low-fat diet promotes weight gain. Alternatively, overweight children have been found to underreport energy intake more than their leaner peers.[34] Longitudinal studies where dietary information is collected before weight gain are necessary for understanding the relationship. However, the results from these studies are far from conclusive. In the CARDIA study, dietary fat consumption predicted greater weight gain,[28] while no relationship between dietary fat and weight gain was found in the GUTS[27] or the Dortmund Nutritional and Anthropometric Longitudinally Designed (DONALD) study.[35] Differences in analytic approaches may explain the discrepancies, but it is also possible that these discrepancies are the result of differences in the association between specific fat type and weight gain. For instance, among adult women, Field et al.[36] observed that saturated and trans fat promoted weight gain, whereas, vegetable fat was unrelated to weight gain. Similar types of analyses have yet to be conducted among children and young adults.

Calcium

The role of calcium intake in weight regulation is another controversial topic. Although Zemel et al.[37,38] have reported that high-calcium intake protects against weight gain, the results have not been confirmed by many other researchers (see Chapter 14). Neither Phillips et al.[39] nor Berkey et al.[40] observed an association between dairy food or calcium intake and weight gain among adolescents in two different prospective cohort studies. Moreover, in a small intervention among girls by Lappe et al.,[41] no differences in body fat or weight gain were found between a high-calcium diet group and a usual diet group. However, in a prospective study of 52 eight-year-old white children and their mothers, Skinner et al.[42] observed an inverse relationship between dietary calcium and percent body fat (as measured by dual energy x-ray absorptiometry [DXA]). In addition, calcium was observed to have an inverse association with change in body fat in a prospective study of preschool students[43] and another prospective study of young adult women.[44] It would be prudent to continue promoting calcium intake for bone health, but not necessarily for the prevention of excessive weight gain.

Glycemic Index

The role of glycemic index or glycemic load in weight gain is debatable, but gaining in acceptance. Glycemic index is a property of carbohydrate-containing food that describes the increase in blood glucose following a meal (also see Chapter 14). Foods that are digested and absorbed rapidly, such as potatoes and refined grains, have a high glycemic index.[45,46] In controlled studies, rapid increases in blood glucose and insulin levels are seen after oral administration of glucose or foods with a high glycemic index. This is followed in many individuals by a period of reactive hypoglycemia with continued modest elevation in insulin levels and ultimately results in hunger and increased food intake.[47]

It is unclear whether a low-glycemic diet helps to prevent the development of obesity or excessive weight gain. In a cross-sectional study of 485 ten-year-old children and 364 sixteen-year-old children in Denmark, among 10-year-old children there was no association between body fatness and either glycemic load or glycemic index; however, among the older children, glycemic index and glycemic load were positively related to sum of four skinfold measurements.[48] In contrast, among the 6149 female and 4620 male preadolescents and adolescents in the GUTS, no association was seen between glycemic index or load and weight.[27] In a small randomized study of 14 obese youth, Ebbeling et al.[49] observed that that a low-glycemic load diet was more effective than an energy-restricted low-fat diet in treating obesity; however, in a 12-month intervention of 23 young adults, following a low-glycemic load diet resulted in a similar amount of weight loss (8.4%) as adhering to an energy-restricted low-fat diet (7.8%) and both groups remained below their baseline weight at one year follow-up.[50] Thus, it appears that a low-glycemic diet might be helpful for the treatment of obesity, but more research is needed to understand how effective the strategy is compared to other treatment options.

There are not enough large prospective studies on the topic among preadolescents and adolescents to reach any firm conclusions; however, there are at least several possible explanations for the discrepancy in results. It is possible that a low-glycemic diet is more effective for weight loss and weight loss maintenance than prevention of weight gain and the development of obesity. In addition, since the beneficial effect of a low-glycemic diet appears to be small, studies that use food-frequency questionnaires and other self-reported instruments to measure diet might not be able to detect a true small association due to measurement error.

Eating Patterns: Food Purchased Away from Home

There has recently been a shift towards studying dietary patterns instead of intake of specific macro- or micronutrients as predictors of weight gain. There are several advantages to studying eating patterns instead of nutrients, including that it is easier for the general population to understand recommendations based on buying patterns and servings of foods, as opposed to nutrients. One pattern of interest is purchasing food away from home. Guthrie et al.[51] found that between 1977-1978 and 1994-1996, consumption of foods prepared away from home increased by 14% to 32% of total calories. Portion sizes of foods purchased away from home tend to be larger than when the same foods are prepared at home and thus contain more calories. In addition, many of the serving sizes have been getting larger over time.[52,53] Moreover, many of these foods are high in fat, particularly unhealthy fats such as saturated fat and trans fat.

The consumption of fast food and other fried foods has been the focus of several recent studies. Two large studies have observed that fast food intake was positively associated with caloric intake,[54,55] suggesting that fast-food consumption could lead to consuming more calories than a child expends and therefore promote obesity. In the GUTS, Taveras et al.[55] observed that cross-sectionally the frequency of eating fried foods away from home was positively associated with intake of calories, trans fat, and sugar-sweetened beverages. One prospective study found that children who increased their consumption of foods fried away from home from less than weekly to four to seven times a week over the 1-year follow-up had larger increases in BMI than their peers. Moreover, in a 15-year follow-up of the CARDIA cohort, Pereira et al.[56] observed that both baseline frequency of eating fast food and change in frequency of consuming fast food were independently associated with changes in weight among blacks and whites; however, the association was stronger among whites. Although some studies have not observed a relationship between fast food intake and weight status,[57] several other studies, including longitudinal studies, support the hypothesis that consumption of fast food can promote excessive weight gain and the development of obesity.

Snack Food and Soda

There are numerous reasons that snack-food intake might increase the risk of becoming or remaining overweight. For example, snack foods may contribute to excessive caloric intake by being consumed in addition to regular meals, instead of as a replacement. Despite an ecological association between increasing prevalence of pediatric obesity and intake of snack foods over the past two decades,[3,58] the relationship between snack food intake and weight change is not well understood. It is widely believed that the two are positively associated, although the data are not conclusive. Among 173 Caucasian girls followed from ages 5 to 9, Francis et al.[59] observed an association between weight gain and snack food consumption among children with at least one overweight parent. However, in two other longitudinal studies, no meaningful association between intake of snack food and change in BMI was observed.[60,61] Unlike Francis et al., Field et al.[60] observed that offsprings of overweight mothers gained more weight than their peers, but that there was not an independent association of snack-food intake and weight change among children of lean mothers or overweight mothers. One limitation of all of these studies is that they did not assess snacking patterns, including snacking on items other than *snack foods*, such as cereal, smoothies, sandwiches, or breakfast foods or main dishes that contain at least as many calories as many snack-food items. Therefore, more longitudinal studies that assess snacking behaviors and foods consumed as snacks are needed to better understand the relationship between snacking and excessive weight gain.

Several recent prospective studies have observed that intake of sugar-sweetened beverages predicted greater weight gain.[62-64] Although the effect was relatively small in two of these studies, the lack of a stronger association should not be misinterpreted to mean that these foods and beverages, which are of low nutritional value but may be high in calories, do not need to be targeted as part of obesity-prevention efforts. Overall, the results suggest that overconsumption of any type of food or beverage should result in weight gain since weight gain is a result of energy intake that is higher than energy expenditure. Since there are a variety of healthy food and beverage options that contain more nutrients and minerals for the same or fewer calories per serving, it would be wise to target reducing foods and beverages that contain empty calories, such as snack foods and sugar-sweetened beverages, in an effort to reduce total caloric intake and prevent the development of obesity.

Physical Activity

When studying modifiable predictors of obesity in children, it is important to study physical activity as well as diet since change in weight reflects energy intake not being in equilibrium with energy output. However, the results of studies on the role of activity in the prevention of weight gain have not been consistent. Some studies have found a protective effect, while others have not.[27,65] Some studies have found that activity is protective against weight gain only among females, while other studies have seen the protective effect only among males.

Cross-sectional studies can be difficult to interpret since overweight children might try to become more active in order to lose weight; thus it is best to focus on the results from prospective studies. Although Gordon-Larsen et al.[66] assessed whether baseline activity levels and change in activity levels predicted overweight status at follow-up in the National Longitudinal Study of Adolescent Health (Add Health), they did not control for baseline BMI or weight status. Therefore, it is difficult to know whether the associations are cross-sectional or due to changes in overweight status. They found that among the 12,759 adolescent girls and boys, level of moderate-to-vigorous activity at baseline was protective against obesity at the young adult follow-up and that among the boys, but not the girls, increases in moderate-to-vigorous activity also decreased the odds of being obese at follow-up.

The results from prospective studies are more consistent for females than males, but the results are not as strong and consistent as many would assume given the importance of energy expenditure in the weight equilibrium equation. Some studies have focused on changes in BMI, while others have focused on changes in fatness, such as skinfolds. This difference in outcome may explain some of the inconsistencies in the literature.

In an analysis of the GUTS, low level of activity predicted larger BMI changes among the girls, but there was no association among the boys.[27] The lack of an association among the boys might reflect that activity may lead to loss of fat mass but increases in muscle mass, which BMI does not distinguish between. Alternatively, activity may be protective against weight gain only if it is coupled with decreases in caloric intake. Stronger support for the role of activity comes from a study of 222 boys and 214 girls in northern France.[67] Although baseline activity level was not related to adiposity in boys or girls, girls who decreased their level of moderate activity over 2 years increased their BMI, percent body fat, skinfolds, and waist circumference the most. Among the boys, changes in vigorous activity were strongly related to changes in adiposity. In the National Growth and Health Study (NGHS), a prospective cohort study of 1,152 black and 1135 white girls, there were marked decline in activity and increases in the prevalence of obesity over the 10 years of follow-up.[68,69] Girls who decreased their activity gained more weight and had larger increases in their skinfold thickness than their more active peers. At the end of follow-up, active girls were almost two to three BMI units lighter than their inactive peers.[70] However, in the Girls Health Enrichment Multisite Studies (GEMS) pilot study of 126 African American girls, aged 8 to 10 years, there was no association between physical activity and change in BMI.[65] The lack of association could be due to the small sample size and the shorter follow-up period, which resulted in modest statistical power to detect moderate associations. Large prospective studies of adolescent males and females that include measures of BMI, fatness, and dietary intake are needed to better understand the role of activity in preventing excessive weight gain.

Inactivity

Inactivity is the time people spend engaging in sedentary activities such as watching television, sitting, or being on the computer; however, in many studies time spent watching television is the only form of inactivity studied. Physical activity and inactivity are not related constructs; one can be low on both or high on both, but it is thought that one way inactivity promotes obesity is by limiting the time one can be active. Time spent watching television is one of the strongest modifiable predictors of weight gain in children and adolescents.[71,72] The most successful interventions to prevent obesity in youth[17,65] have included components to decrease television viewing. It is thought that television viewing promotes obesity by encouraging viewers to eat the highly caloric, nutrient-dense foods advertised, by motivating the viewers to buy or ask their mothers to buy the energy-dense foods advertised on television, and by limiting the time viewers are active. Given the robust findings, it would be prudent for all obesity-prevention efforts to encourage youth to limit their television viewing.

Physical Health Consequences

Although there has been some concern that the increasing attention to childhood overweight, including the use of BMI report cards by some school districts, might increase weight concerns and disordered eating and should therefore be curtailed, it is important to remember the health consequences of pediatric obesity. Overweight children and adolescents are likely to become overweight or obese adults[12-14] and therefore be at risk for developing a variety of chronic diseases, such as cardiovascular disease (CVD),[73] certain cancers,[74,75] diabetes,[76] and asthma.[77] In addition, overweight adults have an elevated mortality rate.[78] The health outcomes of pediatric obesity have been less studied.

Cardiovascular Disease

Overweight adolescents are more likely than their leaner peers to develop heart disease in adulthood. Few studies have followed children for a long enough time to be able to study the relationship between childhood weight status and adult chronic diseases, but among the 508 men and women in the Harvard Growth Study, those who had been overweight as adolescents were more likely than their peers to have a coronary event in adulthood.[79]

High blood pressure (i.e., hypertension) is a common and highly treatable condition that is strongly related to body weight. If left untreated though, it has severe consequences, as hypertension is a strong predictor of more severe CVD. There is a strong positive relation between body weight and blood pressure among children, adolescents, and adults. Among 783 people, initially 13 to 17 years and then followed up when they were 27 to 31 years of age, Srinivasan et al.[80] observed that those who had been overweight as adolescents were eight times more likely than their leaner peers to have hypertension and high cholesterol. They observed that males were more likely than females to develop elevated systolic blood pressure and that overweight youth were approximately four times more likely than children with a BMI between the 25th and 50th percentile to develop elevated systolic blood pressure. In addition, they observed a significant, but weaker, association between overweight and elevated diastolic blood pressure. Similar results were observed by Field et al.[14] among 314 children who were 8 to 15 years old at baseline and were followed up 8 to 12 years later, and among 9,167 children, 5 to 17 years of age, in the Bogalusa Heart

Study.[15] In addition, in the Bogalusa Heart Study and the NGHS, overweight children were observed to have elevated triglyceride levels.

Diabetes

It is believed that type 2 diabetes is becoming more common among adolescents and young adults;[81] however, the exact prevalence is not known among children and adolescents. A recent estimate by Duncan,[82] who assessed the current prevalence of diabetes and impaired fasting glucose among adolescents in the NHANES population, found 0.5% (95% CI: 0.24 to 0.76) reported having diabetes. Of those with diabetes, 29% (95% CI: 14 to 44) had type 2 diabetes and of those adolescents who did not report having diabetes, 11% (95% CI: 8 to 14) had impaired fasting glucose levels. If these estimates are correct, they would generalize to 39,005 adolescents in the United States having type 2 diabetes.

The strong association between BMI and incident cases of type 2 diabetes is well established among adults,[83,84] but not as well studied in youth. Nevertheless, it is believed that excessive weight in childhood and adolescence increases the risk of type 2 diabetes through insulin resistance, the same mechanism responsible for the association in adults.[85]

High BMI in childhood has been found to be associated with insulin levels (OR = 12.6, 95% CI: 10 to 16) among the 9,167 children in the Bogalusa Heart Study, thus supporting that childhood weight status is a risk factor for type 2 diabetes.[15]

In addition to weight status, weight gain is associated with risk. Weight gain in childhood appears to confer the greatest risk of developing diabetes among children who were small at birth or early childhood. Among 13,517 Finnish men and women, Barker et al.[86] observed that BMI at age 11 was predictive of developing diabetes in adulthood. Although the highest risk in all strata was among the participants who had a BMI > 17.6 kg/m² at age 11, the association was significant only among the participants who had been in the leanest strata of birth weight. Similar results were seen by Bhargava et al.,[87] who observed that among 1,492 young-adults, those who were low weight at age two but made large increases in their BMI between ages 2 and 12 were at increased risk of developing impaired glucose tolerance and diabetes.

It also appears that weight in adolescence and young adulthood is related to developing diabetes. In the Nurses' Health Study, it has been observed that recalled weight at age 18 (late adolescence) is strongly related to diabetes. Colditz et al.[88] observed that among 114,281 female nurses, 30 to 55 years of age, BMI at age 18 had a strong association with the development of type 2 diabetes in adulthood. Women with a BMI between 25 and 27 kg/m² were three times more likely (relative risk [RR] = 3.3) and women with a BMI greater than or equal to 35 kg/m² were 13 times more likely (RR = 13.5) than women with a BMI 22 kg/m² at age 18 to develop diabetes.

Cancers

There are limited data on the association between childhood weight and the development of cancer. Much of the data comes from participants who were asked to recall their weight or shape at earlier time periods. For example, in a large population-based case-control study in Sweden, recalled body shape at age 7 was inversely related to postmenopausal breast cancer.[89] In both the Swedish case-control study[89] and a large case-control study in the United States,[90] as well as the Nurses' Health Study,[75] BMI at age 18 was observed to be a weak inverse predictor of postmenopausal breast cancer. The inverse association was also seen with BMI at age 14 among 117,415 Danish women.[91] The decrease in risk may be due to a higher prevalence of menstrual irregularities and their associated low estrogen levels in overweight women.

Although less studied than the relationship between BMI and breast cancer, a couple of studies suggest that a high BMI in late adolescence increases the risk of ovarian cancer.[92,93] An analyses of 109,445 women in the Nurses' Health Study who were followed for 20 years found that the doubling in risk seen among women who were overweight at age 18 was seen only with premenopausal ovarian cancer.[93]

Asthma

Most,[94-96] but not all,[97] cross-sectional analyses have observed an association between childhood overweight and asthma; however, the results have been difficult to interpret because the temporal order of the association was unclear. Results from prospective studies have been more consistent.[77,98] Among 3,792 participants in the Children's Health Study in southern California who were assessed annually between 1993 and 1998, overweight and obese children were significantly more likely than their leaner peers to develop asthma.[77] Similarly, among 9,828 children examined annually over 5 years in six U.S. cities, the risk of developing asthma was associated with BMI at baseline and BMI changes during the study.[98] And among 2,399 adolescents, girls, but not boys, who were overweight were two times more likely to develop a wheeze.[99] Taken together the results suggest that the most common chronic disease in childhood, obesity, is a risk factor for one of the other most common chronic diseases of childhood, asthma.

Social and Psychosocial Consequences

Although many of the physical health consequences of childhood overweight, other than hypertension and type 2 diabetes, do not often become apparent until adulthood, many of the social and psychosocial consequences of childhood overweight occur during childhood and adolescence. Despite the rapid increase in the prevalence of overweight, westernized societies value thinness and fitness. It appears that this cultural value is adopted by children at young ages. Some studies suggest that parents play a role in the transmission of these cultural values.[100,101]

Among 178 nine-year-old girls and their parents, Davison and Birch[102] observed that negative stereotypes of overweight people were common. Further evidence of the bias against overweight individuals by children comes from Latner and Stunkard,[103] who studied 458 fifth and sixth graders in public schools across the United States. They were asked to rank drawings of obese, disabled, or *healthy* same-sex children, according to how much they liked each child. As in a similar study conducted in 1961, the children liked the obese child least, with dislike of the overweight child being greater among the girls than the boys. Moreover, in a study of 5-year-old girls, heavier girls were perceived to have a lower cognitive ability.[104] In addition, in large studies of adolescents overweight youth have been found to be more socially isolated than lean adolescents.[105,106] There are numerous other negative social consequences for overweight adolescents, particularly overweight females. Overweight adolescent females are less likely to be accepted to college[107] and less likely to marry.[108] Gortmaker et al.[108] followed a nationally representative sample of 10,039 young-adults who were 16 to 24 years of age for over 8 years. They observed that compared to women who had not been overweight as adolescents, those who had been overweight completed fewer years of school (0.3 years less), were 20%

less likely to have married, and had household income that was an average of $6,710 less than their leaner peers. Among males, fewer consequences were observed; however, overweight males were 11% less likely than their nonoverweight peers to be married at follow-up.

Eating Disorders

Children and adolescents, particularly girls, who are overweight are more likely to have higher weight concerns and to engage in binge eating and purging behaviors (i.e., using laxatives and self-induced vomiting to control weight) than their average-weight peers.[109-112] In studies of clinical populations, bulimics frequently report a history of being overweight.[113,114] Because many individuals with bulimia have been symptomatic for at least several years before seeking treatment,[115] reports of having been overweight could be due to a distorted self-perception, which is a symptom of an eating disorder, rather than accurate recall. Two case-control studies by Fairburn et al.[116,117] observed that a recalled history of childhood obesity was associated with having a diagnosis of anorexia nervosa or bulimia nervosa in adulthood. However, it is unclear whether the association is real or the result of confounding since only univariate associations were presented. An independent association between weight status and risk of eating disorder development was not observed in one 3-year prospective study.[118] Moreover, in the GUTS, Field et al.[119] observed that boys who engaged in binge eating gained significantly more weight that their peers over a 3-year period, independent of their BMI at baseline. In addition, severity of binge eating has been found to decrease with weight loss,[120] thus suggesting that a recalled or cross-sectional association between weight status and binge eating may be due to weight gain caused by, rather than causing, bulimia. More longitudinal studies are needed to better understand the association between weight status and eating disorder development.

Teasing and Bullying

Teasing and being bullied are other negative social consequences to being overweight in childhood. In a large cross-sectional study of adolescents in Minnesota, overweight adolescents were more likely than their average-weight peers to be teased about their weight.[121] Among the overweight adolescents, a higher percentage of those who were teased reported binge eating and unhealthy weight maintenance behaviors. Hayden-Wade et al.[122] studied history of teasing among 156 overweight and nonoverweight children, 10 to 14 years of age, and observed that overweight youth are more likely to be bullied. Among overweight youth, appearance-related teasing was more frequent and upsetting, and was found to be associated with bulimic behaviors. Within a sample of 5,749 Canadian 11- to 16-year-old boys and girls[123] that assessed the relationship of weight status to being bullied and bullying others, obese girls and boys were significantly more likely than their leaner peers to be the victim of peer aggression.

Self-esteem

The relationship between overweight and self-esteem is controversial. Some cross-sectional studies have reported lower levels of self-esteem among overweight or obese children compared to leaner children;[124,125] however other studies have not observed this association.[126] The results from longitudinal studies suggest that the association may vary by gender and race/ethnic group. Strauss[124] did not observe a cross-sectional association at baseline between obesity and global self-esteem among 1,520 children, 9 to 10 years of age, enrolled in the National Longitudinal Study of Youth. However, over a 4-year period the self-esteem levels of obese white and Hispanic girls significantly decreased compared to their nonobese white and Hispanic peers. Among black girls, the decrease was not significant. A cross-sectional difference in levels of self-esteem among obese and nonobese white and Hispanic girls was observed at ages 13 to 14 as a result of the decreases in self-esteem. Among boys, the decrease in self-esteem was also significant, but less striking than among the girls. In a 5-year prospective analysis of 1,166 white and 1,213 black girls ages 9 to 10 at baseline enrolled in the NGHS, Brown et al.[127] found that self-worth remained stable over the ages of 9 to 14 in black girls ($P = .09$), but decreased significantly among white girls. During this time period, physical appearance ratings decreased in both white and black girls. As BMI increased, self-worth, physical appearance, and social acceptance scores decreased, with greater decreases in physical appearance among white girls as BMI increased. In a more recent analysis of the cohort with additional follow-up data of the girls, from ages 9 to 22, Biro et al.[128] found that regardless of age and race, girls with a BMI greater than one standard deviation above the mean had the lowest self-esteem. Race and BMI were important predictors of self-esteem, with increased BMI associated with decreased self-esteem.

Quality of Life

There is a growing body of research that demonstrates the impact obesity has on many aspects of quality of life among both children and adults (also see Chapter 12). In a cross-sectional study among 4,743 children and adolescents ages 7 to 12 years, Swallen et al.[129] observed that overweight and obese adolescents reported significantly worse health. In addition, obese adolescents were more likely to report functional limitations. Similarly, among 371 preadolescents, ages 8 to 11 years, children who were overweight scored significantly lower than their average-weight peers on physical functioning and psychosocial health summaries.[130] However, the most striking results come from a study of 106 children and adolescents by Schwimmer et al.,[131] who observed that health-related quality of life was lower among obese children and adolescents than their nonoverweight peers and similar to that of children and adolescents diagnosed with cancer. Taken together, the results demonstrate that overweight children and adolescents have a low quality of life due to social stigma and the health consequences of obesity.

Measurement

In reviewing the literature on childhood overweight, it is important to take methodological issues into consideration. Not only should results from prospective studies be given greater consideration, readers should also consider the implications of measurement errors that are common when studying the determinants and consequences of pediatric obesity.

Weight (BMI, Adiposity)

There are several possible reasons for the lack of strong associations between dietary intake and physical activity with subsequent weight gain. First, while BMI does a good job at distinguishing underweight from overweight children and adults, it is not a perfect measure because it does not differentiate body fat from muscle mass. In fact, some individuals may be classified as overweight based on their BMI, but have low body fat. Many studies, however, rely on BMI to classify participant weight since more accurate methods, such as underwater weighing and skinfold measurements, are expensive and labor intensive, which make them cost prohibitive for many studies. Second, among children, unlike adults, weight gain is not necessarily unhealthy. In fact, most children should be gaining some weight. Therefore, the challenge is to separate healthy from unhealthy or excessive weight gain. One reason for the lack of consistent findings in predictors of weight gain and the development of obesity is the fact that dietary intake and physical activity may be predictive of both healthy and unhealthy weight gain. Furthermore, due to gender-specific changes in fat mass during adolescence, studies that do not account for maturational stage may be misclassifying participants if they include both males and females in their analyses since body fat increases among females but decreases among males during adolescence.

Dietary Data

An important issue to consider is the difficulty in assessing dietary intake among children. Children must have the ability to think abstractly to provide information on average dietary intake; thus children younger than approximately 9 to 10 years of age may provide information that is not sufficiently accurate for the purpose of identifying predictors of weight gain. Moreover, although dietary methods such as 24-hour recalls do not require children to provide information on average intake, there is a consensus that young children are not reliable reporters on intake even when it is framed in terms of concrete meals consumed recently.[132] Therefore, regardless of the method used to accurately capture the dietary patterns of young children, information from multiple informants (i.e., parents, teacher, and child) is necessary. Given that relatively few studies of early childhood diet include dietary assessments completed by multiple informants, it is not surprising that the literature on dietary intake and weight gain is inconsistent; there may be too much measurement error to identify true predictors of excessive weight gain.

Another measurement issue that is important to consider is the fact that the dietary assessment tools used in most studies assessing childhood dietary intake were not developed to assess long-term dietary patterns that predict weight gain. The most accurate methods, such as 24-hour recalls, might do a good job at capturing diet on any given day, but since there is considerable day-to-day variation in dietary intake,[133,134] a considerable number of nonconsecutive days including both weekdays and weekends would be necessary to assess long-term dietary patterns as predictors of weight gain. Owing to logistical and financial reasons, very few studies are able to collect an adequate number of 24-hour recalls to capture average dietary intake with sufficient precision to predict subsequent weight gain. Methods such as food-frequency questionnaires do a better job at capturing average diet, but the methodology is appropriate only for children who are at least 9-10 years of age. Nevertheless, food-frequency questionnaires may not be sensitive enough to capture the small imbalances between energy intake and expenditure that result in weight gain. Another important methodological issue is that overweight children have been found to underreport their dietary intake[135] and children in overweight prevention interventions have been found to have a tendency to report a desirable diet rather than their true diet at follow-up.[136] Thus, it is likely that some true associations between dietary intake and weight gain are missed due to the dietary methods that are used and that those that have been consistently identified most likely underestimate the true associations.

Activity

The limitations in assessing physical activity are even more pronounced than those for assessing dietary intake. Although questionnaires and 24-hour recalls have been used in many studies, they do a better job at ranking participants rather than estimating with precision the amount of time children engage in activity since children tend to overestimate the time they spend being active.[137,138] The most accurate methods for assessing total activity, such as tritrac monitoring, are expensive thus they have not been used in many of the largest studies due to cost and other logistical issues. Moreover, the information collected from such monitors is difficult to interpret in terms of minutes/day or week being active, which is how the Healthy People 2010 goal is framed.[139,140] The combination of measurement error in the assessments of both dietary intake and activity make it difficult to identify true associations unless the associations are very strong. Adding to the complexity is the challenge of distinguishing healthy from unhealthy weight gain in analyses identifying predictors of obesity in youth, which means that there is the potential for considerable measurement error. Given the lack of precision in both the outcome and the predictors, it is not surprising that few dietary factors of activity patterns have been consistently identified as predictors of obesity. It does not mean that predictors do not exist, but more refined tools may need to be designed in order to capture these more subtle associations.

Conclusion

The prevalence of overweight in children and adolescents in the United States, as well as other Westernized countries, is rising rapidly. We can expect the rates of chronic diseases, such as CVD, hypertension, diabetes, asthma, and certain cancers to rise over the next several decades. Despite the health risks of obesity and the societal pressures to be thin, particularly for girls, the prevalence of pediatric overweight continues to rise.

Although weight gain should be the result of consuming more calories than one expends, the relationship of dietary intake and obesity remains poorly understood. Better methods of assessing dietary intake and physical activity are needed to better understand the modifiable determinants of excessive weight gain. The data on relationships with specific micro and macronutrients is conflicting, suggesting that more effort should be spent on preventing unhealthy dietary patterns, such as consuming sugar-sweetened beverages, and purchasing foods outside the home, particularly fast food, since those associations are stronger and the messages are easier for people to understand. In addition, children and adolescents should be encouraged to engage in physical activity and to limit the amount of time they watch television. Activity is helpful for maintaining weight loss and preventing excessive weight gain, thus, children and adolescents should be encouraged to be active regardless of their weight.

References

1. Ogden CL, Carroll MD, Curtin LR, McDowell MA, Tabak CJ, Flegal KM. Prevalence of overweight and obesity in the United States, 1999-2004. *JAMA*. 2006;295:1549-1555.
2. Flegal KM, Carroll MD, Kuczmarski RJ, Johnson CL. Overweight and obesity in the United States: prevalence and trends, 1960-1994. *Int J Obes Relat Metab Disord*. 1998;22:39-47.
3. Ogden CL, Flegal KM, Carroll MD, Johnson CL. Prevalence and trends in overweight among US children and adolescents, 1999-2000. *JAMA*. 2002;288:1728-1732.

4. Hedley AA, Ogden CL, Johnson CL, Carroll MD, Curtin LR, Flegal KM. Prevalence of overweight and obesity among US children, adolescents, and adults, 1999-2002. *JAMA*. 2004;291:2847-2850.

5. Wang Y, Monteiro C, Popkin BM. Trends of obesity and underweight in older children and adolescents in the United States, Brazil, China, and Russia. *Am J Clin Nutr*. 2002;75:971-977.

6. Himes JH, Dietz WH. Guidelines for overweight in adolescent preventive services: recommendations from an expert committee. The Expert Committee on Clinical Guidelines for Overweight in Adolescent Preventive Services. *Am J Clin Nutr*. 1994;59:307-316.

7. Cole TJ, Bellizzi MC, Flegal KM, Dietz WH. Establishing a standard definition for child overweight and obesity worldwide: international survey. *BMJ*. 2000;320:1240-1243.

8. CDC. 2000 CDC Growth Charts: United States. http://www.cdc.gov/growthcharts/. 2002. Available at: http://www.cdc.gov/growthcharts/. Accessed December 15, 2003.

9. Guo SS, Wu W, Chumlea WC, Roche AF. Predicting overweight and obesity in adulthood from body mass index values in childhood and adolescence. *Am J Clin Nutr*. 2002;76:653-658.

10. Williams S. Overweight at age 21: the association with body mass index in childhood and adolescence and parents' body mass index. A cohort study of New Zealanders born in 1972-1973. *Int J Obes Relat Metab Disord*. 2001;25:158-163.

11. Magarey AM, Daniels LA, Boulton TJ, Cockington RA. Predicting obesity in early adulthood from childhood and parental obesity. *Int J Obes Relat Metab Disord*. 2003;27:505-513.

12. Serdula MK, Ivery D, Coates RJ, Freedman DS, Williamson DF, Byers T. Do obese children become obese adults? A review of the literature. *Prev Med*. 1993;22:167-177.

13. Whitaker RC, Wright JA, Pepe MS, Seidel KD, Dietz WH. Predicting obesity in young adulthood from childhood and parental obesity. *N Engl J Med*. 1997;337:869-873.

14. Field AE, Cook NR, Gillman MW. Weight status in childhood as a predictor of becoming overweight or hypertensive in early adulthood. *Obes Res*. 2005;13:163-169.

15. Freedman DS, Khan LK, Dietz WH, Srinivasan SR, Berenson GS. Relationship of childhood obesity to coronary heart disease risk factors in adulthood: the Bogalusa Heart Study. *Pediatrics*. 2001;108:712-718.

16. Gortmaker SL, Cheung LW, Peterson KE, et al. Impact of a school-based interdisciplinary intervention on diet and physical activity among urban primary school children: eat well and keep moving. *Arch Pediatr Adolesc Med*. 1999;153:975-983.

17. Gortmaker SL, Peterson K, Wiecha J, et al. Reducing obesity via a school-based interdisciplinary intervention among youth: Planet Health. *Arch Pediatr Adolesc Med*. 1999;153:409-418.

18. Baranowski T, Baranowski JC, Cullen KW, et al. The Fun, Food, and Fitness Project (FFFP): the Baylor GEMS pilot study. *Ethn Dis*. 2003;13(Suppl 1):S30-S39.

19. Beech BM, Klesges RC, Kumanyika SK, et al. Child- and parent-targeted interventions: the Memphis GEMS pilot study. *Ethn Dis*. 2003; 13(Suppl 1):S40-S53.

20. Story M, Sherwood NE, Himes JH, et al. An after-school obesity prevention program for African-American girls: the Minnesota GEMS pilot study. *Ethn Dis*. 2003;13 (Suppl 1):S54-S64.

21. James J, Kerr D. Prevention of childhood obesity by reducing soft drinks. *Int J Obes*. 2005;2:54-57.

22. Rochon J, Klesges RC, Story M, et al. Common design elements of the Girls health Enrichment Multi-site Studies (GEMS). *Ethn Dis*. 2003;13(Suppl 1):S6-S14.

23. Rimm EB, Ascherio A, Giovannucci E, Spiegelman D, Stampfer MJ, Willett WC. Vegetable, fruit, and cereal fiber intake and risk of coronary heart disease among men. *JAMA*. 1996;275:447-451.

24. Willett WC. Diet and health: what should we eat? *Science*. 1994;264:532-537.

25. Koh-Banerjee P, Franz M, Sampson L, et al. Changes in whole-grain, bran, and cereal fiber consumption in relation to 8-y weight gain among men. *Am J Clin Nutr.* 2004;80:1237-1245.

26. Howarth NC, Huang TT, Roberts SB, McCrory MA. Dietary fiber and fat are associated with excess weight in young and middle-aged US adults. *J Am Diet Assoc.* 2005;105:1365-1372.

27. Berkey CS, Rockett HR, Field AE, et al. Activity, dietary intake, and weight changes in a longitudinal study of preadolescent and adolescent boys and girls. *Pediatrics.* 2000;105:E56.

28. Ludwig DS, Pereira MA, Kroenke CH, et al. Dietary fiber, weight gain, and cardio-vascular disease risk factors in young adults. *JAMA.* 1999;282:1539-1546.

29. Faith M, Dennison BA, Edmunds L, Stratton H. Fruit juice intake predicts increased adiposity gain in children from low-income families: weight status-by-environment interaction. *Pediatrics.* 2006;118:2066-2075.

30. Dennison BA, Rockwell HL, Baker SL. Excess fruit juice consumption by preschool-aged children is associated with short stature and obesity. *Pediatrics.* 1997;99:15-22.

31. O'Connor T, Yang S, Nicklas T. Beverage intake among preschool children and its effect on weight status. *Pediatrics.* 2006;118:1010-1018.

32. Field AE, Gillman MW, Rosner B, Rockett HR, Colditz GA. Association between fruit and vegetable intake and change in body mass index among a large sample of children and adolescents in the United States. *Int J Obes Relat Metab Disord.* 2003;27:821-826.

33. Garemo M, Palsdottir V, Strandvik B. Metabolic markers in relation to nutrition and growth in healthy 4-y-old children in Sweden. *Am J Clin Nutr.* 2006;84:1021-1026.

34. Fisher J, Johnson R, Lindquist C, Birch L, Goran M. Influence of body composition on the accuracy of reported energy intake in children. *Obes Res.* 2000;8:597-603.

35. Alexy U, Sichert-Hellert W, Kersting M, Schultze-Pawlitschko V. Pattern of long-term fat intake and BMI during childhood and adolescence—results of the DONALD Study. *Int J Obes Relat Metab Disord.* 2004;28:1203-1209.

36. Field A, Willett W, Lissner L, Colditz G. Dietary fat and weight gain among women in the nurses' health study. *Obesity.* 2007;15:967-976.

37. Zemel M. The role of dairy foods in weight management. *J Am Coll Nutr.* 2005; 24:537-546.

38. Zemel M, Shi H, Greer B, Dirienzo D, Zemel P. Regulation of adiposity by dietary calcium. *FASEB J.* 2000;14:1132-1138.

39. Phillips SM, Bandini LG, Cyr H, Colclough-Douglas S, Naumova E, Must A. Dairy food consumption and body weight and fatness studied longitudinally over the adolescent period. *Int J Obes Relat Metab Disord.* 2003;27:1106-1113.

40. Berkey CS, Rockett HR, Willett WC, Colditz GA. Milk, dairy fat, dietary calcium, and weight gain: a longitudinal study of adolescents. *Arch Pediatr Adolesc Med.* 2005;159:543-550.

41. Lappe JM, Rafferty KA, Davies KM, Lypaczewski G. Girls on a high-calcium diet gain weight at the same rate as girls on a normal diet: a pilot study. *J Am Diet Assoc.* 2004;104:1361-1367.

42. Skinner JD, Bounds W, Carruth BR, Ziegler P. Longitudinal calcium intake is negatively related to children's body fat indexes. *J Am Diet Assoc.* 2003;103:1626-1631.

43. Carruth BR, Skinner JD. The role of dietary calcium and other nutrients in moderating body fat in preschool children. *Int J Obes Relat Metab Disord.* 2001;25:559-566.

44. Lin YC, Lyle RM, McCabe LD, McCabe GP, Weaver CM, Teegarden D. Dairy calcium is related to changes in body composition during a two-year exercise intervention in young women. *J Am Coll Nutr.* 2000;19:754-760.

45. Foster-Powell K, Miller JB. International tables of glycemic index. *Am J Clin Nutr.* 1995;62:871-890.

46. Wolever TM, Jenkins DJ, Jenkins AL, Josse RG. The glycemic index: methodology and clinical implications. *Am J Clin Nutr.* 1991;54:846-854.

47. Ludwig DS, Majzoub JA, Al-Zahrani A, Dallal GE, Blanco I, Roberts SB. High glycemic index foods, overeating, and obesity. *Pediatrics.* 1999;103:E26.

48. Nielsen B, Bjornsbo K, Tetens I, Heitmann B. Dietary glycaemic index and glycaemic load in Danish children in relation to body fatness. *Br J Nutr.* 2005;94:992-997.

49. Ebbeling CB, Leidig MM, Sinclair KB, Hanger JP, Ludwig DS. A reduced-glycemic load diet in the treatment of adolescent obesity. *Arch Pediatr Adolesc Med.* 2003;157(8):773-779.

50. Ebbeling CB, Leidig MM, Sinclair KB, Seger-Shippee LG, Feldman HA, Ludwig DS. Effects of an ad libitum low-glycemic load diet on cardiovascular disease risk factors in obese young adults. *Am J Clin Nutr.* 2005;81:976-982.

51. Guthrie J, Lin B, Frazao E. Role of food prepared away from home in the American diet, 1977-78versus 1994-96: changes and consequences. *J Nutr Educ Behav.* 2002;34:140-150.

52. Briefel RR, Johnson CL. Secular trends in dietary intake in the United States. *Annu Rev Nutr.* 2004;24:401-431.

53. Young LR, Nestle M. The contribution of expanding portion sizes to the US obesity epidemic. *Am J Public Health.* 2002;92:246-249.

54. Bowman SA, Gortmaker SL, Ebbeling CB, Pereira MA, Ludwig DS. Effects of fast-food consumption on energy intake and diet quality among children in a national household survey. *Pediatrics.* 2004;113:112-118.

55. Taveras EM, Berkey CS, Rifas-Shiman SL, et al. Association of consumption of fried food away from home with body mass index and diet quality in older children and adolescents. *Pediatrics.* 2005;116:518-524.

56. Pereira MA, Kartashov AI, Ebbeling CB, et al. Fast-food habits, weight gain, and insulin resistance (the CARDIA study): 15-year prospective analysis. *Lancet.* 2005;365:36-42.

57. French SA, Story M, Neumark-Sztainer D, Fulkerson JA, Hannan P. Fast food restaurant use among adolescents: associations with nutrient intake, food choices and behavioral and psychosocial variables. *Int J Obes Relat Metab Disord.* 2001;25:1823-1833.

58. Jahns L, Siega-Riz AM, Popkin BM. The increasing prevalence of snacking among US children from 1977 to 1996. *J Pediatr.* 2001;138:493-498.

59. Francis LA, Lee Y, Birch LL. Parental weight status and girls' television viewing, snacking, and body mass indexes. *Obes Res.* 2003;11:143-151.

60. Field AE, Austin SB, Gillman MW, Rosner B, Rockett HR, Colditz GA. Snack food intake does not predict weight change among children and adolescents. *Int J Obes Relat Metab Disord.* 2004;28:1210-1216.

61. Phillips SM, Bandini LG, Naumova EN, et al. Energy-dense snack food intake in adolescence: longitudinal relationship to weight and fatness. *Obes Res.* 2004;12:461-472.

62. Berkey CS, Rockett HR, Field AE, Gillman MW, Colditz GA. Sugar-added beverages and adolescent weight change. *Obes Res.* 2004;12:778-788.

63. Ebbeling CB, Feldman HA, Osganian SK, Chomitz VR, Ellenbogen SJ, Ludwig DS. Effects of decreasing sugar-sweetened beverage consumption on body weight in adolescents: a randomized, controlled pilot study. *Pediatrics.* 2006;117:673-680.

64. Schulze MB, Manson JE, Ludwig DS, et al. Sugar-sweetened beverages, weight gain, and incidence of type 2 diabetes in young and middle-aged women. *JAMA.* 2004;292:927-934.

65. Robinson TN, Killen JD, Kraemer HC, et al. Dance and reducing television viewing to prevent weight gain in African-American girls: the Stanford GEMS pilot study. *Ethn Dis.* 2003;13(Suppl 1):S65-S77.

66. Gordon-Larsen P, Adair LS, Popkin BM. Ethnic differences in physical activity and inactivity patterns and overweight status. *Obes Res.* 2002;10:141-149.

67. Kettaneh A, Oppert JM, Heude B, et al. Changes in physical activity explain paradoxical relationship between baseline physical activity and adiposity changes in adolescent girls: the FLVS II study. *Int J Obes (London).* 2005;29:586-593.

68. Kimm SY, Barton BA, Obarzanek E, et al. Obesity development during adolescence in a biracial cohort: the NHLBI Growth and Health Study. *Pediatrics*. 2002;110:54-58.
69. Kimm SY, Glynn NW, Kriska AM, et al. Decline in physical activity in black girls and white girls during adolescence. *N Engl J Med*. 2002;347:709-715.
70. Kimm SY, Glynn NW, Obarzanek E, et al. Relation between the changes in physical activity and body-mass index during adolescence: a multicentre longitudinal study. *Lancet*. 2005;366:301-307.
71. Gortmaker SL, Must A, Sobol AM, Peterson K, Colditz GA, Dietz WH. Television viewing as a cause of increasing obesity among children in the United States, 1986-1990. *Arch Pediatr Adolesc Med*. 1996;150:356-362.
72. Robinson TN. Reducing children's television viewing to prevent obesity: a randomized controlled trial. *JAMA*. 1999;282:1561-1567.
73. Manson JE, Colditz GA, Stampfer MJ, et al. A prospective study of obesity and risk of coronary heart disease in women. *N Engl J Med*. 1990;322:882-889.
74. Shoff SM, Newcomb PA. Diabetes, body size, and risk of endometrial cancer. *Am J Epidemiol*. 1998;148:234-240.
75. Huang Z, Hankinson SE, Colditz GA, et al. Dual effects of weight and weight gain on breast cancer risk. *JAMA*. 1997;278:1407-1411.
76. Field AE, Coakley EH, Must A, et al. Impact of overweight on the risk of developing common chronic diseases during a 10-year period. *Arch Intern Med*. 2001;161:1581-1586.
77. Gilliland FD, Berhane K, Islam T, et al. Obesity and the risk of newly diagnosed asthma in school-age children. *Am J Epidemiol*. 2003;158:406-415.
78. Manson JE, Willett WC, Stampfer MJ, et al. Body weight and mortality among women. *N Engl J Med*. 1995;333:677-685.
79. Must A, Jacques PF, Dallal GE, Bajema CJ, Dietz WH. Long-term morbidity and mortality of overweight adolescents. A follow-up of the Harvard Growth Study of 1922 to 1935. *N Engl J Med*. 1992;327:1350-1355.
80. Srinivasan SR, Bao W, Wattigney WA, Berenson GS. Adolescent overweight is associated with adult overweight and related multiple cardiovascular risk factors: the Bogalusa Heart Study. *Metabolism*. 1996;45:235-240.
81. Bloomgarden ZT. Type 2 diabetes in the young: the evolving epidemic. *Diabetes Care*. 2004;27:998-1010.
82. Duncan G. Prevalence of diabetes and impaired fasting glucose levels among US adolescents: National Health and Nutrition Examination Survey, 1999-2002. *Arch Pediatr Adolesc Med*. 2006;160:523-528.
83. Colditz GA, Willett WC, Stampfer MJ, et al. Weight as a risk factor for clinical diabetes in women. *Am J Epidemiol*. 1990;132:501-513.
84. Field AE, Manson JE, Laird N, Williamson DF, Willett WC, Colditz GA. Weight cycling and the risk of developing type 2 diabetes among adult women in the United States. *Obes Res*. 2004;12:267-274.
85. Mahler RJ, Adler ML. Clinical review 102: type 2 diabetes mellitus: update on diagnosis, pathophysiology, and treatment. *J Clin Endocrinol Metab*. 1999;84:1165-1171.
86. Barker DJ, Eriksson JG, Forsen T, Osmond C. Fetal origins of adult disease: strength of effects and biological basis. *Int J Epidemiol*. 2002;31:1235-1239.
87. Bhargava SK, Sachdev HS, Fall CH, et al. Relation of serial changes in childhood body-mass index to impaired glucose tolerance in young adulthood. *N Engl J Med*. 2004;350:865-875.
88. Colditz GA, Willett WC, Rotnitzky A, Manson JE. Weight gain as a risk factor for clinical diabetes mellitus in women. *Ann Intern Med*. 1995;122:481-486.
89. Magnusson C, Baron J, Persson I, et al. Body size in different periods of life and breast cancer risk in post-menopausal women. *Int J Cancer*. 1998;76:29-34.
90. Shoff SM, Newcomb PA, Trentham-Dietz A, et al. Early-life physical activity and postmenopausal breast cancer: effect of body size and weight change. *Cancer Epidemiol Biomarkers Prev*. 2000;9:591-595.

91. Ahlgren M, Melbye M, Wohlfahrt J, Sorensen T. Growth patterns and the risk of breast cancer in women. *Int J Gynecol Cancer.* 2006;16:569-575.

92. Lubin F, Chetrit A, Freedman LS, et al. Body mass index at age 18 years and during adult life and ovarian cancer risk. *Am J Epidemiol.* 2003;157:113-120.

93. Fairfield KM, Willett WC, Rosner BA, Manson JE, Speizer FE, Hankinson SE. Obesity, weight gain, and ovarian cancer. *Obstet Gynecol.* 2002;100:288-296.

94. von Kries R, Hermann M, Grunert VP, von Mutius E. Is obesity a risk factor for childhood asthma? *Allergy.* 2001;56:318-322.

95. von Mutius E, Schwartz J, Neas LM, Dockery D, Weiss ST. Relation of body mass index to asthma and atopy in children: the National Health and Nutrition Examination Study III. *Thorax.* 2001;56:835-838.

96. Kwon H, Ortiz B, Swaner R, Shoemaker K, Jean-Louis B, Harlem Children's Zone Asthma Initiative. Childhood asthma and extreme values of body mass index: the Harlem Children's Zone Asthma Initiative. *J Urban Health.* 2006;83:421-433.

97. To T, Vydykhan TN, Dell S, Tassoudji M, Harris JK. Is obesity associated with asthma in young children? *J Pediatr.* 2004;144:162-168.

98. Gold DR, Damokosh AI, Dockery DW, Berkey CS. Body-mass index as a predictor of incident asthma in a prospective cohort of children. *Pediatr Pulmonol.* 2003;36:514-521.

99. Tollefsen E. Female gender is associated with higher incidence and more stable respiratory symptoms during adolescence. *Respir Med.* 2007;101:896-902.

100. Hill AJ, Franklin JA. Mothers, daughters and dieting: investigating the transmission of weight control. *Br J Clin Psychol.* 1998;37:3-13.

101. Lowes J, Tiggemann M. Body dissatisfaction, dieting awareness and the impact of parental influence in young children. *Br J Health Psychol.* 2003;8:135-147.

102. Davison KK, Birch LL. Predictors of fat stereotypes among 9-year-old girls and their parents. *Obes Res.* 2004;12:86-94.

103. Latner J, Stunkard A. Getting worse: the stigmatization of obese children. *Obesity.* 2003;11:452-456.

104. Davison KK, Birch LL. Weight status, parent reaction, and self-concept in five-year-old girls. *Pediatrics.* 2001;107:46-53.

105. Falkner NH, Neumark-Sztainer D, Story M, Jeffery RW, Beuhring T, Resnick MD. Social, educational, and psychological correlates of weight status in adolescents. *Obes Res.* 2001;9:32-42.

106. Strauss RS, Pollack HA. Social marginalization of overweight children. *Arch Pediatr Adolesc Med.* 2003;157:746-752.

107. Canning H, Mayer J. Obesity-its possible effect on college acceptance. *N Eng J Med.* 1966;275:1172-1174.

108. Gortmaker SL, Must A, Perrin JM, Sobol AM, Dietz WH. Social and economic consequences of overweight in adolescence and young adulthood. *N Engl J Med.* 1993;329:1008-1012.

109. Field AE, Camargo CA Jr, Taylor CB, et al. Overweight, weight concerns, and bulimic behaviors among girls and boys. *J Am Acad Child Adolesc Psychiatr.* 1999;38:754-760.

110. Ackard DM, Neumark-Sztainer D, Story M, Perry C. Overeating among adolescents: prevalence and associations with weight-related characteristics and psychological health. *Pediatrics.* 2003;111:67-74.

111. Boutelle K, Neumark-Sztainer D, Story M, Resnick M. Weight control behaviors among obese, overweight, and nonoverweight adolescents. *J Pediatr Psychol.* 2002;27: 531-540.

112. Neumark-Sztainer D, Story M, Hannan PJ, Perry CL, Irving LM. Weight-related concerns and behaviors among overweight and nonoverweight adolescents: implications for preventing weight-related disorders. *Arch Pediatr Adolesc Med.* 2002;156:171-178.

113. Beumont PJ, George GC, Smart DE. "Dieters" and "vomiters and purgers" in anorexia nervosa. *Psychol Med.* 1976;6:617-622.

114. Garner DM, Garfinkel PE, O'Shaughnessy M. The validity of the distinction between bulimia with and without anorexia nervosa. *Am J Psychiatr.* 1985;142:581-587.

115. Herzog DB, Keller MB, Lavori PW, Ott IL. Short-term prospective study of recovery in bulimia nervosa. *Psychiatr Res.* 1988;23:45-55.

116. Fairburn CG, Welch SL, Doll HA, Davies BA, O'Connor ME. Risk factors for bulimia nervosa. A community-based case-control study. *Arch Gen Psychiatr.* 1997;54:509-517.

117. Fairburn CG, Cooper Z, Doll HA, Welch SL. Risk factors for anorexia nervosa: three integrated case-control comparisons. *Arch Gen Psychiatr.* 1999;56:468-476.

118. Patton GC, Selzer R, Coffey C, Carlin JB, Wolfe R. Onset of adolescent eating disorders: population based cohort study over 3 years. *BMJ.* 1999;318:765-768.

119. Field AE, Austin SB, Taylor CB, et al. Relation between dieting and weight change among preadolescents and adolescents. *Pediatrics.* 2003;112:900-906.

120. Stunkard AJ, Allison KC. Two forms of disordered eating in obesity: binge eating and night eating. *Int J Obes Relat Metab Disord.* 2003;27:1-12.

121. Neumark-Sztainer D, Falkner N, Story M, Perry C, Hannan PJ, Mulert S. Weight-teasing among adolescents: correlations with weight status and disordered eating behaviors. *Int J Obes Relat Metab Disord.* 2002;26:123-131.

122. Hayden-Wade H, Stein R, Ghaderi A, Saelens B, Zabinski M, Wilfley D. Prevalence, characteristics, and correlates of teasing experiences among overweight children vs. non-overweight peers. *Obesity Res.* 2005;13:1381-1392.

123. Janssen I, Craig WM, Boyce WF, Pickett W. Associations between overweight and obesity with bullying behaviors in school-aged children. *Pediatrics.* 2004;113:1187-1194.

124. Strauss RS. Childhood obesity and self-esteem. *Pediatrics.* 2000;105:15.

125. Kimm SY, Barton BA, Berhane K, Ross JW, Payne GH, Schreiber GB. Self-esteem and adiposity in black and white girls: the NHLBI Growth and Health Study. *Ann Epidemiol.* 1997;7:550-560.

126. French SA, Story M, Perry CL. Self-esteem and obesity in children and adolescents: a literature review. *Obes Res.* 1995;3:479-490.

127. Brown K, McMahon R, Biro F, Crawford P, Schreiber G, Similo S. Changes in self-esteem in black and white girls between the ages of 9 and 14 years. The NHLBI Growth and Health Study. *J Adolesc Health.* 1998;23:7-19.

128. Biro F, Striegel-Moore R, Franko D, Padgett J, Bean J. Self-esteem in adolescent females. *J Adolesc Health.* 2006;39:501-507.

129. Swallen K, Reither E, Haas S, Meier A. Overweight, obesity, and health-related quality of life among adolescents: the National Longitudinal Study of Adolescent Health. *Pediatrics.* 2005;115:340-347.

130. Friedlander SL, Larkin EK, Rosen CL, Palermo TM, Redline S. Decreased quality of life associated with obesity in school-aged children. *Arch Pediatr Adolesc Med.* 2003;157:1206-1211.

131. Schwimmer JB, Burwinkle TM, Varni JW. Health-related quality of life of severely obese children and adolescents. *JAMA.* 2003;289:1813-1819.

132. Matheson D, Hanson K, McDonald T, Robinson T. Validity of children's food portion estimates: a comparison of 2 measurement aids. *Arch Pediatr Adolesc Med.* 2002;156:867-871.

133. Beaton G, Milner J, McGuire V, Feather T, Little J. Source of variance in 24-hour dietary recall data: implications for nutrition study design and interpretation. Carbohydrate sources, vitamins, and minerals. *Am J Clin Nutr.* 1983;37:986-995.

134. Tarasuk V, Beaton G. The nature and individuality of within-subject variation in energy intake. *Am J Clin Nutr.* 1991;54:464-470.

135. Maffeis C, Schutz Y, Zaffanello M, Piccoli R, Pinelli L. Elevated energy expenditure and reduced energy intake in obese prepubertal children: paradox of poor dietary reliability in obesity? *J Pediatr.* 1994;124:348-354.

136. Harnack L, Himes J, Anliker J, Clay T, Gittelsohn J, Jobe J. Intervention-related bias in reporting of food intake by fifth-grade children participating in an obesity prevention study. *Am J Epidemiol.* 2004;160:1117-1121.

137. Wong S, Leatherdale S, Manske S. Reliability and validity of a school-based physical activity questionnaire. *Med Sci Sports Exerc.* 2006;38:1593-1600.

138. Treuth M, Sherwood N, Butte N, McClanahan B, Obarzanek E, Zhou A. Validity and reliability of activity measures in African-American girls for GEMS. *Med Sci Sports Exerc.* 2003;35:532-539.

139. CDC. Healthy People 2010: National Health Promotion and Disease prevention Objectives. 2000. Available at: http://www.healthypeople.gov/Document/HTML/Volume2/22Physical.htm. Accessed August 3, 2002.

140. Koplan JP, Liverman CT, Kraak VI. Preventing childhood obesity: health in the balance: executive summary. *J Am Diet Assoc.* 2005;105:131-138.

21

Genetic Predictors of Obesity

Frank B. Hu

The search for human obesity genes began several decades ago, but efforts have intensified in recent years with the completion of the Human Genome Project and advances in molecular biology, genotyping technology, and genetic epidemiologic methods. Several genetic factors responsible for rare monogenic forms of obesity have been identified; however, genes for common forms of obesity remain largely elusive. Nonetheless, there is hope that rapid advances in genomics technology and genetic association studies of complex diseases will provide new tools and an impetus for progress in the identification of susceptibility genes for common forms of obesity.

This chapter begins with a review of the genetic factors underlying monogenic and syndromic forms of obesity. We then describe the genetics of common obesity, with a particular focus on results from genome-wide linkage and candidate gene association studies. We also discuss recent findings using the genome-wide association (GWA) approach. Finally, several methodological problems that commonly plague genetic association studies, especially the inability to replicate findings, are addressed. A detailed description of the physiological basis of weight regulation is beyond the scope of this chapter, but would nonetheless facilitate a better understanding of the role that genetics play in the development of obesity. Information on this topic can be found in other excellent reviews.[1-3]

Genetics of Monogenic Forms of Obesity

Over the past several decades, animal models, human linkage studies, and detailed genotyping and phenotyping of severely obese patients have greatly enhanced understanding of single mutations that contribute to the development of monogenic obesity.[4-8] These rare forms of severe obesity, typically beginning in childhood, result from spontaneous mutations in single genes, and display a Mendelian pattern of inheritance. Several genetic mutations responsible for monogenic obesity have been identified, many of which alter the leptin and melanocortin pathways (Fig. 21.1).[5]

Leptin is an adipocyte-secreted hormone transported across the blood-brain barrier to bind receptors that transmit satiety signals to the hypothalamic centers, where a complex network of neuropeptides regulate long-term energy homeostasis and weight control.[9] Leptin signals through catabolic and anabolic pathways, each consisting of distinct classes

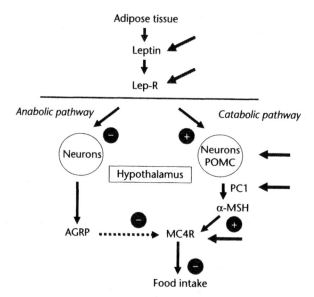

Figure 21.1 Leptin and melanocortin pathways. Lep-R, leptin receptor; POMC, proopiomelan-ocortin; α-MSH, α-melanocyte-stimulating hormone; AGRP, agouti-related protein; MC4R, melanocortin-4 receptor; PC1, proconvertase 1; →, location of mutations responsible for monogenic obesity in man; →, AGRP is a natural antagonist of MC4R; +, pathway activated; −, pathway inhibited. Reproduced with permission from Clement K. Genetics of human obesity. *Proc Nutr Soc.* 2005;64:133-142.[5]

of neurons.[2] The catabolic pathway includes the anorexigenic peptides proopiomelano-cortin (POMC) and cocaine- and amphetamine-related transcript (CART), which reduce appetite and food intake. Increased leptin secretion stimulates the production of POMC, which is converted to α-melanocortin-stimulating hormone (α-MSH) through procon-vertase 1 (PC1). The actions of melanocortins are mediated by a family of melanocor-tin receptors. The melanocrotin 4 receptor (MC4R) is largely expressed in the brain and central nervous system; activation of MC4R inhibits appetite and increases energy expenditure. The anabolic pathway includes neuropeptide-Y (NPY) and agouti-related protein (AGRP). Activation of NPY/AGRP neurons promotes positive energy balance by increasing appetite and food intake and decreasing energy expenditure. Reduced leptin secretion activates NPY/AGRP signaling and reduces MC4R signaling, thus stimulating food intake and promoting weight gain. Ghrelin, a gastrointestinal peptide hormone produced mainly by the stomach, opposes the action of leptin through disinhibition of NPY/AGRP, thereby stimulating short-term food intake and decreasing energy expen-diture.[10] Rare genetic mutations on the leptin and melanocortin pathways can disrupt both production and function of catabolic and anabolic neuropeptidies, leading to severe early-onset obesity and a variety of neuroendocrine abnormalities. In the following sec-tions, we briefly review the major genetic mutations within these pathways that con-tribute to monogenic obesity (Table 21.1). For further information, readers can refer to several comprehensive reviews.[4-7]

LEP Gene Mutations

Leptin, a hormone produced by adipose tissue and the product of the obese (*ob*) gene, plays a key role in regulating food intake and energy homeostasis. *Ob/ob* mice with a

Table 21.1 Mutations in Human Obesity Affecting the Leptin and the Melanocortin Pathways

Gene	Transmission	Obesity	Associated Phenotypes
Leptin (*LEP*)	Recessive	Severe, from the first days of life	Leptin deficiency, gonadotropic, thyrotropic, insufficiency
Leptin receptor (*LEPR*)	Recessive	Severe, from the first days of life	Gonadotropic, thyrotropic and somatotropic insufficiency, high leptin
Proopiomelanocortin (*POMC*)	Recessive	Severe, from the first month of life	Adrenocorticotropin insufficiency, mild hypothyroidism, ginger hairs
Proconvertase 1 (*PC1*)	Recessive	Severe, from the first month of life	Gonadotropic and corticotropic insufficiency, hyperinsulinemia, other dysfunctions of gut peptides
Melanocortin-4 receptor (*MC4R*)	Dominant	Early onset, variable severity, large size	No other phenotype

Adapted from Clement K. Genetics of human obesity. *C R Biol.* 2006;329:608-622.[6]

homozygous *LEP* gene mutation exhibit complete leptin deficiency and early-onset severe obesity and diabetes.[9] In 1997, Montague et al.[11] reported on two leptin-deficient children from a consanguineous family of Pakistani origin who presented with early-onset severe obesity and hyperphagia. Both patients were homozygous for a single-nucleotide deletion at position 398 of the *LEP* gene, resulting in a frameshift of the leptin-coding region after Gly132 and a premature termination of peptide synthesis. Consistent with an autosomal recessive inheritance of the disorder, other family members, who were heterozygous for this mutation, were not severely obese. In a subsequent study, daily subcutaneous injections of recombinant human leptin for up to 4 years dramatically reduced body weight in three morbidly obese children with congenital leptin deficiency.[12]

LEPR Gene Mutations

Leptin receptors exist in several isoforms and play a part in modulating the availability and biological function of leptin.[13,14] Mutations in *LEPR* in *db/db* mice produce the same phenotype as in *ob/ob* mice. Rather than displaying leptin deficiency, however, *db/db* mice are characterized by leptin resistance. A mutation in the human *LEPR* was first reported by Clement et al.[15] in three morbidly obese sisters (13 to 19 years of age) from a consanguineous family of Algerian origin. The patients were homozygous for a single nucleotide substitution at a splice site in exon 16 of the *LEPR* gene, resulting in leptin receptor deficiency, and consequently, elevated serum leptin levels. They developed hyperphagia and severe obesity within a few months of birth. In that heterozygous parents and siblings of these affected patients were not severely obese, the disorder was characterized as an autosomal recessive trait. In a recent study, Farooqi et al.[8] reported that pathogenic *LEPR* mutations were present in up to 3% of individuals with severe early-onset obesity. They identified five nonsense and four missense mutations in eight probands. All of the missense mutations were shown to either impair or completely prevent leptin receptor signaling. Interestingly, serum leptin levels in these patients were not substantially elevated.

PC1 Gene Mutations

Proconvertases are required for processing of POMC into its constituent peptides. Loss-of-function mutations in *PC1* gene have been shown to cause obesity.[3] Congenital deficiency of PC1 was first described by Jackson et al.[16] in a case report of a middle-aged woman presenting with severe, early-onset of obesity, impaired glucose tolerance, hypogonadism, hypoadrenalism, and reactive hypoglycemia. This woman was compound heterozygous for two mutations in the *PC1* gene: a Gly483Arg missense mutation in *PC1* resulting from a G→A substitution in exon 13 and an A→C substitution in the intron 5 donor splice site, which led to reduced production of functional *PC1*. The affected woman's four children were heterozygous for one of the two mutations but of normal weight. Subsequently, Jackson et al.[17] reported a second case of human *PC1* deficiency, also due to compound heterozygosity for the two mutations. That patient shared the obesity phenotype with the first one, but also suffered from severe small-intestinal absorptive dysfunction.

POMC Gene Mutations

POMC-derived peptides play a critical role in regulating energy homeostasis and body weight through their actions at melanocortin receptors in the hypothalamus.[5] Krude et al.[18] described mutations in the *POMC* gene in a 5-year-old girl and a 5-year-old boy from unrelated families who developed early-onset obesity with hyperphagia. Both had pale skin, red hair, and adrenocorticotropin (ACTH) deficiency during infancy. The girl was compound heterozygous for two mutations (G7013T, C7133delta) in exon 3 of *POMC*, which resulted in loss of ACTH and α-MSH production. The boy was homozygous for a C3804A substitution in the 5′ untranslated region of *POMC* that abolished POMC translation. Additional loss-of-function mutations in the *POMC* gene have been identified in other severely obese children presenting with POMC deficiency.[19] In POMC deficiency, obesity results from insufficient POMC-derived hormones and neuropeptides, ligands for the melanocortin receptors that are critical for body weight regulation.[20]

MC4R Gene Mutations

The MC4R is found in hypothalamic nuclei that regulate body weight by decreasing food intake and increasing energy expenditure.[21] Homozygous *MC4R* knockout mice exhibit multiple metabolic phenotypes, including obesity, hyperphagia, hyperinsulinaemia, and hyperglycemia, while heterozygous mice present an intermediate obesity phenotype.[22] In 1998, two independent studies reported multiple heterozygous frameshift mutations in the human *MC4R* gene that were associated with dominantly inherited obesity.[23,24] Since then, more than 90 different mutations in this gene have been reported in obese subjects from various ethnic groups.[4] These include frameshift, inframe deletion, nonsense, and missense mutations across the gene. Most of these mutations follow a dominant pattern of inheritance and result in partial or complete loss of receptor function.[25,26] The prevalence of *MC4R* mutations ranges from 0.5% to 6% in severe cases of early-onset obesity.[4] The prevalence of *MC4R* mutations in the general population, however, is very low. After screening 528 subjects for *MC4R* mutations by direct sequencing, Jacobson et al.[27] detected six missense and six silent variants, but none were significantly associated with obesity or related phenotypes.

In a German population of 1003 severely obese adults, nonsynonymous *MC4R* mutations that cause impaired receptor function occurred in only 2 subjects.[28] Among 769 adult patients with a body mass index (BMI) of at least 35 kg/m^2, the prevalence of obesity-specific *MC4R* mutations was 2.6%.[29] Ma et al.[30] sequenced the coding region of the *MC4R* gene in 426 full heritage, non-first-degree-related adult Pima Indians. They detected only three coding variations as heterozygotes in 12 of the 300 severely obese subjects in this population. Taken together, these studies suggest that although many pathogenic *MC4R* mutations have been identified, their prevalence in the general population is very low, and therefore, they account for only a small fraction of obesity.

Genetic Syndromes of Obesity

In a recent review of monogenic obesity in humans, Farooqi and O'Rahilly[7] described approximately 30 rare syndromes of obesity caused by genetic mutations or chromosomal abnormalities. These syndromes are characterized by severe obesity and frequently accompanied by mental retardation. Prader-Willi Syndrome (PWS) is the most common, with 1 in 25,000 births affected.[31] PWS is an autosomal-dominant disorder typically caused by a paternally inherited deletion at the chromosomal region 15q11.2-q12. It is characterized by obesity, hyperphagia, short status, mental retardation, and hypogonadotropic hypogonadism. Patients with PWS also have elevated circulating ghrelin, which may contribute to increased hunger and hyperphagia.[32]

Bardet-Biedl syndrome (BBS) is a very rare autosomal recessive disorder characterized by central obesity, mental retardation, hypogonadism in males, renal abnormalities, and pigmentary retinopathy.[7] Eight BBS genes have been identified in various pedigrees through positional cloning and candidate gene studies, but their molecular functions have not been completely elucidated.[33] Recently, a study in a French population showed an age-dependent association between common obesity and variants in BBS2, BBS4, and BBS6.[34]

Genetics of Common Obesity

Heritability of Obesity

The degree of genetic contribution to a trait such as obesity can be quantified by narrow-sense heritability, which is defined as the percent of total phenotypic variation that can be attributed to additive genetic effects ($h^2 = V_G/V_P$, where V_G is the additive genetic variance and V_P is the phenotypic variance).[35] Findings from family and twin studies suggest that obesity and obesity-related traits have a substantial heritable component. Studies comparing monozygotic (MZ) and dizygotic (DZ) twins have been especially informative. MZ twins share all genes, and DZ twins an average of half, making twin studies a useful way to estimate genetic heritability of obesity. Such analyses are based on the "equal environment" assumption that degree of environmental sharing among MZ co-twins is the same as that among DZ co-twins, and thus, any difference in shared phenotype between MZ and DZ twins is due to genetic factors.[35] On the basis of data from more than 25,000 twin pairs and 50,000 biological and adoptive family members, Maes et al.[36] estimated that the mean correlations for BMI were 0.74 for MZ twins, 0.32 for DZ twins, 0.25 for siblings, 0.19 for parent-offspring pairs, 0.06 for adoptive relatives, and 0.12 for spouses. The stronger correlations among MZ twins than DZ twins, siblings, or parent-offspring pairs suggest a strong genetic influence on BMI.

In 1977, the National Heart, Lung, and Blood Institute (NHLBI) Twin Study demonstrated genetic heritability of obesity and other cardiovascular risk factors.[37] Since then, numerous twin studies have produced heritability estimates ranging from 25% to 90% for BMI.[38] Heritability estimates have ranged from 65% to 75% for fat mass and percentage of body fat;[39-41] 46% to 90% for waist circumference;[42-44] 48% to 69% for skinfolds (total, extremity, and trunk)[44]; and 38% to 73% for serum leptin.[45,46] Similar heritability estimates ranging from 50% to 70% have been obtained for BMI in MZ twins reared apart.[47] While the classic twin study requires the equal environment assumption, studies of twins reared apart have the advantage of co-twins raised in uncorrelated environments through random replacement.

While adoptive parents and their adopted offspring share only environmental sources of variance, adoptees and their biological parents share only genetic sources. This makes adoption studies another useful approach for separating genetic and environmental influences on obesity traits. Data from these studies suggest that genetic factors account for 20% to 60% of variation in BMI.[35] In a study of over 3,500 subjects from the Danish Adoption Register, a strong relationship was observed between the BMI of adoptees and biological parents across a wide range of body fatness.[48] In contrast, no significant relationship was observed between adoptees and adoptive parents.

In summary, common obesity is clearly a heritable trait, although the exact degree of genetic heritability is still debatable. Nonetheless, the strong genetic basis of obesity has spurred intensive efforts to identify *obesity genes* over the past two decades. Unlike monogenic obesity, common obesity is likely to be caused by many genes. Linkage analysis and candidate-gene associations have been the primary approaches to identifying common obesity susceptibility genes. A description of these two approaches, including their strengths and weaknesses, is presented later. Recent findings from GWA studies are also discussed.

Linkage Analysis and "Positional Cloning"

Linkage analyses map genetic loci using data from related individuals, including siblings, nuclear families, and large pedigrees.[49] In genome-wide linkage analyses, a series of anonymous markers across the entire genome is used without *a priori* hypotheses to identify regions of the genome that may harbor disease susceptibility genes. Evidence for linkage is evaluated by a logarithm of the odds (LOD) score first proposed by Morton in 1955.[50] Larger LOD scores indicate greater evidence for linkage. *Significant linkage* is commonly defined as an LOD score >3.6, while *suggestive linkage* is defined as a score >2.2.[51] These criteria, however, are arbitrary and a modest LOD score (e.g., in the range of 1.5 to 2.2) does not necessarily exclude linkage. Nonetheless, applying the stringent criterion of at least 3.6 (equivalent to the genome-wide type 1 error rate of 0.05) is intended to minimize false-positive results.[52]

Although linkage analysis was initially used for mapping genes that underlie monogenic obesity, this method has also been widely applied to map common obesity genes. According to the Human Obesity Gene Map,[53] 253 quantitative trait loci (QTL) have been identified in 61 genome-wide scans performed in various populations, including Caucasians, African Americans, Mexican Americans, and Asians. Scans have also been performed in isolated populations, such as Pima Indians and the Old Order Amish. A wide variety of obesity measures or biomarkers have been evaluated, including BMI, fat mass; fat-free mass; skinfold thickness; intra-abdominal fat; waist circumference;

adipocyte size; percentage of body fat; respiratory quotient; and levels of insulin, leptin, glucose, and adiponectin.

Despite large numbers of linkage studies on common obesity, few obesity susceptibility genes have been identified and replicated. This limited success is likely due to multiple factors. First, the pathogenesis of common obesity, unlike monogenic obesity, is likely to involve a large number of genes, with each contributing only a modest effect. Most family-based linkage studies are underpowered to detect these effects.[54] Second, common obesity is a complex and heterogeneous phenotype. A variety of obesity-related quantitative traits, such as BMI and measures of body composition, have been used in linkage analysis. Since obesity is significantly related to energy metabolism, some intermediate phenotypes (e.g., leptin levels, resting metabolic rate, and respiratory quotient) have also been used to search for obesity QTL.[55] However, different genes may regulate different obesity-related traits, leading to heterogeneity of linkage regions across various studies. Third, obesity linkage studies have been conducted in populations that live in diverse obesogenic environments. Environmental factors may modify genetic influences (Chapter 22). However, most linkage analyses do not take gene-environment interactions into account, a factor that may also contribute to heterogeneous results. Finally, because genes that influence early-onset obesity may differ from those that contribute to weight gain in later life, linkage studies in children and adults may implicate different genomic regions.

Linkage analysis is only the first step in the gene discovery process. Once a genomic region is identified, the next step is to *clone* the gene through fine mapping, association studies, and functional analyses—the so-called *positional cloning* technique. This technique has recently led to the identification of several novel genes that may contribute to common obesity. In a 1998 genome-wide scan of 158 obese French Caucasian families, Hager et al.[56] reported significant evidence for linkage of obesity to a region of chromosome 10p. Replication studies in other populations have confirmed the linkage.[57] Subsequently, Boutin et al.[58] conducted fine mapping of the chromosome 10p locus by assessing 16 polymorphic markers around the linkage peak in 620 individuals from 188 nuclear families. Further analysis narrowed the linkage signal to one marker located in intron 7 of the glutamate decarboxylase 2 (*GAD2*) gene. Association tests in two independent case-control studies suggested a relationship between several single-nucleotide polymorphisms (SNPs) in *GAD2* gene (−243 A>G, +61450 C>A, and +83897 T>A) and risk of morbid obesity (BMI > 40 kg/m^2). The −243 A>G SNP, which was associated with 30% increased obesity risk, was also associated with significantly higher hunger and disinhibition scores. In addition, functional data showed a sixfold increase in *GAD2*-promoter activity for the risk allele of the −243 A>G SNP. *GAD2* encodes the glutamic acid decarboxylase enzyme, which catalyzes the formation of gamma-aminobutyric acid (GABA). GABA interacts with NPY to stimulate hunger and food intake.[59] *GAD2* is therefore considered a strong positional and biological candidate gene for obesity. Attempts to replicate these associations, however, have produced mixed results. A large family study and two independent case-control samples showed no associations between the −243 A>G SNP or two other *GAD2* SNPs and morbid obesity.[60] In contrast, a second study by Meyre et al.[61] confirmed the association of the *GAD2* −243 A>G SNP with early-onset severe obesity among French children [odds ratio (OR), 1.25; $P = .04$].

In a genome-wide linkage scan of Finnish obese nuclear families, Ohman et al.[62] reported linkage to chromosome Xq24. Suviolahti et al.[63] further investigated this locus in 218 obese Finnish sibling pairs by genotyping 9 microsatellite markers and 36 SNPs for 11 candidate genes spanning the 15-Mb linkage region. This approach led to significant associations between SNPs in *AGTR2*, *SLC6A14*, and *SLC25A5* and obesity.

A follow-up study of 117 cases and 182 controls from the Finnish population reported significant associations between obesity and SNPs 22510 C>G (rs20718772) and 20649 C>T (rs2011162) in *SLC6A14*. In a second study of Swedish-Finnish subjects, Tiwari et al.[64] also reported an association between SNP 22150 C>G and obesity, but in the opposite direction. More recently, Durand et al.[65] examined SNPs 20649 C>T and 22510 C>G in a French population of 1267 obese and 649 nonobese, normoglycemic subjects. Results confirmed the initial findings by Suviolahti et al.[63] (OR: 1.23 for 20649T and 1.36 for 22510G). However, no relationship between either SNP and childhood obesity was observed. Potential reasons for the discrepant findings from these studies will be discussed later in the chapter.

Candidate Gene Association Studies

Candidate gene association studies test the relationships between polymorphic markers within selected candidate genes and the obesity phenotype. Candidate genes are typically selected on the basis of locations within genomic regions (positional candidates) implicated by linkage analysis to the obesity phenotypes or biological functions (functional candidates).[66] *GAD2* and *SLC6A14* are good examples of positional candidate genes. Functional candidates can be derived from animal models of obesity, in vitro characteristics of gene variants related to energy metabolism, or genes that have been implicated in monogenic obesity (discussed earlier).

Once candidate genes are selected, the next step is to choose genetic markers within those genes. Genetic variation can occur in many forms, including SNPs, copy number variants, microsatellites, and deletions of entire genes or regions of a chromosome. SNPs are the most common form of genetic variation, accounting for more than 90% of the total variation in the human genome. Because SNPs are widespread across the genome (>10 million SNPs have been identified) and are easily genotyped by a number of genotyping platforms, these have been the most commonly used markers in association studies. Four criteria have been commonly used to choose SNPs for genotyping: (a) the prior probability of being functional (e.g., exonic SNPs are more likely to be functional than intronic SNPs); (b) the degree of linkage disequilibrium (LD) among the SNPs; (c) missense variants detected by sequencing; and (d) the availability of high-throughput and low-cost SNP arrays that cover the whole genome.[66]

Most of the candidate gene association studies discussed later have evaluated only one or few SNPs in a candidate gene. A comprehensive approach should genotype all common (>5% frequency) nonsynonymous coding SNPs as well as other candidate SNPs in the regulatory region and splicing-sites. Selections can be based on purported function or earlier reported association with obesity or an obesity-related phenotype. In addition, a small number of "tagging SNPs" can serve as efficient surrogates for most remaining common SNPs of unknown function.[67] The choice of these surrogate SNPs has been facilitated by the completion of Phase II of the HapMap,[68] a comprehensive survey of LD patterns in samples from three major continental populations: Africans, East Asians, and Europeans. A simple and effective algorithm can be used to choose a set of tagging SNPs to capture any other SNPs in the region that have high pairwise correlations with one of the tagging SNPs.[69,70] This algorithm has been implemented in the program Haploview (http://www.broad.mit.edu/mpg/haploview/), which can also be used to visualize LD patterns among a set of SNPs.

Because of their simplicity, case-control studies of unrelated individuals are the most common type of association studies. Such studies compare the frequency of variant alleles of selected candidate genes in obese versus nonobese individuals and determine whether there is an association between the alleles and obesity phenotype. Association studies can be also carried out in multiple families.[71] For example, the Transmission Disequilibrium Test (TDT), using parent/affected offspring trios, assesses whether the transmission of an allele from heterozygous parents to affected children deviates from that expected by chance (50%).[71] The main advantage of family-based association studies is that they are not affected by population stratification bias (discussed later), but they suffer from several other disadvantages that prevent their widespread use.[66] Not only is it difficult to recruit family trios, but selectively recruiting subjects and their parents introduces potential bias towards early-onset disease. Moreover, the power of TDT is low because only the heterozygous parents are informative. In contrast, case-control studies of unrelated individuals are easier to conduct and more powerful. For these reasons, association studies of unrelated individuals have been the most popular method for genetic association studies.

To date, a large number of obesity candidate genes have been tested in association studies in various populations. Most of the genes were selected based on their potential functions related to appetite control, food intake, energy metabolism, and adipocyte differentiation. According to the Human Obesity Gene Map,[53] 426 findings of positive associations with 127 candidate genes have been reported from genetic association studies. The vast majority of these findings have not been replicated. Only 22 genes have been confirmed by at least five positive studies, with varying degrees of statistical significance. However, these positive studies were offset by an equal or even higher number of negative studies. Therefore, careful meta-analyses of all published genetic associations are often required to synthesize the evidence about reported associations. In the following sections, we briefly review obesity candidate genes that have been subject to meta-analyses. The results of these meta-analyses are summarized in Table 21.2.

β3-Adrenergic Receptor Gene W64R Polymorphism

β3-Adrenergic receptors (ADRB3) are mainly expressed in adipose tissue and play a key role in regulating lipolysis and thermogenesis.[72] In 1995, several studies examined the association between obesity and a tryptophan (W) to arginine (R) substitution at amino acid position 64 in the ADRB3 gene.[73-75] Kadowaki et al.[74] reported a significantly higher BMI for Japanese with the RR genotype compared to those with the WW genotype (24.7 kg/m² vs. 22.1 kg/m²), while Widen et al.[75] found the R allele to be significantly associated with an elevated WHR in Finns. Subsequently, dozens of studies have been published on the relationship between this polymorphism and obesity or obesity-related traits. Three meta-analyses have been published with somewhat contradictory results. The first was conducted by Allison et al.[76] in 1998 and included results from 23 studies. No significant association between the W64R polymorphism and BMI was observed. These findings contrasted with the meta-analysis by Fujisawa et al.[77] published in the same year in which pooled results from 31 studies showed a significantly higher mean BMI (mean difference 0.30 kg/m²) among the R allele carriers than among noncarriers. In 2001, Kurokawa et al.[78] performed a meta-analysis of 27 studies in Japanese populations and found a significant mean difference in BMI of 0.26 kg/m² between R allele carriers and noncarriers. The frequency of the variant was higher in Japanese than in Caucasians, which may have improved the power to detect a small effect of the polymorphism on BMI when meta-analysis was restricted to studies of Japanese populations. However, subsequent studies conducted in other Japanese populations have produced mixed results,[79,80] underscoring the need for further investigations.

Table 21.2 Summary of Meta-Analyses of Candidate Gene Variants Associated with BMI or Obesity-Related Phenotypes

Author (Year)	Gene, Variations	Number of Studies	Findings
Allison et al. (1998)[76]	β3-Adrenergic receptor (ADRB3), W64R	23 studies (n = 7399)	Not significantly associated with BMI
Fujisawa et al. (1998)[77]	ADRB3, W64R	31 studies (n = 9236)	The carriers had significantly higher BMI, with a mean difference of 0.30 (0.13–0.47)
Kurokawa et al. (2001)[78]	ADRB3, W64R	27 studies (n = 6582; all Japanese)	The carriers had significantly higher BMI, with a mean difference of 0.26 (0.18–0.42)
Heo et al. (2002)[87]	Leptin receptor (LEPR), K109R, Q223R, and K656N	9 studies (n = 3263)	None of the three variants was significantly associated with BMI or waist circumference
Masud et al. (2003)[85]	Peroxisome proliferator-activated receptor-γ (PPARG2), P12A	30 studies (n = 19 136)	A12 allele was significantly associated with greater BMI only among those with BMI ≥ 27, with a mean difference of 0.11 between the carriers and noncarriers
Geller et al. (2004)[100]	MC4R, V103I	14 studies (n = 7713)	Significantly associated with lower risk of obesity, OR = 0.69, 95% CI 0.50–0.96
Sookoian et al. (2005)[94]	Tumor Necrosis Factor-α (TNF), −308G>A	Obesity, 8 studies (n = 3562); BMI, 18 studies (n = 5009); WHR, 13 studies, (n = 3910); and leptin level, 4 studies (n = 845)	Associated with increased risk of obesity, OR = 1.23, 95% CI 1.04–1.45; associated with elevated BMI (P = .034) but not waist-to-hip ratio or leptin levels
Paracchini et al. (2005)[86]	Leptin receptor (LEPR), Q223R, K109R, and K656N; PPARG2, P12A	Q223R, 10 studies (n = 2972); K109R, 7 studies (n = 1696); and K656N, 7 studies (n = 2064); and PPARG2, 6 studies (n = 4022) (all healthy subjects)	None of the variants was significantly associated with obesity risk: Q223R, OR = 1.13, 95% CI 0.98–1.30; K109R, OR = 1.05, 95% CI 0.89–1.23; K656N, OR = 1.02, 95% CI 0.86–1.21; and P12A, OR = 1.13, 95% CI 0.98–1.29
Marti et al. (2006)[91]	Glucocorticoid receptor gene (GR or NR3C1), N363S	13 studies (n = 5909)	Carriers had slightly elevated BMI (0.18, 95% CI 0–0.35) than noncarriers. Not significantly associated with obesity risk, OR = 1.02, 95% CI 0.56–1.87
Qi et al. (2007)[99]	Interleukin 6 (IL6), −174G>C	19 studies (n = 26 944)	The genotypes were not significantly associated with BMI, waist circumference, or waist-to-hip ratio

Peroxisome Proliferator Activated Receptor-γ Gene P12A Polymorphism

Peroxisome proliferator activated receptor-γ (*PPARG*) is an attractive obesity candidate gene because it regulates adipocyte differentiation, lipid metabolism, and insulin sensitivity.[81,82] The most frequently studied *PPARG* variant is the proline (P) to alanine (A) substitution at amino acid 12 which reduces *PPARG* activity and improves insulin sensitivity.[83,84] Masud et al.[85] carried out a meta-analysis using 40 datasets from 30 independent studies to examine the effect of the P12A polymorphism on BMI. There was a negligible difference in mean BMI (0.07 kg/m^2) between the A allele carriers and noncarriers. However, stratified analysis revealed significant differences only among obese subjects (mean difference of 0.11 kg/m^2). Recently, Paracchini et al.[86] summarized data from six case-control studies and reported a borderline significant increased risk of obesity associated with the A allele (OR: 1.13, 95% CI: 0.98 to 1.29).

LEPR Gene Polymorphisms

In addition to rare mutations in *LEPR* causing monogenic obesity, several common SNPs on this gene may be relevant to the common form of obesity. Three SNPs resulting in amino acid substitutions, including Q223R, K109R, and K656N, have been extensively examined with respect to obesity. The R223 and R109 variants occur more frequently among Asians than other ethnic groups, while the N656 variant is more frequent among Caucasians.[86] In an earlier meta-analysis, Heo et al.[87] summarized data from 9 studies yielding a total of 3263 related and unrelated subjects from diverse ethnic background. They found no significant relationships between the three *LEPR* alleles and BMI or waist circumference in the overall population or subgroups defined by age, sex, and ethnicity. A more recent meta-analysis of case-control studies yielded similar results.[86] The pooled ORs for obesity were 1.13 (95% CI: 0.98 to 1.30) for Q223R (10 studies), 1.05 (95% CI: 0.89 to 1.23) for K109R (7 studies), and 1.02 (95% CI: 0.86 to 1.21) for K656N (7 studies).

Glucocorticoid Receptor Gene N365S Polymorphism

Increased cortisol production has been implicated in the development of visceral obesity (see Chapter 18). The glucocorticoid receptor belongs to a nuclear receptor subfamily and is involved in the regulation of the transcription of glucocorticoid-responsive genes.[88] The glucocorticoid receptor gene (*GRL*) is located on chromosome 5q31.3 and contains a common asparagine (N) to serine (S) substitution at codon 363 of exon 2. The S variant increases the transactivating capacity and has been shown to be associated with an increased sensitivity to glucocorticoids.[89,90] This variant has been associated with increased BMI, but the results have been inconsistent. Marti et al.[91] conducted a meta-analysis to assess the association between the N363S polymorphism and obesity risk. The analysis, including 5909 subjects from 12 published and 3 unpublished studies, found that carriers of the S allele had a modest but significantly higher BMI than noncarriers (mean difference of 0.18 kg/m^2). However, the association between this variant and obesity risk was not statistically significant.

Tumor Necrosis Factor-α Gene −308G>A Polymorphism

Tumor necrosis factor-α (TNFA) is an inflammatory cytokine that stimulates production of other cytokines and regulates glucose and lipid metabolism and insulin resistance.[92] Adipose tissue is a major source of endogenous TNFA production, and elevated levels of TNFA are associated with increased adiposity and insulin resistance in humans. The G to A substitution at position −308 in the promoter region of the *TNFA* gene has been shown in vitro to enhance nuclear factor binding, resulting in increased transcriptional activity.[93] Sookoian et al.[94] summarized association studies on this polymorphism in relation to obesity, insulin resistance, and hypertension (n = 3,562). There was an increased risk of obesity associated with the combined GA and AA genotypes compared with the GG genotype (OR: 1.23). Mean BMI and WHR, however, were not significantly different between the two genotype groups.

Interleukin-6 Gene −174G>C Polymorphism

Interleukin-6 (IL6) is a proinflammatory cytokine secreted by adipose tissue, immune cells, and muscles. Circulating levels of IL6 are elevated in obesity and predict development of both insulin resistance and type 2 diabetes.[95,96] A −174G>C polymorphism within the *IL6* promoter region has been associated with plasma IL6 levels, fasting insulin levels, measures of insulin sensitivity, and glucose homeostasis.[97,98] However, a recent meta-analysis of 26,944 individuals from 19 studies found no significant association between this SNP and measures of adiposity (BMI, WHR, or waist circumference).[99]

MC4R Gene V103I Polymorphism

Genetic variability in *MC4R* has not only been implicated in monogenic obesity but also the common form of obesity. The V103I polymorphism on this gene has been extensively studied in regard to obesity risk. In a meta-analysis of 7,713 individuals from 14 studies, the pooled OR of obesity for the I allele carriers was 0.69 (95% CI: 0.50 to 0.96).[100] A more recent study of 7,937 participants also reported a significantly inverse association between this variant and obesity risk.[101]

Taken together, meta-analyses suggest modest, if any, associations between widely studied polymorphisms and various measures of obesity. There appears to be more consistent evidence to support associations with genetic variations in *GRL*, *MC4R*, and *TNFA*, but the evidence is far from conclusive. While this review has focused on the main effects of polymorphisms, whether these candidate loci interact with the environment to modulate risk of obesity must also be considered. The topic of gene-environment interactions is further discussed in Chapter 22.

Genome-Wide Association Studies

Although the candidate gene approach has had some successes in identifying susceptible genes for common diseases, it has been hampered by the modest contribution of each SNP to overall heritability, the limited scope in surveying the large number of SNPs in the whole genome, and variability in criteria used for selecting candidate genes and SNPs.[102] The candidate gene approach is also limited by our incomplete understanding of biological mechanisms of the disease. Instead of relying on selecting the correct genes, the GWA approach surveys the entire genome for causal genetic variants in a comprehensive and unbiased manner. Recent advances in genotyping technology have made this approach feasible.[103] Commercially available products commonly used in GWA studies to simultaneously assay hundreds of thousands of loci include the Affymetrix and Illumina SNP chips. The SNPs available on these chip sets are selected either at random across the genome (earlier Affymetrix products) or based on LD from the HapMap (Illumina products and more recent Affymetrix products). These high-density SNP arrays can capture >80% of common variations (minor allele frequency >10%) in the human genome.[104]

Multistage approaches have been commonly used to screen and replicate promising leads from GWA scans.[105] In a two-stage design, a subset of available subjects are genotyped on a genome-wide SNP panel, then a much smaller subset of the most significant markers are genotyped on the remaining subjects. Such a study, if designed and analyzed appropriately, can have nearly as much power at a much lower cost than a single-stage design in which all subjects are genotyped on the genome-wide panel.[106,107] Recently, the GWA approach has identified several common SNPs associated with chronic diseases in unexpected genes. The first successful example was the association between complement factor H variants and age-related macular degeneration.[108] Subsequent GWA studies have identified several novel loci for type 2 diabetes,[109-112] coronary heart disease,[113-115] and other conditions.[116] These findings demonstrate the potential of GWA analyses to identify new susceptibility genes for complex diseases.

The first GWA study specifically on obesity was conducted by Herbert et al.[117] After genotyping 694 participants from the Framingham Heart Study offspring cohort for 116,204 SNPs, the authors found that only SNP rs7566605 G>C near the insulin-induced gene 2 (*INSIG2*) was significantly associated with obesity. The rs7566605 CC genotype was associated with obesity in three replication studies of family-based samples, as well as three of four case-control studies of unrelated individuals. A meta-analysis of all the case-control samples showed that the CC genotype was significantly associated with obesity under a recessive model, with an OR of 1.22. Because *INSIG2* is involved in fatty acid and cholesterol synthesis,[118] it is a plausible obesity candidate gene. However, subsequent replications have been inconsistent.[119-122]

More recently, a GWA scan identified a common variant in the *FTO* gene that was associated with type 2 diabetes risk; this association was entirely mediated through its association with obesity.[123] The association between SNP rs9939609 T>A and BMI, initially discovered in the GWA scan, was replicated in 13 cohorts with 38,759 participants. Adults with the AA genotype (16%) weighed about 3 kg more and had 67% increased risk of obesity compared to those with the TT genotype. Further analysis of two large birth cohorts suggested that the *FTO* SNP was not associated with changes in fetal growth, but was associated with childhood adiposity. The association between *FTO* variants and obesity has been confirmed in several additional studies.[124,125] So far, these variants represent the most replicated genetic markers for common forms of obesity, although biological function of the *FTO* gene remains unknown.[126]

Methodological Problems in Obesity Association Studies

Association studies are commonly used to identify genetic variants that affect polygenic traits such as obesity. Such designs have had some success but have been plagued by lack of reproducibility. In a systematic review, Hirschhorn et al.[127] found that of 166 putative associations studied three or more times, only six were reproduced at least 75% of the time. There are many potential reasons for the lack of reproducibility and these have been discussed extensively.[66,128-130] In the following section we briefly discuss a few of these.

False-Positive Findings and the Winner's Curse

False-positives (type 1 errors) can arise from a number of sources, including chance findings or statistical fluctuation, multiple testing, and publication bias. Most nonreplicated findings in the literature were initially positive, but could not be reproduced in subsequent studies. In most situations, the association in the first positive report exceeded the genetic effect estimated by meta-analysis in subsequent studies, a phenomenon referred to as the *winner's curse*.[131,132] Most of the genetic associations for common obesity reviewed in this chapter follow the *winner's curse* pattern. Thus, the genetic associations identified in the first positive study cannot typically be used to estimate the overall or true genetic effect.[131]

Multiple Testing

With advances in genotyping technology, it is now feasible to assess a large number of SNPs simultaneously, which can increase the risk for false-positives due to multiple testing. This is becoming a growing concern, particularly with the advent of GWA, where hundreds of thousands of markers are assessed simultaneously. For these analyses, the standard significance threshold of $\alpha = 0.05$ (producing one false-positive result for every 20 independent tests) is considered too liberal. Conversely, procedures that maintain strong control of the family-wide error rate (i.e., the probability of any false-positives), such as the Bonferroni correction, which is roughly equivalent to 0.05 divided by the total number of markers tests, are likely to be too conservative, and can increase the number of false-negative results. They are also inappropriate for GWA studies since the extensive LD in the genome ensures that many SNPs are correlated.[133] An appropriate strategy to correct for multiple testing should, therefore, balance the risk of false-positives and false-negatives. Permutation testing is a nonparametric resampling approach that is used to control the family-wide type 1 error rate.[134] Because this approach retains the correlations among SNPs present in the actual data, it is less conservative than the Bonferroni correction. In addition, the false discovery rate (FDR) method has been increasingly used to address the multiple testing issue; it controls the expected proportion of false-positives among all positive results, instead of controlling any chance of false-positive findings (as Bonferroni correction does).[135] This procedure can reduce false-positive results while attaining greater power to detect true discoveries. Ultimately, replication of genetic associations across different populations is the best protection against false-positive findings resulting from multiple testing or other sources.

Genotyping Errors

Though typically low in most modern genotyping platforms, genotyping errors are inevitable in large association studies. They can lead not only to reduced power but also false-positive results.[136] There are many causes of genotyping errors, including DNA contamination, calling of inappropriate alleles, and nonspecificity of experimental assays. The accuracy of genotyping is critical in association studies of complex diseases because a small genetic effect can be easily masked or exaggerated by even a small amount of genotyping error.[137] By genotyping case and control samples together and blinding researchers and technicians to case-control status, systematic genotyping errors can be minimized. Because deviance from Hardy-Weinberg equilibrium (HWE) usually hints at genotyping errors, HWE tests should be performed for each SNP in the control samples before conducting genetic association tests.[138] In GWA studies, stringent quality control procedures are necessary to minimize sample handling errors and remove poor-quality DNAs and SNPs before conducting the association analyses.[110-112]

Population Stratification

Population stratification can arise from disproportionate selection of cases and controls from genetically mixed populations.[139] This particular form of confounding occurs when ethnicity or ancestry distort the relationship between a genetic marker and disease risk.[140] One classic example of population stratification is a strong negative association between the Gm haplotype Gm3;5,13,14 and type 2 diabetes. Although initially observed in a sample of 4920 Pima Indians, it disappeared after adjustment for European ancestry.[141] Because Gm3;5,13,14 is a marker for Caucasian admixture, overrepresentation of European ancestry in the controls led to an artificial inverse association between the marker and diabetes. In the literature, such clear examples of large biases created by population stratification are rare,[142] and several simulation and empirical studies have found little evidence of bias due to stratification in carefully matched case-control designs.[140,143] Potential bias from population stratification can be minimized by selecting cases and controls from an ethnically and racially homogeneous population and controlling for ancestry in the analyses. Prospective cohorts with cases and controls selected from a clearly defined source population are less susceptible to population stratification bias than retrospective studies.

Although large population stratification biases rarely occur between cases and controls, small biases due to subtle differences in genetic background are still of potential concern in association studies, even those with European-derived populations.[144] Devlin and Roeder[145] proposed a genomic control (GC) approach to control for population stratification in association studies. On the basis of the assumption that population stratification often leads to an inflated χ^2 test that too often rejects the null hypothesis, the inflation factor lambda estimated from a set of randomly selected *null* loci are used to statistically correct for observed genetic associations. A drawback of this approach is that it may lead to overcorrection for markers that do not differ in frequency across subpopulations.

More recently, Price et al.[146] proposed a principal component analysis-based method to adjust for population stratification. In this approach, several principal components are derived from genome-wide genotype data to capture population structure. These components are then included in the regression model as covariates to adjust for population structure. Typically, the first few components that capture most ancestry or ethnic differences between cases and controls are included as covariates to adjust for potential population stratification. There is some evidence that this approach is more powerful and provides better control of the type 1 error rate than the GC method.[146]

False-Negative Findings (Type 2 Errors)

False-negative results, usually arising from small underpowered studies, can also contribute to lack of replication in genetic association studies. Because most genetic variants have low penetrance and only modest effects on complex traits such as obesity, a large sample size (often in the range of thousands of cases and controls) is required for power to achieve even nominal significance.[66] One good example is the association between the *PPARG2* P12A variant and risk of type 2 diabetes. An initial study found a strong effect with an OR of 4.35 ($P = .028$) for the PP genotype,[147] but four of five subsequent studies failed to confirm the association. A meta-analysis of more than 3,000 individuals found a modest (1.25-fold) but significant ($P = .002$) increase in diabetes risk associated with the more common P allele.[84] The nonreplication in earlier individual studies is likely due to small sample size and insufficient power. Indeed, recent association studies with much larger sample sizes have further replicated the association.[148,149] This example illustrates that meta-analysis can substantially improve the power of genetic analyses and help reconcile divergent findings from multiple association studies. However, meta-analysis is not a substitute for large and well-designed association studies.

The frequency of the polymorphism is also an important determinant of the power of an association study. Most studies are designed to test the hypothesis that the genetic risk for a complex trait is due to disease predisposing alleles or haplotypes with relatively high frequencies (>5%) on the basis of the *common disease-common variant* hypothesis.[131] A meta-analysis of 25 different reported associations has provided some support for this hypothesis,[131] and several recent studies[150,151] have suggested that a limited number of common haplotypes account for most of the variation in a candidate gene. However, there is also evidence that rare alleles or haplotypes contribute to complex traits. For example, the *GRL* N365S and *MC4R* V103I polymorphisms associated with obesity (discussed earlier) have <5% frequency of the variant allele. Testing the alternative hypothesis that rare alleles or haplotypes are responsible for common obesity will require much larger samples and genotyping efforts than most of the published studies.

Phenotype and/or genotype measurement errors are another consideration in power estimation in association studies[152] because such errors may significantly reduce the power to identify a genetic association. Commonly used measures of obesity, such as BMI and waist circumference, are imperfect measures of adiposity and body fat distribution. In addition, self-reported measures are susceptible to differential misreporting according to actual obesity status (see Chapter 5). These errors, although relatively modest, can lead to diminished power and inconsistent associations in the literature, especially when the true genetic association is small.

Genuine Heterogeneity

Genuine heterogeneity in genetic associations may exist across different studies, although it is often difficult to distinguish it from nonreplications due to biases or inadequate power. As previously mentioned, epidemiologic studies have used BMI, waist circumference, percent body fat, weight change, and plasma leptin concentrations to assess adiposity. Although these measures are highly correlated, they reflect different aspects of fatness that may not be regulated by the same genetic mechanism. Moreover, while some studies have used moderate overweight as the phenotypic outcome, others have focused on morbid obesity. It is possible that the genetic loci contributing to morbid obesity differ from those for mild obesity.

Reduced exposure to environmental pressure may mean that genetics play a larger part in childhood obesity than in late-onset obesity.[4] Thus, obese children are promising target populations for both linkage scans and association studies. In some studies, the magnitude of genetic associations for obesity appears to differ between samples of children and adults.[65] These divergent results may be due to chance, but they may also represent real heterogeneity in the genetics of early-onset and late-onset obesity. Different genetic or environmental backgrounds in diverse populations are another source of genuine heterogeneity. To date, most genetic association studies of obesity and other complex traits have been conducted in white populations. For individual studies and meta-analyses, it is desirable to have ethnically homogenous samples that reduce potential bias due to population stratification. However, different genetic architecture and allele frequencies in different ethnic groups make it important to replicate these associations in other racial and ethnic groups. The evidence for causality is strengthened if the same variant is found to be associated with the disease in multiple ethnic groups. However, lack of replication in other ethnic or racial groups does not necessarily invalidate the observed genetic associations because some genetic risk may be ethnic-specific.

Gene-environment interactions can also contribute to genuine heterogeneity in genetic associations. The premise of such interactions is that the genetic association is contingent on the environmental context of the populations. Thus, a genetic effect may manifest in one population but not the other, depending on background dietary and lifestyle factors. Although gene-environment interactions are widely believed to explain many of the inconsistent results in the literature, the search for such interactions has been challenging both conceptually and methodologically. In the next chapter, we will discuss the role of gene-environmental interactions in the development of obesity.

Summary

Efforts to map monogenic forms of obesity have been met with great success. Most monogenic obesity cases discovered so far appear to be caused by genetic alterations of the leptin and melanocortin pathways, including rare mutations on the *LEP*, *LEPR*, *PC1*, *POMC*, and *MC4R* genes. These genes play critical roles in appetite control, food intake, and energy homeostasis. Disruption of the functions of these genes causes childhood onset of severe forms of obesity. However, the number of obesity cases caused by single-gene mutations is extremely small. To date, less than 200 human obesity cases caused by single-gene mutations in 11 different genes have been reported in the literature,[53] but these mutations do not appear to contribute to common forms of obesity.

Mapping genes for common forms of obesity has proven more difficult than initially anticipated. Despite a strong hereditary component of common obesity, the contributions of individual genes have not been clearly elucidated and most genetic associations have not been reproduced. Meta-analyses have been conducted for several commonly studied polymorphisms (Table 21.2). Overall, there is suggestive evidence to support the associations for the *GRL* N365S, *MC4R* V103I, and *TNF* −308 G>A polymorphisms, but the genetic effects are small and additional confirmation in large samples is clearly needed.

GWA scans have recently emerged as a comprehensive and powerful approach to identify genetic variants related to complex diseases. Using this approach, several common genetic variants associated with chronic disease have been uncovered in unexpected genes. The association between *FTO* variants and obesity identified through a diabetes GWA scan has been replicated in multiple populations. Because many GWA studies on chronic diseases have been conducted or are underway, and virtually all have collected anthropometric information, the data generated by these studies will provide a tremendous resource for identifying obesity susceptibility genes. Pooled analyses of these GWA studies are necessary to improve power and reduce false negative results.

Similar to other complex diseases, the puzzle of common obesity genetics cannot be solved through a single approach. Future studies will need to harness the resources from large, well-powered population-based studies for initial discovery, replication, and mining of gene-gene and gene-environment interactions for common types of obesity. Although GWA studies will become the mainstay of genetic epidemiology, functional and positional candidate genes will continue to be investigated in genetic association studies of obesity. The identified associations need to be replicated in different ethnic and racial groups. Furthermore, fine mapping and functional studies are required to identify the causal variants. Animal models of obesity, gene expression studies, and advances in genomics technology will continue to provide new insights into biological mechanisms of obesity as well as new tools for genetic epidemiologic research.

References

1. Hofbauer KG. Molecular pathways to obesity. *Int J Obes Relat Metab Disord.* 2002;26(Suppl 2):S18-S27.
2. Cummings DE, Schwartz MW. Genetics and pathophysiology of human obesity. *Annu Rev Med.* 2003;54:453-471.
3. Clement K, Ferre P. Genetics and the pathophysiology of obesity. *Pediatr Res.* 2003;53:721-725.
4. Bell CG, Walley AJ, Froguel P. The genetics of human obesity. *Nat Rev Genet.* 2005;6:221-234.
5. Clement K. Genetics of human obesity. *Proc Nutr Soc.* 2005;64:133-142.
6. Clement K. Genetics of human obesity. *C R Biol.* 2006;329:608-622.
7. Farooqi IS, O'Rahilly S. Monogenic obesity in humans. *Annu Rev Med.* 2005;56: 443-458.
8. Farooqi IS, Wangensteen T, Collins S, et al. Clinical and molecular genetic spectrum of congenital deficiency of the leptin receptor. *N Engl J Med.* 2007;18:237-247.
9. Zhang Y, Proenca R, Maffei M, Barone M, Leopold L, Friedman JM. Positional cloning of the mouse obese gene and its human homologue. *Nature.* 1994;372:425-432.
10. Horvath TL, Diano S, Sotonyi P, Heiman M, Tschop M. Minireview: ghrelin and the regulation of energy balance—a hypothalamic perspective. *Endocrinology.* 2001;142:4163-4169.
11. Montague CT, Farooqi IS, Whitehead JP, et al. Congenital leptin deficiency is associated with severe early-onset obesity in humans. *Nature.* 1997;387:903-908.
12. Farooqi IS, Matarese G, Lord GM, et al. Beneficial effects of leptin on obesity, T cell hyporesponsiveness, and neuroendocrine/metabolic dysfunction of human congenital leptin deficiency. *J Clin Invest.* 2002;110:1093-1103.
13. Chen H, Charlat O, Tartaglia LA, et al. Evidence that the diabetes gene encodes the leptin receptor: identification of a mutation in the leptin receptor gene in db/db mice. *Cell.* 1996;84:491-495.
14. Chua SC Jr, Chung WK, Wu-Peng XS, et al. Phenotypes of mouse diabetes and rat fatty due to mutations in the OB (leptin) receptor. *Science.* 1996;271:994-996.
15. Clement K, Vaisse C, Lahlou N, et al. A mutation in the human leptin receptor gene causes obesity and pituitary dysfunction. *Nature.* 1998;392:398-401.
16. Jackson RS, Creemers JW, Ohagi S, et al. Obesity and impaired prohormone processing associated with mutations in the human prohormone convertase 1 gene. *Nat Genet.* 1997;16:303-306.
17. Jackson RS, Creemers JW, Farooqi IS, et al. Small-intestinal dysfunction accompanies the complex endocrinopathy of human proprotein convertase 1 deficiency. *J Clin Invest.* 2003;112:1550-1560.
18. Krude H, Biebermann H, Luck W, Horn R, Brabant G, Gruters A. Severe early-onset obesity, adrenal insufficiency and red hair pigmentation caused by POMC mutations in humans. *Nat Genet.* 1998;19:155-157.
19. Krude H, Biebermann H, Schnabel D, et al. Obesity due to proopiomelanocortin deficiency: three new cases and treatment trials with thyroid hormone and ACTH4-10. *J Clin Endocrinol Metab.* 2003;88:4633-4640.
20. Krude H, Biebermann H, Gruters A. Mutations in the human proopiomelanocortin gene. *Ann NY Acad Sci.* 2003;994:233-239.

21. Mountjoy KG, Mortrud MT, Low MJ, Simerly RB, Cone RD. Localization of the melanocortin-4 receptor (MC4-R) in neuroendocrine and autonomic control circuits in the brain. *Mol Endocrinol*. 1994;8:1298-1308.
22. Huszar D, Lynch CA, Fairchild-Huntress V, et al. Targeted disruption of the melanocortin-4 receptor results in obesity in mice. *Cell*. 1997;88:131-141.
23. Yeo GS, Farooqi IS, Aminian S, Halsall DJ, Stanhope RG, O'Rahilly S. A frameshift mutation in MC4R associated with dominantly inherited human obesity. *Nat Genet*. 1998;111:2.
24. Vaisse C, Clement K, Guy-Grand B, Froguel P. A frameshift mutation in human MC4R is associated with a dominant form of obesity. *Nat Gene*. 1998;20:113-114.
25. Farooqi IS, Yeo GS, Keogh JM, et al. Dominant and recessive inheritance of morbid obesity associated with melanocortin 4 receptor deficiency. *J Clin Invest*. 2000;106:271-279.
26. Tao YX. Molecular mechanisms of the neural melanocortin receptor dysfunction in severe early onset obesity. *Mol Cell Endocrinol*. 2005;239:1-14.
27. Jacobson P, Ukkola O, Rankinen T, et al. Melanocortin 4 receptor sequence variations are seldom a cause of human obesity: the Swedish Obese Subjects, the HERITAGE Family Study, and a Memphis cohort. *J Clin Endocrinol Metab*. 2002;87:4442-4446.
28. Hinney A, Bettecken T, Tarnow P, et al. Prevalence, spectrum, and functional characterization of melanocortin-4 receptor gene mutations in a representative population-based sample and obese adults from Germany. *J Clin Endocrinol Metab*. 2006;91:1761-1769.
29. Lubrano-Berthelier C, Dubern B, Lacorte JM, et al. Melanocortin 4 receptor mutations in a large cohort of severely obese adults: prevalence, functional classification, genotype-phenotype relationship, and lack of association with binge eating. *J Clin Endocrinol Metab*. 2006;91:1811-1818.
30. Ma L, Tataranni PA, Bogardus C, Baier LJ. Melanocortin 4 receptor gene variation is associated with severe obesity in Pima Indians. *Diabetes*. 2004;53:2696-2699.
31. Goldstone AP. Prader-Willi syndrome: advances in genetics, pathophysiology and treatment. *Trends Endocrinol Metab*. 2004;15:12-20.
32. DelParigi A, Tschop M, Heiman ML, et al. High circulating ghrelin: a potential cause for hyperphagia and obesity in Prader-Willi syndrome. *J Clin Endocrinol Metab*. 2002;87:5461-5464.
33. Sheffield VC. Use of isolated populations in the study of a human obesity syndrome, the Bardet-Biedl syndrome. *Pediatr Res*. 2004;55:908-911.
34. Benzinou M, Walley A, Lobbens S, et al. Bardet-Biedl syndrome gene variants are associated with both childhood and adult common obesity in French Caucasians. *Diabetes*. 2006;55:2876-2882.
35. Bouchard C, Perusse L, Rice T, Rao DC. Chapter 9: Genetics of human obesity. In: Bray GA, Bouchard C, eds. *Handbook of Obesity: Etiology and Pathophysiology*. 2nd ed. New York: Marcel Dekker; 2004.
36. Maes HH, Neale MC, Eaves LJ. Genetic and environmental factors in relative body weight and human adiposity. *Behav Genet*. 1997;27:325-351.
37. Feinleib M, Garrison RJ, Fabsitz R, et al. The NHLBI twin study of cardiovascular disease risk factors: methodology and summary of results. *Am J Epidemiol*. 1977;106:284-285.
38. Bouchard C, Perusse L. Genetic aspects of obesity. *Ann NY Acad Sci*. 1993;699:26-35.
39. Hanisch D, Dittmar M, Hohler T, Alt KW. Contribution of genetic and environmental factors to variation in body compartments—a twin study in adults. *Anthropol Anz*. 2004;62:51-60.
40. Nguyen TV, Howard GM, Kelly PJ, Eisman JA. Bone mass, lean mass, and fat mass: same genes or same environments? *Am J Epidemiol*. 1998;147:3-16.
41. Faith MS, Pietrobelli A, Nunez C, Heo M, Heymsfield SB, Allison DB. Evidence for independent genetic influences on fat mass and body mass index in a pediatric twin sample. *Pediatrics*. 1999;104(1 Pt):61-67.

42. Rose KM, Newman B, Mayer-Davis EJ, Selby JV. Genetic and behavioral determinants of waist-hip ratio and waist circumference in women twins. *Obes Res.* 1998;6:383-392.

43. Selby JV, Newman B, Quesenberry CP Jr, et al. Genetic and behavioral influences on body fat distribution. *Int J Obes.* 1990;14:593-602.

44. Schousboe K, Visscher PM, Erbas B, et al. Twin study of genetic and environmental influences on adult body size, shape, and composition. *Int J Obes Relat Metab Disord.* 2004;28:39-48.

45. Li HJ, Ji CY, Wang W, Hu YH. A twin study for serum leptin, soluble leptin receptor, and free insulin-like growth factor-I in pubertal females. *J Clin Endocrinol Metab.* 2005;90:3659-3664.

46. Narkiewicz K, Szczech R, Winnicki M, et al. Heritability of plasma leptin levels: a twin study. *J Hypertens.* 1999;17:27-31.

47. Allison DB, Kaprio J, Korkeila M, Koskenvuo M, Neale MC, Hayakawa K. The heritability of body mass index among an international sample of monozygotic twins reared apart. *Int J Obes Relat Metab Disord.* 1996;20:501-506.

48. Stunkard AJ, Sorensen TI, Hanis C, et al. An adoption study of human obesity. *N Engl J Med.* 1986;314:193-198.

49. Dawn Teare M, Barrett JH. Genetic linkage studies. *Lancet.* 2005;366:1036-1044.

50. Morton NE. Sequential tests for the detection of linkage. *Am J Hum Genet.* 1955;7:277-318.

51. Lander E, Kruglyak L. Genetic dissection of complex traits: guidelines for interpreting and reporting linkage results. *Nat Genet.* 1995;11:241-247.

52. Khoury MJ, Beaty TH, Cohen BH. *Fundamentals of Genetic Epidemiology.* New York: Oxford University Press; 1993.

53. Rankinen T, Zuberi A, Chagnon YC, et al. The human obesity gene map: the 2005 update. *Obesity (Silver Spring).* 2006;14:529-644.

54. Risch NJ. Searching for genetic determinants in the new millennium. *Nature.* 2000;405:847-856.

55. Comuzzie AG, Allison DB. The search for human obesity genes. *Science.* 1998;280:1374-1377.

56. Hager J, Dina C, Francke S, et al. A genome-wide scan for human obesity genes reveals a major susceptibility locus on chromosome 10. *Nat Genet.* 1998;20:304-308.

57. Saar K, Geller F, Ruschendorf F, et al. Genome scan for childhood and adolescent obesity in German families. *Pediatrics.* 2003;111:321-327.

58. Boutin P, Dina C, Vasseur F, et al. GAD2 on chromosome 10p12 is a candidate gene for human obesity. *PLoS Biol.* 2003;1:E68.

59. Zheng H, Corkern M, Stoyanova I, Patterson LM, Tian R, Berthoud HR. Peptides that regulate food intake: appetite-inducing accumbens manipulation activates hypothalamic orexin neurons and inhibits POMC neurons. *Am J Physiol Regul Integr Comp Physiol.* 2003;284:R1436-R1444.

60. Swarbrick MM, Waldenmaier B, Pennacchio LA, et al. Lack of support for the association between GAD2 polymorphisms and severe human obesity. *PLoS Biol.* 2005;3:e315.

61. Meyre D, Boutin P, Tounian A, et al. Is glutamate decarboxylase 2 (GAD2) a genetic link between low birth weight and subsequent development of obesity in children? *J Clin Endocrinol Metab.* 2005;90:2384-2390.

62. Ohman M, Oksanen L, Kaprio J, et al. Genome-wide scan of obesity in Finnish sibpairs reveals linkage to chromosome Xq24. *J Clin Endocrinol Metab.* 2000;85:3183-3190.

63. Suviolahti E, Oksanen LJ, Ohman M, et al. The SLC6A14 gene shows evidence of association with obesity. *J Clin Invest.* 2003;112:1762-1772.

64. Tiwari HK, Allison DB. Do allelic variants of SLC6A14 predispose to obesity? *J Clin Invest.* 2003;112:1633-1636.

65. Durand E, Boutin P, Meyre D, et al. Polymorphisms in the amino acid transporter solute carrier family 6 (neurotransmitter transporter) member 14 gene contribute to polygenic obesity in French Caucasians. *Diabetes.* 2004;53:2483-2486.

66. Newton-Cheh C, Hirschhorn JN. Genetic association studies of complex traits: design and analysis issues. *Mutat Res.* 2005;573:54-69.

67. Neale BM, Sham PC. The future of association studies: gene-based analysis and replication. *Am J Hum Genet.* 2004;75:353-362.

68. International HapMap Consortium. A haplotype map of the human genome. *Nature.* 2005;437:1299-1320.

69. de Bakker PI, Yelensky R, Pe'er I, Gabriel SB, Daly MJ, Altshuler D. Efficiency and power in genetic association studies. *Nat Genet.* 2005;37:1217-1223.

70. Carlson CS, Eberle MA, Rieder MJ, Yi Q, Kruglyak L, Nickerson DA. Selecting a maximally informative set of single-nucleotide polymorphisms for association analyses using linkage disequilibrium. *Am J Hum Genet.* 2004;74:106-120.

71. Spielman RS, McGinnis RE, Ewens WJ. Transmission test for linkage disequilibrium: the insulin gene region and insulin-dependent diabetes mellitus (IDDM). *Am J Hum Genet.* 1993;52:506-516.

72. Krief S, Lonnqvist F, Raimbault S, et al. Tissue distribution of beta 3-adrenergic receptor mRNA in man. *J Clin Invest.* 1993;91:344-349.

73. Clement K, Vaisse C, Manning, B St. J., et al. Genetic variation in the beta3-adrenergic receptor and an increased capacity to gain weight in patients with morbid obesity. *N Engl J Med.* 1995;333:352-354.

74. Kadowaki H, Yasuda K, Iwamoto K, et al. A mutation in the beta 3-adrenergic receptor gene is associated with obesity and hyperinsulinemia in Japanese subjects. *Biochem Biophys Res Commun.* 1995;215:555-560.

75. Widen E, Lehto M, Kanninen T, Walston J, Shuldiner AR, Groop LC. Association of a polymorphism in the beta 3-adrenergic-receptor gene with features of the insulin resistance syndrome in Finns. *N Engl J Med.* 1995;10:348-351.

76. Allison DB, Heo M, Faith MS, Pietrobelli A. Meta-analysis of the association of the Trp64Arg polymorphism in the beta3 adrenergic receptor with body mass index. *Int J Obes Relat Metab Disord.* 1998;22:559-566.

77. Fujisawa T, Ikegami H, Kawaguchi Y, Ogihara T. Meta-analysis of the association of Trp64Arg polymorphism of beta 3-adrenergic receptor gene with body mass index. *J Clin Endocrinol Metab.* 1998;83:2441-2444.

78. Kurokawa N, Nakai K, Kameo S, Liu ZM, Satoh H. Association of BMI with the beta3-adrenergic receptor gene polymorphism in Japanese: meta-analysis. *Obes Res.* 2001;9:741-745.

79. Oizumi T, Daimon M, Saitoh T, et al. Genotype Arg/Arg, but not Trp/Arg, of the Trp64Arg polymorphism of the beta(3)-adrenergic receptor is associated with type 2 diabetes and obesity in a large Japanese sample. *Diabetes Care.* 2001;24:1579-1583.

80. Matsushita Y, Yokoyama T, Yoshiike N, et al. The Trp(64)Arg polymorphism of the beta(3)-adrenergic receptor gene is not associated with body weight or body mass index in Japanese: a longitudinal analysis. *J Clin Endocrinol Metab.* 2003;88:5914-5920.

81. Berger J, Moller DE. The mechanisms of action of PPARs. *Annu Rev Med.* 2002;53:409-435.

82. Ristow M, Muller-Wieland D, Pfeiffer A, Krone W, Kahn CR. Obesity associated with a mutation in a genetic regulator of adipocyte differentiation. *N Engl J Med.* 1998;339:953-959.

83. Stumvoll M, Haring H. The peroxisome proliferator-activated receptor-gamma2 Pro12Ala polymorphism. *Diabetes.* 2002;51:2341-2347.

84. Altshuler D, Hirschhorn JN, Klannemark M, et al. The common PPARgamma Pro12-Ala polymorphism is associated with decreased risk of type 2 diabetes. *Nat Genet.* 2000;26:76-80.

85. Masud S, Ye S, SAS Group. Effect of the peroxisome proliferator activated receptor-gamma gene Pro12Ala variant on body mass index: a meta-analysis. *J Med Genet.* 2003;40:773-780.

86. Paracchini V, Pedotti P, Taioli E. Genetics of leptin and obesity: a HuGE review. *Am J Epidemiol.* 2005;162:101-114.

87. Heo M, Leibel RL, Fontaine KR, et al. A meta-analytic investigation of linkage and association of common leptin receptor (LEPR) polymorphisms with body mass index and waist circumference. *Int J Obes Relat Metab Disord.* 2002;26:640-646.

88. van Rossum EF, Russcher H, Lamberts SW. Genetic polymorphisms and multifactorial diseases: facts and fallacies revealed by the glucocorticoid receptor gene. *Trends Endocrinol Metab.* 2005;16:445-450.

89. Huizenga NA, Koper JW, De Lange P, et al. A polymorphism in the glucocorticoid receptor gene may be associated with and increased sensitivity to glucocorticoids in vivo. *J Clin Endocrinol Metab.* 1998;83:144-151.

90. Lin RC, Wang WY, Morris BJ. High penetrance, overweight, and glucocorticoid receptor variant: case-control study. *BMJ.* 1999;319:1337-1338.

91. Marti A, Ochoa MC, Sanchez-Villegas A, et al. Meta-analysis on the effect of the N363S polymorphism of the glucocorticoid receptor gene (GRL) on human obesity. *BMC Med Genet.* 2006;7:50.

92. Hotamisligil GS, Spiegelman BM. Tumor necrosis factor alpha: a key component of the obesity-diabetes link. *Diabetes.* 1994;43:1271-1278.

93. Kroeger KM, Carville KS, Abraham LJ. The -308 tumor necrosis factor-alpha promoter polymorphism effects transcription. *Mol Immunol.* 1997;34:391-399.

94. Sookoian SC, Gonzalez C, Pirola CJ. Meta-analysis on the G-308A tumor necrosis factor alpha gene variant and phenotypes associated with the metabolic syndrome. *Obes Res.* 2005;13:2122-2131.

95. Pickup JC, Mattock MB, Chusney GD, Burt D. NIDDM as a disease of the innate immune system: association of acute-phase reactants and interleukin-6 with metabolic syndrome X. *Diabetologia.* 1997;40:1286-1292.

96. Hu FB, Meigs JB, Li TY, Rifai N, Manson JE. Inflammatory markers and risk of developing type 2 diabetes in women. *Diabetes.* 2004;53:693-700.

97. Fernandez-Real JM, Broch M, Vendrell J, et al. Interleukin-6 gene polymorphism and insulin sensitivity. *Diabetes.* 2000;49:517-520.

98. Kubaszek A, Pihlajamaki J, Punnonen K, Karhapaa P, Vauhkonen I, Laakso M. The C-174G promoter polymorphism of the IL-6 gene affects energy expenditure and insulin sensitivity. *Diabetes.* 2003;52:558-561.

99. Qi L, Zhang C, van Dam RM, Hu FB. Interleukin-6 genetic variability and adiposity: associations in two prospective cohorts and systematic review in 26,944 individuals. *J Clin Endocrinol Metab.* 2007;92:3618-3625.

100. Geller F, Reichwald K, Dempfle A, et al. Melanocortin-4 receptor gene variant I103 is negatively associated with obesity. *Am J Hum Genet.* 2004;74:572-581.

101. Heid IM, Vollmert C, Hinney A, et al. Association of the 103I MC4R allele with decreased body mass in 7937 participants of two population based surveys. *J Med Genet.* 2005;42:e21.

102. Hirschhorn JN, Daly MJ. Genome-wide association studies for common diseases and complex traits. *Nat Rev Genet.* 2005;6:95-108.

103. Altshuler D, Daly M. Guilt beyond a reasonable doubt. *Nat Genet.* 2007;39(7):813-815.

104. Pe'er I, de Bakker PI, Maller J, Yelensky R, Altshuler D, Daly MJ. Evaluating and improving power in whole-genome association studies using fixed marker sets. *Nat Genet.* 2006;38:663-667.

105. Kraft P. Efficient two-stage genome-wide association designs based on false positive report probabilities. *Pac Symp Biocomput.* 2006:523-534.

106. Wang H, Thomas DC, Pe'er I, Stram DO. Optimal two-stage genotyping designs for genome-wide association scans. *Genet Epidemiol.* 2006;30:356-368.

107. Skol AD, Scott LJ, Abecasis GR, Boehnke M. Joint analysis is more efficient than replication-based analysis for two-stage genome-wide association studies. *Nat Genet.* 2006;38:209-213.

108. Klein RJ, Zeiss C, Chew EY, et al. Complement factor H polymorphism in age-related macular degeneration. *Science.* 2005;308:385-389.

109. Sladek R, Rocheleau G, Rung J, et al. A genome-wide association study identifies novel risk loci for type 2 diabetes. *Nature.* 2007;445:881-885.

110. Zeggini E, Weedon MN, Lindgren CM, et al. Replication of genome-wide association signals in UK samples reveals risk loci for type 2 diabetes. *Science.* 2007;316:1336-1341.

111. Diabetes Genetics Initiative of Broad Institute of Harvard and MIT, Lund University and Novartis Institutes of BioMedical Research, Saxena R, et al. Genome-wide association analysis identifies loci for type 2 diabetes and triglyceride levels. *Science.* 2007;316:1331-1336.

112. Scott LJ, Mohlke KL, Bonnycastle LL, et al. A genome-wide association study of type 2 diabetes in Finns detects multiple susceptibility variants. *Science.* 2007;316:1341-1345.

113. McPherson R, Pertsemlidis A, Kavaslar N, et al. A common allele on chromosome 9 associated with coronary heart disease. *Science.* 2007;316:1488-1491.

114. Helgadottir A, Thorleifsson G, Manolescu A, et al. A common variant on chromosome 9p21 affects the risk of myocardial infarction. *Science.* 2007;316:1491-1493.

115. Samani NJ, Erdmann J, Hall AS, et al. Genomewide association analysis of coronary artery disease. *N Engl J Med.* 2007;357:443-453.

116. Wellcome Trust Case Control Consortium. Genome-wide association study of 14,000 cases of seven common diseases and 3,000 shared controls. *Nature.* 2007;447:661-678.

117. Herbert A, Gerry NP, McQueen MB, et al. A common genetic variant is associated with adult and childhood obesity. *Science.* 2006;312:279-283.

118. Yabe D, Brown MS, Goldstein JL. Insig-2, a second endoplasmic reticulum protein that binds SCAP and blocks export of sterol regulatory element-binding proteins. *Proc Natl Acad Sci USA.* 2002;99:12753-12758.

119. Dina C, Meyre D, Samson C, et al. Comment on "A common genetic variant is associated with adult and childhood obesity." *Science.* 2007;315:187.

120. Loos RJ, Barroso I, O'rahilly S, Wareham NJ. Comment on "A common genetic variant is associated with adult and childhood obesity." *Science.* 2007;315:187.

121. Rosskopf D, Bornhorst A, Rimmbach C, et al. Comment on "A common genetic variant is associated with adult and childhood obesity." *Science.* 2007;315:187.

122. Lyon HN, Emilsson V, Hinney A, et al. The association of a SNP upstream of INSIG2 with body mass index is reproduced in several but not all cohorts.*PLoS Genet.* 2007;3(4):e61.

123. Frayling TM, Timpson NJ, Weedon MN, et al. A common variant in the FTO gene is associated with body mass index and predisposes to childhood and adult obesity. *Science.* 2007;316:889-894.

124. Scuteri A, Sanna S, Chen WM, et al. Genome-wide association scan shows genetic variants in the FTO gene are associated with obesity-related traits. *PLoS Genet.* 2007;3:e115.

125. Dina C, Meyre D, Gallina S, et al. Variation in FTO contributes to childhood obesity and severe adult obesity. *Nat Genet.* 2007;39:724-726.

126. Groop L. From fused toes in mice to human obesity. *Nat Genet.* 2007;39(6):706-707.

127. Hirschhorn JN, Lohmueller K, Byrne E, Hirschhorn K. A comprehensive review of genetic association studies. *Genet Med.* 2002;4:45-61.

128. Hattersley AT, McCarthy MI. What makes a good genetic association study? *Lancet.* 2005;366:1315-1323.

129. Cordell HJ, Clayton DG. Genetic association studies. *Lancet.* 2005;366:1121-1131.

130. Kathiresan S, Newton-Cheh C, Gerszten RE. On the interpretation of genetic association studies. *Eur Heart J.* 2004;25:1378-1381.

131. Lohmueller KE, Pearce CL, Pike M, Lander ES, Hirschhorn JN. Meta-analysis of genetic association studies supports a contribution of common variants to susceptibility to common disease. *Nat Genet.* 2003;33:177-182.

132. Ioannidis JP, Ntzani EE, Trikalinos TA, Contopoulos-Ioannidis DG. Replication validity of genetic association studies. *Nat Genet.* 2001;29:306-309.

133. Nyholt DR. A simple correction for multiple testing for single-nucleotide polymorphisms in linkage disequilibrium with each other. *Am J Hum Genet.* 2004;74:765-769.

134. Dudbridge F. A note on permutation tests in multistage association scans. *Am J Hum Genet.* 2006;78(6):1094-1095.

135. Benjamini Y, Drai D, Elmer G, Kafkafi N, Golani I. Controlling the false discovery rate in behavior genetics research. *Behav Brain Res.* 2001;125:279-284.

136. Hao K, Li C, Rosenow C, Hung Wong W. Estimation of genotype error rate using samples with pedigree information—an application on the GeneChip Mapping 10K array. *Genomics.* 2004;84:623-630.

137. Xu J, Turner A, Little J, Bleecker ER, Meyers DA. Positive results in association studies are associated with departure from Hardy-Weinberg equilibrium: hint for genotyping error? *Hum Genet.* 2002;111:573-574.

138. Hosking L, Lumsden S, Lewis K, et al. Detection of genotyping errors by Hardy-Weinberg equilibrium testing. *Eur J Hum Genet.* 2004;12:395-399.

139. Redden DT, Allison DB. Nonreplication in genetic association studies of obesity and diabetes research. *J Nutr.* 2003;133:3323-3326.

140. Wacholder S, Rothman N, Caporaso N. Population stratification in epidemiologic studies of common genetic variants and cancer: quantification of bias. *J Natl Cancer Inst.* 2000;92:1151-1158.

141. Knowler WC, Williams RC, Pettitt DJ, Steinberg AG. Gm3;5,13,14 and type 2 diabetes mellitus: an association in American Indians with genetic admixture. *Am J Hum Genet.* 1988;43:520-526.

142. Cardon LR, Palmer LJ. Population stratification and spurious allelic association. *Lancet.* 2003;361:598-604.

143. Ardlie KG, Lunetta KL, Seielstad M. Testing for population subdivision and association in four case-control studies. *Am J Hum Genet.* 2002;71:304-311.

144. Campbell CD, Ogburn EL, Lunetta KL, et al. Demonstrating stratification in a European American population. *Nat Genet.* 2005;37:868-872.

145. Devlin B, Roeder K. Genomic control for association studies. *Biometrics.* 1999;55:997-1004.

146. Price AL, Patterson NJ, Plenge RM, Weinblatt ME, Shadick NA, Reich D. Principal components analysis corrects for stratification in genome-wide association studies. *Nat Genet.* 2006;38:904-909.

147. Deeb SS, Fajas L, Nemoto M, et al. A Pro12Ala substitution in PPARgamma2 associated with decreased receptor activity, lower body mass index and improved insulin sensitivity. *Nat Genet.* 1998;20:284-287.

148. Florez JC, Burtt N, de Bakker PI, et al. Haplotype structure and genotype-phenotype correlations of the sulfonylurea receptor and the islet ATP-sensitive potassium channel gene region. *Diabetes.* 2004;53:1360-1368.

149. Weedon MN, McCarthy MI, Hitman G, et al. Combining information from common type 2 diabetes risk polymorphisms improves disease prediction. *PLoS Med.* 2006;3:e374.

150. Johnson GC, Esposito L, Barratt BJ, et al. Haplotype tagging for the identification of common disease genes. *Nat Genet.* 2001;29:233-237.

151. Daly MJ, Rioux JD, Schaffner SF, Hudson TJ, Lander ES. High-resolution haplotype structure in the human genome. *Nat Genet.* 2001;29:229-232.

152. Gordon D, Finch SJ. Factors affecting statistical power in the detection of genetic association. *J Clin Invest.* 2005;115:1408.

22

Gene-Environment Interactions and Obesity

Frank B. Hu

Compelling evidence indicates that the escalating obesity epidemic is largely driven by changes in diet and lifestyle within a relatively short period of time (i.e., the past several decades). Migrant studies have shown that when people migrate from developing countries with a low prevalence of obesity to Western countries, their risk of obesity increases substantially.[1] Aboriginal populations that undergo Westernization of diet and lifestyle, such as North American Indians[2] and Western Samoans,[3,4] have also experienced dramatic increases in obesity and type 2 diabetes. However, ethnic differences in obesity rates cannot be explained by diet and lifestyle factors alone, and there is strong evidence from family and twin studies that genetic predisposition plays an important role in the development of obesity (see Chapter 21). In addition, convincing evidence demonstrates tremendous interindividual variability of weight change in response to identical dietary or lifestyle interventions. Such variability may be related to undetermined genetic factors.

In his seminal paper, Neel[5] proposed the *thrifty gene* hypothesis—that obesity and diabetes are caused by exaggerated expressions of genotypes for efficient metabolism, which confer advantage in times of nutrient scarcity but contribute to excess energy storage and increased risk of obesity in an energy-abundant environment when combined with an increasingly inactive lifestyle.[1] This hypothesis, postulating an interaction between our ancestral genes and modern environment, has been widely used to explain the very high prevalence of obesity and diabetes in certain populations, such as Pima Indians.[6]

Despite the conceptual appeal of the *thrifty gene* hypothesis, the identification of specific genes and gene-environment interactions related to obesity has been challenging. In this chapter, we discuss several aspects of gene-environment interactions, beginning with conceptual and statistical models, followed by various study designs for identifying gene-environment interactions. Then we summarize results from both intervention and observational studies of gene-environment interactions on obesity and weight change. Finally, we discuss methodological issues in the study of gene-environment interactions, including sample size requirements, the problem of multiple comparisons, lack of replication, and study designs.

Conceptual Models of Gene-Environment Interactions

The idea of gene-environment interactions is not new. As early as 1938, Scottish geneticist J. B. S. Haldane[7] first proposed the conceptual model of "interaction of nature and nurture." In 1942, Tryon[8] conducted a classic experiment demonstrating that the maze-running ability of mice was both genetically and environmentally determined, with the genetic effect dependent on certain environmental conditions. It has become clear over the past decades that many human traits or diseases are products of gene-environment interactions. A classic example is phenylketonuria (PKU), a recessive trait that results from mutations in the gene coding the enzyme phenylalanine hydroxylase (PAH).[9] A defect in the enzyme that leads to an accumulation of phenylalanine in the blood can cause neurological damage and mental retardation. PKU can be screened in newborn infants, and the disease can be treated with a strict low-phenylalanine diet.

PKU is an obvious example of a disease that requires both a genetic defect and an environmental factor (i.e., dietary phenylalanine). For common forms of obesity and other chronic diseases, the interactions between genes and environmental factors are much more subtle and complicated, and practical implications for prevention and treatment are also much less clear. Loos and Bouchard[10] theorized four scenarios of genetic susceptibility to obesity, given an increasingly obesogenic environment (Fig. 22.1). Besides rare monogenic obesity caused by single gene mutations (see Chapter 21), the three additional scenarios include strong predisposition, slight predisposition triggered by changes in lifestyle (e.g., diet and exercise), and genetic resistance, even in a highly obesogenic environment. Most people probably have some genetic predisposition to obesity, depending on ethnicity and family history. However, a change in environment (diet and lifestyle) is necessary to trigger the expression of the obesity-related phenotypes. As an example, the Pima Indians living in the remote Mexican Sierra Madre Mountains have much lower prevalence of obesity and diabetes than those living in Arizona,[11] despite their common genetic background. It is likely that among Pima Indians living in Arizona, their genetic predisposition to obesity is greatly magnified by the change from a traditional lifestyle to a modern environment.

Thus, obesity is a multifactorial disease produced by the interplay between genetic and environmental factors. Unlike the rare genetic mutations that cause monogenic diseases, genetic factors that underlie individual susceptibility to common forms of obesity most likely have only modest effects that are amplified in the presence of certain triggering environmental factors.[12] On the other hand, given the same dietary and lifestyle factors, some individuals may be more prone to weight gain and obesity than others because of different genetic background. Thus, a better understanding of the etiology of obesity requires a careful investigation of gene-environment interactions.

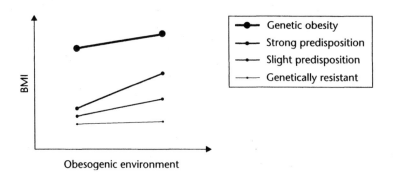

Figure 22.1 Four levels of genetic susceptibility to obesity relative to differences in obesogenic conditions: genetic obesity; strong predisposition; slight predisposition; and genetic resistance, even in a highly obesogenic environment. Reproduced with permission from Loos RJ, Bouchard C. Obesity—is it a genetic disorder? *J Intern Med.* 2003;254:401-425.[10]

However, most genetic association studies lack detailed information on such interactions or nongenetic exposures, especially diet—a factor that may account for substantial heterogeneity in findings, and, thus, lack of replication.[13] Failure to account for gene-environment interactions may also decrease the power to identify disease susceptibility genes and lead to underestimation of effects conferred by genetic and environmental factors. Conversely, a better understanding of gene-environment interactions can help to obtain more accurate estimates of the impact of environmental factors on genetically susceptible individuals and identify high-risk populations for targeted prevention and intervention.

Statistical Models of Gene-Environment Interactions

In general, the term *interaction* means interdependence of two or more variables in influencing a trait or phenotype.[14] Biological interactions occur when two or more factors interact physiologically or chemically in a causal pathway that involves the mechanism of a disease. Statistical interactions (also termed "effect modifications") occur when the value of a second factor alters or modifies the association between an exposure variable and a trait. While biological interactions do not necessarily imply statistical interactions, the latter typically require biological interactions to explain underlying mechanisms.

Gene-environment interaction can be defined as "a different effect of an environmental exposure on disease risk in persons with different genotypes," or, alternatively, "a different effect of a genotype on disease risk in persons with different environmental exposures."[14] The presence and extent of gene-environment interactions depends on the scale used to assess the effect. When a ratio measure is used, the interaction is assessed on the multiplicative scale; when a difference measure is used, the interaction is assessed on the additive scale. While multiplicative models often make useful contributions to the understanding of disease etiology, departure from additivity may be more relevant for public health concerns.[15] In most situations, the purpose of analyses is to discover new genetic markers, most of which have no clinical utility in terms of genetic testing. Therefore, multiplicative models are more appropriate. However, in situations where an interaction may have both public health and etiology implications, it is important to assess both multiplicative and additive models.

Botto and Khoury[16] developed a simple 2×4 table to evaluate joint effects of a genotype and an exposure (both dichotomous) and gene-environment interactions (Table 22.1). The odds ratios (ORs) for the genotype and environmental exposure can be independently assessed and a multiplicative or additive interaction demonstrated if $A/(B \times C) \neq 1$ or $A - (B + C - 1) \neq 0$, respectively. In addition, a case-only OR (ag/ce) can be easily derived and used as a comparison with findings from case-only studies. The case-only design is an efficient and valid way to evaluate gene-environment interactions, if one assumes that the exposure and genetic factors occur independently, and that the disease is rare[17] (see later).

One disadvantage of the 2×4 table is that it allows an assessment only of dichotomous genotypes and environmental exposures. In addition, it does not allow for adjustments for multiple covariates. Regression models are typically used to overcome these limitations. In regression analyses, genotypes can be recoded to reflect dominant, recessive, and additive genetic influences (i.e., dominant model: AA = 1, Aa = 1, aa = 0; recessive: AA = 1, Aa = 0, aa = 0; additive: AA = 1, Aa = 0.5, aa = 0) depending on the biological hypotheses. Multiplicative interactions (specifically, tests of departure from joint effects of exposed genotypes and environmental factors from the product of

Table 22.1 Layouts for a Case-Control Study Assessing the Effect of a Genotype and an Environmental Factor

G*	E*	Cases	Controls	Odds Ratio		Contrast	Main Information
+	+	a	b	ah/bg	A	A vs. D	Joint genotype and environmental factor vs. none
+	−	c	d	ch/dg	B	B vs. D	Genotype alone vs. none
−	+	e	f	eh/fg	C	C vs. D	Environmental factor alone vs. none
−	−	g	h	1	D		Common reference

Other Measures	Odds Ratio	Main Information
Case-only odds ratio	ag/ce	Departure from multiplicative model of interaction
Control only odds ratio	bh/df	Independence of factors in the population
Multiplicative interaction	A/(B × C)	Deviation from multiplicative model of interaction
Additive interaction	A − (B + C − 1)	Deviation from additive model of interaction

Reproduced with permission from Botto LD, Khoury MJ. Commentary: facing the challenge of gene-environment interaction: the two-by-four table and beyond. *Am J Epidemiol.* 2001;153:1016-1020.[16]

ORs for exposure to each individual factor) can be evaluated using the likelihood ratio test (Chapter 4).

Departure from additivity can be evaluated by the synergy index, S (see Chapter 4). S and its corresponding confidence interval can be calculated by using estimated OR and covariances derived from logistic regression models.[18] $S > 1$ indicates departure from additive effects of the gene and environmental factors. Another measure, relative excess risk due to interaction (RERI), has also been used to assess additive interactions.[19]

Study Designs for Evaluating Gene-Environment Interactions

Observational association studies and randomized clinical trials are two main types of study designs for testing the effects of gene-environment interactions on obesity (Table 22.2). Association studies are conducted either in families or in unrelated individuals. There are two main types of family-based association studies: case-parent trio and affected relative pair;[20] both can be used to evaluate gene-environment interactions. The case-parent trio design uses the parents of case subjects as controls, and ORs of the genotype are calculated according to strata of an environmental exposure, thus allowing estimation of gene-environment interactions. The advantage of such a design is immunity to population stratification bias. However, it can be difficult to implement because of difficulty in collecting DNA samples from parents, especially for late onset disease.[21] Also, family-based studies generally have less power than case-control studies of unrelated individuals with the same number of subjects. The affected relative pair study, also known as the affected sibpair method, allows researchers to assess linkage between a locus and disease as well as departure from multiplicative effects of environmental and genetic factors. However, it cannot assess the effects of either exposure or specific alleles.[20]

Table 22.2 Characteristics of Family-Based, Case-Control, Cohort, Case-Only, and Intervention Studies

Characteristic	Family-Based	Case-Control	Cohort	Case-Only	Intervention
Potential for population stratification bias	Nil if appropriately analyzed	Varies; able to be minimized via good design, genomic control	Varies but generally less than retrospective case-control study; able to be minimized via good design, genomic control	Moderate; can be minimized by study design	Similar to cohort study
Potential for recall bias	Moderate to high	Moderate to high	Nil	Moderate to high	Nil
Potential for survivor bias	Moderate to high	Moderate to high	Nil to moderate if DNA is not obtained on all cases and controls at baseline	Moderate to high	Nil
Ability to use plasma phenotypes in cases	No	No	Yes	No	Yes
Required sample sizes achievable?	Common disease: yes	Common disease: yes	Common disease: yes with adequate follow-up	Common disease: yes	Common phenotype such as weight loss: yes
	Rare disease: yes	Rare disease: yes	Rare disease: no, unless multiple studies are pooled	Rare disease: yes	Rare disease: no

Adapted from Kraft P, Hunter D. Integrating epidemiology and genetic association: the challenge of gene-environment interaction. *Philos Trans R Soc Lond B Biol Sci.* 2005;360:1609-1916.[13]

The retrospective case-control study is the most commonly used design for studying main genetic effects as well as gene-environment interactions.[13] In case-control studies, researchers identify subjects with a certain disease or condition (e.g., morbidly obese people) and compare them to unaffected individuals (controls). Although such studies are relatively easy to conduct, there are several potential sources of bias. First, selection bias can result from differences in source populations of cases and controls. In other words, controls may not represent the population from which cases were selected, resulting in noncomparability of the cases and controls with respect to demographic and other characteristics. Second, survival bias can occur when subjects who could have been interviewed or genotyped die from the disease of interest before they can be enrolled in the study. Third, recall bias can occur when subjects report past behaviors (e.g., diet, exercise) or exposures differently than they would have, had they not been diagnosed with the disease. Such bias can lead to nondifferential misclassification and reduced power to detect gene-environment interactions. Finally, population stratification bias can occur if cases and controls differ in ethnicity/ancestry and the genetic markers of interest also vary by ethnicity (see Chapter 21). In most situations, major bias due to population stratification can be eliminated by careful matching of ethnicity/ancestry.[22]

Prospective cohort studies collect data on environmental exposures at baseline, before the occurrence of the disease, and ideally, at repeated follow-up intervals. This approach can minimize or eliminate recall, selection, and survivor biases. In addition, potential population stratification bias is diminished because the study base or source population is clearly defined, but careful matching on ethnicity/ancestry between cases and controls is still required in nested case-control studies. Prospective studies require that large numbers of subjects be enrolled at baseline and that there be adequate follow-up to ensure a sufficient number of cases for reliable analysis.

The case-only design is simple and efficient when used to assess gene-environment interactions.[20] In this method, case subjects are used to assess the association between the exposure of interest and the genotype in a 2×2 table. Under the assumption that the genotype and exposure are independent, the estimated OR is equivalent to the synergy index on a multiplicative scale derived from a regular case-control study. The validity of the case-only method is highly dependent on the assumption of independence between the genetic and environmental factors in the population.[23] Another limitation of the case-only design is that it cannot assess the main effects of either the genotype or the exposure.

Randomized clinical trials have also been widely used to investigate the effects of gene-environment interactions on obesity. Such studies typically use weight change over a few weeks or months as the outcome. Randomized trials offer the advantage of control over the dietary or lifestyle intervention, which allows for a more precise measure of the environmental exposure. In addition, random allocation of dietary interventions largely eliminates confounding by other factors. Such studies, however, are typically small and short-term. Also, compliance with dietary interventions is usually poor and dropouts are common. These problems may complicate the interpretations of results on gene-environment interactions.

Observational Studies of Gene-Diet Interactions on Obesity

Most observational studies have focused on the modulation effects of dietary fat on common variations in genes regulating adipocyte metabolism (Table 22.3). In 592 nondiabetic men and women, Luan et al.[24] found that the ratio of dietary polyunsaturated fat to saturated fat (P:S) strongly interacted with peroxisome proliferator-activated receptor-γ 2 (*PPARG2*) Pro12Ala (P12A) in relation to body mass index (BMI). Subjects who carried the A allele were protected against obesity if they also consumed a diet with a high P:S ratio (*P* for gene-diet interaction = .0038). They found a similar interaction between P:S ratio and the genotype on fasting insulin levels (*P* = .0097).

Two subsequent studies have generally confirmed the effect of interactions between dietary fat and the *PPARG2* gene on adiposity. In one study, Memisoglu et al.[25] found a significant interaction between dietary fat and the *PPARG2* P12A genotype in relation to obesity risk among 2141 healthy women from the Nurses' Health Study. Among individuals homozygous for the P allele , those in the highest quintile of total fat intake had a significantly higher mean BMI compared with those in the lowest quintile (27.3 kg/m² vs. 25.4 kg/m², respectively; *P* for trend < .0001). Among carriers of the variant A allele, no

Table 22.3 Observational Studies of Gene-Diet Interactions

Authors (Year)	Study Design, Subjects	Genes	Dietary Factors	Major Findings
Luan (2001)[24]	Population-based, 592 nondiabetic subjects	PPARG2	Ratio of polyunsaturated fat to saturated fat (P:S ratio)	BMI in 12A allele carriers was greater than that in P homozygotes when dietary P:S ratio was low; but when the P:S ratio was high, the opposite was seen
Nieters (2002)[30]	Case-control, 154 BMI > 35 kg/m² and 154 matched controls	PPARA, PPARG2, UCP1, UCP2, UCP3, ADRB2, ADIPOQ, LEP, SORBS1, HSL, and TNF	Linoleic acid (C18:2 n-6) and ararchidonic acid (C20:4 n-6)	LEP (−2548G > A), TNF (−307G > A), PPARG2 (P12A) interacted with linoleic acid in relation to obesity risk
Marti (2002)[34]	Case-control, 159 obese and 154 normal weight controls	PPARG2	Carbohydrate (CHO)	Carrying 12A was associated with significantly increased risk of obesity only in those with high CHO intake (>49% of total energy)
Robitaille (2003)[26]	Family-based, 720 subjects	PPARG2	Total and saturated fat	P12A interacted with intakes of total or saturated fat in relation to BMI and waist circumference
Martinez (2003)[35]	Case-control, 154 obese (BMI > 30) subjects and 154 controls (BMI < 25)	ADRB2	Carbohydrate (CHO)	High CHO intake was associated with obesity risk only among 27E carriers, but not among 27Q homozygotes
Memisoglu (2003)[25]	Population based, 2141 nondiabetic women	PPARG2	Total fat and monounsaturated fat	P12A significantly modified the relations between intakes of total and monounsaturated fats and BMI and weight gain. A positive association was observed between total fat intake and obesity and BMI in the 12PP genotype, but not among the 12A allele carriers
Miyaki (2005)[36]	Cross-sectional, 295 Japanese men	ADRB3	Total energy	High energy intake (highest quartile) was associated with obesity risk (circumference >85 cm) in the carriers of the 64R allele but not among noncarriers
Robitaille (2006)[31]	Population based, 340 nondiabetic subjects	PPARD	Fat intake	Lower fat intake was associated with lower risk of metabolic syndrome in −87C carriers but not among noncarriers

(continued)

467

Table 22.3 continued

Authors (Year)	Study Design, Subjects	Genes	Dietary Factors	Major Findings
Robitaille (2007)[32]	Population based, 351 nondiabetic subjects	CPT1	Fat intake	Fat intake (34.4% of energy as cutoff) significantly modified the relations between the 531 Glu/Lys variant and body weight, BMI, and waist circumference
Santos (2006)[39]	Case-only study, 549 obese women	26 genes and 42 SNPs	Fiber, P:S ratio, and fat intake	Significant interactions were found between LIPC −514C > T and fiber, ADIPOQ −11377 and PPARG3 −681C > G and fat intake in relation to obesity, but not for other variants
Corella (2007)[33]	Population based, 1703 men and 1207 women	APOA5	Fat intake	BMI increased as fat intake increased only among subjects with the −1131TT genotype. −1131C carriers had a lower risk of obesity and overweight compared to those with the TT genotype only when fat intake was high but not when it was low
Vaccaro (2007)[37]	Cross-sectional, 342 diabetics	PPARG2	Total energy intake	BMI was similar in 12A carriers and noncarriers in the lower quartile of energy intake but significantly higher in A carriers in the upper quartile. Relative to noncarriers, A carriers had a significantly lower energy intake per kg body weight
Song (2007)[38]	Cross-sectional, 285 nondiabetic Japanese men	IL6R	Total energy intake	An association between waist circumference and energy intake was observed among 358D carriers but not among subjects homozygous for the 358A allele

significant trend was detected between dietary fat intake and BMI. While there was no association between intake of monounsaturated fat and BMI among women homozygous for the P allele, an inverse association was observed among carriers of the A allele (P for interaction = .003). Similar interactions were found between dietary fat intake and the genotype for weight gain since age 18.

In a second study, Robitaille et al.[26] investigated whether dietary fat interacted with the PPARG2 P12A polymorphism to influence BMI and waist circumference in a cohort of 720 adults participating in the Quebec Family Study. Significant interactions between total fat and saturated fat intake and PPARG2 genotype were observed for BMI, waist circumference, and several components of the metabolic syndrome. Intake of total fat and saturated fat were significantly correlated with BMI and waist circumference in P homozygotes, but not among carriers of the A allele.

The mechanism underlying the interaction between the *PPARG2* genotype and dietary fatty acids on adiposity is not well understood. In animal experiments, heterozygous null mice (lacking one copy of the *PPARG2* gene) gained significantly less weight than their corresponding wild-type controls when fed a high fat diet.[27] Similarly, reduction in PPARγ activity through PPARγ-specific antagonist treatment confers resistance to high-fat-diet-induced weight gain in mice.[28] PPARγ is the target of the thiazolidinedione class of antidiabetic drugs, which improve insulin sensitivity. In vivo ligands for PPARγ are thought to include a variety of unsaturated fatty acids,[29] and thus the interactions between dietary fatty acids and the P12A variant observed in the studies mentioned earlier are consistent with the biological role of unsaturated fatty acids in activating the *PPARG2* gene.

It appears that other adipose-related genes may also interact with unsaturated fats in the development of obesity.[30-33] Robitaille et al.[31] observed that total and saturated fat modulated the *PPARD* −87T > C polymorphism and *PPARA* Leu162Val (L162V) polymorphism in relation to waist circumference and other components of the metabolic syndrome. In French-Canadians, dietary fat intake was found to interact with variants in the gene encoding the carnitine palmitoyltransferase I (*CPT1*), a key enzyme in beta-oxidation of fatty acids.[32] Measures of obesity, such as BMI and waist circumference, were higher on a high fat diet only among subjects heterozygous for a *CPT1B* Glu531Lys (E531K) polymorphism or homozygous for a *CPT1A* 275 T > A polymorphism. No relationship between BMI and fat intake was observed among those carrying other genotypes.

Corella et al.[33] determined whether dietary intake modifies the association between SNPs in the apolipoprotein A5 (*APOA5*) gene and body weight among participants of the Framingham Offspring Study. An interaction between a −1131 T > C SNP and total fat intake on BMI was observed. The C allele carriers had a lower risk of obesity and overweight compared to those with the TT genotype only when total fat intake was high but not when it was low.

In addition to interactions between SNPs and dietary fat intake on obesity, several studies have examined interactions between genotypes and other components of the diet. Carbohydrates have been found to interact with *PPARG2*[34] and *ADRB2*[35] in determining obesity risk. Moreover, an interaction between high energy intake and the *ADRB3* Trp64Arg (W64R) polymorphism in relation to obesity was observed in a Japanese study.[36] In addition, Vaccaro et al.[37] found an interaction between the *PPARG2* P12A SNP and habitual energy intake on BMI in diabetic subjects; BMI was similar in the A carriers and noncarriers when energy intake was lower, but it was significantly higher in A carriers among those with higher energy intake. The interleukin-6 receptor (*IL6R*) Asp358Ala (N358A) polymorphism has also been found to interact with energy intake to predict abdominal obesity in Japanese men.[38]

Recent studies have taken a more comprehensive approach to assessing gene-diet interactions on obesity. Santos et al.[39] evaluated 42 polymorphisms of 26 candidate genes for gene-diet interactions in a case-only study of 549 obese European women. Candidates were chosen from a number of pathological pathways implicated in obesity, including appetite regulation (e.g., *SL6A14, CART, GAD2, GHRL*), energy expenditure (UCPs), adipocyte differentiation and function (e.g., *PPARGC1A, PPARG2, PPARG3*), lipid and glucose metabolism (e.g., *LIPC, IGF2, KCNJ11, ENPP1*), and adipokine production (e.g., *ADIPOQ, IL6, TNFA*). Dietary variables of interest included fiber intake (grams per day), the P:S ratio, and the percentage of energy derived from fat in the diet as calculated from a weighted 3-day food record. Overall, most interaction tests were not significant. However, a significant interaction was observed between fiber intake and the hepatic lipase (*LIPC*) −514C > T polymorphism in relation to obesity. There was also suggestive evidence that the adiponectin (*ADIPOQ*) −11377G > C and *PPARG3*−681C >G polymorphisms interact with fat intake, but results were not adjusted for multiple testing. In a matched case-control study of 154 obese (BMI > 35 kg/m²) and 154 normal weight European men and women, Nieters et al.[30] genotyped 14 SNPs from 11 candidate genes. Gene-diet interactions were observed for the *LEP*-2548 G > A, *TNFA* −308G > A and *PPARG2* P12A polymorphisms. With increasing intake of linoleic acid, individuals with the *LEP* A allele had a reduced risk, while individuals with the *TNFA* A allele had an increased risk of obesity compared to their corresponding homozygous wildtypes. Carriers of the *PPARG2* A variant had an increased risk of obesity with increasing arachidonic acid consumption compared to individuals with the wild genotype.

Observational Studies of Gene-Physical Activity Interactions

The protective effects of physical activity against obesity and weight gain have been documented in numerous studies (see Chapter 7). Because several obesity candidate genes are involved in energy expenditure, it can be postulated that these genes interact with physical activity to influence body weight. However, only a few studies have examined gene-exercise interactions (Table 22.4). Meirhaeghe et al.[40] found that higher physical activity levels counterbalanced the effect of a β2-adrenergic receptor gene (*ADRB2*) polymorphism Gln27Glu (Q27E) on adiposity measures. In particular, they observed a significant positive association between the polymorphism and BMI and waist circumference among inactive men, but not among active men. A Spanish case-control study also showed an interaction between the Q27E polymorphism and physical activity on BMI; carriers of the 27E allele benefited less from physical activity than did noncarriers.[41] Moreover, the same investigators demonstrated an interaction between the W64R polymorphism of the *ADRB3* gene and exercise.[42] Physical activity appeared to abolish a positive association between the polymorphism and obesity risk.

Genes that encode uncoupling proteins (UCPs) have been extensively investigated as modifiers of weight loss response. UCPs are a family of carrier proteins located in the inner membranes of the mitochondria that play a critical role in energy homeostasis and body-weight regulation.[43] Thus, the *UCP1*, *UCP2*, and *UCP3* genes are considered good candidate genes for obesity. Given the role of UCPs in energy metabolism, several studies have examined obesity risk related to potential interactions between *UCP* genetic variants and physical activity. In a French population, Otabe et al.[44] found an association between the C > T polymorphism in the 5′ sequence of the *UCP3* gene and BMI. The benefits of physical activity were observed only in the group with a wild CC genotype, indicating that the polymorphism modified the association between physical activity and obesity. Alonso et al.[45] also observed an interaction between this polymorphism and physical activity in a Spanish population, but the direction was not consistent with the previous study. While physically active carriers of the *UCP3* −55C > T polymorphism had a lower risk of obesity, sedentary individuals did not. In contrast, Berentzen et al.[46] found no effects of genetic variants in *UCP2* and *UCP3* genes on BMI or weight gain in two cohorts of Danish men. There was also no interaction observed between these variants and physical activity on weight gain over time.

Peroxisome proliferator-activated receptor-gamma coactivator-1 alpha (*PPARGC1A*) is a transcriptional coactivator implicated in energy homeostasis and glucose metabolism. A recent meta-analysis suggested that the common *PPARGC1A* polymorphism,

Table 22.4 Observational Studies of Gene-Physical Activity Interactions

Authors (Year)	Study Design, Subjects	Genes	Lifestyle Factors	Major Findings
Meirhaeghe (1999)[40]	Population based, 1152 subjects	ADRB2	Physical activity	Q27E significantly interacted with physical activity in relation to body weight, BMI, waist circumference, hip circumference, and WHR
Otabe (2000)[44]	Case-control, 401 obese and 231 control subjects	UCP3	Physical activity (tertiles)	BMI was negatively associated with physical activity in −55CC homozygotes but not in other genotypes
Marti (2002)[42]	Case-control study, 159 obese (BMI > 30) and 154 controls (BMI < 25)	ADRB3	Physical activity (ratio of METs h/wk to the time spent sitting down during leisure time, M/S)	W64R was significantly associated with obesity only among those with sedentary lifestyle but not among those who were active
Corbalan (2002)[41]	Case-control study, 139 obese female (BMI > 30) and 113 control women (BMI <25)	ADRB2	Physical activity (same as the above)	Significant interaction between the Q27E polymorphism and activity in relation to BMI in obese women
Berentzen (2005)[46]	Longitudinal study, 1285 subjects	UCP2 and UCP3	Physical activity (inactive, moderately, active)	No significant gene-physical activity interaction on 10-y weight change
Alonso (2005)[45]	Case-control, 150 obese (BMI > 30) and 150 control subjects (BMI < 25)	UCP3	Recreational physical activity	−55C > T polymorphism was associated with lower risk of obesity only in those with higher physical activity
Ridderstrale (2006)[48]	Population based, 1801 subjects	PPARGC1A	Leisure-time physical activity (2 h/wk as cutoff)	Carrying 482S was associated with increased risk of obesity only in elderly males with a low physical activity
Andreasen (2007)[50]	Population based, 17 508 subjects	FTO	Physical activity (physically passive, light or medium, hard or very hard)	rs9939609 AA was associated with higher BMI than TT only among physically inactive subjects

Gly482Ser (G482S), was associated with a small increased risk of type 2 diabetes.[47] Although this SNP has not been directly associated with obesity risk, there is some evidence that it may modify the effects of physical activity on obesity. In a Swedish study, Ridderstrale et al.[48] found a significant positive association between this polymorphism and obesity in physically inactive men, but not among those with a high level of physical activity.

The *FTO* gene was initially shown to be associated with BMI in a genome-wide association (GWA) study of type 2 diabetes[49] and since then this association has been replicated in multiple populations (see Chapter 21). More recently, Andreasen et al.[50] confirmed the increased risk of obesity associated with FTO rs9939609 T > A in a Danish population, but further reported a significant gene-physical activity interaction. Significant differences in BMI between the AA and TT genotypes were observed only among physically inactive subjects, but not among those who were physically active. These results suggest that higher physical activity may attenuate the adverse effects of the *FTO* variant on obesity.

Gene-Diet Interactions on Obesity from Intervention Studies

In 1990, Bouchard et al.[51] published a seminal study (Quebec Overfeeding Study) showing tremendous between-person variability in weight and fat gain in response to overfeeding. In this study, 12 male monozygotic (MZ) pairs were overfed by 1000 kcal/day beyond the energy cost for weight maintenance for 100 days. In response to energy surplus, there was at least three times more variance between pairs than within pairs for weight gain (Figure 22.2). In a subsequent study, seven pairs of young adult MZ twins completed a negative energy balance protocol during which they exercised on cycle ergometers twice

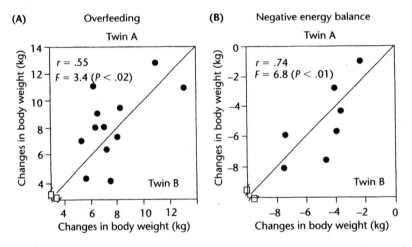

Figure 22.2 Intrapair resemblance in the response of identical twins to long-term changes in energy balance. (A) Twelve pairs of identical twins received an 84 000 kcal energy intake surplus over 100 d. (B) Seven pairs underwent an exercise-induced negative energy balance protocol. The energy deficit was 58 000 kcal over 93 d. Reproduced with permission Bouchard C, Tremblay A, Despres JP, et al. The response to long-term overfeeding in identical twins. *N Engl J Med.* 1990;322:1477-1482;[51] Bouchard C, Tremblay A, Despres JP, et al. The response to exercise with constant energy intake in identical twins. *Obes Res.* 1994;2:400-410.[52]

a day over a period of 93 days, while maintaining a constant daily energy intake.[52] The average weight loss was 5.0 kg (range 1.0 to 8.0 kg). Again, the data showed much larger between-pair than within-pair differences in weight loss (Fig. 22.2).

Findings from these intervention studies in MZ twins indicate considerable heterogeneity in individual responses to chronic energy imbalance. The remarkable intrapair resemblance in response to energy surplus or energy deficit suggests that genetic factors may determine the way individuals respond to the obesogenic environment. However, the exact genetic markers that determine the responsiveness to positive energy balance have not been identified. Using the 12 MZ twin pairs from the Quebec Overfeeding Study, Ukkola and Bouchard[53] examined the role of 40 candidate genes in response to overfeeding. Results showed that variations in several genes—including resistin (*RETN*, IVS2 + 39C > T); adipsin (*CFD*, HINC II); alpha(2A)-adrenergic receptor (*ADRA2A*, DRA I); *ADRB2* (BAN I, Gln27Glu, Arg16Gly); glucocorticoid receptor (*GRL*, Bcl I); insulin-like growth factor-II (*IGF2*, Apa I); and *LPL* (Bam HI, Hind III, and Pvu II)—were significantly related to changes in body weight, total fat mass, or subcutaneous fat. However, the study was limited by a very small sample size.

As discussed in the earlier chapter, ADRB3 plays a role in adipocyte metabolism and body-weight regulation. A common polymorphism in this gene, W64R, has been associated with greater weight gain, especially in Japanese subjects. Several studies have examined whether this polymorphism modulates the effects of weight loss interventions (Table 22.5). In two Japanese studies of obese nondiabetic[54] and diabetic[55] patients, the W64R variant modified the magnitude of weight loss following a 12-week diet and exercise intervention program. In particular, the R allele carriers tended to lose less weight and have a lower resting metabolic rate than noncarriers. This finding was confirmed by a subsequent Japanese study[56] in which a total of 76 perimenopausal women underwent a 3-month behavioral intervention study using a combination of diet and exercise programs. The data showed that while women with the wild genotype experienced significant reductions in body weight and waist circumference, the change was minimal among women with the W64R mutation. Xinli et al.[57] assessed whether the W64R genotype modified weight gain in response to a dietary intervention in obese children in China aged 8-11 years. Thirty-six subjects received a dietary intervention (a diet low in cholesterol and saturated fat), the remaining 11 served as controls. After 3 months, children with the WW genotype, but not the R allele, experienced lower weight gain and BMI increase relative to controls. Taken together, these findings from Asian populations suggest that individuals with the variant R allele may be resistant to diet-induced weight change.

The results of studies among Caucasians, however, have been inconsistent. Rawson et al.[58] found that obese postmenopausal white women who carried the W64R variant in *ADRB3* had changes in body composition and energy expenditure similar to those in noncarriers of the variant in response to weight loss intervention through caloric restriction, and, thus, the presence of the W64R variant did not appear to hinder weight loss. In a similar study, obese postmenopausal white women participating in a ~13-month calorie-restricted weight loss program experienced reductions in body weight and body fat regardless of *ADRB3* genotype.[59] However, loss of visceral adipose tissue was 43% lower in carriers of the R allele as compared to noncarriers. The discrepancy between these reports and the three earlier Japanese studies suggests that the modifying effects of the W64R mutation on diet-induced weight loss may be ethnic-specific, similar to the main effects of this mutation on body weight (see Chapter 21).

Findings regarding the relationship between the *PPARG2* P12A polymorphism and metabolic responses to weight loss have also been mixed. In the Finnish Diabetes Prevention

Table 22.5 Intervention Studies of Gene-Diet Interactions on Obesity/Weight Gain

Authors (Year)	Study Design	Follow-up	Genes	Intervention	Main Results
Yoshida (1995)[54]	88 obese and 100 nonobese women	3 mo	ADRB3	Low-calorie diet and exercise	Weight loss in the carriers of 64R was less than that in the noncarriers among the obese
Fumeron (1996)[63]	163 overweight subjects (BMI > 27 kg/m²)	2.5 mo	UCP1 and ADRB3	Low-calorie diet	Carriers of Allele 1 of UCP1 variation had less weight loss than noncarriers. ADRB3 W64R was not associated with weight loss
Sakane (1997)[55]	61 obese type 2 diabetic women	3 mo	ADRB3	Low-calorie diet and exercise	Carriers of 64R had smaller decreases in body weight, BMI, and WHR than noncarriers
Kogure (1998)[64]	113 obese women	3 mo	ADRB3 and UCP1	Low-calorie diet and exercise	UCP1GG carriers had less weight loss than AA carriers; carriers of both UCP1 GG and ADRB3 64R had less weight loss than carriers of either genotype alone
Tchernof (2000)[59]	24 postmenopausal women (BMI > 27 kg/m²)	13 ± 3 mo	ADRB3	AHA Step 2 diet (1200 kcal/d)	No differences in body weight and body fat reductions. Loss of visceral adipose tissue was significantly lower in 64R carriers compared with noncarriers
Xinli (2001)[57]	47 obese children aged 8-11 years 36 received intervention, 11 served as controls	3 mo	ADRB3	Diet low in cholesterol and saturated fat (NCEPA Step 1 diet) No caloric restriction	Children with the 64WW genotype, but not the 64R allele, experienced lower weight gain and BMI increase relative to controls
Nicklas (2001)[61]	70 postmenopausal women	6 mo intervention + 12 mo follow-up	PPARG2	Hypocaloric diet (250-350 kcal/d deficit)	No difference in weight loss; Carriers of 12A allele had greater weigh regain than 12P homozygotes
Mammes (2001)[68]	289 normal weight and 277 overweight (BMI > 27 kg/m²)	2.5 mo	LEPR	Low calorie (25% reduction)	Overweight women who carried +70T > C lost more weight in response to diet intervention than those who did not carry this polymorphism
Rawson (2002)[58]	34 obese postmenopausal women	13.5 mo	ADRB3	AHA Step 2 diet (1200 kcal/d)	W64R was not related to changes in body mass, BMI, percent body fat, fat-free mass, and fat mass

Study	Subjects	Duration	Genes	Intervention	Findings
Lindi (2002)[60]	522 overweight subjects with IGT	3 y	*PPARG2*	Reduction in the intake of total and saturated fat, and increase in fiber intake and moderate exercise	Subjects with the 12AA genotype lost more weight than subjects with other genotypes
Shiwaku (2003)[56]	85 healthy women	3 mo	*ADRB3*	Low caloric diet (10% reduction) and exercise (taking > 7000 steps/d)	Carriers of 64R were more resistant to weight loss than noncarriers
Ukkola (2004)[53]	12 pairs of monozygotic twins	100 d	>40 candidate genes	Overfeeding, 1000 kcal above baseline intake	Variations in genes *RETN* (IVS2 + 39C > T); *CFD* (*Hinc II*); *ADRA2A* (*Dra I*); *ADRB2* (*Ban I*, Q27E; R16G); *GRL* (*Bcl I*); *IGF2* (*Apa I*) and *LPL* (*Bam HI*, *Hind III*, *Pvu II*) interacted with intervention on body weight, fat mass, or subcutaneous fat
Corella (2005)[74]	150 obese	1 y	*PLIN*	Low-energy diet	Women carrying 11482G > A were resistant to weight loss compared with noncarriers
Sesti (2005)[76]	167 morbid obese subjects (BMI > 40 or > 35 and had comorbidities)	6 mo	*IL6, UCP2, IRS1,* and *PPARG2*	Hypocaloric diet and laparoscopic adjustable gastric banding	*IL6* −174GG homozygotes lost more weight than allele C carriers; *UCP2* −866AA homozygotes had less weight loss than G carriers
Aberle (2005)[71]	606 overweight and hyperlipaemic men	3 mo	*APOA5*	Reduced fat intake (−40 to −50 g/d)	Carriers of polymorphism −1131C allele had significantly greater reduction in BMI than TT homozygotes
Salopuro (2005)[67]	507 individuals with IGT	3 y	*LEPR*	Reduction in the intakes of total and saturated fat, and increase in fiber intake and moderate exercise	Participants carrying the Del/Del genotype were heavier than those with the insertion allele; no gene-intervention interaction on weight change
Vogels (2005)[72]	150 overweight subjects (BMI > 25)	6-wk diet and 1-y weight maintenance	*PPARG2, GRL,* and *CNTF*	VCDL (500 kcal/d)	Individuals carrying *PPARG2* Pl2A and *GRL* intron 2C > G polymorphism were more likely to be successful in weight maintenance

(continued)

Table 22.5 continued

Authors (Year)	Study Design	Follow-up	Genes	Intervention	Main Results
Cha (2006)[66]	214 overweight female Koreans	1 mo	UCP3	Low-energy diet (700 kcal/d)	Changes in BMI and body fat mass were associated with haplotypes possessing polymorphisms −55 C > G, −143 G > C, Y99Y, −47 G > A, −498 C > T, and Y210Y
Sorensen (2006)[75]	771 obese subjects	10 wk	26 genes and 42 SNPs	Hypoenergetic (~600 kcal/d) diets with a targeted fat energy of 20%–25% or 40%–45%	No significant gene-intervention interaction on weight change
Goyenechea (2006)[70]	67 obese subjects	10 wk intervention and 1 y follow-up	PPARG2 and IL6	Low-energy diet (500 kcal lower than the resting energy expenditure)	Carrier of the −174C allele of IL6 gene had less weight regain after weight loss than noncarriers; carriers of both −174C and PPARG2 12A allele improved weight maintenance
de Luis (2006)[69]	67 obese subjects	3 mo	LEPR	Mediterranean hypocaloric diet (1520 kcal/d) and aerobic activity (1 h, 3 d/wk)	BMI, weight, and waist circumference decreased, regardless of genotype. Fat mass decreased in 656K homozygotes but not in 656N carriers
Franks (2007)[78]	3356 subjects at high risk for diabetes	1 y	PPARG	Metformin, troglitazone, or lifestyle modification (~7% weight loss and ~150 min physical activity/wk)	In the metformin and lifestyle groups, weight loss occurred across genotypes, but was significantly greater in 12A carriers. Troglitazone treatment induced weight gain, which tended to be greater in 12A carriers
Santoro(2007)[73]	184 obese children	12 mo	MC3R	Hypocaloric diet (60% of recommended dietary allowances), physical activity and behavioral therapy	Higher prevalence of 17A heterozygotes than 17C homozygotes was observed among subjects who lowered their BMI z score <1.5. (No 17A homozygotes were reported)

Study,[60] subjects with the AA genotype lost significantly more weight during the 3-year intervention period than subjects with other genotypes. Conversely, Nicklas et al.[61] found that although the A variant did not affect weight loss following a 6-month hypocaloric diet intervention, weight regain was significantly greater in women with the A allele (5.4 ± 0.9 kg) than in those homozygous for the P allele (2.8 ± 0.4 kg). The *PPARG2* genotype appeared to be the best predictor of weight regain. These results indicate that genetic factors may have different effects on weight loss and weight maintenance.[62]

Several studies suggest that genetic variants of *UCPs* modify the response to weight loss interventions. In a French study, Fumeron et al.[63] found that an A to G transition in the 5'-untranslated region (also referred to as the BclI polymorphism) of *UCP1* modified weight change in response to a 10-week low-calorie diet (25% energy restriction). G homozygotes lost less weight (−4.6 kg) than the A homozygotes (−7.1 kg). This finding was confirmed in a Japanese study[64] of 113 obese women participating in a combined diet and exercise program for 12 weeks. Women with the GG genotype lost significantly less weight (−4.3 kg) than those with the AA genotype (−7.4 kg). The resistance to weight loss was even greater among G homozygotes who also carried the W64R mutation of the *ADRB3* gene (−3.3 kg). The synergistic effects between *UCP1* and *ADRB3* variants were also found in a small intervention study using a very-low-calorie diet (VLCD).[65] These data suggest that a combination of the W64R mutation in *ADRB3* and the A to G polymorphism in *UCP1* was associated with faster weight gain after a VLCD. In a Korean study, Cha et al.[66] examined the effects of *UCP3* haplotypes on weight change following a 1-month low-calorie diet in 214 overweight women. Data showed that the haplotypes modified diet-induced weight loss and fat mass, but not changes in fat-free mass.

The role of several other adiposity-related genes has also been examined in the context of weight loss or maintenance intervention studies. These genes include the *LEPR*,[67-69] *IL6*,[70] *APOA5*,[71] glucocorticoid receptor (*GRL*),[72] melanocortin receptor 3 (*MC3R*),[73] and perilipin (*PLIN*).[74] These studies showed that one or more common genetic variants influenced the magnitude of weight loss in response to dietary interventions. For example, in a 1-year trial, Corella et al.[74] demonstrated that obese subjects carrying a *PLIN* 11482G > A polymorphism lost significantly less weight following an energy-restricted diet than did those with the wildtype. In addition, the −1131T > C polymorphism in the *APOA5* gene was found to interact with a short-term fat restriction so that the reduction of BMI was significantly greater in the C allele carriers than in the T allele carriers.[71]

In a recent randomized intervention trial, Sorensen et al.[75] examined whether 42 SNPs from 26 obesity-related genes (e.g., *UCP2*, *UCP3*, *GAD2*, *PPARG2*, *IL6*, and *TNFA*) influenced weight loss in 648 obese individuals who completed a 10-week dietary intervention of hypoenergetic (−600 kcal/day) diets with a targeted fat intake of 20 to 25% or 40 to 45% of total caloric intake. After adjusting for multiple testing, there were no significant associations between SNPs and magnitude of weight loss in either intervention. The authors concluded that genetic variants in this panel of obesity-related candidate genes were unlikely to play a major role in modulating weight loss induced by a moderate hypoenergetic low- or high-fat diet.

In response to the growing obesity epidemic, surgical and pharmacological treatments have become more widely available. Several recent studies have examined whether the success of these interventions is modified by genetic polymorphisms. One study investigated the impact of common genetic variants on weight loss in morbidly obese subjects after laparoscopic adjustable gastric banding and hypocaloric diet.[76] At the 6-month follow-up, subjects with the *IL6* −174GG genotype lost more weight than those with the −174GC or CC genotype (*P* = .037), and subjects with the *UCP2* −866AA genotype lost more weight than those with the −866GG (*P* = .018) and −866GA (*P* = .035) genotypes. Weight loss was smaller in subjects with the insulin receptor substrate-1 gene (*IRS1*) Gly972Arg (G972R) genotype than those with G972G, but the difference was not statistically significant (*P* = .06).

Hauner et al.[77] investigated whether genetic variants modified the effects of a weight loss drug, Sibutramine (a centrally acting noradrenaline and serotonin reuptake inhibitor), in 111 subjects participating in a randomized placebo-controlled clinical trial. They found that the G-protein β3 subunit gene (*GNB3*) 825C > T polymorphism was highly predictive of weight loss induced by sibutramine treatment. Specifically, a 15 mg sibutramine treatment was more effective in individuals with the CC genotype than in subjects with the TT/TC genotypes (weight loss: 7.2 ± 2.2 kg vs. 4.1 ± 2.1 kg, *P* = .0013, sibutramine vs. placebo).

More recently, Franks et al.[78] examined whether the *PPARG2* P12A polymorphism modified obesity-related traits in a 1-year randomized trial of treatment with metformin, troglitazone or lifestyle modification relative to placebo for diabetes prevention in high-risk individuals. In the metformin and lifestyle groups, weight loss occurred across genotypes, but was significantly greater in the A allele carriers. Troglitazone treatment induced weight gain, which tended to be greater in the A allele carriers (*P* = 0.08). This study suggests that genetic variability may modify adverse responses (i.e., weight gain) of diabetes treatment.

Methodological Issues

Similar to the literature on the main genetic variants predisposing to obesity, lack of replication is a common problem in studies on gene-environment interactions of obesity and its related phenotypes. Replication is more challenging for gene-environment interactions than main effects because such studies involve the assessment of joint effects of genetic variants that typically have modest marginal effects and environmental variables that are often difficult to measure. The problem of multiple testing is exacerbated in gene-environment studies because numerous subgroups can be compared. In addition, most studies are small and underpowered. In the subsequent sections, we discuss several common methodological issues in gene-environment studies.

Sample Size Requirement

Inadequate sample size has been a major limiting factor in genetic epidemiologic studies, especially those on gene-environment interactions. A rule of thumb is that the sample size necessary to test departure from a multiplicative gene-environment interaction is at least four times that needed to evaluate the main genetic or environmental associations.[79] Larger samples are needed to compensate for measurement error associated with environmental exposures.[80] Inadequate power has been a common problem with many genetic studies—an important reason for the high number of false-positives and non-reproducible findings.[81] Hunter[82] estimated that in most scenarios, thousands of cases and controls are needed to detect multiplicative interactions with ORs ranging from 1.5 to 2, even under the assumption of a common variation (minor allele frequency >5%) and sizable genetic and environmental effects (an OR of 1.5 for both). Unfortunately, most observational studies have been limited to a sample size of a few hundred subjects. The sample size for most of the intervention trials has been even smaller. Small underpowered studies contribute to both false-positive and false-negative findings. Thus, there is an urgent need for large, well-powered, and carefully designed observational studies to examine gene-environment interactions in the development of obesity. Larger and longer-term intervention studies are also needed to test the effects of gene-diet interactions on weight loss and maintenance.

Multiple Testing

Multiple testing is one of the most serious concerns in genetic association studies (Chapter 21). This is particularly true in gene-environment interactions because numerous genetic markers can be tested. In addition, multiple environmental factors and different definitions of these risk factors can be included in the analyses. Further, one can also test multiple models of interaction, depending on whether continuous or categorical environmental variables are used. Thus, the standard significance threshold alpha = 0.05 (producing one false-positive result for every 20 independent tests) is often too liberal, especially in studies testing a large number of candidate genes. Although correction for multiple testing is now increasingly used in studies that focus on main genetic effects, few studies on gene-environment interactions have considered the multiple testing problem. As discussed in Chapter 21, the standard Bonferroni correction is too conservative in most situations. Alternative approaches to address the multiple testing problem include permutation-adjusted P values,[83] false discovery rates (FDR),[84] the Bayesian inference-based method,[85] and nonparametric methods, such as multiple dimensionality reduction (MDR).[86] Nonetheless, replication across populations remains the strongest safeguard against false-positive results. Thus, collaborations among research groups are crucial in identifying genuine genetic markers and gene-environment interactions.

Study Designs

Choice of study design can affect validity of gene-environment interaction studies. In the retrospective case-control or cross-sectional design, data on environmental exposures and samples are obtained after diagnosis of disease. Such studies are prone to selection and recall biases. These biases can lead to biased estimates of genetic and environmental factors and reduced power to detect gene-environment interactions. Prospective studies can minimize selection and recall biases because the study base is well defined and exposure data are collected before the diagnosis of the disease. In addition, long-term weight changes can be evaluated as an outcome when measures on adiposity and environmental exposures are periodically updated. Many large prospective cohort studies have begun to collect repeated anthropometric, diet, and lifestyle measures. This approach provides a unique opportunity to test marginal and joint effects of both genetic and environmental factors on the development of obesity and weight gain.

In randomized clinical trials, the environmental variable (i.e., dietary intervention) is precisely measured and randomly assigned. In theory, this approach eliminates confounding by other lifestyle factors and provides the strongest tests for gene-environment interactions that affect weight loss and maintenance. However, most of the existing randomized clinical trials are small, short-term, and underpowered. Compliance with dietary interventions is always a challenge, especially in long-term studies. Thus, randomized intervention trials cannot replace observational studies in testing gene-environment interactions on obesity. Another consideration is that most intervention trials have focused on weight loss and weight maintenance. Genetic determinants of these outcomes, however, may differ from those involved in weight gain and the development of obesity.

Summary and Future Prospects

Obesity and its related metabolic diseases are complex conditions affected by many genetic and environmental factors. In most situations, neither genetic nor environmental factors alone are sufficient or necessary to cause the phenotypic traits. Thus, there has been growing interest in evaluating the interactive or joint effects of genes and environmental factors on risk of obesity and its associated metabolic complications. Recent advances in genomics, genotyping technology, and genetic epidemiologic methods have dramatically improved our ability to identify these interactions. Ultimately, this information will enable us to better understand the genetic and environmental basis of obesity, and hopefully, lead to more effective prevention and treatment of the disease.

Evidence from intervention trials among MZ twins indicates that the individual response to chronic positive or negative energy balance is strongly determined by genetic factors. However, genetic variants that modulate the effects of dietary factors on obesity, weight loss, or maintenance have not been clearly identified. Among the many candidates studied, several genetic variants appear promising (e.g., *ADRB3* W64R, *PPARG2* P12A, and *UCP1* −3826A > G), although evidence on the role of these polymorphisms is still limited. Lack of replication remains the biggest challenge in the field. Replicating gene-diet interactions is difficult because of differences in study designs, dietary assessment methodology, durations of follow-up, and variation in endpoints (e.g., BMI vs. waist circumference, weight gain vs. weight loss). In addition, the heterogeneity of study populations in age, sex, and ethnicity can also contribute to different results across studies. Although the identification of gene-environment interactions could eventually yield targeted screening and interventions in susceptible individuals, current evidence does not justify individually tailored dietary or exercise recommendations.

Calls for greater collaboration and coordination among various research groups to facilitate data pooling and rapid replications of genetic associations are increasing.[87] Because of the high risk of false-positives or false-negatives in analyses of gene-environment interactions, cooperative efforts are considered all the more important.[82] Pooling of original data analyses from multiple cohorts increases power and minimizes publication bias. Another advantage is the use of standard approaches to define dietary and lifestyle exposures and analyze gene-environment interactions. However, such cooperative approaches are costly and require great effort to coordinate data management and analyses.

As discussed in the earlier chapter, GWA studies have emerged as a powerful and comprehensive approach to testing genetic associations. Although gene-environment interaction tests could be incorporated into GWA studies,[13] that might greatly magnify a multiple testing problem. GWA scans have been conducted for a variety of diseases, and most datasets contain data for BMI. Current genetic analyses focus on the main or marginal effects of genetic variants, which are typically modest. If sizeable effects only occur in the presence of certain environmental exposure(s), then the current GWA approach, which focuses on single-locus effects, may miss many important genetic factors. Thus, it is desirable to incorporate searches for stratum-specific effects or gene-environment interactions into GWA studies. Such analyses need to take into consideration both marginal effects of the genes and interactive effects between the genes and environmental factors.[88]

It remains to be seen whether current advances in genomics, genetic epidemiologic study designs, and genotyping technology will lead to more successful identification of genetic markers of obesity and gene-environment interactions. Many in the field are optimistic that these advances will eventually uncover susceptibility genes for most chronic diseases, and thus, have important clinical and public health repercussions.[89,90] Others, however, are skeptical about the search for numerous genetic factors with small effect sizes in complex combinations, unsure whether the efforts will be fruitful or even worthwhile.[91] Common forms of obesity will be a particularly important area in which to test the usefulness of modern genetic methods in uncovering the role of gene-environment interactions in the development of complex diseases.

References

1. Schulze MB, Hu FB. Primary prevention of diabetes: what can be done and how much can be prevented? *Annu Rev Public Health.* 2005;26:445-467.
2. Gohdes D, Kaufman S, Valway S. Diabetes in American Indians. An overview. *Diabetes Care.* 1993;6:239-243.
3. Collins VR, Dowse GK, Toelupe PM, et al. Increasing prevalence of NIDDM in the Pacific island population of Western Samoa over a 13-year period. *Diabetes Care.* 1994;17:288-296.
4. Hodge AM, Dowse GK, Toelupe P, Collins VR, Imo T, Zimmet PZ. Dramatic increase in the prevalence of obesity in Western Samoa over the 13 year period 1978-1991. *Int J Obes Relat Metab Disord.* 1994;18:419-428.
5. Neel JV. Diabetes mellitus: a "thrifty" genotype rendered detrimental by "progress"? *Am J Hum Genet.* 1962;14:353-362.
6. Ravussin E, Lillioja S, Knowler WC, et al. Reduced rate of energy expenditure as a risk factor for body-weight gain. *N Engl J Med.* 1988;318:467-472.
7. Haldane JBS. *Heredity and Politics.* New York: W.W. Norton Company; 1938.
8. Tryon RC. Individual differences. In: Moss FA, ed. *Comparative Psychology* (Rev. Ed). New York: Prentice-Hall; 1942.
9. National Institutes of Health Consensus Development Panel. National Institutes of Health Consensus Development Conference Statement: phenylketonuria: screening and management, October 16-18, 2000. *Pediatrics.* 2001;108:972-982.
10. Loos RJ, Bouchard C. Obesity—is it a genetic disorder? *J Intern Med.* 2003;254:401-425.
11. Ravussin E, Valencia ME, Esparza J, Bennett PH, Schulz LO. Effects of a traditional lifestyle on obesity in Pima Indians. *Diabetes Care.* 1994;17:1067-1074.
12. Tiret L. Gene-environment interaction: a central concept in multifactorial diseases. *Proc Nutr Soc.* 2002;61:457-463.
13. Kraft P, Hunter D. Integrating epidemiology and genetic association: the challenge of gene-environment interaction. *Philos Trans R Soc Lond B Biol Sci.* 2005;360:1609-1916.
14. Ottman R. Gene-environment interaction: definitions and study designs. *Prev Med.* 1996;25:764-770.
15. Rothman KJ, Greenland S, Walker AM. Concepts of interaction. *Am J Epidemiol.* 1980;112:467-470.
16. Botto LD, Khoury MJ. Commentary: facing the challenge of gene-environment interaction: the two-by-four table and beyond. *Am J Epidemiol.* 2001;153:1016-1020.
17. Piegorsch WW, Weinberg CR, Taylor JA. Non-hierarchical logistic models and case-only designs for assessing susceptibility in population-based case-control studies. *Stat Med.* 1994;12:153-162.
18. Skrondal A. Interaction as departure from additivity in case-control studies: a cautionary note. *Am J Epidemiol.* 2003;158:251-258.
19. Andersson T, Alfredsson L, Kallberg H, Zdravkovic S, Ahlbom A. Calculating measures of biological interaction. *Eur J Epidemiol.* 2005;20:575-579.
20. Khoury MJ, Flanders WD. Nontraditional epidemiologic approaches in the analysis of gene-environment interaction: case-control studies with no controls! *Am J Epidemiol.* 1996;144:207-213.
21. Umbach DM, Weinberg CR. The use of case-parent triads to study joint effects of genotype and exposure. *Am J Hum Gene.* 2000;66:251-261.
22. Cardon LR, Palmer LJ. Population stratification and spurious allelic association. *Lancet.* 2003;361:598-604.
23. Gatto NM, Campbell UB, Rundle AG, Ahsan H. Further development of the case-only design for assessing gene-environment interaction: evaluation of and adjustment for bias. *Int J Epidemiol.* 2004;33:1014-1024.
24. Luan J, Browne PO, Harding AH, et al. Evidence for gene-nutrient interaction at the PPARgamma locus. *Diabetes.* 2001;50:686-689.

25. Memisoglu A, Hu FB, Hankinson SE, et al. Interaction between a peroxisome prolif-erator-activated receptor gamma gene polymorphism and dietary fat intake in relation to body mass. *Hum Mol Genet.* 2003;12:2923-2929.

26. Robitaille J, Despres JP, Perusse L, Vohl MC. The PPAR-gamma P12A polymorphism modulates the relationship between dietary fat intake and components of the metabolic syndrome: results from the Quebec Family Study. *Clin Genet.* 2003;63:109-116

27. Kubota N, Terauchi Y, Miki H, et al. PPAR gamma mediates high-fat diet-induced adipocyte hypertrophy and insulin resistance. *Mol Cell.* 1999;4:597-609.

28. Yamauchi T, Waki H, Kamon J, et al. Inhibition of RXR and PPARgamma amelio-rates diet-induced obesity and type 2 diabetes. *J Clin Invest.* 2001;108:1001-1013.

29. Krey G, Braissant O, L'Horset F, et al. Fatty acids, eicosanoids, and hypolipidemic agents identified as ligands of peroxisome proliferator-activated receptors by coactiva-tor-dependent receptor ligand assay. *Mol Endocrinol.* 1997;11:779-791.

30. Nieters A, Becker N, Linseisen J. Polymorphisms in candidate obesity genes and their interaction with dietary intake of n-6 polyunsaturated fatty acids affect obesity risk in a sub-sample of the EPIC-Heidelberg cohort. *Eur J Nutr.* 2002;41:210-221.

31. Robitaille J, Gaudet D, Perusse L, Vohl MC. Features of the metabolic syndrome are modulated by an interaction between the peroxisome proliferator-activated receptor-delta −87T>C polymorphism and dietary fat in French-Canadians. *Int J Obes (Lond).* 2006;31(3):411-417.

32. Robitaille J, Houde A, Lemieux S, Perusse L, Gaudet D, Vohl MC. Variants within the muscle and liver isoforms of the carnitine palmitoyltransferase I (CPT1) gene interact with fat intake to modulate indices of obesity in French-Canadians. *J Mol Med.* 2007;85:129-137.

33. Corella D, Lai CQ, Demissie S, et al. APOA5 gene variation modulates the effects of dietary fat intake on body mass index and obesity risk in the Framingham Heart Study. *J Mol Med.* 2007;85(2):119-128.

34. Marti A, Corbalan MS, Martinez-Gonzalez MA, Forga L, Martinez JA. CHO intake alters obesity risk associated with Pro12Ala polymorphism of PPARgamma gene. *J Physiol Biochem.* 2002;58:219-220.

35. Martinez JA, Corbalan MS, Sanchez-Villegas A, Forga L, Marti A, Martinez-Gonzalez MA. Obesity risk is associated with carbohydrate intake in women carrying the Gln27Glu beta2-adrenoceptor polymorphism. *J Nutr.* 2003;133:2549-2554.

36. Miyaki K, Sutani S, Kikuchi H, et al. Increased risk of obesity resulting from the interaction between high energy intake and the Trp64Arg polymorphism of the beta3-adrenergic receptor gene in healthy Japanese men. *J Epidemiol.* 2005;15:203-210.

37. Vaccaro O, Lapice E, Monticelli A, et al. Pro12Ala polymorphism of the PPAR-gamma2 locus modulates the relationship between energy intake and body weight in type 2 diabetic patients. *Diabetes Care.* 2007;30(5):1156-1161.

38. Song Y, Miyaki K, Araki J, Zhang L, Omae K, Muramatsu M. The interaction between the interleukin 6 receptor gene genotype and dietary energy intake on abdominal obesity in Japanese men. *Metabolism.* 2007;56(7):925-930.

39. Santos JL, Boutin P, Verdich C, et al. Genotype-by-nutrient interactions assessed in European obese women: a case-only study. *Eur J Nutr.* 2006;45:454-462.

40. Meirhaeghe A, Helbecque N, Cottel D, Amouyel P. Beta2-adrenoceptor gene polymor-phism, body weight, and physical activity. *Lancet.* 1999;353:896.

41. Corbalan M, Marti A, Forga L, Martinez-Gonzalez MA, Martinez JA. The 27Glu polymorphism of the beta2-adrenergic receptor gene interacts with physical activity influencing obesity risk among female subjects. *Clin Genet.* 2002;61:305-307.

42. Marti A, Corbalan MS, Martinez-Gonzalez MA, Martinez JA. TRP64ARG polymor-phism of the beta 3-adrenergic receptor gene and obesity risk: effect modification by a sedentary lifestyle. *Diabetes Obes Metab.* 2002;4:428-430.

43. Ricquier D, Bouillaud F. Mitochondrial uncoupling proteins: from mitochondria to the regulation of energy balance. *J Physiol.* 2000;529(Pt 1):3-10.

44. Otabe S, Clement K, Dina C, et al. A genetic variation in the 5' flanking region of the UCP3 gene is associated with body mass index in humans in interaction with physical activity. *Diabetologia.* 2000;43:245-249.

45. Alonso A, Marti A, Corbalan MS, Martinez-Gonzalez MA, Forga L, Martinez JA. Association of UCP3 gene −55C>T polymorphism and obesity in a Spanish population. *Ann Nutr Metab.* 2005;49:183-188.

46. Berentzen T, Dalgaard LT, Petersen L, Pedersen O, Sorensen TI. Interactions between physical activity and variants of the genes encoding uncoupling proteins -2 and -3 in relation to body weight changes during a 10-y follow-up. *Int J Obes (Lond).* 2005;29:93-99.

47. Barroso I, Luan J, Sandhu MS, et al. Meta-analysis of the Gly482Ser variant in PPARGC1A in type 2 diabetes and related phenotypes. *Diabetologia.* 2006;49:501-505.

48. Ridderstrale M, Johansson LE, Rastam L, Lindblad U. Increased risk of obesity associated with the variant allele of the PPARGC1A Gly482Ser polymorphism in physically inactive elderly men. *Diabetologia.* 2006;49:496-500.

49. Frayling TM, Timpson NJ, Weedon MN, et al. A common variant in the FTO gene is associated with body mass index and predisposes to childhood and adult obesity. *Science.* 2007;316:889-894.

50. Andreasen CH, Stender-Petersen KL, Mogensen MS, et al. Low physical activity accentuates the effect of the FTO rs9939609 polymorphism on body fat accumulation. *Diabetes.* 2007 (in press).

51. Bouchard C, Tremblay A, Despres JP, et al. The response to long-term overfeeding in identical twins. *N Engl J Med.* 1990;322:1477-1482.

52. Bouchard C, Tremblay A, Despres JP, et al. The response to exercise with constant energy intake in identical twins. *Obes Res.* 1994;2:400-410.

53. Ukkola O, Bouchard C. Role of candidate genes in the responses to long-term overfeeding: review of findings. *Obes Rev.* 2004;5:3-12.

54. Yoshida T, Sakane N, Umekawa T, Sakai M, Takahashi T, Kondo M. Mutation of beta 3-adrenergic-receptor gene and response to treatment of obesity. *Lancet.* 1995;346:1433-1434.

55. Sakane N, Yoshida T, Umekawa T, Kogure A, Takakura Y, Kondo M. Effects of Trp64Arg mutation in the beta 3-adrenergic receptor gene on weight loss, body fat distribution, glycemic control, and insulin resistance in obese type 2 diabetic patients. *Diabetes Care.* 1997;20:1887-1890.

56. Shiwaku K, Nogi A, Anuurad E, et al. Difficulty in losing weight by behavioral intervention for women with Trp64Arg polymorphism of the beta3-adrenergic receptor gene. *Int J Obes Relat Metab Disord.* 2003;27:1028-1036.

57. Xinli W, Xiaomei T, Meihua P, Song L. Association of a mutation in the beta3-adrenergic receptor gene with obesity and response to dietary intervention in Chinese children. *Acta Paediatr.* 2001;90(11):1233-1237.

58. Rawson ES, Nolan A, Silver K, Shuldiner AR, Poehlman ET. No effect of the Trp64Arg beta(3)-adrenoceptor gene variant on weight loss, body composition, or energy expenditure in obese, Caucasian postmenopausal women. *Metabolism.* 2002;51:801-805.

59. Tchernof A, Starling RD, Turner A, et al. Impaired capacity to lose visceral adipose tissue during weight reduction in obese postmenopausal women with the Trp64Arg beta3-adrenoceptor gene variant. *Diabetes.* 2000;49(10):1709-1713.

60. Lindi VI, Uusitupa MI, Lindstrom J, et al. Association of the Pro12Ala polymorphism in the PPAR-gamma2 gene with 3-year incidence of type 2 diabetes and body weight change in the Finnish Diabetes Prevention Study. *Diabetes.* 2002;51:2581-2586.

61. Nicklas BJ, van Rossum EF, Berman DM, Ryan AS, Dennis KE, Shuldiner AR. Genetic variation in the peroxisome proliferator-activated receptor-gamma2 gene (Pro12Ala) affects metabolic responses to weight loss and subsequent weight regain. *Diabetes.* 2001;50:2172-2176.

62. Moreno-Aliaga MJ, Santos JL, Marti A, Martinez JA. Does weight loss prognosis depend on genetic make-up? *Obes Rev.* 2005;6:155-168.

63. Fumeron F, Durack-Bown I, Betoulle D, et al. Polymorphisms of uncoupling protein (UCP) and beta 3 adrenoreceptor genes in obese people submitted to a low-calorie diet. *Int J Obes Relat Metab Disord.* 1996;20:1051-1054.

64. Kogure A, Yoshida T, Sakane N, Umekawa T, Takakura Y, Kondo M. Synergic effect of polymorphisms in uncoupling protein 1 and beta3-adrenergic receptor genes on weight loss in obese Japanese. *Diabetologia.* 1998;41:1399.

65. Fogelholm M, Valve R, Kukkonen-Harjula K, et al. Additive effects of the mutations in the beta3-adrenergic receptor and uncoupling protein-1 genes on weight loss and weight maintenance in Finnish women. *J Clin Endocrinol Metab.* 1998;83:4246-4250.

66. Cha MH, Shin HD, Kim KS, Lee BH, Yoon Y. The effects of uncoupling protein 3 haplotypes on obesity phenotypes and very low-energy diet-induced changes among overweight Korean female subjects. *Metabolism.* 2006;55:578-586.

67. Salopuro T, Pulkkinen L, Lindstrom J, et al. Genetic variation in leptin receptor gene is associated with type 2 diabetes and body weight: The Finnish Diabetes Prevention Study. *Int J Obes (Lond).* 2005;29:1245-1251.

68. Mammes O, Aubert R, Betoulle D, et al. LEPR gene polymorphisms: associations with overweight, fat mass and response to diet in women. *Eur J Clin Invest.* 2001;31:398-404.

69. de Luis RD, de la Fuente RA, Sagrado MG, Izaola O, Vicente RC. Leptin receptor Lys656Asn polymorphism is associated with decreased leptin response and weight loss secondary to a lifestyle modification in obese patients. *Arch Med Res.* 2006;37(7):854-859.

70. Goyenechea E, Dolores Parra M, Alfredo Martinez J. Weight regain after slimming induced by an energy-restricted diet depends on interleukin-6 and peroxisome-proliferator-activated-receptor-gamma2 gene polymorphisms. *Br J Nutr.* 2006;96:965-972.

71. Aberle J, Evans D, Beil FU, Seedorf U. A polymorphism in the apolipoprotein A5 gene is associated with weight loss after short-term diet. *Clin Genet.* 2005;68:152-154.

72. Vogels N, Mariman EC, Bouwman FG, Kester AD, Diepvens K, Westerterp-Plantenga MS. Relation of weight maintenance and dietary restraint to peroxisome proliferator-activated receptor gamma2, glucocorticoid receptor, and ciliary neurotrophic factor polymorphisms. *Am J Clin Nutr.* 2005;82:740-746.

73. Santoro N, Perrone L, Cirillo G, et al. Effect of the melanocortin-3 receptor C17A and G241A variants on weight loss in childhood obesity. *Am J Clin Nutr.* 2007;85:950-953.

74. Corella D, Qi L, Sorli JV, et al. Obese subjects carrying the 11482G>A polymorphism at the perilipin locus are resistant to weight loss after dietary energy restriction. *J Clin Endocrinol Metab.* 2005;90:5121-5126.

75. Sorensen TI, Boutin P, Taylor MA, et al. Genetic polymorphisms and weight loss in obesity: a randomised trial of hypo-energetic high- versus low-fat diets. *PLoS Clin Trials.* 2006;1:e12.

76. Sesti G, Perego L, Cardellini M, et al. Impact of common polymorphisms in candidate genes for insulin resistance and obesity on weight loss of morbidly obese subjects after laparoscopic adjustable gastric banding and hypocaloric diet. *J Clin Endocrinol Metab.* 2005;90:5064-5069.

77. Hauner H, Meier M, Jockel KH, Frey UH, Siffert W. Prediction of successful weight reduction under sibutramine therapy through genotyping of the G-protein beta3 subunit gene (GNB3) C825T polymorphism. *Pharmacogenetics.* 2003;13:453-459.

78. Franks PW, Jablonski KA, Delahanty L, et al.; Diabetes Prevention Program Research Group. The Pro12Ala variant at the peroxisome proliferator-activated receptor gamma gene and change in obesity-related traits in the Diabetes Prevention Program. *Diabetologia.* 2007 (in press).

79. Smith PG, Day NE. The design of case-control studies: the influence of confounding and interaction effects. *Int J Epidemiol.* 1984;13:356-365.

80. Wong MY, Day NE, Luan JA, Chan KP, Wareham NJ. The detection of gene-environment interaction for continuous traits: should we deal with measurement error by bigger studies or better measurement? *Int J Epidemiol.* 2003;32:51-57.

81. Hattersley AT, McCarthy MI. What makes a good genetic association study? *Lancet.* 2005;36:1315-1323.
82. Hunter DJ. Gene-environment interactions in human diseases. *Nat Rev Genet.* 2005;6:287-298.
83. Doerge RW, Churchill GA. Permutation tests for multiple loci affecting a quantitative character. *Genetics.* 1996;142:285-294.
84. Benjamini Y, Yekutieli D. Quantitative trait loci analysis using the false discovery rate. *Genetics.* 2005;171:783-790.
85. Wacholder S, Chanock S, Garcia-Closas M, El Ghormli L, Rothman N. Assessing the probability that a positive report is false: an approach for molecular epidemiology studies. *J Natl Cancer Inst.* 2004;96:434-442.
86. Hahn LW, Ritchie MD, Moore JH. Multifactor dimensionality reduction software for detecting gene-gene and gene-environment interactions. *Bioinformatics.* 2003;19:376-382.
87. Ioannidis JP, Gwinn M, Little J, et al. A road map for efficient and reliable human genome epidemiology. *Nat Genet.* 2006;38:3-5.
88. Kraft P, Yen YC, Stram DO, Morrison J, Gauderman WJ. Exploiting gene-environment interaction to detect genetic associations. *Hum Hered.* 2007;63:111-119.
89. Merikangas KR, Low NC, Hardy J. Commentary: understanding sources of complexity in chronic diseases—the importance of integration of genetics and epidemiology. *Int J Epidemiol.* 2006;35:590-592.
90. Khoury MJ, Gwinn M. Genomics, epidemiology, and common complex diseases: let's not throw out the baby with the bathwater! *Int J Epidemiol.* 2006;35:1363-1364.
91. Buchanan AV, Weiss KM, Fullerton SM. Dissecting complex disease: the quest for the Philosopher's Stone? *Int J Epidemiol.* 2006;35:562-571.

Index

Note: Page numbers in *italics* refer to illustrations and tables.